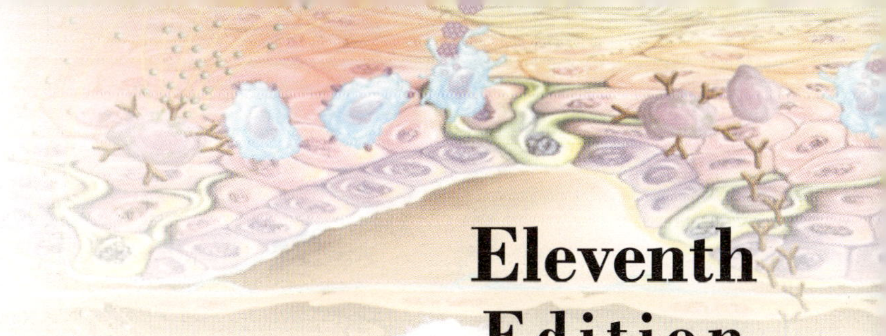

Eleventh Edition

Practice of Dermatology

Eleventh Edition

Practice of Dermatology

PN Behl MBBS, FCRP (Edin), FICAI
Director, Skin Institute and School of Dermatology, New Delhi; Director, Behl Institute, Dasna (UP)
Founder, PN Behl Foundation; Director, Rural-cum-Industrial Skin and Health Institute
Director, Dr PN Behl Wholistic Health Centre, Ashok Vihar, New Delhi
President, Skin Institute and Public Services Charitable Trust
Chief Editor, *Dermatology Times* and *Asian Clinics in Dermatology*

Govind Srivastava MBBS, MD, MNAMS
Dean and Senior Consultant Dermatologist, Skin Institute and School of Dermatology, New Delhi
Deputy Director and Senior Consultant Dermatologist, Dr PN Behl Wholistic Health Centre
Ashok Vihar, New Delhi
Editor, *Dermatology Times* and *Asian Clinics in Dermatology*

Asok Aggarwal MBBS, MD
Senior Consultant Dermatologist and Former Dean and Professor
Skin Institute and School of Dermatology, New Delhi
Editor, *Dermatology Times* and *Asian Clinics in Dermatology*

Gautam Srivastava MBBS, MS
Clinical Dermatologist, Faculty of Life Sciences and Education
University of South Wales, United Kingdom

CBSPD

CBS Publishers & Distributors Pvt Ltd

New Delhi • Bengaluru • Chennai • Kochi • Kolkata • Lucknow • Mumbai
Hyderabad • Jharkhand • Nagpur • Patna • Pune • Uttarakhand

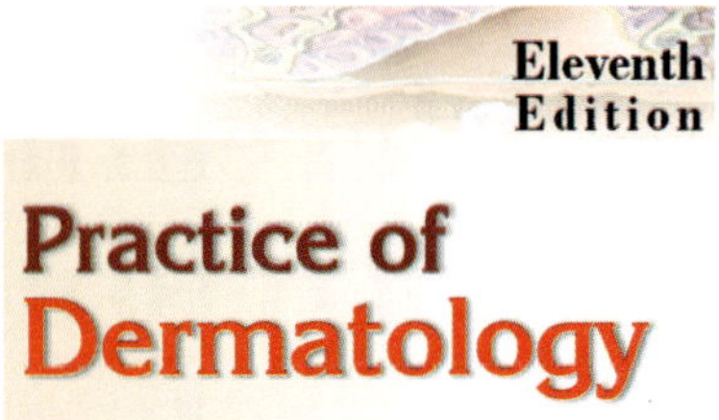

Disclaimer

Science and technology are constantly changing fields. New research and experience broaden the scope of information and knowledge. The authors have tried their best in giving information available to them while preparing the material for this book. Although all efforts have been made to ensure optimum accuracy of the material, yet it is quite possible some errors might have been left uncorrected. The publisher, the printer and the authors will not be held responsible for any inadvertent errors, omissions or inaccuracies.

ISBN: 978-93-5466-628-5

Eleventh Edition 2024

Reprint **2025**
First Edition 1962
Second Edition 1972
Third Edition 1975
Fourth Edition 1976
Fifth Edition 1982
Sixth Edition 1987
Seventh Edition 1990
Eighth Edition 1998
Ninth Edition 2002
Tenth Edition 2005

Published by Satish Kumar Jain and produced by Varun Jain for
CBS Publishers & Distributors Pvt Ltd
4819/XI Prahlad Street, 24 Ansari Road, Daryaganj, New Delhi 110 002, India
Ph: 011-23289259, 23266838 Website: www.cbspd.com
e-mail: delhi@cbspd.com

Corporate Office: 204 FIE, Industrial Area, Patparganj, Delhi 110 092, India
Ph: 011-49344934 Fax: 011-49344935
e-mail: publishing@cbspd.com; publicity@cbspd.com

Branches

- **Bengaluru:** Seema House 2975, 17th Cross, K.R. Road, Banasankari 2nd Stage, Bengaluru 560 070, Karnataka, India
  Ph: +91-80-26771678/79 Fax: +91-80-26771680 e-mail: bangalore@cbspd.com
- **Chennai:** 18/8B, Subbarayan Street, Shenoy Nagar, Chennai 600 030, Tamil Nadu, India
  Ph: +91-44-42032115, 26681266 e-mail: chennai@cbspd.com
- **Kochi:** 42/1325, 1326, Power House Road, Opp KSEB, Ernakulum, Kochi 682 018, Kerala, India
  Ph: +91-484-4059061-65,67 Fax: +91-484-4059065 e-mail: kochi@cbspd.com
- **Kolkata:** 147, Hind Ceramics Compound, 1st Floor, Nilgunj Road, Belghoria, Kolkata-700056, West Bengal, India
  Ph: 033-25633055/56 e-mail: kolkata@cbspd.com
- **Lucknow:** Basement, Khushnuma Complex, 7 Meerabai Marg (Behind Jawahar Bhawan), Lucknow-226001, UP, India
  Ph: +91-522-4000032 e-mail: tiwari.lucknow@cbspd.com
- **Mumbai:** PWD Shed, Gala no 25/26, Ramchandra Bhatt Marg, Next to JJ Hospital Gate no. 2, Opp. Union Bank of India, Noorbaug, Mumbai-400009, Maharashtra, India
  Ph: +91-22-66661880/89 e-mail: mumbai@cbspd.com

Representatives

- **Hyderabad** 0-9885175004
- **Jharkhand** 0-9811541605
- **Nagpur** 0-8692091830
- **Patna** 0-9334159340
- **Pune** 0-9664372571
- **Uttarakhand** 0-9716462459

Printed at HT Media Ltd, Greater Noida, UP, India

to

Revered Late Professor PN Behl

Father of Dermatology and Dermatosurgery in India

On whose Ideals

this book is Based

Preface

Over the span of more than six decades, the inaugural edition of the textbook *Practice of Dermatology* came into existence and was subsequently published. It has significantly flourished in the early years of the new millennium. Throughout this prolonged period, notable advancements have been achieved in the field of medicine encompassing dermatology, and vast experiences have been accumulated from various corners of the globe, be it urban, rural, or tribal settings. The outcomes of these efforts have become readily apparent, as ideas have matured and gained greater clarity. Consequently, a clear distinction can be drawn between valuable insights and mere trivialities, between practical application and theoretical suppositions, all while employing investigative tools.

Moreover, it is crucial to establish a sense of proportion in approaching the subject matter with a greater emphasis on addressing common day-to-day dermatological issues rather than focusing excessively on uncommon and obscure ones. By doing so, dermatology practitioners can undoubtedly provide effective solutions to alleviate the suffering of their patients. Regrettably, there appears to be a lamentable reality wherein practitioners seem to possess limited knowledge, expertise, and enthusiasm when it comes in terms of managing common dermatoses but become entirely engrossed when confronted with a rare and incurable ailment.

The current landscape of scientific journals, conferences, symposia, and educational initiatives presumably plays a significant role in shaping this situation. In the practical realm, one is disheartened to observe that the afflicted patient often confronts the harsh truth and becomes disenchanted with contemporary medicine. The misuse of drugs and the commodification of the once venerable medical profession only serve to exacerbate this already troubling state of affairs.

The tenth iteration of the book made its debut back in the year 2005, arriving a few years subsequent to the sorrowful passing of the esteemed Prof (Dr) PN Behl. The ardent aspiration he held of upholding the academic legacy has been triumphantly realized by those who succeeded him over the years. And at present, after a substantial passage of time, the eleventh edition of the book has been meticulously crafted with due consideration for the emerging cohort of medical practitioners.

In order to bestow upon the book an all-encompassing nature and to pique the interest of contemporary educators, a more elaborate exploration of certain uncommon dermatoses has been undertaken. This book is characterized by its lucid and accessible language, providing comprehensive elucidations of facts, and giving due prominence to practical approaches in management—a distinctive set of qualities that sets it apart.

The authors express profound gratitude to the diverse publishers for their generous permissions enabling the inclusion of copyrighted material in the form of pictures and photographs. While we diligently strived to maintain accuracy, we acknowledge that inadvertent errors, if present, may have arisen during the printing process. Hence, any such unfortunate oversights are sincerely regretted. In earnest pursuit of excellence, we earnestly welcome any constructive feedback or suggestions from our esteemed readers.

With sanguine anticipation, it is our fervent hope that this eleventh edition of *Practice of Dermatology* shall profoundly aid students, medical practitioners, and dermatologists alike in comprehending the expansive domain of skin diseases, thereby equipping them to administer adept, efficient, and compassionate care to the marginalized and frequently overlooked patients. To cater to the pragmatic concerns of medical economics, we have duly emphasized relevant aspects, and have thoughtfully incorporated a dermatological formulary. For the pursuit of knowledge pertaining to rare diseases, detailed discussions, and comprehensive references, we kindly direct readers to larger volumes and research monographs, which shall cater to their inquisitive pursuit with greater intricacy.

Lastly, we deem it imperative to express our profound gratitude and heartfelt appreciation to Mr Satish Kumar Jain of CBS Publishers & Distributors, whose unwavering support and collaboration have been instrumental in bringing this edition to fruition, thereby enabling us to accomplish our undertaking with utmost satisfaction.

Govind Srivastava
Asok Aggarwal
Gautam Srivastava

Contents

Part I

Basic Information

Chapter

1

Introduction

Diseases of the skin are a common occurrence. There are not many statistics to prove the exact frequency of skin diseases in this country, but general impression is 10–20% of patients seeking medical advice suffer from skin diseases. While infections are more common in the tropics, chemical and psychogenic dermatoses are common in Western countries.

Diseases of the skin account for a great deal of misery, suffering, incapacity and economic loss. Besides this, they are a great handicap in the society, because they are visible. Fortunately, however, due to recent advances, cutaneous scars can be successfully removed by plastic planing, laser therapy and skin grafting.

There is a popular adage that skin patients are never cured and never die. Like all generalizations, this is quite untrue. Admittedly, skin diseases are seldom fatal; but, we assure you, the cure rate in skin diseases compares quite favourably with the cure rate in any other speciality, and cases which cannot be cured outright are often positively influenced by the control of troublesome complaints. Contrary to the popular belief, only a few skin diseases are really contagious. Besides, the presence of ubiquitous and tropical diseases, and the problems created by poverty and illiteracy in tropical countries, climatic factors too create special problems in the treatment of skin diseases. A physician practising in the tropics, therefore, must also take them into account.

Since the subject matter of dermatology is superficial, and so available for observation, the practice of dermatology pertinently requires an acute observation with an ability to pay attention to details; it requires recognition of trifles from which deductions can often be made. It has been appropriately said that, especially in the diagnosis of contact dermatitis and eczema, the dermatologist should be a good detective with powers of observation and deduction almost like those of Sherlock Holmes. The diagnosis of cutaneous diseases is essentially objective, and attention to details of eruptions, occupational stigmas, bearing of the patient and clothing is important. Laboratory tests and instrumental aids do not afford any shortcuts to diagnosis.

In chalking out a practical line of treatment, one must never omit reassurance and explanation. Reassurance is the stock-in-trade of faith healers and quacks. It goes a long way towards the ultimate recovery of the patient and it is a pity that qualified doctors often lose sight of it. A mysterious approach produces anxiety; an explanation of the disease helps to prevent this unhealthy reaction. The practice of dermatology demands a good background of general medicine which, far from being alien, is closely allied to dermatology. However superficial its subject matter, dermatology is not merely skin-deep. Its scope includes the whole range of life from the human mind to the various microorganisms, vast external environments and complex endocrine and metabolic

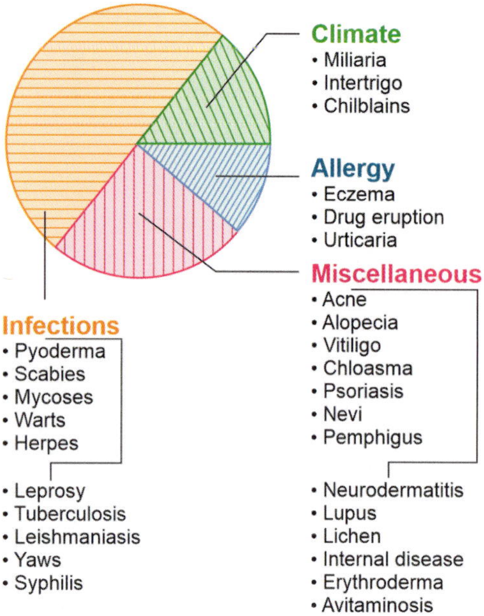

Fig. 1.1: Pattern of dermatology

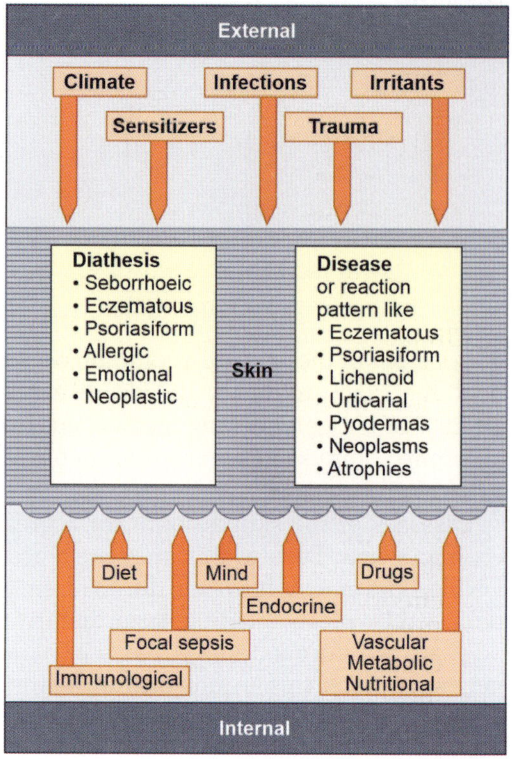

Fig. 1.2: Scope of dermatology—reaction patterns

transactions within the body **(Fig. 1.1)**. In the practice of dermatology, undue stress should not be laid on giving diagnostic labels; time would be more usefully spent if an emphasis was given to establish the cause or causes of the malady in question.

A skin disease, seen in practice, is often a reaction pattern resulting from the effects of different etiological stresses on a particular diathesis **(Fig. 1.2)**. In the past, undue stress has been laid on unnecessary and often conflicting jungle of terminology at the cost of understanding the disease and the patient. For proper treatment, emphasis should be on tackling the cause, and less stress on managing the reaction pattern along with palliative treatment.

Last of all, the line of treatment should be simple but sure; one should not play with potent, powerful drugs without knowing their specific side-actions. It is a strange fact of modem practice that a large percentage of diseases are man-made; undoubtedly, there should be a strong plea for the prevention of such man-made dermatoses. This could be achieved to a great extent by the timely realization of the dangers involved in the use of potent drugs and the promotion of healthy teamwork in medical practice. Economy is important, more so in thesedays of rising cost of medical practice. It involves austerity in the use of drugs, cheaper effective drugs and medicaments, only essential laboratory investigations, cutting down the period of morbidity and quicker return of work, so that the least working time is lost. Medical economics plays an important role in practice, more so in the under-developed countries **(Fig. 1.3)**.

Dermatoses in the Tropics

A. Skin of Persons in the tropics.

- Pigment is more
- Low threshold for itching and scratching
- Tendency to
  - Lichenification
  - Keloid formation
  - Pigmentation, hypopigmentation and depigmentation

B. Climate

- Strong sun—photo-sensitization
- Heat-predisposes to infection:
  - Bacterial
  - Fungal
  - Parasitic
- Hyperhidrosis—causes maceration; further sweat exerts a bleaching effect on clothes and footwear.
- Prickly heat becoming eczematized
- Contact or infective eczema
- Intertriginous eczema in the summer and the monsoon
- Eczema crackle in winter and in leprosy patients
- Seasonal aggravation

C. Environment

- Most of the tropical countries are not so advanced as the non-tropical countries, hence the environment affects the skin.
- Illiteracy, quackery, poverty and malnutrition.
- Social customs—massages, baths
- Unhygenic conditions—parasites, scabies, bugs, cockroach
- Use of the drugs for tropical ailments
- With industrializations, more instances of contact dermatitis due to industrial chemicals.

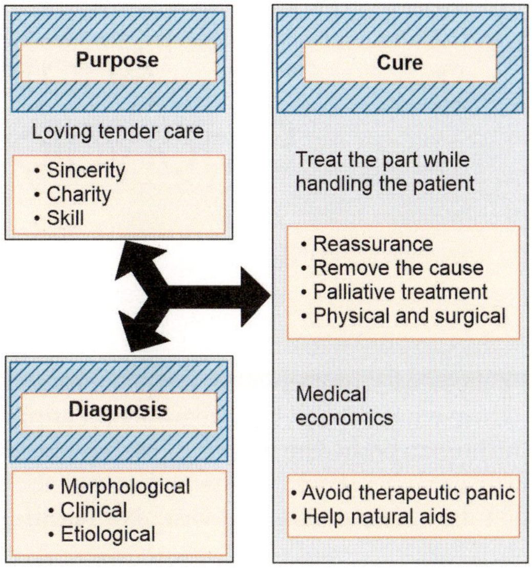

Fig. 1.3. Essentials of the practice of dermatology

Chapter

2 Anatomy, Physiology, Embryology, Bacteriology and Pathology

The skin is a protective covering of the body. It, with all its specialized derivatives, makes up what is called the integument (Latin: a covering) which covers the entire surface of the human body. The human skin shows wide regional variations in structure like scalp, face, ear lobes, back, palms and soles, etc. Thickness varies; the number of sebaceous glands, collagen fibre and vasculature differ in different parts of the integument.

ANATOMY

The skin is composed of a superficial epithelial layer—the Epidermis, and an underlying connective tissue layer, the dermis or corium. Beneath the corium is another connective tissue layer, rather loose in texture—the hpodermis, or subcutaneous layer **(Figs 2.1 and 2.2)**. The free surface of the epidermis is marked by a network of linear furrows and ridges or variable sizes. On the fingers, these have a constant pattern differing in each individual; a person, therefore, can be identified by his fingerprints (dermatoglyphics).

Structure of Epidermis

The epidermis is formed of non-vascular stratified epithelium. Its usual thickness is between 0.07 mm and 0.12 mm. But in certain parts, like the soles of the feet and the palms of the hand, it is very thick, ranging from 0.8 mm to 1.4 mm. Squamous epithelium is 10–12 cells thick in the palms and soles and 3–4 cells over the eyelids and forearms. As viewed in three-dimensional manner, the downward projections of epidermis are now referred to as rete ridges and not rete pegs. They are actually ridges of dermis. The epidermis is mainly divisible into two main systems, viz. keratinising or malpighian system (keratinocytes) which forms the bulk and the pigmentary system (melanocytes) which produces the pigment. Melanin is transferred to the keratinocytes through the dendrites of melanocytes (cytocrine secretion).

ln addition to four types of cells viz., keratinocytes, melanocytes, Langerhans cell, and indeterminate cell in the epidermis, another unique cell known as Merkel cell (or Haascheiben) or touch cells are found at the base of epidermal rete ridges which are in contact with nerve fibrils. They are mostly present in palms, soles, nail beds, oral and genital epithelium, and act as slow touch receptors. Merkel cell trabecular carcinoma has occasionally been reported.

The following are the main layers of the epidermis which can be made out microscopically in a section perpendicular to the skin surface:

1. **Stratum germinativum or basal cell layer.** This is the deepest portion of the epidermis and is composed of columnar cells placed perpendicular to the skin surface. The

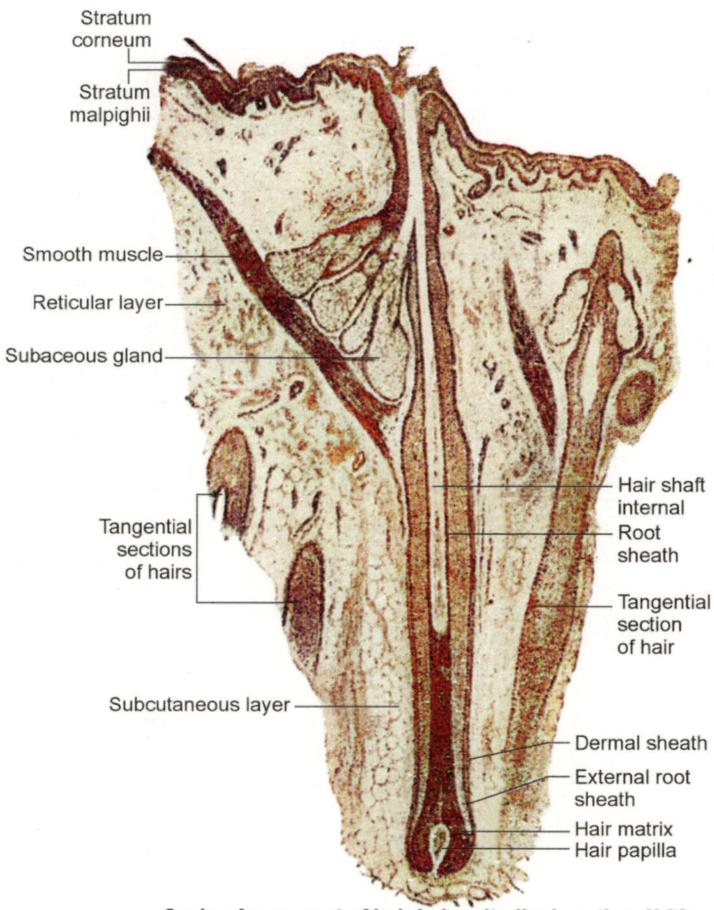

Scalp of man, root of hair in longitudinal section, X 32

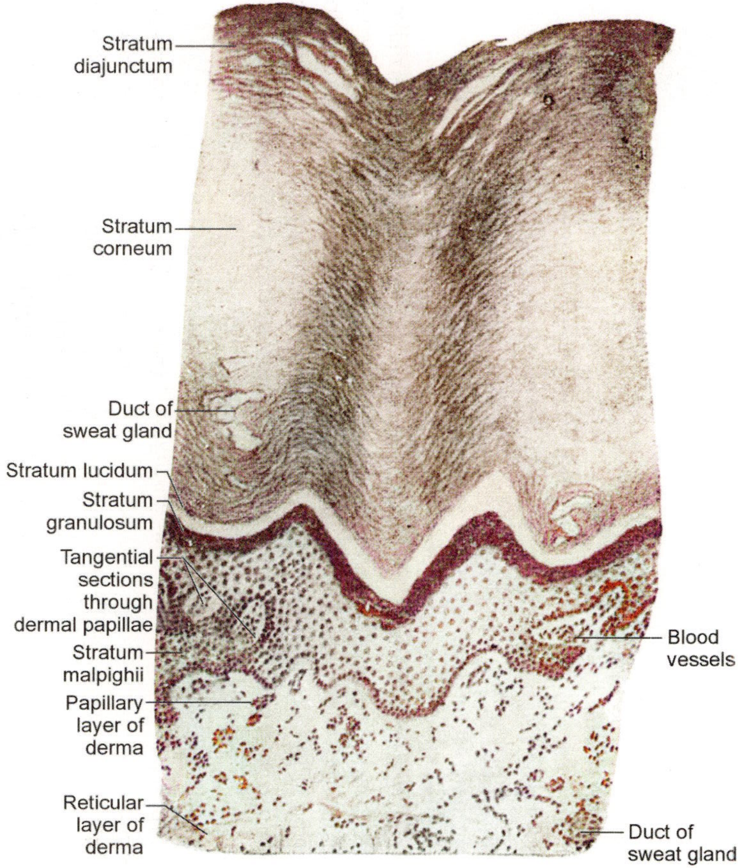

Section of skin of human sole, perpendicular to free surface X 100

Figs 2.1 and 2.2: Anatomy of skin (*Courtesy:* WB Saunders Company, Philadelphia from Histology by Maximow & Bloom, VI Ed.)

whole of the epidermis germinates from this stratum hence the name "stratum germinativum". Any trauma to this layer would result in scarring; trauma above the level of this layer heal without scarring. This basal layer contains many mitotic figures signifying the occurrence of cellular multiplication. More and more cells are formed and pushed off to the superficial layers. Some of the cells of the stratum genninativum contain granules of pigment called melanin. Besides, melanoblasts or melanocytes are found in this layer; these have branching processes ramifying between the other cells. These appear to be non-pigmented.

2. **Stratum malpighii or the prickle cell layer.** It is superficial to the basal cell layer. and is composed of several layers of polyhedral cells connected to each other by intercellular bridges. Electron microscopic studies have revealed that adjacent epidermal cells have at their point of contact areas of thickened membranes. These are called desmosomes. Between the desmosomes of the two cells, there appears to be a structureless cement like substance, giving an appearance of bridges. All keratinocytes adhere together by desmosomes. Half size desmosomes also occur on the under-surface of basal cells which play an important part in anchoring the epidermis to the dermis via dermoepidermal junction.
3. **Stratum granulosum.** It is superficial to the stratum malpighii. It is composed of flat, fusiform cells which are one to three layers thick. These cells contain irregular granules of keratohyalin and lysosomal enzymes and cystine rich proteins. Above the top of the prickle cell layer, near the granular cells layer; lamellar granules (keratinosomes) also known as Odland bodies are found. These Odland bodies take part in the barrier function of the epidermal permeability. Granular contents of the Odland bodies are discharged into the intercellular space below the cornified cell layer and form an effective waterproof barrier.
4. **Stratum lucidum.** Superficial to the stratum granulosum is the pale, wavy-looking layer known as stratum lucidum. It is formed by many layers of flattened and closely packed cells whose outlines have become quite indistinct and the nuclei have disappeared. This layer contains refractile droplets of eleidin.
5. **Stratum corneum.** This is the most superficial layer, the outer surface of which is exposed to the atmosphere. It consists of many layers of non-nucleated, flattened, cornified cells. Almost all the cellular structure is lost. It is this layer which becomes thicker with the application of intermittent mechanical pressure. This layer is thickest on the palms of the hands and the soles of the feet, but thinnest on the outer aspect of the lips, on the glans penis and the eyes. When interior of the keratinocytes are studied with the help of electron microscope, they reveal filaments in the cytoplasm (tonofilaments) which form bundles (tonofibrils) which are inserted in the cell membrane at the desmosomes. In the stratum malpighii, the cytoplasmic organelles are diminished, the centrioles absent and tonofibrils increased, whereas in the basal layer (stratum germinativum) full complement of cytoplasmic organelles and centrioles are present. At the level of the stratum granulosum, most of the organelles have disappeared, tonofibrils have increased and dense keratohyalin granules are seen surrounding the tonofibrils. Then there is an abrupt change to the cells of the stratum corneum—no organelles, no nuclei but tonofibrils are seen embedded in a dense structureless matrix. These tonofibrils at the final stage are considered as mature fibrous protein keratin; early prickle (spinous/malpighii) cells contain tonofibrils

which contain sulphahydril and disulfide bonds, which are precursors of keratin. Keratohyalin granules do not contain sulphahydril groups. Epidermal horny layer, because of content of keratohyalin cement is referred to as soft keratin. Hard keratin is present in the nails and the hair.

6. **Dendritic cells of epidermis.** These are melanocytes, Langerhans cells and indeterminate cells. The melanocytes are the pigment-producing cells and are derived in foetal life from neural crest; their numbers are subject to regional variation. They are normally present in the ratio of 1:5 to 1: 10 to the epidermal basal cells. Melanocytes can be stained by the silver impregnation method and dopa stain.

   The cells of Langerhans are found about the middle of epidermis; they can be identified by histochemical methods and electron microscopy. These cells are dopa negative and contain hydrolytic enzyme, adenosine triphosphatase. These cells are also stained by gold chloride method. Recent work indicates that probably they are phagocytes of mesenchymal origin, and play an important part in antigen transport between the surface of the epidermis and regional lymph nodes. The indeterminate dendritic cells are also seen in the epidermis which can be only visualized by electron microscopy. The exact function of these cells is being elucidated.

   The junction of epidermis and dermis is formed by basement membrane zone. Electron microscopy has shown that it is composed of several components. From the plasma membrane of basal cells come extensions called half desmosomes which anchor basal cells to basal lamina. Extending from the basal cell membrane are anchoring dermal filaments. Pemphigoid antigen and laminin are located between the basal cell and basal lamina. This area is 35–45 nm wide and is also referred as lamina lucida. The basement membrane is considered to be a porous semipermeable filter which permits exchange of fluid and cells between the epidermis and dermis. It is made up by type IV collagen. It is a PAS-positive membrane. Electron microscopy and immunoperoxidase tests have made it possible to locate defects precisely in BMZ in a variety of dermatoses.

Time of Maturation of Epidermal Cells

Basal germinal cells are continuously producing daughter cells by normal mitotic division. The mitotic activity may be increased during stress, inflammation and in psoriasis. Normally, from basal cells to the final maturation stage of horny cells take 4–5 weeks. It may be as short as 72 hours to up to 7 days; time varies according to the stimulus.

Structure of Dermis (Cutis Vera or Corium)

Dermis is profusely supplied with blood vessels. Dermis is divided into papillary and reticular dermis. It contains connective tissue fibres, various cells and all dermal appendages. Connective tissue is formed by three main components (1) collagen fibres (2) elastic fibres (3) ground substance. The most abundant dermal constituent is collagen. All these are produced by master cell fibroblast. There are at least 13 known type of connective tissue collagen of which seven are detected in human skin. Type I collagen accounts for 80% of total collagen in skin and type III makes up another 15% of total collagen. Collagen is a protein and constitutes about 70% of dry weight of dermis. A single collagen bundle 1.0 mm in diameter can sustain a load of 10–40 kg without breaking. Collagen molecule is termed as "tropocollagen". It consists of three polypeptide chains. Each chain consists of hydroxyproline, hydroxylysine and glycine. Elastic fibres are smaller and offer extensibility to the skin. In the papillary dermis, the fibres are vertically oriented. Its deeper parts merge imperceptibly into the hypodermis. Beneath the basement membrane are distributed many blood vessels forming a capillary network which sends up loops into the dermal papillae. These papillae are microscopic finger-like processes projecting into the epidermis, which is moulded over and attached to them.

The connective tissue cells in the dermis are spindle-shaped and are more numerous in the superficial layers than in the deeper ones. Thickness of dermis is 1–3 mm. In a microscopic section passing through the dermis, besides the structures mentioned above, are also seen hair follicles, various types of sebaceous and sweat glands, plain muscle fibres, sensory end-organs like Pacinian and Meissner's corpuscles and adipose tissue; the latter is present mostly in the deeper parts. There are a few round cells, an occasional fibrocyte and a few pigment-carrying histiocytes called melanophores.

Within the skin, the blood supply and drainage lie along well-determined pathways. There are rich capillary beds in the papillae and around the appendages and in sub-papillary plexus; deep reticular plexus is much less rich **(Figs 2.3)**. In the deeper layer of the dermis, there is arteriovenous anastomosis surrounded by sphincter-like group of smooth muscles under autonomic control. Skin is richly innervated by myelinated and non-myelinated sensory fibres and via non-myelinated autonomic fibres supplying blood vessels and appendages. Conspicuous nerve supply consists of plexuses in the papillae, Meissner's corpuscles, Pacinian corpuscles, Merkel's discs and nerve endings in the basal layer of the epidermis.

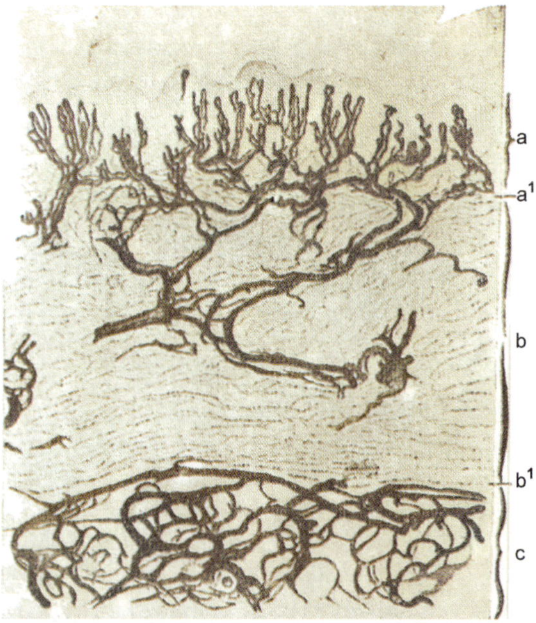

Fig. 2.3: Section of skin with blood vessels injected: (a) Papillary layer of dermis. (a^1) Subpapillary plexus. (b) Reticular layer of dermis. (b^1) Subdermic plexus. (c) Vessels of adipose tissue (*Courtesy:* Longmans, Green & Co. Ltd., London from Essentials of Histology by Schafers, XIV Ed.)

In addition to superficial and deep plexuses of rich vascular supply, arteriovenous anastomoses are present in the skin. These specialised segments are known as Sucquet–Hoyer canal. They are surrounded by ovoid-shaped smooth cells known as glomus cells. They are under the control of sympathetic nervous system. A small nerve twig is associated with every glomus, and they respond to variety of pharmacologic agents and cause vasoconstriction. Thermoregulation is an important function of the skin vasculature.

Sebaceous Glands

They are scattered all over the integument in association with the hair follicles. They are absent from the hairless portions of the body like the palms of the hands, the soles and sides of the feet. These glands, however, occur independently of hair follicles at certain places like the eyelids, margins of lips, external auditory meatus, nipples, anus and around the external genitalia, and at these sites the glands are more superficial. The sebaceous glands are numerous and large on the scalp, forehead, ears, face, the sternal and interscapular regions. In the hairy portions of the skin, the ducts of these glands open into the hair follicles, while in the non-hairy portions, they open directly on the surface of the skin. One or more sebaceous glands may be attached to one hair follicle. Meibomian glands, mammary glands and smegma glands of the penis are modified sebaceous glands. Perspiration in hot climate and in hot weather stimulates the production of sebum. Further, the sebaceous glands are more active at and after puberty, during menstruation and pregnancy.

Structurally, these are small glands composed of a number of rounded sacs, the alveoli **(Fig. 2.4)**. Adjacent alveoli form a mass like a bunch of grapes. All these alveoli open into a short duct near the hair follicle. An alveolar wall is formed by a basement membrane supported by a thin layer of fibrillar connective tissue. Lining the inner surface of this basement membrane is a single layer of thin, secretory cells with round nuclei. During secretory activity, most of these cells become polyhedral and large, and are filled with fat droplets. Large cells distended with fat, with shrinking nuclei, can be seen in the centre of the alveoli. The nuclei disappear and the cells break down into fatty detritus which mixes with the horny scales of other cells. This oily secretion of glands is then thrown out into the hair follicles and upon the surface of the epidermis.

The ducts of the sebaceous glands are lined by stratified squamous epithelium which is continuous with the external root sheath of the hair, and with the malpighian layer of the epidermis.

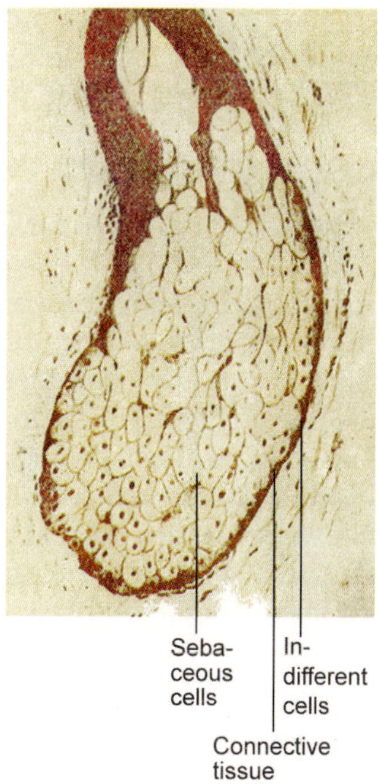

Fig. 2.4: Section of human sebaceous gland. X120 (*Courtesy:* WB Saunders Company, Philadelphia from Histology by Maximow & Bloom, VI Ed.)

Sweat Glands

These are of two types:

Eccrine glands: They are the ordinary, small-sized (0.3–0.4 mm) sweat glands which are distributed all over the skin except on the beds of nails, margins of lips and the glans penis **(Fig. 2.5)**. Over 3 million sweat units are present at birth. The glandular portion is a simple tube folded by a number of unequal twists into the shape of a ball. This tube is composed of a thick, connective tissue basement membrane which is lined by a single layer of cubical or columnar cells. These cells secrete sweat. Between the basement membrane and the secretory cells are longitudinally or obliquely placed spindle-shaped cells called the myo-epithelial cells. These cells are contractile and are supposed to help in the discharge of sweat.

The sweat gland opens into the sweat duct which has an epithelial lining consisting of two or three layers of cells. The passage of this duct through the epidermis has no proper wall, but is merely a channel in between the epithelial cells.

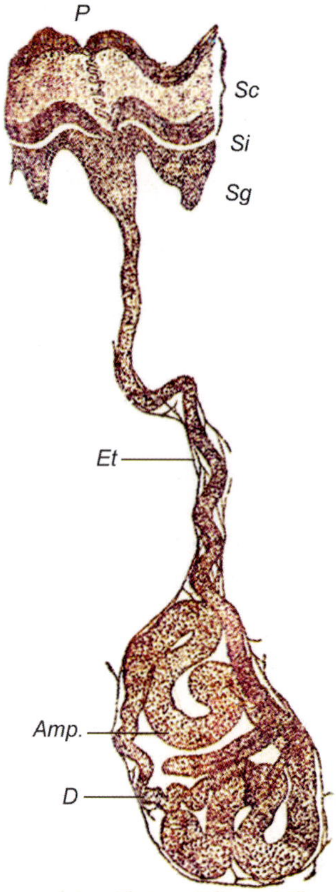

Fig. 2.5: Sweat Glands from volar surface of index finger. The drawing was combined from sections and a teased preparation: (P) Sweat pore. (Sc) Stratum corneum. (SI) Stratum lucidum. (Sg) Stratum germinativum. (EI) Elastic tissue surrounding the duct. (Amp.) Ampulla. (D) Sudoriferous duct. X45 (*Courtesy:* WB Saunders Company, Philadelphia from Histology by Maximow & Bloom, VI Ed.)

Apocrine glands: They occur in the axillae, areola and nipples of breasts, umbilicus, around the anus and the genitalia. Their glandular portion is very large and may measure 3–5 mm in diameter (the eccrine glands being only 0.3–0.4 mm in diameter). The myo-epithelial cells are highly developed and more abundant in these glands. They are specialized sweat glands, and their secretion is odoriferous with a secondary sexual significance (pheromone).

Hair

Hair is found on almost every part of the body surface except on the palms, soles, the dorsal surface of the terminal phalanges, the inner surface of the labia, the inner surface of the prepuce and the glans penis. Hairs differ in length (short or long), thickness (thick or thin) and colour (black, brown or blonde) in different parts of the body and in different races (curly or straight). There are three types of hair:

1. Long, medullated, pigmented hair seen on the scalp.

2. Short, fine, non-medullated and non-pigmented 'lanugo' hair seen in women, children, and on the faces and trunks of adults (vellus hair). Even in bald persons, vellus hair may be present.
3. Thick bristles seen in the nose and the ears.

Hair grows about 1–2 cm. per month. The growth varies in different people, races and also on the different parts of the body. Hair growth and development is under endocrine control. Fine balance of oestrogens, androgens and gonadotrophins determines the pattern in an individual. Hair follicle and its hair can be anatomically divided into three segments:

1. *Infundibulum:* Extends from pilar orifice above to the entrance of sebaceous gland below.
2. *Isthmus:* The short midsection of the follicle bounded superiorly by the sebaceous duct and inferiorly by the insertion of arrector pilorum muscle.
3. *Inferior:* This extends from the insertion of muscle to the base of the follicle. The upper segments of the isthmus and infundibulum are permanent. The entire follicle beneath the isthmus disappears during the involutionary stages of the hair cycle and again reforms during the growth cycle.

The hair follicle and its hair are fundamentally one structure derived partly from undifferentiated cells of the foetal epidermis. It is better to combine hair follicle, hair and sebaceous glands as one functional unit. In post-foetal life following the establishment of hair germ, growth occurs upwards as well as down the dermis. Hair follicles are found at different levels in the dermis. The coarse terminal hair extend up into the subcutaneous fat, fine body hair up to the mid-dermis, and fine vellus hair to superficial dermis.

The lower part of the hair is the site of growth. About half way up the follicle, it becomes the keratinised structure devoid of living cells. The junction of these two zones (Adamson's fringe) is the level up to which keratinophilic fungi infect the hair. Actually living cells are not infected, so no permanent hair loss occurs following ringworm infection of the scalp.

A hair is composed of a root—the part embedded in the skin, and a shaft-the portion projecting from the surface. The root of the hair at its lower end forms a bulbous enlargement which is called the root bulb. The hair is contained in the skin in a series of invaginations called the hair follicles. If the hair root is of considerable length, the follicle may extend even into the hypodermis. The hair follicle extends inwards from the surface of the epidermis, where it is funnel-shaped, either perpendicularly or in a curved fashion-the latter in curly hair. It is dilated at its inner end and is known here as the hairpit. The hair bulb, i.e., the inner-most portion of the hair root, fits into this pit **(Fig. 2.1)**. The hair shaft is a dead cornified structure that extends from the follicle to above the surface of the skin. It has three components—an outer cuticle, a cortex and inner medulla.

The hair follicle consists of two coats—the inner one corresponding to the epidermis, the outer one corresponding to the dermis. The outer one, therefore, consists of a hyaline basement membrane, external to which is a compact layer of connective tissue fibres and spindle cells, arranged circularly around the follicles. The inner coat which is intimately attached to the root of the hair consists further of an internal root sheath and an external root sheath. The internal root sheath is made up of 3 layers: (1) a fine cuticle composed of a single layer of imbricated scales with indistinct or no nuclei,

(2) Huxley's layer consisting of one or two layers of horny and flattened nucleated cells, and (3) Henle's layer consisting of a single layer of cubical cells with flattened nuclei. The external root sheath corresponds to the polyhedral cells of the stratum malpighii. At the bottom of the hair follicle, these cells become continuous with those of the hair bulb.

The hair bulb lies over the vascular papilla and consists of epithelial cells of polyhedral shape. ln the hair root, the cells are elongated; at the periphery, spindle-shaped, and in the centre, polyhedral. One or more sebaceous glands pour their secretion into the upper third of the follicular canal through a short duct.

The growth of the hair is cyclical. There are three phases in the life cycle of hair; growing (anagen), involutionary (catagen) and resting (telogen).

Growth of Hair (Cyclical Patterns)

1. *Anagen phase:* Growing phase—hair root pigmented, papilla and inferior segment present
2. *Telogen phase:* Resting phase—club-shaped, cornified sac of inferior segment. Tip depigmented.
3. *Catagen phase:* Involutionary phase—inferior segment shriveled up.

Anagen begins between the papillae and the undifferentiated cell. As anagen begins, matrix cells generate a new hair which pushes upward and dislodges the old club hair. Mature anagen hair follicle consists of infundibulum, isthmus and inferior segments. During catagen, entire inferior segment of follicle shrivels upward as a thin cord of epithelial cells and is followed upward by the papillae. During telogen the club-shaped hair rests in its comified saç at the level of the hair arrector muscle.

During telogen phase the hair melanocytes cease to synthesize melanin. This function of melanin formation begins again with anagen phase. Therefore the root of the anagen hair is pigmented, whereas the tip of the telogen hair is unpigmented.

Arrector pili muscles are the small bundles of plain muscle fibres which extend from the connective tissue sheath of the hair follicles (below the level of the opening of the duct of the sebaceous gland) to the epidermo-dermal junction. When these contract under the effect of cold or emotions, they move the hair into a more vertical position. They also pull on the epidermis in the adjoining region, thus producing an effect whereby the skin in the region around the follicle appears to be raised, while in the adjoining region, it appears to be depressed. This gives the so-called appearance of "goose flesh". The contraction of these muscle fibres is also thought to squeeze out sebum from the duct of the sebaceous gland.

Nails

These are semi-transparent, plate-like horny structures, covering the dorsal surfaces of the distal phalanges of the fingers and toes.

The proximal edge of the nail is known as the root of the nail. The visible portion of the nail is called the nail plate. It is semi-transparent and looks red due to the abundant vascular supply in the nail bed. The more opaque and rather whitish semi-lunar portion of the nail plate near its root is known as the lunula **(Fig. 2.6)**.

The surface of the skin on which the nail rests is known as the nail bed. The fold of the skin surrounding the lateral and proximal borders of the nail are known as the lateral and posterior nail folds.

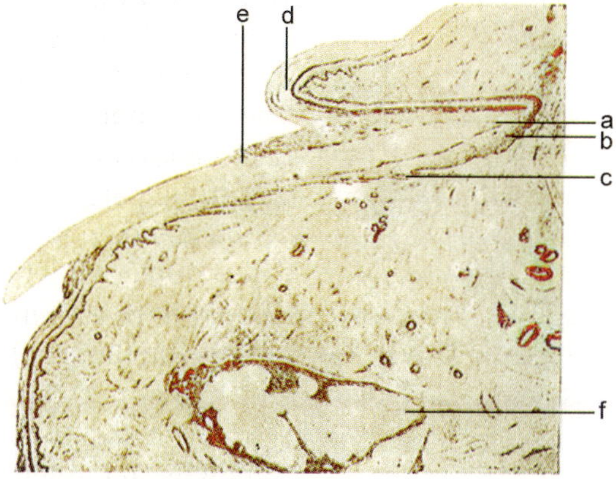

Fig. 2.6: Longitudinal section through root of nail and its matrix. X10 (a) Root of nail. (b) Malpighian layer of matrix. (c) Ridges in cutis and nail bed. (d) Cuticle of skin continuous with eponychium. (e) Eponychium. (f) Bone (terminal phalanx) of finger (*Courtesy:* Longmans, Green & Co. Ltd., London from Essentials of Histology by Schafers, XIV Ed.)

Nails may be object of admiration and beauty; nevertheless, they are homologous to the claws and hooves of lower animals. The material of the true nail develops from the matrix, which is the deeper portion of the proximal or posterior nail fold and the epithelium of the proximal part of the nail bed. The nail plate and the proximal nail fold are joined by a thin cuticle called the eponychium which makes the exterior groove waterproof. Its rupture by enthusiastic manicuring or dissolving of the eponychium, as in the case of washermen (dhobis) results in disease.

Mucous Membranes

There are definite differences between the skin and mucous membranes. In the latter, stratum corneum, lucidum and granulosum are absent. Stratum malpighii has less number of layers. Dermal appendages like hair, sweat and sebaceous glands are absent; on the other hand, mucous glands are present. Pigmentation is minimal. On the lips, transition from skin to mucous membrane is typically seen. The outer vermilion border has more pigment and is somewhat thicker than the inner part. For this reason and also because of the absence of hair follicles, the chances of repigmentation are least in depigmentary disorders.

Lines of Langer denote lines of normal tension of the integument. These pattems are caused by the peculiar arrangement of elastic tissue in the corium, which throws the papillary layer into definite folds. The main significance of these lines is surgical. Incisions along these lines close smoothly, while those across these lines tend to gape and cause wide scars. The pattern of these lines is fairly uniform in all persons.

PHYSIOLOGY

The skin performs a multitude of functions. These are:

1. Protection—self and body
2. Sense organ
3. Secretion and excretion

4. Body temperature regulation
5. Storage of fat, blood
6. Absorption
7. Gaseous exchange.

1. Protective function: As an organ of protection, the skin exhibits a wide range of modifications in the various species of animals. For instance, the skin of the alligator has horny plates, and that of the toad has poisonous glands located in it. In human beings, the tough, horny, and keratinized waterproof epidermis, and appendages like hair and nails, provide a sufficiently strong barrier against injury, epidermal penetration of harmful substances and bacterial invasions; they also protect the underlying structures.

Another protective function of skin is to protect against sunlight by synthesis of melanin pigment.

The stratum corneum has been held as major barrier to penetration. External substances not only are unable to pass through this barrier, but water loss to outside by insensible perspiration is also restrained. There is about 70% of water in the epidermis and about 15% in the horny layer. The horny layer becomes hard and brittle when the water content falls below 10%. The skin looks dry and brittle. It is now appreciated that dry skin is due to lack of water and not due to lack of greasy lipids or fatty substances. Permeability properties of this cornified layer maintain the body's water content and electrolyte concentration. If the injury to the cornified layer is severe and widespread, death may result from dehydration or toxicity.

2. Sense organ: The skin is richly supplied with nerves and various types of specialized sensory end-organs, which provide information regarding environmental changes; the body can then adjust its activities accordingly. In some animals, the hair at certain situations have specialized sensory receptors located at the bases of the hair follicles which serve to enhance sensory appreciation, an example of this being the whiskers of a cat.

3. Secretion and excretion: The skin possesses various types of glands which pour secretions on the surface. The more important ones are the sweat and the sebaceous glands. Their structures have already been dealt with. The eccrine glands which are scattered all over the body surface secrete a thin, transparent, watery fluid, known as true sweat; while the apocrine glands secrete a thicker, rather milky and odoriferous solution; their secretions are meant for sexual attraction in the lower animals, but their importance is lost as we ascend the ladder of evolution. However, they do have some relationship with the menstrual cycle in females. The secretory cells get hypertrophied during the premenstrual period and regress during the menstrual phase.

Sweat in its composition consists of 1.2% solids (organic 0.4% and inorganic 0.8%) and 98.8% water. The important substances excreted in it are sodium chloride, sodium phosphate, sodium bicarbonate, keratin and a small amount of urea. Water and chlorides are by far the most important constituents. In the hot tropical summers, when sweating is profuse, one can lose a large amount of water, and salt. This can give rise to heat cramps and dehydration, which can be rectified by the administration of salts and water.

Man perspires very little at low and moderate temperature, but his perspiration sharply increases at high temperature. Direct studies on the amount of sweat secreted on the surface of the human skin show that sweat glands react very strongly to changes in the atmospheric temperature. This is known as thermal sweating. ln areas like the palms of the hands and soles of the feet, sweating does not increase with the rise of temperature alone. It can also show an increase in the different emotional conditions of fear, anxiety or mental stress. This is called cold sweating or mental sweating, and is under direct cerebral control. This forms one basis of LIE detection. It should be understood, however, that in exercise, sweating is both mental and thermal.

Eating of hot spicy food, causes facial sweating known as "gustatory sweating". Emotional stress, pain, fear or anger causes generalized or localised sweating on the palms, soles, axillae and forehead.

The sweat glands are innervated by cholinergic fibres belonging to the sympathetic nervous system. These nerve fibres are axons of cells located in the sympathetic ganglia. The central efferent mechanisms of perspiration are located segmentally along the entire spinal cord corresponding to the distribution of the neurons from whose axons the sympathetic fibres are formed. Regional disorders in perspiration can, therefore, prove quite important in diagnosing the diseases in the corresponding divisions of the spinal cord.

Besides the substances excreted in sweat in the normal way (water, salts, lactic acid and products of nitrogen metabolism), the skin can also excrete certain drugs administered to the individual, for example mercury, arsenic, iodine, etc. ln certain diseases of disturbed metabolism, a variety of substances have been found in sweat, i.e. cystine in cystinurea, and glucose in diabetes. Elimination of urea and other compounds through the skin, to some extent can compensate for kidney failure. The sebaceous glands of the skin secrete sebum which is composed of fatty acids, cholesterol, alcohols, etc. Fatty acid have a mild fungistatic activity. The sebum acts as a lubricant for the drying effects of the atmosphere. Another advantage of sebum and sweat is that they have a destructive action on streptococci and other organisms through certain fatty acids and enzymes.

Excessive production of sebum is called seborrhoea. Sebaceous glands undergo marked hypertrophy during puberty indicating hormonal control of these glands. Sebaceous gland is an androgen target organ. Sebum may evoke inflammation by action of free fatty acids leading to formation of comedones in acne. Sebaceous gland secretion being androgen dependent, excess or deficiency will cause certain dermatological disorders.

4. Body heat regulation: The vital activity of warm-blooded species like human beings is, in a large measure, independent of the 'temperature conditions of the external environments because of their constant internal temperature. This constancy is achieved by the existence of a heat regulating mechanism which adjusts the body heat loss to the heat generated in it.

The skin plays the most important role in the regulation of heat loss. It loses heat to the external environment in three ways: by conduction, by radiation and by evaporation. Heat loss by the first two mechanisms takes place when the environmental temperature is lower than that of the skin. Heat loss by the evaporation mainly means the amount of heat spent by the body to evaporate the sweat from the surface of the skin. Even when no perspiration is visible, a certain amount of fluid continues to evaporate through the skin. This is known as insensible or invisible perspiration. About 90% of the total heat loss of the body is regulated by the skin. The heat loss through the skin is regulated by various physiological mechanisms which include (1) the reaction of the cutaneous vessels, (2) perspiration, and (3) the reaction of the smooth muscle fibres of the skin.

The temperature of the skin depends upon the amount of blood flowing through the blood vessels in the dermis. Therefore, for all practical purposes, the amount of heat loss by physical means is determined by the condition of these vessels. The most important way of reducing the loss of heat is to reduce the flow of blood through the skin. Thus, in the cold, when we want to conserve heat, it is accomplished by the constriction of the arterioles in the dermal vascular plexuses. Flushing of the skin occurs when the environmental temperature rises and when one takes exercise, thus ensuring greater amount of heat loss.

Perspiration which adjusts the heat loss through evaporation, also depends upon, firstly, the blood flow through the skin, and secondly, the stimulation of the sweat glands through the autonomic nervous system. Insensible perspiration depends mostly upon blood flow through the skin.

Hair also plays a major part in limiting the heat loss in animals. Contraction of the arrector pili occurs at low temperatures. As a result the position of the hair in the fur alters, thus changing the amount of air in the fur and its heat-preserving properties. In human beings, this function hair is largely vestigeal in nature. Man has retained a rudiment of this reaction observed in the form of "goose flesh".

The sensory end-organs of heat (organs of Ruffini) and cold (end bulbs of Krause) are present in the dermis. These, when stimulated, send impulses to the heat regulating centres situated in the hypothalamus, which through its connections with the vasomotor mechanisms brings about vascular adjustments in the dermis by constricting or dilating the vessels, thus regulating the heat loss. It also regulates sweating through the autonomic nerves.

5. Storage function of skin: The dermis in conjunction with the hypodermis has a considerable capacity for storing various materials, of these the best known are fat and blood.

a. Fat is laid down in fat cells as a permanent store of subcutaneous adipose tissue. This provides the reserve stores of body energy. Incidentally, it also prevents heat loss, and is a good shock absorber.
b. Blood is stored in the rich subpapillary plexuses of the dermis. A rough estimate of its capacity in a normal adult comes to near about one litre. Whenever there is a greater requirement of blood by the muscles or other organs, blood is directed from this storehouse to those regions.
c. The skin is also a good storehouse of ergosterol—the provitamin for vitamin D. This ergosteraol is irradiated by the ultraviolet light of the sun and converted into vitamin D (calciferol).
d. The other type of storage which occurs in the skin is a storage by inundation. This, in fact, is the storage of extracellular fluid in the interstitial spaces. This fluid represents an escape from the blood capillaries whenever the hydrostatic pressure in the capillaries increases. The extra fluid is thus held in the dermal and hypodermal layers. In pathological states, this may lead to oedema. Conversely, in dehydration or decrease of plasma volume, the water from such places can be drawn back to the blood.

Certain substances like glucose and chloride may also be stored in the skin temporarily when their level in the blood registers a sudden rise.

Recent studies have shown that cornified layer also acts as a reservoir for topically applied corticosteroids or other hormones which are absorbed slowly for many days from the skin surface. Dermis contains ground substances. The acid mucopolysaccharides, hyaluranic acid, chondroitin sulfate, dermatan sulfate are the major elements of the ground substance. The ground substance has a great capacity to bind water. Examples of these are cases of myxoedema, focal mucinosis, etc.

6. Absorption: It is almost an established fact that the uninjured skin is impermeable to watery solution of salts or other substances. Ions can, however, be made to permeate with the application of an electric current by a process known as iontophoresis. In some measure, the skin can absorb substances dissolved in fatty solvents like vitamins and hormones. This is the principle behind the local application and massaging of various ointments, solutions and cream. Inflammation greatly increases the skin permeability. Substances that are completely insoluble in water and lipids do not penetrate. Current methods of augmenting the penetration of topical medication is to occlude the skin surface with cellophane or wraps. Percutaneous absorption mainly occurs via the pilo-sebaceous apparatus. The dried secretion which blocks the ducts of sebaceous glands, and thus brings about troublesome black-heads and pimples, often seen in adolescents, can be "dissolved out" by the local massage of creams containing fat solvents. Very little penetration occurs through the cornified cells via the intercellular spaces.

Skin without an epidermis, in extensive ulcers, erosions, etc. becomes freely permeable and absorbs substances easily. Boric acid compresses have caused death due to boron poisoning.

7. Gaseous exchange through skin: A small amount of gaseous exchange occurs through the skin. In man, the amount of CO_2 exchanged through the skin is negligible compared to the amount exhaled from the lungs (near about 1/150–1/200 of that exhaled by the lungs). But in a thin-skinned animal like the frog, the absorption of O_2 and the excretion of CO_2 through the skin may be sufficient for the proper oxygenation of its blood, so that it may continue to live even after the removal of its lungs.

EMBRYOLOGY

The whole of the skin—epidermis and dermis—is a unified integrated organ system, but it develops from two different primitive embryonic layers—epidermis from the ectoderm and dermis from the mesoderm.

The general ectoderm of the early human embryo, except for the part that specializes as the neural ectoderm, consists of a single layer of cuboidal cells. By the fifth week of intrauterine life, this becomes double layered. The most superficial layer of flattened cells is called periderm or epitrichium because the hair that grows later from the deeper layer is said not to penetrate through it, but to push it up and cast it off. During the third month of foetal life, three layers of cells are recognizable, the periderm. the intermediate and the basal layer which is close to the dermis. The basal cells multiply rapidly and keep pushing the older cells towards the periderm, and thus, by the fifth month a stratum of these cells (prickle cells) superficial to the basal cells, forms a definite stratum malpighii.

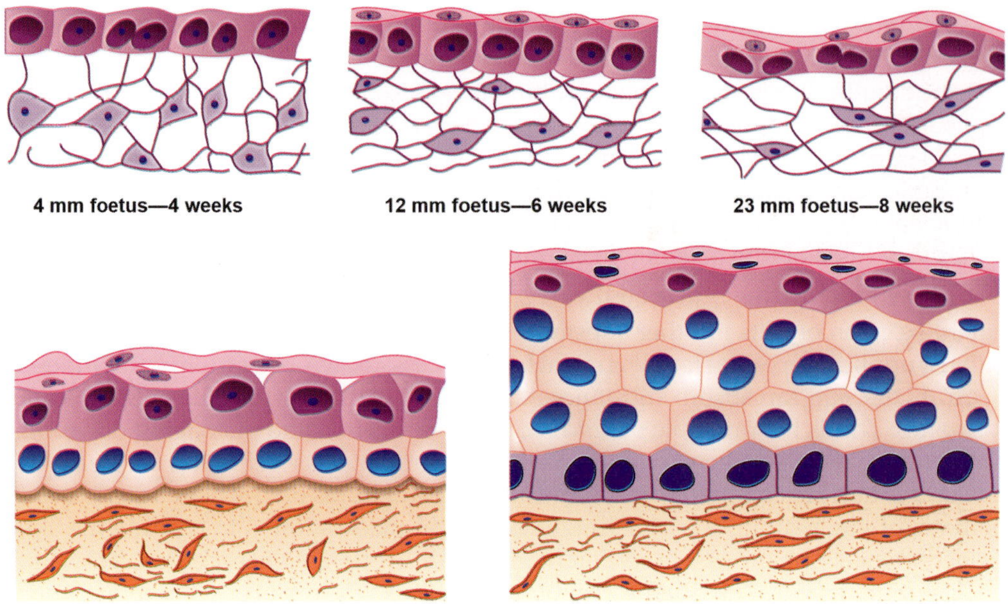

Fig. 2.7: Development of skin

The cells in the zone overlying the stratum malpighii show keratohyalin granules and form the stratum granulosum. As the cells, keep moving outwards owing to new cells being added from the basal layer, the most superficial ones culminate in cornification forming the stratum corneum near the surface. Next to the stratum corneum, a thin, clear zone containing homogeneous semi-fluid eleidin is evident, particularly on the palms and soles, giving rise to the stratum lucidum. The early intermediate layer of cells becomes a part of the stratum germinativum, and the periderm by the end of the fourth month of foetal life is east off as a part of the vernix caseosa **(Figs 2.7 and 2.8)**.

The embryonic stratum germinativum, besides giving rise to the surface epidermis, forms the primary epithelial germ which later develops, by downward prolongations into the mesoderm, into the hair, sebaceous glands and apocrine glands and also forms the eccrine sweat glands. Soon after birth, the cells of the stratum germinativum acquire pigment granules from the melanoblasts which migrate from the primitive neural crest and specialize in melanin pigment formation (Rawles, 1953).

The dermis is derived mostly from the mesenchyme, although some cells from the ventrolateral part of the somite (dermomyotome) may contribute to deeper layers of the corium. Until the end of the second month of intrauterine life, the dermis consists of closely-packed, spindle-shaped mesenchymal cells, and by the third month of intra-uterine life, fine reticulum fibres are demonstrable, which later increase in number and thickness and form the collagenous fibre, the latter, usually during the sixth month of foetal life. The subcutaneous fat is apparent by the end of the third month of intrauterine life, but it becomes abundant only during the later months of foetal life.

The nail starts as an epidermal specialization on the dorsum of the tips of the digits by the third month of foetal life.

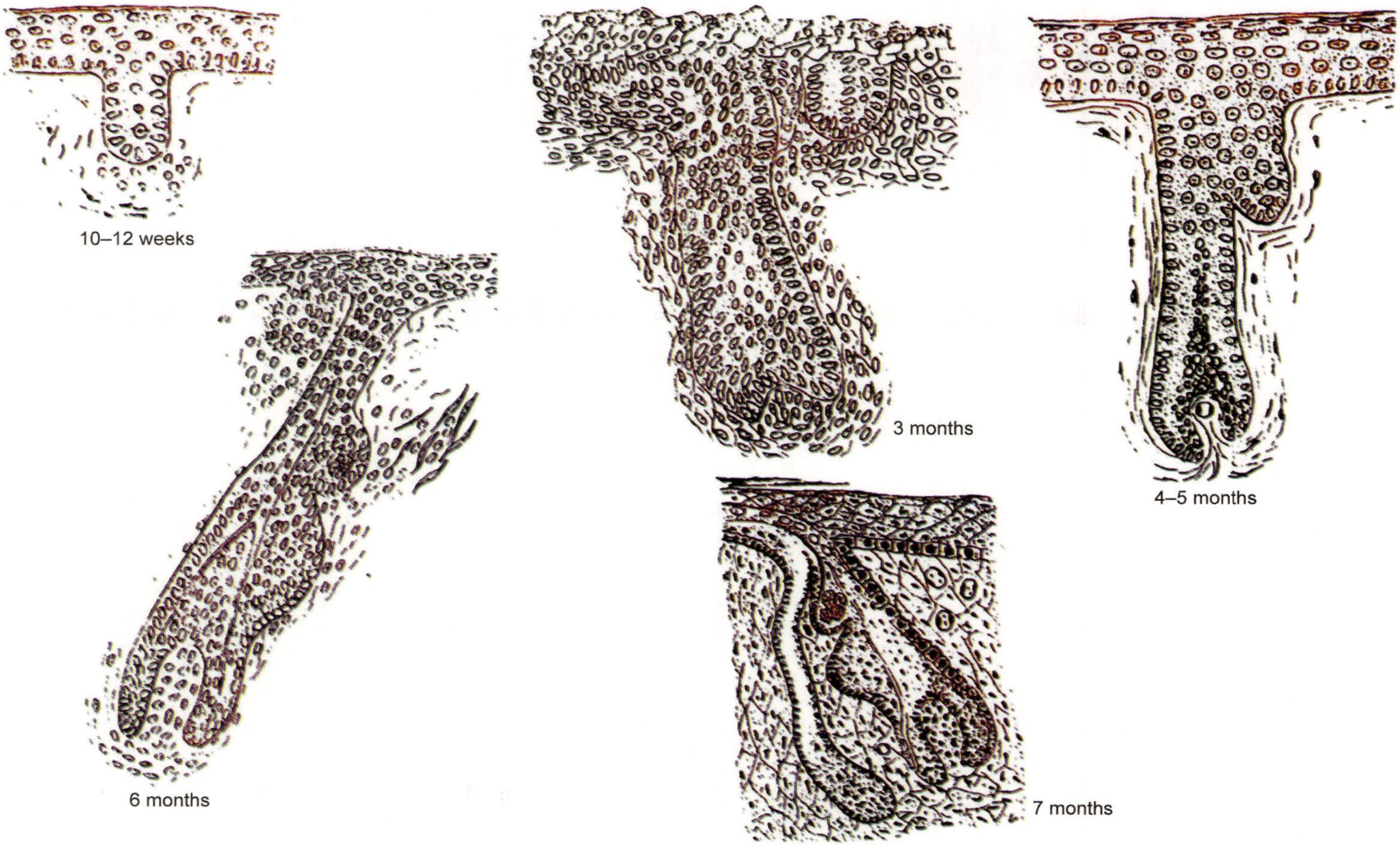

Fig. 2.8: Development of hair and sweat gland

The earliest hair appears on the eyebrows, upper lip and chin at the end of the second month of intrauterine life. By the fourth month, hair appears over the general body surface. This hair is fine, silky, downy, termed lanugo hair and is cast off before birth as a component of the vernix caseosa. The replacing hair develops to some extent from the new hair follicles and is shed thereafter and replaced periodically throughout life. The hair on the face, neck and trunk of the female, and on the face, except for the beard, the flexor aspect of the upper arms and the trunk, in the male, remains apparently of the lanugo type throughout life. Under the influence of sex hormones at puberty, coarser and darker hair appear on the pubis and axillae of both the sexes and on the face and certain regions of the trunk of the male **(Fig. 2.8)**.

Most of the sebaceous glands in the body develop in connection with hair follicles during the fifth month of foetal life, as solid epidermal buds, which later become lobulated. ln certain regions like the upper eyelids, hairless deeper portion of the vestibule of the nose, prepuce, vulva and the anal region, these glands arise from the general epidermis, independent of the hair follicles.

Most of the eccrine sweat glands develop independently as solid down-growths from the epidermis. They first appear on the finger tips, the palms and the soles during the fourth month of intrauterine life. By the sixth month of foetal life, they become simple cords, which later coil and acquire lumina.

Congenital Anomalies of the Integumentary System

As will be seen from the process of development of the integument, congenital anomalies could involve only a local area or the general body surface. They could also affect all the components of the integument or only the appendages of the skin. There are, however, other anomalies which occur at the regions where the ectodermal lines normally fuse in the early embryo. Here, only a short description of a few anomalies is included.

Dermoid cysts occur as a result of epidermal inclusions along the lines of fusion of embryonic structures, e.g., bronchial cysts and cysts along the mid-dorsal and mid-ventral body, wall. The contents of the cyst will naturally show all the derivatives of the integument.

Pilonidal (Latin: pilus-hair, and nidus-nest) cyst: A variety of the dermoid cyst, formed due to the persistent foveola coccygea near the tip of the coccyx at the embryonic site of the terminal attachment of the neural tube to the embryonic skin.

Congenital ectodermal defect: There is an absence of eyebrows, deformed nails and teeth which may be entirely absent; and sometimes., accompanied by the absence of sweat glands. Scalp hair is sparse, the eyes have an upward slant and the nose is saddle-shaped. (Refer to Chapter 27 for details of congenital defects)

BACTERIOLOGY

Normally, the integument harbours several resident organisms like *Staphylococcus albus* and *Corynebacterium acnes* on its surface and crevices. *Pityrosporon ovale*, a saprophytic fungus, is frequently found on the scalp and face. Bacteria like *Streptococcus pyogenes* and *Staphylococcus aureus*, may occasionally be found on the skin as transient flora, though they can often be demonstrated in the nose, mouth and throat. These pathogenic bacteria are also frequently found in the body folds particularly the perineum. Occasionally,

Candida albicans and intestinal bacteria may be seen on the skin particularly near the anus.

Despite the presence of these organisms, normally no harm is done to the skin, because the latter protects itself with its auto-disinfecting defence mechanism, viz. the acidic pH mantle, the fatty acids of the sebum, the continuous desquamation of the stratum corneum and the enzymes of sweat. Daily washing and the sun rays also inhibit the growth of bacteria. The normal resistance of the skin is reduced in debilitating diseases like diabetes; xerodermic skin lacks the defence mechanism and is, therefore, more prone to pyoderma. In the body folds, particularly in obese patients where sweating is increased, pH is high, maceration is more, local temperature is raised, hence the infection is frequent. Seborrhoeic individuals are supposed to have altered sebaceous secretion; hence they are also prone to infections. Resident bacterial flora like Staph. albus which is normally non-pathogenic, may become pathogenic in persons with defective defence mechanism.

PATHOLOGY

The pathological processes in the skin may involve one or more of its constituents, viz. epidermis, dermis or subcutaneous tissue or their component parts or layers. The changes are hypertrophic, atrophic, inflammatory or dystrophic. The physician should be familiar with the meaning of these pathological changes and the terminology used to describe them.

Epidermis

Hyperkeratosis implies hypertrophy of the stratum corneum. In localized form it is seen in corns, warts and keratoses. In diffuse form, it is seen in ichthyosis, keratodermas and pityriasis rubra pilaris.

Parakeratosis implies incompletely cornified but abnormally increased horny layer. The latter is seen as swollen horny cells with oedema and retention of nuclei. Cells are loosely attached. Parakeratosis signifies oedema of prickle cell layer, usually due to an inflammatory process, e.g. psoriasis, eczema, seborrhoeic dermatitis.

Dyskeratosis implies imperfect and premature keratinization taking on various shapes. It may be benign as it is seen in Darier's disease (corps ronds and grains of Darier) and chronic benign pemphigus of Hailey and Hailey, or it may be malignant as in epitheliomas (Bowen's disease, Paget's disease and squamous cell carcinoma).

Acanthosis implies hyperplasia of the prickle cell layer. It is usually a benign process and is seen typically in chronic eczema, psoriasis, lichen planus and warts. In tuberculosis cutis verrucosus and pyoderma vegetans, acanthosis and hyperkeratosis are secondary to the disease process in the corium. Special type of acanthosis is seen in condyloma acuminatum and molluscum contagiosum; the latter exhibits molluscum bodies.

If there is atypical proliferation of prickle cells with hyperchromatic nuclei and mitotic figures (anaplasia) accompanied by loss of intercellular fibrils, malignancy must be suspected.

Spongiosis implies spongy appearance of the epidermis (mainly prickle cell layer) caused by intercellular oedema. With the increase of oedema, collections of fluid result in intraepidermal vesicles or bullae e.g., eczema. Viral affections also produce intraepidermal bullae.

Acantholysis is typically seen in pemphigus. Due to lysis of intercellular fibrils of basal and prickle cell layer, degenerated epidermal cells become detached, shrunken and rounded with swollen, compact, hyperchromatic nuclei (Tzanck cells). Acantholytic bulla is seen in pemphigus.

Atrophy implies thinning of the epidermis with straightened epidermodermal junction along with Ioss of rete ridges e.g., senile atrophy, scleroderma, acrodermatitis atrophicans, lichen sclerosus et atrophicus, leprosy, etc. Basal cell degeneration is seen in discoid lupus erythematosus.

Corium

Infiltration: Polymorphonuclear cell infiltration is seen in acute inflammations, while in chronic inflammations, lymphocytes predominate. Infiltration is mainly around blood vessels (perivascular), pilo-sebaceous apparatus and sweat glands. Epithelioid cells are seen in infective granulomas, mainly tuberculosis, leprosy, sarcoid, etc. A granuloma, histologically speaking, implies circumscribed dermal infiltration which is usually persistent and slowly progressive. Granulomas, are composed of histiocytes, epithelioid cells, giant cells (Langhans', foreign body) and plasma cells.

It is important to establish the different cells of the infiltration process, their location, number and distribution. Since these are differently affected in different disease processes, correct histological reading helps in confirmation of diagnosis.

Bullae: Dermal bullae are seen typically in dermatitis herpetiformis, erythema multiforme and epidermolysis bullosa. ln miliaria profunda, sweat is imprisoned in the upper part of the corium.

Collagen tissue is increased in fibrosis. Increased collagen, accompanied by hyalinization and oedema is seen in scleroderma. Elastic tissue is affected in elastosis, cutis laxa and pseudo-xanthoma elasticum.

Neoplasms in the corium may arise from any of its constituents, viz. fibroma from fibrous tissue, a leiomyoma from smooth muscle of arrector pili, neuromas from nerve fibres, lipomas from fatty tissue, etc. Then there are different types of naevi, malignant melanomas, sarcomas and reticuloses particularly mycosis fungoides, etc. Tumours related to hair follicles are seen in trichoepitheliomas; and syringomas arise from sweat glands.

Cysts: Sebaceous, sweat, etc. may be seen in the corium. Degenerative changes may effect corium- collagen or elastic tissue or both. ln special stained sections, these tissues become basophilic, degenerated lumps or granules. Elastic tissue is more resistant than collagen, hence the latter shows degenerative changes first. Necrobiosis means partial destruction of tissues-nuclei are disintegrated but the cellular structure is preserved. It is typically seen in necrobiosis lipoidica diabeticorum.

Blood vessels of the corium are typically affected in syphilis (panarteritis with perivascular cuffing of plasma cells), Schamberg's disease, nodular vasculitis, angioma, angiokeratoma, etc. Extravasation of red cells is seen in purpura and Schamberg's disease, and in inflammations, etc.

Subcutaneous tissue is affected in panniculitis, erythema nodosum, erythema induratum and Milroy's disease.

Chapter 3

Clinical Features, Case-taking and General Diagnosis

SYMPTOMS

The common symptoms of skin diseases are itching, pain and disturbed sensations in the nature of crawling, sense of heat, stinging, anaesthesia or hyperaesthesia. These subjective symptoms, as much as the apparent rash, are responsible for bringing the patient to the doctor for consultation.

1. *Itching (pruritus):* It is an annoying complaint. Its intensity varies according to the disease and the sensitivity of the individual. It may be continuous or spasmodic, localized or generalized, accompanied or unaccompanied by a rash. The objective evidence of itching is a scratch mark in the form of a linear excoriation. The common causes of itching are:
   - Scabies
   - Pediculoses
   - Ringworm
   - Eczema
   - Urticaria
   - Dermatitis herpetiformis
   - Neurodermatitis
   - Insect bite
2. *Pain:* It may be localized to the skin, as in boils, abscesses, or radiate along a nerve, as in leprotic neuritis and herpes zoster.
3. Crawling sensation (formication) as if insects are crawling under the skin. It is a variety of itching, e.g. acarophobia.
4. *Sense of heat:* In dermatological practice, 'heat in the blood' or sense of heat (SOH) is not an uncommon complaint. It is seen as the first sign or symptom of drug eruption, in urticaria and allergy. Lay patients even call venereal diseases as 'Heat-Garm' (syphilis in Arabic means heat). Ayurveda, Hippocrates and Galen have laid stress on constitution, temperament and elementary qualities like heat, cold, dryness and moisture.

   It is experienced as warm sensation to feeling of burning hot, warm to hot hands and feet, uncomfortable to burning sensation in the sun, and keeping feet and hands outside the covering while sleeping. SOH is very significant in skin diseases esp. of allergic origin. Almost every cause of urticaria, drug rash and disseminated eczema is preceded or accompanied by SOH. This is more in cholinergic and physical urticarias.

SOH, as a matter of fact, is a more useful guide than leucocyte count or allergy tests in urticaria and endogenous eczema. Further, according to our experience, persons with SOH are more prone to skin diseases. May be change in eating and living habits (sattvic vegetarian diet, no spices, chillies, tea, alcohol, etc.) help to reduce the SOH and hence the predisposition to allergic dermatoses.

5. *Stinging sensation* is characteristic of stinging of insect bites.
6. *Hyperaesthesia* signifies increased sensitivity, e.g. post-herpetic neuralgia.
7. *Anaesthesia* signifies loss of sensations. It is noticed in leprosy, syringomyelia, etc. The patient may notice the anaesthesia himself, but usually it is found on physical examination. The sensations tested, pertaining to skin diseases are pain sensation (pin-prick), touch and temperature (hot and cold).

SIGNS

Objective signs are more important in cutaneous diseases than subjective ones since cutaneous lesions are at once noticeable. Quite a few skin diseases are symptomless. Clinical lesions are, basically, of two types:

1. Primary
2. Secondary

In case-taking, primary lesions are the most important. The differential diagnosis centres mostly around them **(Figs 3.1 to 3.7)**. The clinician must look for the primary lesion in the most recently developed eruption or at the periphery of the rash. The history and observation of an intelligent patient will be helpful. With the passage of time, primary lesions either involute or transform or get modified into secondary lesions.

Primary Lesions

1. ***Macule:*** A macule is a small-sized, not raised, circumscribed lesion with alteration in colour **(Fig. 3.1)**. There are two types of macules:
   a. Erythematous
   b. Pigmentary

When of large size, this alteration in colour is called a patch or sheet of erythema or pigmentation. A macule must be palpated for infiltration or induration which is typical of granulomatous diseases and reticuloses. Further, erythematous macules must be differentiated from purpuric macules. In the former, erythema disappears under pressure, while in the latter, the redness is brighter, and does not fade under pressure.

Pigmentary macules are further differentiated into hyperpigmented or depigmented types. The common examples of macular eruptions are:

Erythematous Macules

Dermatitis	Tinea circinata
Exanthemata	Psoriasis
Drug eruption	Pityriasis rosea
Macular syphilide	Leprosy
Erythema multiforme	

Hyperpigmentary Macules

Chloasma	Freckles

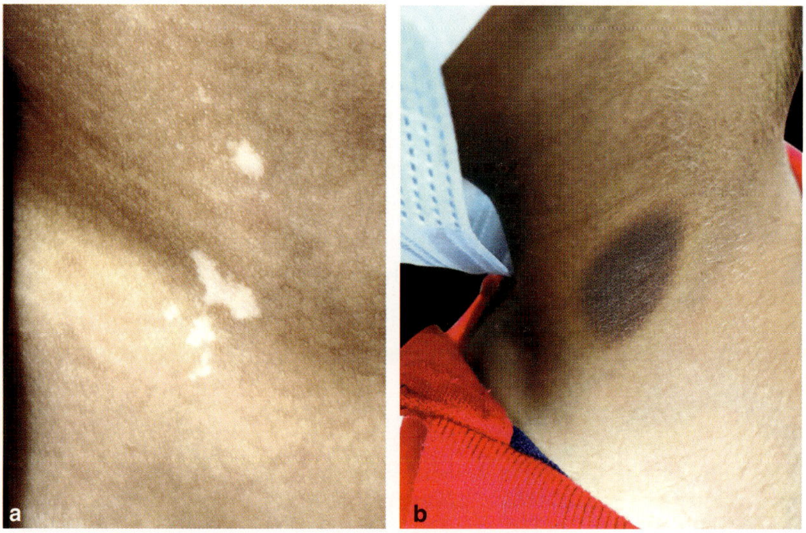

Fig. 3.1: (a) Depigmented macules of vitiligo; (b) Hyperpigmented macule of fixed drug eruption

Fixed drug eruption
Melanodermas
Addison' s disease
Naevi
Lentigines

Hypopigmentation

Leprosy
Tinea versicolor
Pityriasis alba

Depigmentation

Leucoderma
Vitiligo

2. ***Papule:*** It is a solid, raised lesion about the size of a split pea or smaller. A similar lesion, but larger in size, is called a nodule (as big as a hazel nut, or smaller), or tumour (bigger than a hazel nut). A papule may be a static lesion or a transition to other lesions; hence in practice, a dermatologist may come across papulovesicular, papulopustular and erythematopapular lesions. When dealing with papules, the points to be studied are their size, shape, colour, whether they be discrete or grouped, whether they be follicular or interfollicular, inflammatory or non-inflammatory in nature. Further, an attempt should be made to distinguish epidermic from dermic and mixed papules. An epidermic papule is usually superficial, dry, solid and flesh-coloured; and dermic papule is deeper, elastic and reddish. The common examples of papules are:

   Warts
   Epidermal and dermal naevi
   Drug eruptions
   Syphilis
   Chickenpox and smallpox
   Psoriasis
   Lichen planus
   Lichen scrofulosorum
   Lichen spinulosum
   Eczema and eczematides
   Acne vulgaris
   Rosacea
   Prickly heat
   Tumours

Papules in Lines

Warts
Insect bites
Psoriasis
Lichen planus

Examples of Nodules

Naevi
Neurofibromatosis
Skin cancer
Dermal leishmaniasis
Leprosy
Syphilis
Tuberculosis cutis
Sarcoid
Erythema nodosum
Xanthomatosis
Mycosis fungoides

Examples of Tumours

Epithelioma
Lymphosarcoma
Mycosis fungoides
Gumma
Keloid
Xanthoma
Naevi
Lipomas
Neurofibromas
Secondary carcinomatosis
Sarcoid

3. Vesicle: It is a circumscribed, serum- or plasma-containing elevation of the integument. When ruptured, the contents ooze out. The size of a vesicle varies from the size of a pin-head to that of a small pea. A similar lesion, but larger in size, Is called a bulla. The following characters of vesicles must be studied: Their shape and size; Is there uniformity or irregularity of shape or size? Are they tense or flaccid, grouped or discrete? What is the mode of evolution? As a rule, vesicles are transitory and of short duration; they either rupture and ooze, or their contents coagulate to form crusts, or enlarge to form bullae, or transform into pustules, or their roofs get rubbed off to leave behind a moist, raw surface. On the palms of the hands, they are situated rather deeply, hence, their contents are discharged with difficulty. On the mucous membranes, their roofs get rubbed off very easily producing erosions.

The common examples of vesicles are:

Eczema, cheiropompholyx
Herpes simplex
Impetigo
Scabies
Smallpox
Chickenpox
Dermatitis herpetiformis
Herpes zoster
Miliaria crystallina and rubra
Tinea
Drug eruptions
Insect bites

The common examples of bullae are:

Impetigo contagiosa
Erythema multiforme
Pemphigus
Dennatitis herpetiformis
Insect bites
Epidermolysis bullosa
Hydroa aestivale
Drug eruptions

4. Wheal: It is a flat, evanescent swelling of the skin caused by the local dilatation of blood vessels and increased permeability resulting in localized oedema. The temporary, evanescent nature of a wheal and its duration (from a few hours to a maximum of 24 hours or so) is characteristic; it helps distinguish a wheal from a persistent granulomatous lesion. Wheals disappear without leaving any trace of stains, scars or atrophy. A wheal is usually pale in the centre and red at the periphery, but it may be uniformly whitish or reddish. Common examples of weals are:

Urticaria
Trauma
Insect bites
Urticaria pigmentosa
Drug rashes

Occasionally, a weal may be surmounted by a vesicle, e.g. papular urticaria of childhood, or accompanied by bulla formation, e.g. urticaria bullosa.

5. Pustule: It differs from a vesicle or a bulla in the nature of its contents. It is a purulent, fluid-containing elevation. It may arise as such, or it may be a transformation from a papule, or more so, a vesicle. The following characters should be studied: the size, shape, number. Is the pustule discrete or confluent, epidermal or follicular, superficial or deep? An example of a superficial, epidermal pustule is impetigo, and of a deep, epidermal pustule is ecthyma. When a pustule is in the upper part of a hair follicle, it is called folliculitis. When it is in the deeper part of a hair follicle and involves the root of the hair which comes out as the core, it is called furunculosis (boil). When a conglomeration of boils forms a deep, dermic abscess with multiple holes on the skin through which pus is discharged, it is called a carbuncle **(Fig. 3.2)**. Pustules terminate by rupture, or desiccate to form irregular yellow crusts.

Common examples of pustules are:

Impetigo
Bacterids
Sycosis barbae
Furunculosis
Carbuncle
Scabies
Drug eruptions (iodides and bromides)
Anthrax
Tuberculides
Acne vulgaris
Smallpox and chickenpox

Secondary Lesions

1. Scale or squama: It is a dry exfoliation of the skin due to increased or abnormal formation of stratum corneum (hyper- or parkeratosis). It results from erythema or inflammation of the skin or increased dryness. Study the following characters: the colour, shape; whether the scale is dry or greasy; whether it is thin or thick, loose or adherent, whether powdery or squamous, etc.

In certain cutaneous diseases they are very characteristic, hence, of diagnostic value, e.g., the silvery layer-upon-layer scales of psoriasis, the greasy scales of seborrheic dermatitis, the cigarette-paper-like centripetal scaling of pityriasis rosea the furfuraceous (powdery) scaling of pityriasis versicolor and the adhesive scale, with its nutmeg-like under-surface of lupus erythematosus. In other disorders, the diagnosis is based upon the primary lesion to which the secondary feature of scaling has been added.

The important causes of scaling are:

Dermatitis and eczema
Seborrhoeic dermatitis
Psoriasis
Pityriasis versicolor

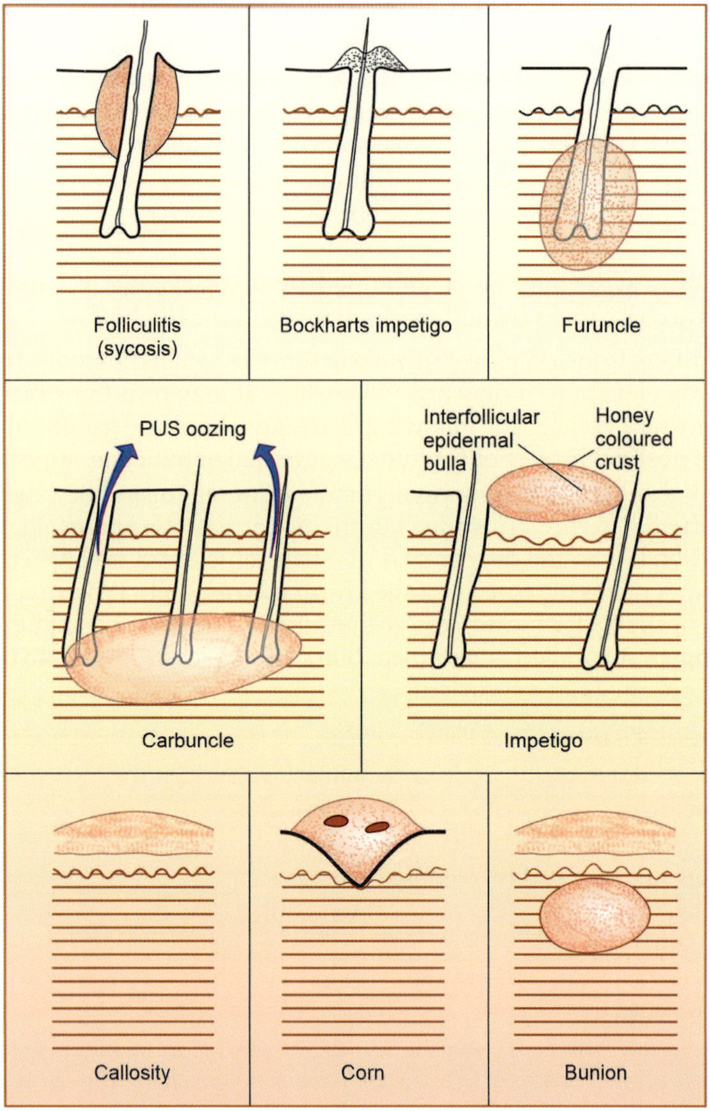

Fig. 3.2: Diagrammatic representation of pustular lesions, callosity, corn and bunion (*Courtesy:* Mr P Chaturvedi)

Exfoliative dermatitis	Tinea corporis
Pityriasis rubra pilaris	Drug eruptions
Tinea capitis	Ichthyosis
Syphilis	Lichen planus
Lupus erythematosus	Malnutrition-pellagra
Exanthemata following scarlet fever	Pityriasis rosea

2. Crust or scab: It represents a dried-up mass of oozing and other products of inflammatory tissues particularly epithelial debris. Scabs form on vesicles, pustules, bullae, ulcers, erosions and excoriations. The colour, thickness, adhesiveness, consistency and odour of a crust should be studied, also its underlying surface, visible only after the crust has been removed. These characters of the crust, its underlying surface and the primary lesion which the crust has supplemented, are all helpful in the making of an accurate diagnosis.

The common causes of crusts are:

Impetigo contagiosa, ecthyma
Sycosis
Seborrhoeic dermatitis
Eczema and dermatitis
Exanthemata—chickenpox and smallpox
Herpes zoster
Ulcers
Kaposi' s varicelliform eruption
Drugs—iodides, bromides and heavy metals
Syphilis—Rupial and noduloulcerative
Scratch marks (blood crusts)

3. Excoriations: They are superficial, linear lesions characterized by the removal of the epidermis by scratching or by abrasion. An excoriation may be superficial or deep.

It gets covered by a crust—simple, blood or impetiginous.

It is produced by trauma; an excoriation is an evidence of pruritus; a search should be made for its cause.

4. Fissure: It is a linear crack in the integrity of the skin reaching down to the papillary layer of the dermis, or deeper. It has length but unlike an ulcer, no breadth. A fissure is usually accompanied by pain which interferes with the use of the affected part. Because of the loss in integrity, there is risk of secondary infection.

Common examples of fissures are:

- Chapping of hands as in extreme dryness
- Chronic eczema of the palms and soles
- Menopausal keratoderma
- Syphilitic fissures
- Fissure in ano
- Intertrigo
- Angular stomatitis

5. Ulcer: It is a circumscribed lesion starting from a break in the skin, reaching up to the level of the dermis. It has definite length, also breadth as opposed to a fissure. A clinician should study its size, contour, depth, edge, covering crust, contents, odour and the surrounding area of skin.

The common causes of ulcers are:

Traumatic
Pyogenic
Tuberculosis
Syphilis
Dermal leishmaniasis
Leprosy
Tropical ulcer
Veldt sore
Actinomycosis
Neoplastic ulcers
Varicose ulcer
Trophic ulcers
Peripheral vascular disorders
Metabolic disorders
Syringomyelia and tabes
Frost-bite

Causes of ulcers in the mouth

Stomatitis
Dental irritation
Pemphigus
Tuberculosis
Syphilis
Epithelioma

6. Scar: It represents a healed destructive lesion of the dermis and deeper parts. Whenever any inflammatory or traumatic lesion destroys the basal layer of the epidermis and the underlying corium, a scar is formed. Superficial epidermal lesions heal without scarring; these are important points to be remembered in surgery and in the treatment of cutaneous lesions. A patient can be forewarned about whether or not a scar will be produced- a question asked by most patients with problems on the exposed parts of their bodies. In people with dark skins, Indians and Negroes, scars have a tendency to be keloidal. So, due precautions should be taken in surgery and in the treatment of burns.

Certain scars are very characteristic, viz. the tissue-paper-like scars of lupus vulgaris, the wrinkled, achromic scars of leprosy, the depressed, pigmented scars of cutaneous leishmaniasis, pock marks of smallpox. The clinician should study the size, shape, colour, texture, depression or elevation of the scar-whether it is attached or free, whether there is any accompanying deformity and loss of sensations, hair, sebaceous or sweat secretion.

The common causes of scars are:

- Traumatic
- Ecthyma, acne necrotica and conglobata
- Exanthemata—smallpox and chickenpox
- Herpes zoster
- Granulomata—tuberculosis, syphilis, leprosy, leishmaniasis, yaws and fungi
- Varicose ulcer
- Neoplasms

Certain Dermatological Terms (Special Lesions)

Alopecia: It implies loss of hair resulting in a bald patch. Defluvium capillorum means fall or thinning of hair without areas of complete baldness. It must be remembered that the hair occur in three states: Growing, stationary and falling. The last state comprises a very small percentage. For the causes of baldness, see Chapter 32.

Atrophy: It means wasting away of the skin, which appears thin. There is loss of elasticity, wrinkling with diminished or complete loss of hair, sweat and sebum. All destructive disease processes of the corium with intact epidermis (i.e. without ulceration) leave behind atrophy. An atrophic patch may or may not be accompanied by scaling, pigmentation and telangiectasia.

Burrow: It is a straight or tortuous, slightly elevated, flesh-coloured or slightly darker line found on the wrist, hand or genitalia in scabies. It represents the path or tunnel of the *Acarus scabiei* (*Sarcoptes scabiei*) in the stratum corneum of the skin. At the deeper end of the burrow an *Acarus* can be demonstrated.

Cyst: It is a circumscribed collection of fluid or semi-solid substances in the skin surrounded by well-defined walls. Its size, shape, consistency, translucency, depth, and whether or not it is adherent to the skin and underlying structures, should be studied.

The common causes of cutaneous cysts are:
- Sebaceous cyst
- Milia
- Mucous cyst
- Implantation cyst
- Dermoid cyst
- Benign cystic epithelioma
- Pilonidal cyst
- Hydrocystoma

Comedones (blackheads): It represents a plug at the pilo-sebaceous opening. It consists of dried sebum and epithelial debris. To begin with, it is white. With the passage of time, the sulphur of sebum is converted into sulphide and the colour becomes black. Comedones are usually found on the face, shoulders, sternal region and back in acne vulgaris and acneiform eruptions due to iodides and bromides **(Fig. 3.3)**. Tar, chlorine and oils, by contact, produce comedones on exposed parts like the face, arms and legs.

Circinata: It implies a circular lesion-shaped like a coin or disc. If there is central clearing and spreading at the periphery, the lesions are called annular **(Fig. 3.4)**.

Common examples are:

Tinea circinata
Impetigo
Discoid dermatitis
Lupus erythematosus
Psoriasis
Infective eczema
Erythema multiforme
Granuloma annulare

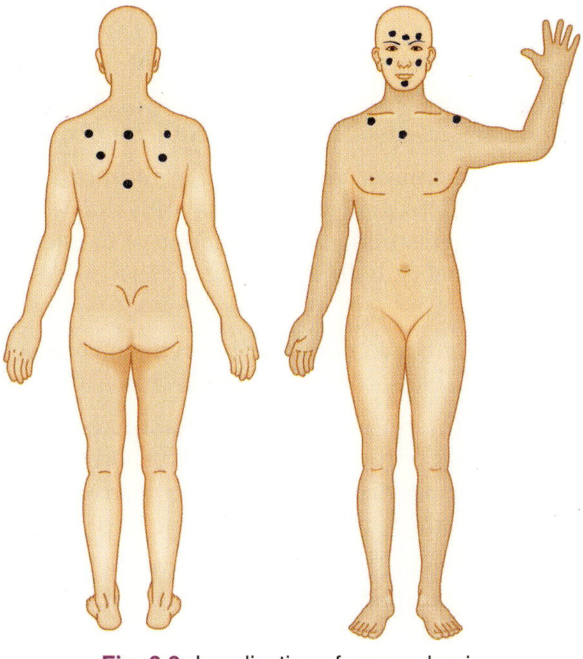

Fig. 3.3: Localization of acne vulgaris

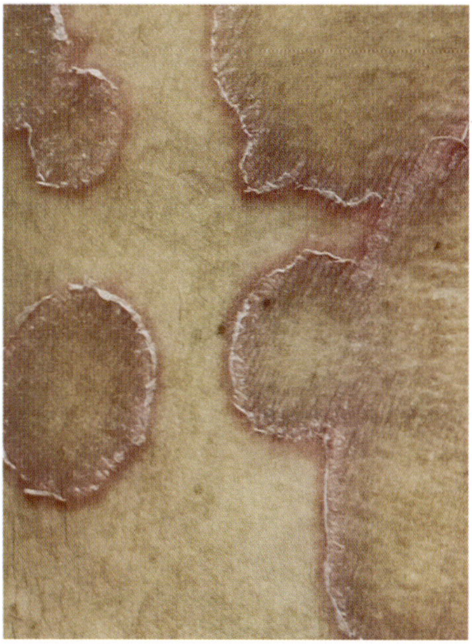

Fig. 3.4: Circinate/annular lesions of tinea corporis

Syphilides	Seborrhoea corporis
Leprosy	Drug eruption
Lichen planus annularis	Pityriasis rosea

Further special configurations may occur in different skin diseases, viz. half circle (arciform), multiple circles joined together (polycyclic) or circular with central dots (iris).The latter is typically seen in erythema multiforme.

Erythema: It implies redness of the skin due to dilatation of blood vessels. It is a common early sign of most cutaneous diseases, but may be difficult to make out in dark people.

Erythroderma: It implies generalized redness and infiltration of the integument as is evident in pityriasis rubra pilaris, generalized dermatitis due to drugs and reticuloses. When accompanied by marked scaling and exfoliation of the skin, the term exfoliative dermatitis is employed. In reality, both terms mean more or less the same thing. (For details, *see* Chapter 20).

Erythematosquamous: It means a combination of erythema and scaling, e.g. psoriasis, tinea, syphilis, lichen planus, parapsoriasis, pityriasis rosea and exfoliative dermatitis.

Elephantiasis: It is a clinical term signifying elephant-like swelling due to extreme lymphoedema and fibrous hypertrophy of a part of the body. The common causes are: filariasis, streptococcal lymphangitis, congenital lymphoedema. The parts commonly affected are the feet, legs and the genitalia.

Granuloma: It is a chronic swelling usually in the form of a well-defined, deep-seated, dermic nodule. Clinically it is marked by chronic induration and scarring; histologically, histiocyte infiltration in the corium is its special feature. They are very common in the tropics. There are several causes of granulomas:

Infective

- Tuberculosis
- Syphilis, granuloma inguinale and lymphogranuloma inguinale
- Leprosy
- Yaws
- Leishmaniasis

PRÉCIS OF CASE-TAKING IN DERMATOLOGY

History

A. Name, age, sex, occupation: Exact nature with list of substances handled in occupational dermatoses only: Duration:

B. Complaints:
  1.
  2.
  3.

C. History of present illness; emphasis on:
  1. Site of onset
  2. Primary lesion
  3. Manner of spread
  4. Eruption—active or quiescent
  5. Subjective symptoms, if any; also whether the symptoms preceded or followed the eruption
  6. Patient's own idea of cause and aggravating factors
  7. History of any illness preceding or accompanying the skin disorder

D. Personal history—hobbies, special habits, etc.

E. Past history of any skin disorder, duration and response

F. Family history of skin and allied disorders

G. General health-Any specific disorder and its relationship to the skin ailment

H. Treatment tried—in order of use, and the response to it.

I. Special history, in particular ailments to find out the cause.
  1. Use of drugs (habit or temporary), tonics, sleeping tablets, cough medicines, opening medicines, etc.
  2. Emotional stress
  3. Contacts in contact eczema
  4. Any other relevant fact

Examination

A. Local:
  1. Inspection: Clinical nature of lesions: Primary, secondary, special term
     Distribution: Regional, general or local; grouped or polymorphous. Particular examination of scalp, mouth, nails, genitalia and feet
  2. Palpation, scraping, diascopy, sensations, etc.

B. General physical examination: Patient ill, toxic, conscious, cyanotic, febrile, anaemic, debilitated or not. Mental make-up, bearing, clothes, mannerisms. Relative examination of heart, lungs, abdomen, glands, etc.

Laboratory Aids

- Septic
- Deep fungi-like actinomycosis, etc.
- Sarcoid

Drugs
- Bromides
- lodides

Neoplastic
- Epitheliomas
- Secondary metastases
- Reticuloses Iike mycosis fungoides, Hodgkin's disease, etc.

Keratosis: It is a circumscribed hyperplasia of the stratum corneum (horny layer) of the skin, e.g. senile keratosis, arsenical keratosis, seborrhoeic keratosis. Keratoses have a predisposition to malignancy. Follicular keratoses is seen in lichen spinulosus, keratosis follicularis, vitamins A, C or fatty acid deficiencies. pityriasis rubra pilaris, Darier' s disease, lichen planopilaris, lichen scrofulosorum, etc.

Keratoderma: It signifies diffuse plaques of hyperplasia of the stratum corneum of the skin, particularly of the hands and feet, e.g. tylosis, congenital, arsenical, menopausal, chronic eczema, syphilis, psoriasis, avitaminosis, pityriasis rubra pilaris, etc.

Koebner phenomenon: It means linear lesions produced by scratching a primary lesion, which results in new lesions developing along the line of the scratch, e.g. lichen planus, warts and psoriasis.

Lichenoid: Violaceous or purplish, solid, fine papules, resembling lichen planus but not due to it. This term is loosely used till a proper diagnosis is established. Similarly terms like pemphigoid, leucodermoid and psoriasiform have been coined to describe cutaneous lesions morphologically.

Telangiectasia: They represent groups of fine, dilated capillaries. The common causes are rosacea, spider naevus, alcoholism, liver disorder and X-ray burn.

Vegetations: They are cauliflower-like growths in moist areas like the ano-genital region, groins and axillae. If the stratum corneum is absent, vegetations look eroded-erosive vegetations. If the stratum corneum is hypertrophic, the vegetations are termed verrucous vegetations. The common causes are condylomata lata, pemphigus vegetans and pyoderma vegetans.

Zosteriform: Grouped lesions along the course of a nerve, usual1y unilaterally. Common example is herpes zoster. But zosteriform grouping may also be seen in naevi and vitiligo. Further, zosteriform grouping should be distinguished from linear, retiform, Herpetiform and corymbiform grouping.

DIAGNOSIS

Case-taking is an art acquired with experience. A routine case-taking, on the lines suggested above, helps collect all data and removes the likelihood of oversight in any respect. It is very essential for a beginner. But in the actual practice of dermatology, physical examination is done first and then specific questions are asked to confirm the diagnosis, to eliminate resembling diseases, to elicit the cause, and to establish the prognostic criteria. After all, these are the important tasks of a clinician, and the short-circuit method recommended above helps save time and unnecessary questioning. But in every atypical case, the routine precis of case-taking should be strictly followed before any deduction is made.

As the skin is available for dose examination, the examiner must have a sharp eye, an acute power of observation and a dear, imaginative mind for the correct analysis of facts. The examination should be done in natural light; where this is not possible, an examination under daylight bulb or fluorescent tube lighting should be insisted upon. It is advisable to wear gloves while examining a skin patient, particularly in cases of suspected infections like syphilis. Regardful of his complaint, ask the patient to take off all his clothes, and then examine him from head to foot, paying special attention to the scalp, mouth, nails, genitalia and feet. A magnifying lens is useful in the study of individual lesions. Diascopy is another technique employed in the scrutiny of lesions. It consists of pressure by a glass slide which drains away the blood from the lesion. It is useful in picking out apple-jelly nodules in lupus vulgaris, and in the study of haemangiomas.

Scraping with a pointed, dissection forceps, helps to study the scaling process in scaling lesions, particularly those of pityriasis versicolor and the silvery scales of psoriasis, etc.

Three Important steps in Dermatological Diagnosis

1. Morphological diagnosis—based on morphological study, localization and distribution.
2. Clinical diagnosis—establishment of disease entity based on history and signs.
3. Etiological diagnosis—establishment of cause or causes in the individual patient.

The ultimate aim of the treating physician should be to establish the etiological diagnosis. Having established the diagnosis, information regarding activity, severity and acuity of the disease process (prognostic criteria) be elicited and collected before treatment is prescribed.

Localization of Common Dermatoses

Acne vulgaris: Face, shoulders, upper back and chest.

Atopic dermatitis **(Fig. 3.5)***:* Eyes, face, neck, front of elbows and back of knees.

Chilblains: Fingers and toes.

Contact dermatitis: Site of suspected contact.

Dermatitis herpetiformis **(Fig. 3.6)***:* Scapular region, lower back, chest and forearms.

Dermal leishmaniasis: Exposed parts: face, hands and elbows.

Erythema multiforme: Hands, forearms, face and mouth.

Erythema nodosum: Front of legs.

Herpes simplex: Lips and genitalia.

Herpes zoster: Unilateral lesions—trunk, face, neck and extremities.

Intertrigo-flexures: Groins, axillae, inframammary region.

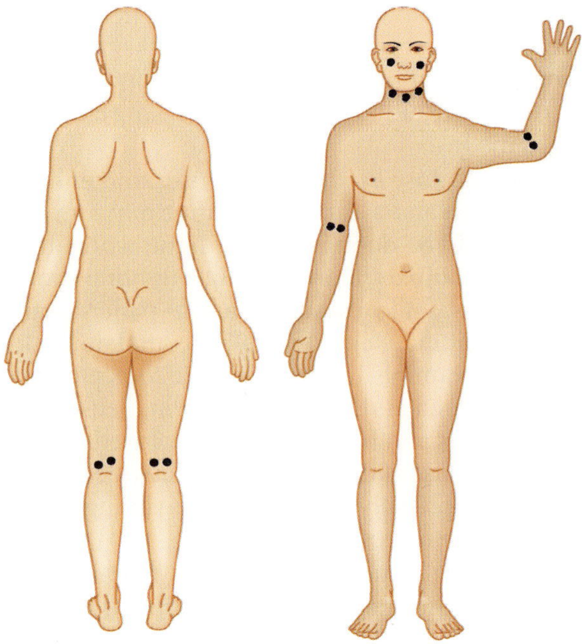

Fig. 3.5: Atopic dermatitis

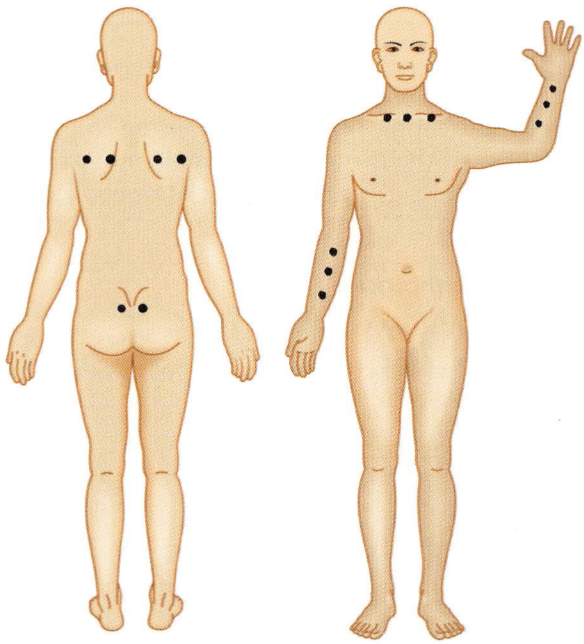

Fig. 3.6: Dermatitis herpetiformis

***Lupus erythematosus (chronic)* (Fig. 3.7):** Butterfly distribution-face.

Lichen planus: Legs, wrists, forearms, genitalia and mouth.

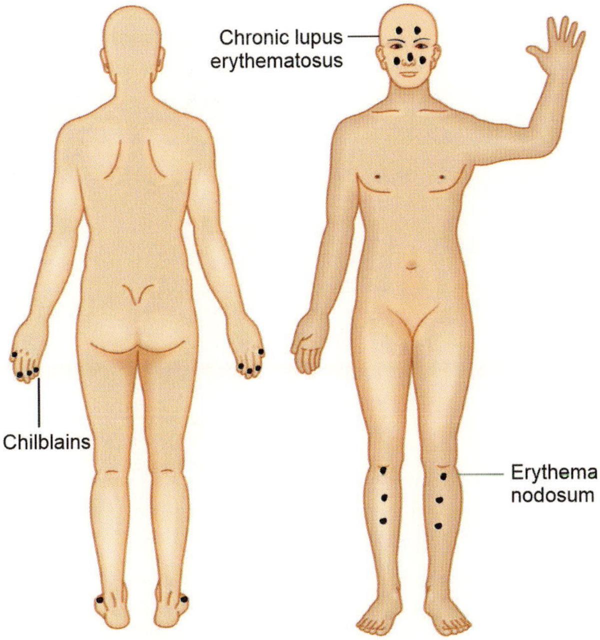

Fig. 3.7: Miscellaneous

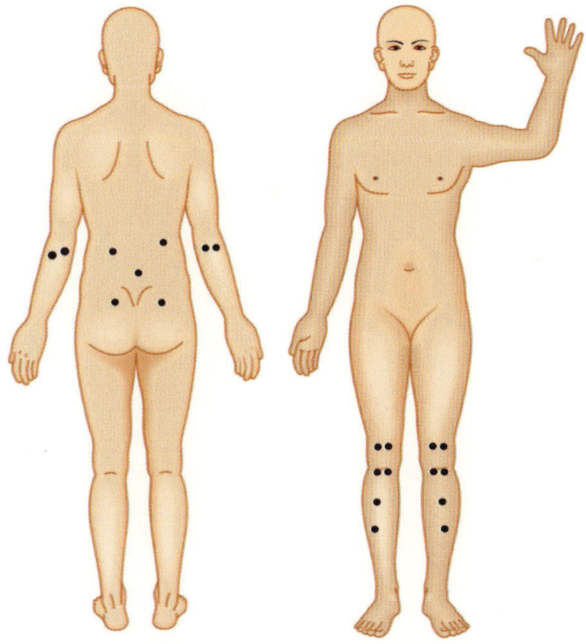

Fig. 3.8: Psoriasis

Neurodermatitis: Back of neck, forearms, legs, ankles and anogenital region.

Psoriasis (Fig. 3.8)*:* Scalp, elbows, knees, back, legs and nails.

Pityriasis versicolor (Fig. 3.9)*:* Chest, back and upper parts of arms.

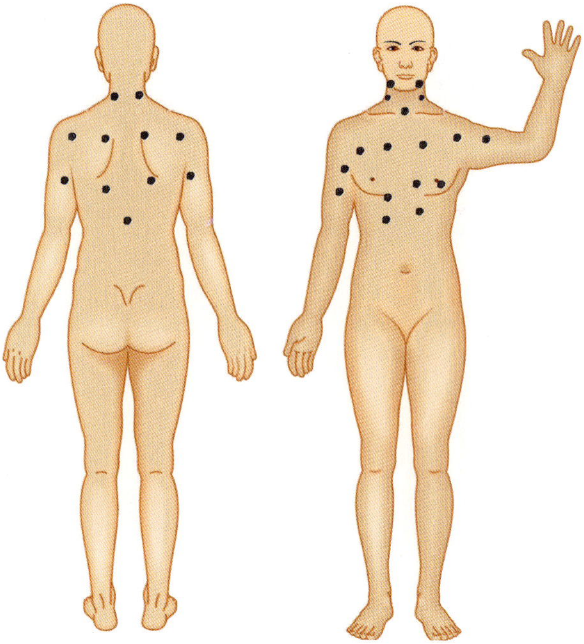

Fig. 3.9: Pityriasis versicolor

Pediculoses: Scalp, trunk and pubic region (according to variety).

Rosacea: Central part of face.

Scabies (Fig. 3.10)*:* Hands (interdigital spaces, palms), front of wrists, elbows, penis, buttocks, and abdomen.

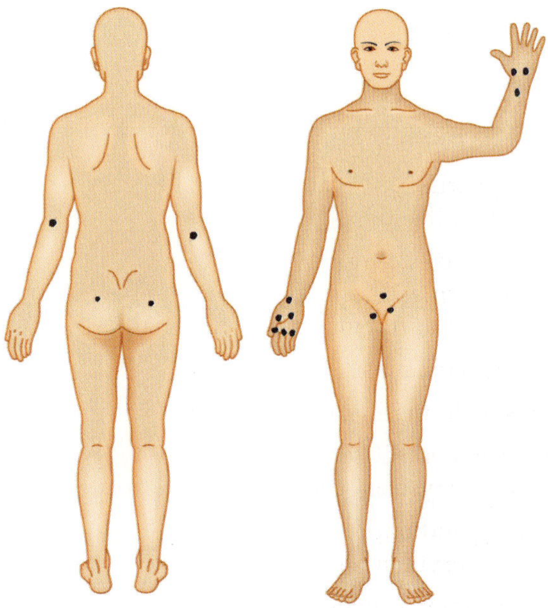

Fig. 3.10: Scabies

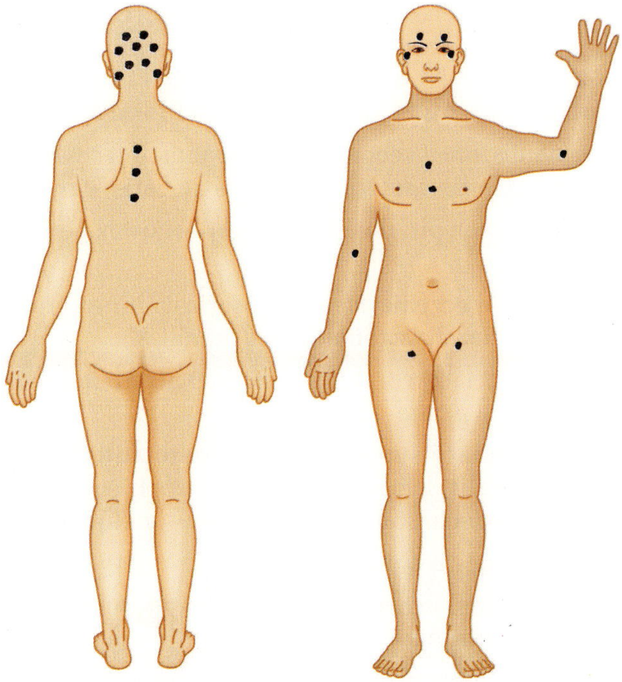

Fig. 3.11: Seborrhoeic dermatitis

Seborrhoeic dermatitis (Fig. 3.11)*:* Scalp, retroauricular region, eyebrows and eyelids, sternal region, interscapular region and flexures, sycosis barbae: Beard region.

Tinea pedis: Interdigital spaces of feet, soles.

Tinea cruris: Inner sides of thighs near the groins, scrotum.

Varicose ulcer: Ankles (inner surface).

Regional Differential Diagnosis of Common Dermatoses

Scalp: Pityriasis capitis, psoriasis, seborrhoeic dermatitis, infective eczema, tinea capitis, pediculoses and diseases of the hair.

Face: Contact dermatitis and eczema, sycosis, impetigo, rosacea, acne vulgaris, atopic dermatitis, seborrhoeic dermatitis, herpes simplex and zoster, lupus vulgaris (LV), dermal leishmaniasis, lupus erythematosus (LE), chloasma, vitiligo.

Nose: Rosacea, dermal leishmaniasis, LE, LV, chloasma, rhinoscleroma.

Ear: Leprosy, seborrhoeic dermatitis, infective eczema.

Neck: Back: Sycosis nuchae, contact dermatitis, neurodermatitis. Front contact dermatitis, pityriasis versicolor, actinomycosis, pyoderma, scrofuloderma.

Lips: Cheilitis, cheilitis glandularis, deficiency diseases, contact dermatitis, angular stomatitis, syphilis, lupus erythematosus, lichen planus.

Mouth: Stomatitis, pemphigus, lichen planus, epithelioma, syphilis, tuberculosis, deficiency diseases.

Back: Pityriasis versicolor, pityriasis rosea, seborrhoeic dermatitis, pediculosis corporis, acne, herpes zoster, dermatitis herpetiformis, pemphigus. Pityriasis versicolor, pityriasis rosea (along the ribs), psoriasis, seborrhoeic dermatitis (interscapular region), acne vulgaris (upper part), herpes zoster, dermatitis herpetiformis, pemphigus.

Armpits: Contact dermatitis, tinea, seborrhoeic dermatitis, infective. eczema, hidradenitis suppurativa, Fox–Fordyce's disease, trichomycosis axillaris, flexural psoriasis.

Abdomen: Pityriasis versicolor, pityriasis rosea, herpes zoster, pemphigus, tinea, lichen planus, pediculosis pubis.

Groins: Intertrigo, infective eczema, flexuraI psoriasis, tinea cruris, scrofuloderma, lymphogranuloma inguinale, chancroidal bubo, moniliasis.

Anal region: Condylomata lata, condyloma acuminatum, neurodermatitis, contact eczema, pruritus ani, fissure in ano.

Genitalia: Chancre, secondary syphilis, contact dermatitis, granuloma inguinale, chancroid, herpes progenitalis, lichen sclerosus et atrophicus, leukoplakia, kraurosis vulvae, epithelioma, phagedena, scabies, lichen planus, neurodermatitis, pediculoses.

Arms: Tinea versicolor, herpes zóster.

Forearms: Discoid dermatitis, lichen planus, erythema multiforme, psoriasis, tinea circinata, dermatitis herpetiformis.

Elbows: Atopic dermatitis (front), psoriasis (back), dermal leishmaniasis, lupus vulgaris.

Hands: Dyshidrosis (palms), id eruption, contact eczema, infective dermatitis, Nummular eczema, pustular bacterides, psoriasis, tinea, drug allergy, keratoderma, syphilis, chilblains, Raynaud's disease, leprosy, warts, tuberculosis verrucosus.

Thighs: Contact dermatitis, tinea, folliculitis.

Knees: Atopic dermatitis (back), psoriasis (front), lupus vulgaris.

Legs: Psoriasis, lichen planus, neurodermatitis, discoid dermatitis, folliculitis, Henoch–Schönlein purpura, erythema nodosum, Bazin's disease.

Feet: Tinea, contact dermatitis, dyshidrosis, bacterides, discoid dermatitis, leprosy, actinomycosis madurae, post-traumatic infective eczema, warts, varicose ulcer, neurodermatitis, chilblains, Raynaud's disease, Buerger's disease, keratoderma, tuberculosis cutis verrucosus.

ECOLOGY

Environment, living habits, nutritional status, financial position, education, development or backwardness, occupation and climate play an important role in the predisposition, development and aggravation of dermatoses. Further, because of these factors, certain diseases are more prevalent than others in a particular area. A disease or reaction pattern is usually the manifestation of genetic or constitutional diathesis and environments. Hence ecological study of an individual as well as a community is very important in practice.

Dark asiatic skin has a predisposition to keloids, lichenification and itching.

Pigmentary anomalies are also common, more so after surgery, trauma and burn. White Western skin is predisposed to neoplasms. Shift from squatting at home and at work, to standing and sitting on the chairs has increased the incidence of vascular disorders: stasis ulcers, dermatitis and Schamberg's disease. Climate affects the incidence of different dermatoses in a particular area in a particular season, e.g. dermal leishmaniasis and Veldt sore are in dry, hot climate of North India; post-dermal leishmanoid, filariasis and tropical ulcer in moist, humid climate of eastern states like West Bengal, Odisha and Assam; tinea, pyodermas, infective eczema, dyshidrosis and miliaria are common in the summer and monsoon; seborrhoeic dermatitis and acne in the autumn and spring; discoid dermatitis, ichthyosis and psoriasis in winter. In developed communities, contact dermatitis, allergies and psychosomatic problems are common, while in under-developed backward communities, infections and nutritional problems predominate. So, one can realise the importance of ecology in dermatology.

NATURAL HISTORY OF DISEASE

A good clinician and an intelligent patient are of enormous help in studying natural history of disease, thereby assisting in making a correct diagnosis, because different diseases follow different and varied courses depending, of course, on climate, patient's resistance and virulence of disease process, etc. **(Fig. 3.12)**. A few important examples are listed.

Exanthemata like smallpox, chickenpox, herpes zoster have limited course of 12–15 days unless secondarily infected. Pyodermas are of short duration, unless they become chronic as in folliculitis. Anthrax, tropical ulcer and pyoderma gangrenosum develop rapidly.

In comparison, fungus affections in tropical countries are common in summer and more so in warm, humid season of monsoon. In the cold weather, they become dormant to recur again in the hot weather unless properly treated. History extends over years.

Scabies is more frequently seen in winter, while insect bites in the summer and monsoon on exposed parts.

Warts spread slowly by auto-inoculation except in the beard region (spread fast by shaving) and moist areas (condyloma acuminatum).

History of dermal leishmaniasis is usually in weeks in endemic areas. Syphilitic chancre develops a few weeks after exposure, while herpes progenitalis and gonorrhea within 1–3 days and chancroid in 3–5 days, granuloma venereum in 2–6 days and lympho-granuloma in 1–2 weeks. History of epithelioma on glans penis extends to months and warts only a few weeks. Syphilitic gumma has history of months, white natural history of tuberculosis and leprosy extends over years.

Psoriasis has usually winter aggravation, but some cases do show summer flare-ups when prickly heat becomes psoriasiform. Seborrhoeic dermatitis and lichen planus have sudden or insidious onset depending upon the cause. Drug eruptions are usually acute in onset and short-lived unless caused by heavy metals like arsenic or produce erythroderma-like picture.

Amongst the neoplasms, history of basal cell epitheliomas is in years, squamous cell epitheliomas in months, while malignant melanomas develop in weeks to months.

IMMUNITY AND ALLERGY

During the last three decades, concept of immunity has undergone revolutionary changes and has widened its scope immeasurably. WHO report defines immunity

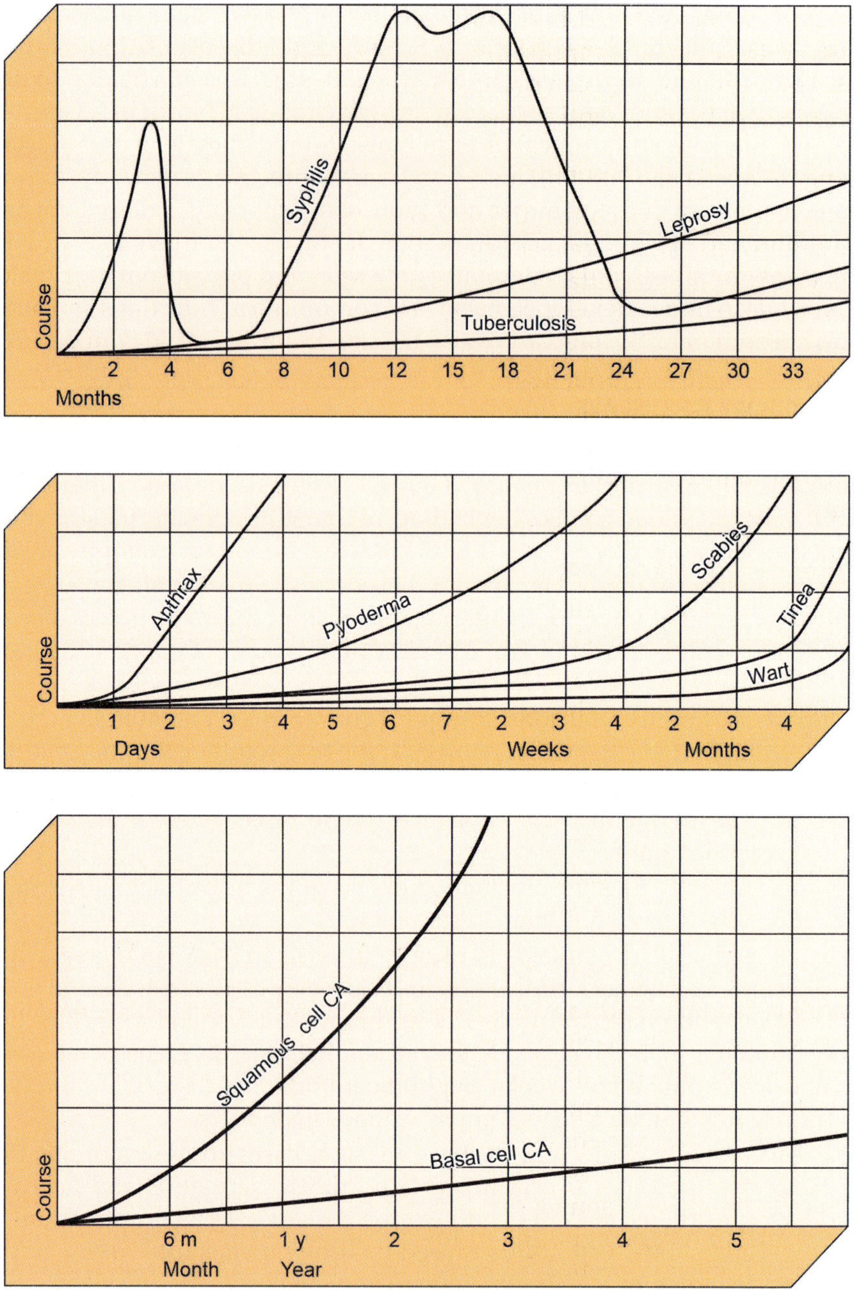

Fig. 3.12: Natural history of disease

as: "'The immune response comprises all the phenomena that result from the specific interaction of cells of the immune system with antigen."

Immunologic response involves two separate mechanisms, mediated by two types of cells-T-lymphocyte (thymus dependent) and B-lymphocyte (bursa of Fabricius). Source of these two types of cells are the precursor stem cells of bone marrow. T-cells migrate to thymus, modified here and released into blood. They are long-lived and comprise 60–80% of the lymphocytes in the circulation. B-cells are independent of thymus. The B-lymphocytes can proliferate, differentiate and mature into plasma cells which synthesize humoral antibodies (immunoglobulins).

Cell-mediated (T-cell) Immunity

Here cells directly approach the antigen wherever it is localized, may destroy it and become sensitized. On a second or continued exposure to the antigen, the sensitized lymphocytes may become attached to it. This form of immunity is responsible for the rejection of foreign cells, resistance to many viral and fungal infections, delayed type of hypersensitivity and rejection of tissue transplants. T-cells have a complex reaction and release soluble factors, lymphokines, which take part in cell-mediated immunity and can destroy antigen, attract leucocytes, slow down the work of macrophages, may be killer ce1ls which are cytotoxic for graft target cells and cooperate with B-lymphocytes to antibody production. Failure of T-cell system will lead to defective cell-mediated immunity.

Humoral (Antibody-mediated) Immunity

On antigenic stimulation, B-cells (lymphocytes) transform to plasma cells which produce antibodies (immunoglobulins) that are released in the circulation. Immunoglobulins are serum proteins and there are five major types—lgG, IgM, IgA, IgD, and IgE.

Any defect which limits the number of B-lymphocytes will lead to deficiency of immunoglobulin synthesis.

Immunoglobulins IgG can pass through the placental barrier and can reach into foetus to neutralize bacterial toxins. IgA prevents adherence of microorganisms to cell surface. Finding of raised IgM in a person's blood indicates previous infection. IgE normally binds with mast cells and basophils and releases histamine, bradykinin, acetylcholine, serotonin and other chemical substances.

Human Leucocyte Antigens (HLA)

The major histocompatibility system of man is referred to as human leucocyte antigen (HLA) system and on the basis of leucocyte typing it appears that there are more than 30 transplantation antigens. Transfer of tissue or cell from one member of species to another always induces an immune response. HLA antigens are present on leucocytes on the cell surface and are richest on lymphoid cells. It is essential to type H antigen of donor and recepient as is done in case of red cell antigens (blood grouping in ABO and Rh system). ln transplantation of skin, kidneys and other organs HL-A antigens have to be matched. Autologous grafting of skin from one site in the body to another site presents no immunologic problem. Rejection of graft principally involves cell-mediated immunity and to some extent also humoral antibody. A detailed discussion is beyond the scope of this book and the interested reader is referred to books dealing on modern immunology and allergy.

Allergy and Hypersensitivity

According to modern immunologists these two terms are synonymous. The concept of hypersensitivity was first introduced by Portier and Richet in 1902. The term allergy was coined by Clemens von Pirquet in Vienna in 1906. Allergy means altered energy (allos-other; ergon-energy). Simple scratching of the skin causes the triple response of Lewis (Sir Thomas Lewis, 1927). This consists of erythema, weal and flare reaction. Flare is due to dilatation of arterioles by a local axon reflex and the liberation of vasodilator substances (histamine-like H-substances, serotonin, bradykinin, acetylcholine, prostaglandin, etc.) from the injured cells like mast cells and basophils, etc.

The manifestation of hypersensitivity may be immediate (anaphylactic) or delayed (late) tuberculin in type. Charles Richet (1902) coined the term anaphylaxis to describe that certain injected substances, diminish instead of increasing the defences of an animal to their harmful effect. Ricket won a Nobel Prize in Medicine in the year 1913, in recognition of his work on anaphylaxis.

Arthus phenomenon is local anaphylaxis. Arthus demonstrated that each successive inoculation of a foreign protein initially harmless, leaves the tissue more sensitized eventually leading to the necrosis of the surrounding tissue.

Cutaneous Allergy

In the skin, there are two important but different allergic reactions. One as in urticaria, the causative antigen reaches the skin through ingestion, inhalation or injection of protein substances and the reacting antibodies circulate in the serum. Allergic reaction takes place in the dermis–dermal reaction. In this type of allergy, Prausnitz–Kustner passive transfer reaction is positive, and only the intradermal (injection or scratch) tests show reactivity. The response is weal formation which occurs in a few minutes.

The second type of allergic cutaneous reaction is epidermal reaction, as is seen in the allergic dermatitis or eczema. Causative substances reach the skin by contact. Intradermal allergic tests are negative; on the contrary, patch tests show reactivity. Prausnitz–Kustner reaction is also negative. Sensitizers vary from simple substances (chromate and nickel) to complex chemicals (plastics) or even bacterial products (streptococci, fungi).

Allergen + epidermal protein conjugation → Antigen formation → Antibodies production (probably in lymph glands) → Circulation → Fixed in epidermal cells.

Next occasion: Allergen + Antibodies → eczematous reaction (in the epidermis).

A severe local reaction may result in auto-intoxication and dissemination of eczematous reaction to distant parts.

Delayed hypersensitivity is believed to produce lymphomas, sarcoid (zirconium reaction, Kligman). Allergy to immunochemically related substances (group sensitizers) has also been proved. Further it is believed that in cases of severe allergic states, a state may develop when the patient becomes hypersensitive to even unrelated substances, e.g. status eczematicus or status urticatus. This is comparable to status asthmaticus in the practice of internal medicine.

Further, it must be realized that epidermal or dermal sensitization affects the entire integument, and this sensitization once acquired, is life long. According to some, a degree of blunting in reactivity may be seen with the passage of time.

To deal with cutaneous reactions of allergy is a challenge to a dermatologist in establishing the offending cause of the allergic reaction. Successful treatment produces dramatic results which are satisfying both to the suffering patient and the treating

Table 3.1: Classification of allergic reactions			
Type	*Time*	*Antibody involved*	*Tissue reaction*
Type I anaphylactic	1–20 minutes	IgE mainly	Urticaria, ANO, asthma, atopic dermatitis, allergic rhinits
Type II	5–30 minutes	IgE, IgM and complements	Haemolysis, agranulocytosis, cytotoxic drug hypersensitivity, autoimmune disorders
Type III arthus reaction	4–6 hours	IgG, IgM and complements	Serum sicknes, SLE, ENL, allergic vasculitis
Type IV tuberculin	1–2 days	Sensitized cells—lymphocytes	Contact dermatitis, homograft reaction

Table 3.2: Stem cell and lymphoid cell				
Stem cell	Erythorocyte	Granulocyte	Monocyte (macrophages)	Megakaryocyte
Lymphoid cell	T-lymphocyte • Suppressor, helper, killer and memory • Cell-mediated immunity delayed hypersensitivity		B-lymphocyte • Plasma cells • Antibody-mediated immunity (immunoglobulins)	

Table 3.3: Allergic reaction and threshold		
Facilitating factors like emotional stress, infection, debility, endocrines. They lower the threshold for reaction		
S P E C I F I C	A L L E R G E N S	Exciting factors—(trigger)—drugs, infection, diet
Predisposing causes like age, climate, heredity and race		

medical practitioner. In tropical countries like India, allergic dermatoses are not so common as in Western countries. The reason for this may either be racial (pigmented skin) or environmental (a less artificial way of life). These allergies are encountered mostly in the sphere of infections, urticarias and drug eruptions **(Tables 3.1 to 3.3)**.

Complement System

It is an important part of humoral immune system. It is composed of nine individual factors which are known as C1, C2, C3 up to C9. These proteins are normally found in an inactive form in the circulation and are activated via two different pathways.

Immunoglobulins like IgG and IgM activate complement system via classical pathway. Endotoxin and trypsin-linked enzyme activate different complement factors via the alternate pathway. During the course of complement activation several biologically active substances are released which are required to destroy or eliminate an antigen.

Immunological Tolerance

Immune system discriminates between self and nonself. Tolerance to one's own tissue is developed in foetal life.

Autoimmunity is a biological paradox in which the cells and tissues of the body itself, by forming auto-antibodies and autosensitized T-cells, react against antigens of the individual's own tissue (self). The exact mechanism of this type of tissue response is not understood. It has been postulated that the tissue is altered by injury or disease so that the individual recognises it as foreign to him, e.g. Hashimoto's disease (thyroid gland involved), autoimmune haemolytic anaemia, primary biliary cirrhosis, collagen disease like DLE, scleroderma, polyarteritis nodosa, etc.

SYSTEMIC DISEASES PRODUCING CUTANEOUS DISORDERS

Cutaneous lesions are occasionally produced by systemic disorders, so they may help in the diagnosis of the latter. On the other hand, a cutaneous disease may affect the internal organs. Important examples of systemic diseases producing cutaneous disorders are:

a. ***Nutritional:*** Pellagra, avitaminosis.

b. ***Metabolic***
   - Diabetes—pruritus, moniliasis, furunculoses, carbuncle, xanthomatosis, necrobiosis lipoidica, trophic ulcers, gangrene **(Fig. 3.13)**.
   - Amyloidosis cutis.
   - Cirrhosis—spider naevi, sallow complexion, pruritus.
   - Porphyrinuria—pigmentation, hydroa aestivale.
   - Xanthomatosis.
   - Bronze diabetes or haemochromatosis.

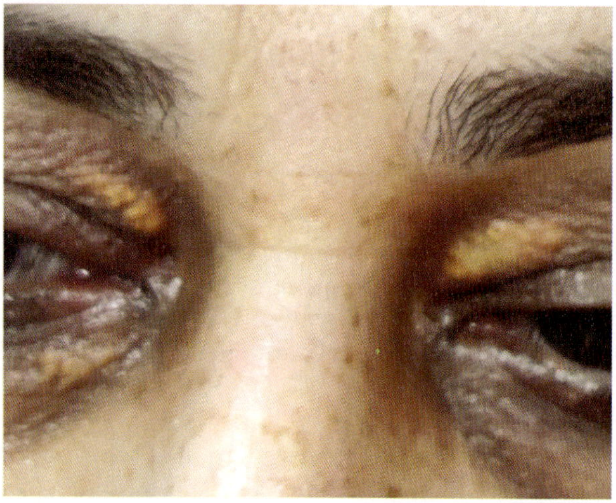

Fig. 3.13: Xanthelasma in a 52-year-old woman

c. ***Endocrine***

- Thyrotoxicosis—pigmentation.
- Myxoedema—alopecia, myxoedematous skin.
- Cushing's disease—flame-shaped stria.
- Pituitary cachexia (Simmond's)—alopecia.
- Addison's disease—pigmentation.
- Menstrual disorders—pigmentation, chloasma, alopecia, hirsutism.

d. ***Focal sepsis*** (in teeth, ears, sinuses, tonsils, lungs, gallbladder, kidneys, prostate, etc.)

- Pyaemic abscesses lupus erythematosus
- Bacterids, Rosacea
- Discoid eczema acne vulgaris
- Urticaria erythema multiforme
- Dermatitis herpetiformis dyshidrosis

e. ***Vascular disorders***

- Raynaud's disease
- Arteriosclerosis

f. ***Carcinomatosis***

- Secondaries in skin pigmentation
- Pruritus acanthosis nigricans.

g. ***Naevi***

- Haemangioma of skin–associated with angioma of brain.
- Adenoma sebaceum–associated with tuberous sclerosis.
- Neurofibromatosis–associated with lesions in bones, nerves and eyes **(Fig. 3.14)**.

h. ***Collagen diseases***

- Lupus erythematosus, scleroderma, dermatomyositis **(Fig. 3.15)**.

i. ***Fever and rashes*** (Chapter 26).

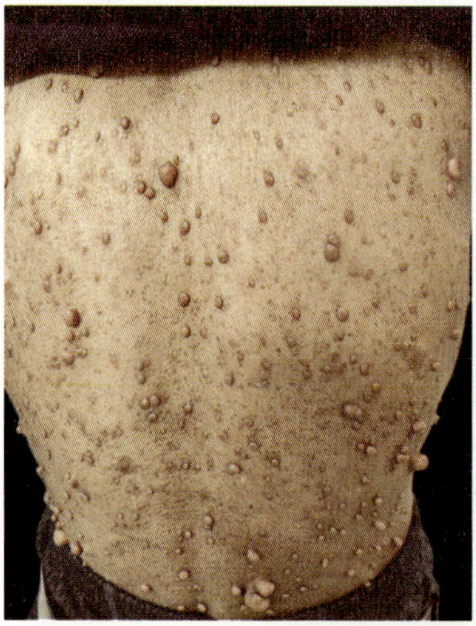

Fig. 3.14: Neurofibromatosis

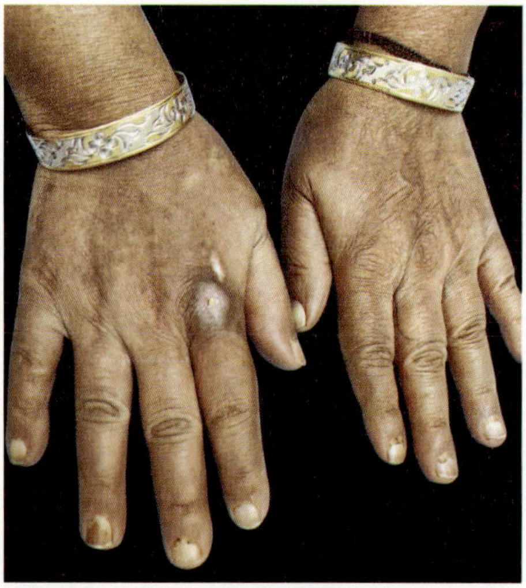

Fig. 3.15: Early scleroderma with swollen and bound-down skin and calcinosis cutis in base of right index finger

Chapter
4
Laboratory and Other Aids

Consider the need, cost and burden on the laboratory. Clinician's clinical acumen are more important than reliance on laboratory aids.

BACTERIOLOGICAL STUDIES

They are useful in finding out the exact causative organisms, both in acute and chronic cases of bacterial infections and infective granulomata (*see* Chapters 10 to 18).

Smears and stains: Discharge from an infected area is smeared on glass slides and stained with Gram's stain for ordinary organisms, and Ziehl–Neelsen stain for acid-fast bacilli **(Fig. 4.1)**. Dark field examination is done to demonstrate *Treponema pallidum* in the primary and secondary lesions of syphilis.

For examination of LD bodies, the edge of the suspected lesion is firmly grasped with the thumb and forefinger of the left hand , and by means of a thin-blade scalpel, a knife point of the tissue from the edge of the lesion is removed and smeared on a slide. The oozing blood is wiped off successfully until clear serum begins to exude. A slide of the serum is also made. With some experience, the serum can be sucked into a pipette from the edge of an intact lesion without the use of a knife. The slides are stained with Giemsa's stain. LD bodies are seen as blue cytoplasm, pink nucleus and deep red kinetoplast.

A nasal smear for lepra bacilli is made by firmly scraping the roof and sides of the anterior part of the nose by means of a swab stick, and smearing the material on a slide the staining with Ziehl–Neelsen stain.

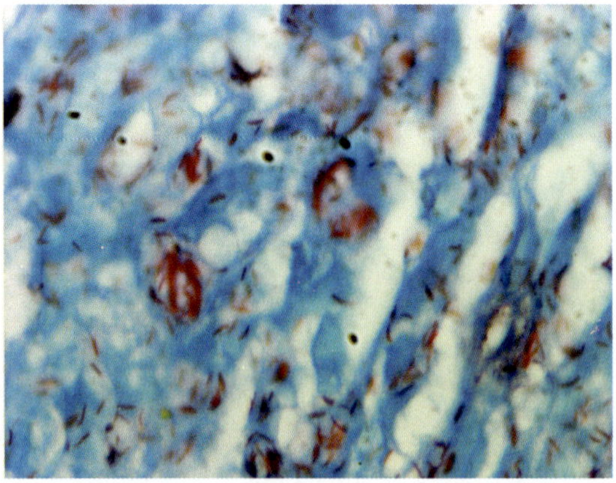

Fig. 4.1: Acid-fast bacilli seen under Ziehl–Neelsen staining

A slit biopsy in leprosy is performed by firmly holding the edge of a suspected cutaneous lesion or ear lobe (posterior surface to conceal the scar of the slit) between the thumb and index finger of the left hand. This will make the part avascular and numb.

Then with the help of a thin blade scalpel, the tissue is slit open superficially. Bleeding should be avoided. The bottom of the slit is scraped along with the oozing serum and smeared on the slide by means of the blunt edge of the scalpel.

Cultures: They are made routinely on blood agar plates to identify the types of organisms; biochemical examinations also may be required for this purpose. With the help of a flamed platinum loop, a specimen of the pus from the lesion is inoculated at one end of the plate and spread. Plates are incubated at 37°C in an incubator for 24 hours or longer.

Tubercle bacilli are grown on a special medium-glycerine egg medium. LD bodies are cultured on NNN medium.

Sensitivity tests: They are extremely useful, both in acute and chronic bacterial infections. Before starting treatment in such cases, the sensitivity of the causative organisms to different antibiotics is determined to save the patient from undue drugging.

Vaccines: They are of two types: stock (ready-made) and autovaccine (made from the organisms grown from the lesions of the same patient—so the same strain of organisms). Curative vaccines are specifically used for chronic bacterial infections like chronic furunculoses, folliculitis and recurrent infectious eczematoid dermatitis. Autovaccines are usually preferable to stock vaccines; in the face of failure to make an autovaccine, a stock vaccine prepared by a reliable manufacturer may be employed.

BCG vaccine is successfully employed to prevent leprosy in children. Staphylococcal toxoid is useful in chronic staphylococcal infections.

Vaccines of inhalants, foods and also drugs are useful in desensitizing allergic cases. Allergens must be so prepared as to retain their allergenic properties. They must also be sterile.

MYCOLOGICAL STUDIES

The most important confirmatory evidence of clinical diagnosis of dermatomycosis can be obtained by scraping the lesion and by the microscopic demonstration of fungus. The procedure is very easy to perform, and does not take much time; preferably, it should be done by the physician himself.

Collection of Material

1. ***Skin*** scrapings are obtained by scraping the growing edge of the suspected lesion where it merges with the normal skin, with a scalpel, the blade of which should neither be too sharp nor too blunt. It is advisable to wet the scalpel blade with a swab of 70% alcohol when the scraping is being done.

   The edge of the scalpel blade is gently agitated in a drop of 10% potassium hydroxide solution taken on a slide to release the scales adherent to it. It is advisable to prepare two coverslip preparations from each lesion, and if there are a number of lesions, it is better if specimens from two or more lesions are obtained. If vesicles are present, the domes should be snipped off with a pair of scissors, and the contents examined in a potassium hydroxide preparation.

2. ***Hair:*** Areas showing thinning or scaling of hair with broken-off stumps should be selected. The stumps of the broken-off hair should be epilated and a coverslip preparation of the material placed in a drop of 10% potassium hydroxide should be microscopically examined.
3. ***Nails:*** All nails which are discoloured or lustreless or ridged with hyperkeratotic debris should be fully examined. The nails are cut away, and the debris from under the nail is removed, placed in a potassium hydroxide solution and examined microscopically.
4. ***Pus*** from granulomata like actinomycosis and sporotrichosis is collected aseptically and examined directly, or a smear is made and stained with Giemsa's or Gram's stain, and then examined under the microscope.

Microscopic Examination

The preparation is gently warmed, or allowed to stand for 20 minutes to half an hour. This helps to soften the keratinous tissue and allows the fungus to stand out more clearly. The preparation is first examined under the low power and then the high power dry objective of the microscope.

In the skin, the fungus appears as a set of parallel septate lines, which show branching at places. In some areas, the fungus may be seen segmented into a number of separate cells all in the same line. Absence of mycelia does not rule out tinea.

It must be clearly understood that this picture is common to all the dermatophytes infecting the skin, and the identification of their species is impossible from a coverslip preparation. Only by culturing, can the different species be identified. In the hair, the fungus appears in the form of rounded spores which may be small or large in size. Furthermore, the spores may be present around the shaft of the hair. When situated thus, they are known as ectothrix spores; when present inside the hair shaft, they are called endothrix spores.

Culture: Sabouraud's medium is the one very commonly used. For culture work, the aim is to reduce bacterial contamination to the minimum.

After the affected area has been cleansed with 70% alcohol, scraping is done with the usual technique; the material so obtained is removed from the scalpel with the point of a straight needle and inoculated on the surface of the medium to be used. At least two Petri dishes and two slopes of the medium prepared in test tubes or screw- capped bottles are used for each case, and about 4 inoculations of the material on each medium is made. The culture is kept at room temperature or best at 26°C and examined every alternate day. No culture should be discarded as sterile unless kept for at least 3 weeks.

Another difficulty to overcome is to know whether a growth which is taking place is saprophytic or pathogenic. A working rule in this connection is: Any growth which takes place within three days and grows rapidly is likely to be saprophytic. The growth, however, should be investigated before being so labelled. With experience in the identification of saprophytes, however, this difficulty could, in due course be overcome.

Staining: The two reagents commonly employed are: lactophenol blue for the staining of fungus smears routinely and Periodic acid-Schiff stain (PAS) for the staining of fungus in tissues.

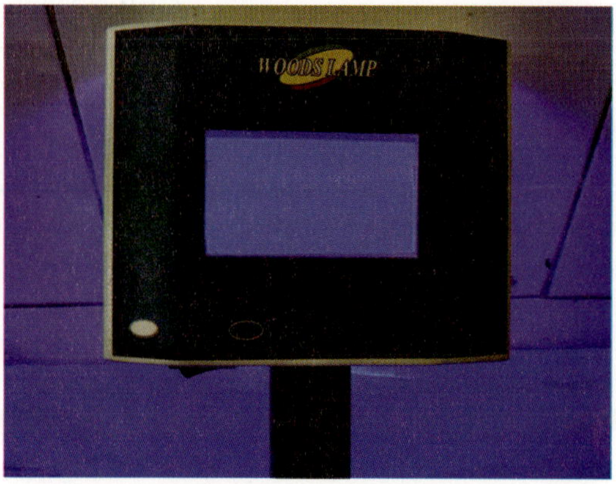

Fig. 4.2: Wood's lamp

WOOD'S LAMP EXAMINATION

A Wood's lamp is a mercury vapour lamp with a special Wood's filter made of nickel oxide and barium silicate **(Fig. 4.2)**. It allows only certain wavelengths of ultraviolet rays (365 nm) to filter through.

In Wood's lamp light, *Microsporum* infection of the hair is visible as a greenish fluorescence. The scalp must be thoroughly washed of all medicaments before it is examined under the Wood's lamp. It helps to pick up early cases of tinea capitis amongst contacts, especially school children, and aids in following up a treated case and declaring it cured.

The colour of the fluorescent light, seen best in a darkened room, is characterised in **Table 4.1**.

SEROLOGICAL TESTS FOR SYPHILIS

The commonly used blood tests for syphilis are: The Kahn test, the VDRL, Wasserman reaction and the Menicke's slide tests. It is advisable to do all these tests for the sake of and to separate the positive from the biologically false-positive reactions. It must be

Table 4.1

Condition	*Fluorescent colours*
Tinea capitis	Bright yellow green
Erythrasma	Coral red or pink
Vitiligo	Milky white
Albinism	Blue white
Leprosy	Blue white
Tuberous sclerosis	Blue white
Pseudomonas infection	Greenish white
Porphyria	Pink/orange
Tinea versicolor	Golden yellow

remembered that these tests can become positive in low titres in leprosy, yaws, chronic malaria, jaundice, etc. (For details, refer to Chapter 18).

HISTOLOGICAL STUDIES

Dermal histology has played an important role in the study of skin disease. A pathologist must be aware of his limitations while interpreting skin biopsy; there should be close cooperation with his clinical colleagues. Biopsy has its inherent limitations. Value of biopsy in skin diseases has been critically analysed. Results vary with different workers. Hela and Pinkus have analysed 1000 cases and found that 65% are of value. Twiston-Davies made a critical analysis of 200 cases. He reports about 80% of cases of some value, but missed 43 cases.

Biopsy should be done whenever possible. It is a very simple procedure. For most tumours and many inflammatory conditions a definite diagnosis may be made with certainty by light microscopy; many diagnosis by the clinical findings alone will be excluded by the histopathological findings.

Technique of Biopsy

It is important to select the right material for a biopsy **(Table 4.2)**; it should either be from a fully developed primary lesion or the edge of such a lesion. Involuting lesions or secondary lesions or secondarily infected lesions should not be selected. It is strongly advisable to do excision biopsies in cases of melanomas. Incision or excision should be arranged along cleavage lines to avoid disfigurement. There are several types of skin biopsy—punch biopsy, incisional biopsy, excisional biopsy, shave biopsy, etc. Incisional biopsy is preferable to punch biopsy. Punch sizes vary from 3 to 8 mm. Punch biopsy of

Table 4.2: Commonly used tissue stains

Tissue	*Stain*	*Result*
Tissue section routine	Haematoxylin and Eosin	Nuclei blue, cytoplasm pink
Collagen and muscle	Van Gieson	Collagen red and muscle fibres yellow; elastic fibres stain black
Elastic fibres	Verhoeff	Elastic fibres black
Reticulin	Gömöri's	Reticulum fibres black
Amyloid	Congo red	Amyloid stains red
Glycogen, fungus and basement membrane	PAS	Glycogen red; fungus purple basement membrane red or black; pale to deed pink
Acid fast bacilli	Fite-Faraco stain (Z–N stain)	Bacilli stain red
Leishmania and mast cells	Giemsa's stain	LD bodies purple
Iron (haemosiderin)	Perl's ferrocyanide reaction (Prussian blue)	Pigment stains blue
Melanin	Mason's ammoniacal	Melanin black
Calcium	Von Kossa	Dark-brown to black

4 mm size is suitable for most purposes. In skin sterilization, only colourless disinfectants are to be used.

The lesion should not be infiltrated with the anaesthetic but only the surroundings. Some persons like to use adrenalin but it is not advisable.

Once the specimen has been removed it is placed epidermis upward on a blotting paper. This is then placed in the jar or plastic container with fixative (10% neutral buffered formalin solution) which being a protein coagulant helps the specimen to stick to the blotting paper and comes to the laboratory unwrinkled. Usually no suture is needed for 4 mm size punch biopsies. After approximately 12 hours fixation, specimen is ready for processing. In colder areas like Kashmir, Shimla and other hilly areas, instead of 10% formalin solution, lillies fixative may be used for skin biopsies, if possible.

Cytological Examination

It is useful in office practice.

LE cell in acute lupus erythematosus: The study is made either with a bone marrow smear, or a smear of the buffy cell layer of centrifuged, heparinized blood. The smear is stained with Leishman's stain. A longer period of staining (10 minutes) is required in this case than in blood smears.

In positive preparations, three features are observed:

1. The LE cell which is a large neutrophil leucocyte, distended by a large, homogeneous, globular inclusion body pushing the cytoplasm and the nucleus into a thin rim at the periphery.
2. Rosettes of polymorphonuclear leucocytes surrounding the LE cell.
3. Extracellular masses which consist of globular masses resembling the inclusion bodies of LE cells lying outside the cells. The LE phenomenon implies demonstration of LE cells in normal blood when the serum from a lupus erythematosus patient has been added to it. LE cells are typically demonstrable in acute and subacute lupus erythematosus (systemic variety).

Tzanck test: It is a simple, cytological procedure employed to demonstrate acantholysis in pemphigus, though similar cells have been seen in other bullous conditions as well. The procedure consists in snipping off the roof of an early vesicle or a bulla with a sterile knife, wiping off the serum, scraping the base and smearing the scraped material on a clean slide. Smears are fixed in methyl alcohol and stained with Giemsa's stain. The pemphigus cell (Tzanck cell) is a separate, detached and rounded cell with a large, pyknotic nucleus and a deeply staining cytoplasm which is pushed to the periphery (thin rim).

Smears in skin cancers: Microscopic examination or smears made from basal and squamous cell epitheliomas is a speedy and inexpensive method of diagnosis in expert hands. Typical cancer cells can be rapidly seen while the biopsy is being undertaken.

Histochemistry

Histochemical methods have been described for detecting many inorganic substances. Formalin fixed and paraffin sections are satisfactory for this purpose.

Stains for mucopolysaccharides, glycogen, lipids, mucins, nucleic acids and various enzymes can be studied by histochemical methods.

Immunofluorescence

Immunofluorescence is a technique for detecting the position and presence of substances in tissue sections.

Unfixed cryostat cut sections are necessary (frozen sections). Certain fluorescent dyes like fluorescein, isothiocyanate, rhodamine B, auramine O or acridine orange, etc. when exposed to ultraviolet light emit fluorescent radiation. By direct and indirect immunofluorescent techniques, Ig class antibodies, other globulins, tissue antigens-bacterial, viral, fungal, protozoal, helminthic, etc. can be identified. In the field of autoimmunity, demonstration of antinuclear antibody in the sera of patients with various collagen diseases by this technique is now possible.

This technique has been used as a diagnostic tool in certain bullous diseases. Bullous pemphigoid can be differentiated from dermatitis herpetiformis and erythema multiforme. Immunofluorescence of the basal lamina can be seen in lupus erythematosus but not in lichen planus.

ALLERGY TESTS

Allergies cover a wide field. Allergy tests can be of great value to a dermatologist in the objective evaluation of an allergic patient. A detailed discussion of these tests procedure and assessment is beyond the scope of this book; the reader should refer to books dealing in detail with the subject.

Tests are selected entirely on the basis of correct history and clinical observations; laboratory results must be assessed on the basis of clinical findings, otherwise a great deal of confusion will arise.

Patch tests: They are done in cases of contact dermatitis to establish the etiological agent or agents. It is simply a reproduction in miniature of a small area of contact dermatitis.

It is artificial and does not necessarily duplicate the clinical exposure in which sweating, maceration and multiple applications play great roles.

Test reading should be taken 20 minutes to 1 hour after removal of patches. This time interval allows pressure effect and erythema from tape removal to subside. The original dermatitis of the patient must be completely under control before the tests are undertaken. The patient should not be taking any immunosuppressive drugs and systemic steroids. The back or the arms are the sites of choice, preferably as close to the original site of the disease as possible. The affected part is cleaned with water and allowed to dry. Patches are placed at distances of 2–3 inches in rows—about 20 patches can be applied at one time. The material for testing should be cut to about 5 mm in diameter and moistened with normal saline or distilled water; liquid contactants can be applied directly. The testing material is covered with a piece of lint one square inch in size and an adhesive tape applied firmly, each patch being labelled or numbered. A control patch of lint dipped in normal saline is also applied.

The patient should be advised to report after 48 hours or earlier if itching starts, and again, after 96 hours. Tests will have to be modified according to tested agents. The reading is done when the patient reports after 48 hours or earlier in case of acute sensitivity.

In every patient, there is mild redness and folliculitis under the adhesive tape. Unless severe, this is a normal reaction to adhesive tape. A binder bandage may be employed for patients allergic to adhesive and scotch tape. The small area in the centre of the patch should be examined and recorded. Be careful about false-positive reactions.

+ Only redness
+ + Marked redness and swelling
+ + + Marked redness, swelling and papules
+ + + + Redness, oedema and vesicles

If there is no reaction in 48 hours, the patches should be reread in 96 hours for delayed positive reaction. Sometimes, the original healed area of contact dermatitis flares up during a test, particularly when there exists a severe degree of hypersensitivity **(Table 4.3)**.

Table 4.3: Standard tray for patch testing

Medicaments, preservatives, perfumes			
• Ammoniated mercury	1%		
• Ethylene diamine dihydrochloride	1%		
• Parabens	15%		
• Wool alcohol	30%		
• Benzocaine	5%		
• Balsam of Peru	25%		
• Lanolin	10%		
• Thimersol	5%		
• Neomycin	20%		
• Quatemium	2%		
• Imidazodinylurea	2%		
• Framycetin	5%		
• Nitrofurazone	1%		
Metals			
• Pot. dichromate	0.5%		
• Nickel sulphate	2.5%		
• Cobalt	5.0%		
Rubber chemicals			
Mercaptobenzothiazole mix	1%		
Thiuram mix	1%		
Naphthyl mix	1%		
PPD mix	0.6%		
Carbol mix	3%		
Others			
Formaldehyde	2%	Garlic	100%
P-phenylene diamine	1%	Parthenium	15%
Expoxy resin	1%	DDT	1%
P-tert-butylphenol	1%	Malathione	0.5%

Primary irritants should be properly diluted before testing. Shampoos, soaps, detergents, shaving creams should be diluted to 1%. Solids can be powdered or cut into small pieces; they show relatively milder reaction.

Ingredients of the standard tray vary with the requirements of each individual clinic. Specific trays are made for each profession. As far as possible, natural contactants should be patch tested in each case.

Intradermal tests for allergies to foods, inhalants and drugs. In the majority of cases, the history of a definite allergy is more important than laboratory tests. Besides, these tests are not very accurate. Hence, they should be undertaken only in a limited number of cases where history and examination does not entirely help. The skin conditions in which these tests are helpful are: urticaria, endogenous eczema, atopic dermatitis and drug sensitivity. The response is a weal reaction.

Foods: An eliminative diet or a diet diary is much more useful than allergic tests, since few positive skin reactions can be correlated with clinical symptoms, and negative skin reactions may appear in the definite allergic patient. But in the hands of experts, the tests do give some vital information, like for instance, the presence of a constitutional allergic diathesis, and thus help to determine the lines along which the diet should be ordered. Scratch tests should be ordered first, and only in cases of negative reactions, intradermal tests should be done to avoid severe complications and fatal reactions in hyperallergic patients.

Inhalants: They cause nasal and respiratory allergic symptoms; only very rarely do they affect the skin. The results of inhalant tests are more reliable than those of food allergy tests.

The important inhalants employed for the tests are:

1. Animal danders—cat, dog, cow, horse, sheep, buffalo
2. House dust, mite, cotton dust, wheat dust
3. Vegetable gums
4. Pollens—grasses, trees, flowers, wood.
5. Moulds, cockroaches, mite, housefly, mosquitoes and moth
6. Miscellaneous—feathers, kapok, oris roots, tobacco, silk, wool.

A properly prepared antigen is scratched into the skin. The reactions are read at the end of 20 minutes, as follows:

+ Erythema less than diameter of 5 mm
++ Erythema more than diameter of 5 mm
+++ Erythema with weal in the centre
++++ Weal with pseudopodia and surrounding erythema

Passive transfer (Prausnitz–Küstner) testing is employed in dermographic patients and uncooperative children. Serum from the patient is used to sensitize the skin of a non-allergic individual and then intracutaneous tests are done on the so sensitized skin.

Sensitivity to drugs is tested by the intradermal injection of a diluted drug (preferably a non-irritant but water soluble one) in the forearm and by reading the reaction 20 minutes later on the same basis as other intradermal tests. The test must always be compared with the control. In the present state of increasing drug eruptions (due particularly to antibiotics), and their severe nature, it is essential to do the test before administering penicillin because of the severe and fatal complications caused by it.

BIOLOGICAL TESTS

Basophil degranulation test (Shelley): It is based on the principle that basophils exhibit degranulation in the presence of antigen–antibody reaction of allergy. Sensitivity to drugs, foods and contactants has been established by this technique; it is also helpful in cases of atopic dermatitis.

Technique consists of mixing basophil leucocytes, the patient's serum, solution of antigen and the stain on a slide. Test is read microscopically 10 minutes later. In case of positive reaction, rapid movement of granules first inside the cell and later out of the cells is seen.

The tuberculin (mantoux) test: This test is made with solutions of old tuberculin (1 in 100,000; 1 in 10,000 and 1 in 1,000) in descending order. The test is helpful as a prognostic, less so diagnostic, index in skin tuberculosis and sarcoidosis. The test is read after 72 hours.

The lepromin test: It is made by the intradermal injection of emulsion of lepra bacilli and tissues. It is a prognostic test and has no value in the diagnosis of leprosy (for details, *see* Chapter 17).

The Frei test: It is an intradermal biological test conducted with Frei's antigen or lygranum in cases of lymphogranuloma inguinale. 0.1 cc is injected, and the test is read 48 hours later.

The Leishmania vaccine test: This is made with the solution of *Leishmania tropica* culture on NNN medium. 0.1 cc of solution is injected intradermally. The test is read 48–96 hours later. Similarly, biological skin tests can be done for filariasis, syphilis and granuloma venereum.

Kveim test: There is doubt regarding its specificity in sarcoidosis for which it is employed. The antigen consists of suspension of ground-up sarcoid lymph node. 0.1 cc is injected intradermally; the test is read after 2 weeks. In positive cases, an infiltrated macule or papule or nodule or even an ulcer may be produced. A biopsy of this nodule will show the typical histology of sarcoid.

Ito–Reenstierna test: Carried out for chancroid, this test is made with a solution of pure culture of Ducrey's bacilli, and read after 48 hours.

HAEMATOLOGICAL, RADIOLOGICAL, ETC.

Haematological studies are important; most of these tests are of a routine nature, viz., haemoglobin, RBC count, total and differential leucocyte count, and erythrocyte sedimentation rate. Others like blood chemistry-proteins, cholesterol and its esters, sugar and vitamin A, calcium and sodium content, cortisol, copper and zinc content are done in certain metabolic disorders. Their relative significance is discussed in subsequent chapters.

Cryoglobulin test: It is positive in several dermatoses particularly systemic lupus erythematosus, lymphogranuloma inguinale, cold sensitivity and purpura. Of course, multiple myelomatosis must be excluded. Cold precipitating serum globulins (cryoglobulins) can be demonstrated as gelatinous precipitate by collecting patient's blood in a warm syringe, separating the serum at 37°C and then cooling in a refrigerator.

Urine analysis: It is important in cases of chronic pruritus, moniliasis and porphyrinurias. The urine should be tested for sugar and albumin whenever diabetes and nephritis are suspected as causing cutaneous symptoms. In endocrine disorders, urine should be examined for 17-ketosteroids.

Stool examination: It is made for ova, amoeba, cysts, cellular reaction and digestive disorders in cases of vitiligo, urticaria, endogenous eczemas, dermatitis enteropathica, etc.

Radiological: Since bony and visceral involvement may be associated with several cutaneous diseases, a radiological investigation may be indicated, viz., syphilis, sarcoidosis, neurofibromatosis, tuberculosis, xanthomatosis and actinomycosis.

IMMUNOGLOBULINS

Immunoglobulins are a group of proteins that have antibody properties. They are synthesized by plasma cells which develop from B-lymphocytes. Immunoglobulins in humans are divided into five groups as IgG, IgA, IgE, IgM and IgD; they are found in different body fluids and secretions like serum, mother's milk, sweat, saliva.

Function of immunoglobulins is to bind specifically to antigen. They also bind to mast cells and release histamine, and mediate complement activation.

Method of test: Radial immune diffusion.

Normal levels	
IgA	1.25–4.25 g/L
IgG	5.0–16.0 g/L
IgM	0.50–1.80 g/L
IgE	20 IU/ml = Atopic genesis is unlikely
IgD	100 IU/ml = Atopic genesis is highly probable

Chapter 5

Management

Remarkable progress has been made in therapeutics. Scientific rational measures are replacing empirical remedies. Management relies essentially on curing the disease by natural aids and correction of cause/causes but not on drug pushing. Treatment must be individualized to suit every patient. Skin is a superficial and being an ectodermal structure takes time to heal. Hence, great care should be exercised in prescribing the right topical remedy and in its mode of application.

Principles of Dermatological Management

1. Correct diagnosis, establishment of the cause and sincere attempts to eliminate or correct causes.
2. Reassurance to the patient and relatives so as to allay their anxiety about infectivity, severity, scarring and chances of recovery.
3. Specific and palliative treatment:
   a. General measures—Diet, rest, environments
   b. Internal—Systemic drugs
   c. Local—Topical measures
   d. Physical treatment and surgery—Discussed in Chapter 6.

GENERAL MEASURES

The integument is a part of the body, so when it is affected, the whole body has to be considered and treated accordingly.

I. Mind

To begin with, a patient's mind should be set at rest. Simply ordering the patient to relax is not enough. Psychogenic stresses and emotional conflicts are responsible for, originally causing and secondarily complicating, quite a few skin diseases. If the cause is simple, bedside psychotherapy is enough. In complicated cases and in psychotic patients, the help of a psychiatrist is very valuable.

II. Diet

It has an important role to play. Spices, hot condiments, non-vegetarian foods, tea, coffee and alcohol (non-*sattvik* foods) predispose to sense of heat and to several dermatoses.

Simple nourishing and wholesome food is recommended in all skin diseases. Other restrictions may be necessary in allergic conditions, seborrhoeic conditions, chronic pyoderma, erythroderma and pemphigus.

Diet in allergic dermatoses (urticaria, allergic and atopic eczema): It is needless to enforce diet restriction in every case of allergic dermatosis. Only when an allergy due to foodstuffs is suspected in history, should a special diet be prescribed, both as a diagnostic and therapeutic measure. It gives more valuable information than even food allergy tests. The single factor eliminative diet and a diet diary are two useful measures. In the former, we start the patient on one foodstuff, like boiled milk. If the disease persists, he is given, to start with, boiled rice and sugar. It is rarely that a patient is sensitive to both rice and milk. If the allergy is due to dietetic factors, the disease should be controlled with this diet alone (mind you, without help of drugs). After the disease has been controlled on boiled milk or rice, every three days, one more foodstuff is added, starting with essential ones like wheat (*chapattis** and bread), fats (butter and *ghee***), mutton, eggs, peas, carrots, bananas, potatoes, lentils, till either an allergic attack develops, meaning that the patient is sensitive to the last added foodstuff, or the normal diet is reached. Usually, patients are sensitive to protein diets or vegetables and fruits, or to the synthetic chemicals used for preserving food; starches, fats and minerals make poor allergens. In underdeveloped countries, adulterated foodstuffs cause a lot of mischief.

Diet diary: A specimen chart **(Table 5.1)** is maintained for a month or two depending upon the case. Every foodstuff taken during the day is marked by a cross (x), and at the

Table 5.1: Specimen of a diet chart

Foodstuff	*Day/date*	*Day/date*	*Day/date*	*Comments*
Chapattis				
Lentils				
Milk				
Rice				
Maize				
Barley				
Mutton				
Chicken				
Eggs				
Fish				
Oranges				
Bananas				
Mangoes				
Apples				
Potatoes				
Peas				
Spinach				
Result: B–Better; W–Worse; N–No lesion; A–Acute flare-up; S–Same				

*A Hindi word for a kind of unleavened bread made of flour, baked on a griddle and roasted over the fire. **A white cooking medium made from melted butter.

bottom of the column, the patient puts down whether he felt better or worse, or suffered from an acute flare-up; the cause can be discovered. The diet diary is a simple and non-cumbersome procedure through which the cause of diet allergies can be found out.

Diet in seborrhoeic conditions (acne vulgaris, seborrhoeic dermatitis and rosacea): Patients are advised to consume more milk, eggs, fish, mutton, chicken, and also to add green vegetables and fresh fruits. They should cut down, and in severe cases strictly avoid, concentrated, strachy and fat-rich fried stuffs like *puries****, white bread, porridge, rice, potatoes, bananas, mangoes, cakes, puddings, pastry, nuts and cheese. Condiments, sauces and pickles should also be avoided. We may add a word of caution: There is no place for a rigid menu since a strict diet never cures a seborrhoeic condition but on the contrary demoralises the patient restricting his social activities unnecessarily. Restricted diets should not be continued for very long periods.

Diet in chronic pyoderma: Recurrent folliculitis and furunculoses do well when there is restriction of sweets, stodgy, concentrated starches and mangoes, etc. on the lines recommended above.

Chronic erythroderma, pemphigus and leprosy: Extra proteins and minerals should be added to the diet to keep up the body's strength and make up for the loss of these from the skin in the form of scales and serum, particularly so in the first two dermatoses.

Disseminated and acute eczemas: They heal quicker on restricted salt and a light, easily digestible diet. In patients with acute and disseminated eczemas, it is customary to give a restricted diet, i.e., milk and rice for at least 3 days. It helps the body to eliminate the toxic products of disease, with the result that the patient recovers more speedily. In endogenous eczemas and urticarias, bland vegetarian diet with restricted tea, coffee and alcohol (*Sattvik* food) is helpful. It should be continued for at least 4–12 weeks.

III. Rest

Complete bed-rest is seldom necessary. Only patients with debilitating disease like pemphigus, erythroderma, generalized eczema, psoriasis and lepromatous leprosy require rest at home, or preferably be hospitalised. Cases of infectious leprosy should be isolated completely- separate room, separate utensils, separate linen and no visitors. Cases of scabies and impetigo contagiosum should be isolated at home till these diseases are completely controlled.

Localized contact dermatitis and eczema warrant local protection with bandages and masks to exclude all irritants and sensitizers till the affected part has healed; these measures also protect the affected part from being scratched. If the eczema is extensive or generalized, it is advisable to isolate the patient in a simple, non-allergenic environment, such as a clean room with simple and limited furniture, without carpets. rugs and the like- no knick-knacks, no flowers, no chemicals, etc. Daily bandages in these patients are cumbersome, expensive and painful to change.

IV. External Environments

A skin patient should be nursed in homely and clean environments; fresh air and mild sunlight help to heal the affected skin. The atmosphere should be free from dust and

***Hindi word for small cakes of fried, unleavened bread made either out of whole wheat or white flour.

chemicals. Atopic eczematous patients must be kept, to start with, in pollen-free rooms unless declared insensitive to pollens; they are "tricky" patients. External temperature plays an important part in the healing of the skin. In tropical countries, the external atmospheric temperature needs to be regulated with an air-conditioner, particularly for chronic illnesses. If air-conditioning is not available, the patient should be removed to a more suitable climate. A climatic change may be the only therapeutic measure available for certain cases of chronic and atopic eczemas, severe ichthyosis and prickly heat. Besides a change in climate, a move to a different place provides a change in mental outlook, and helps the mind to relax.

SYSTEMIC TREATMENT

There has been a considerable addition to the skin pharmacopoeia in the last few decades. A variety of broad-spectrum antibiotics, potent corticosteroids, fungicidal, antiviral and cytotoxic agents have been launched, and used successfully. Retinoids, cyclosporin, interferons, a plethora of biologicals too have found their way in the market, but require a judicial use by expert hards only.

Corticosteroids and Adrenocorticortrophic Hormones

These hormone preparations are very widely used. However, cortisone is no more considered a panacea or a miracle drug for all ailments, as it was once thought when the drug was first introduced to the medical profession by Kendall and Hench. These drugs may be lifesaving for the management of life-threatening dermatoses such as pemphigus vulgaris and systemic lupus erythematosus. They are also useful for acute debilitating dermatoses such as extensive allergic contact dermatitis and drug eruptions. The treatment with corticosteroids must however be individualized with considerable attention to relative risks and benefits.

Corticosteroids are absorbed through the skin if used over large areas, and produce retention of salt and water in the body. Topical use can cause cutaneous atrophy and telangiectasia. There are ever increasing number of worst cases of striae atrophicans induced by injudicious use of corticosteroids, which are more common in the present commercial set-up. Its anti-mitotic effect inferferes with wound healing. Topical steroids are often used with benefit, in combination with topical antibiotics, antiseptics and anti fungal agents.

The dermatologic uses of systemic corticosteroids are enumerated in Table 5.2.

Pulse Therapy

The pulse therapy technique, which dates back to the early 1980s, involves the use as much as one gram of methylprednisolone sodium succinate in 150 ml of 5% dextrose daily for 3–5 dsays. The use of the pulse therapy as an alternative treatment for the usually steroid-responsive dermatoses that have become treatment resistant is believed to have lesser side effects. Pemphigus, pemphigoid, pemphigus foliaceus, refractory febrile neutrophilic dermatosis, erythema multiforme, and toxic epidermal necrolysis may respond to pulse therapy. There are definite risks associated with pulse therapy, and it should be administered only in hospitals. Patients who exhibit decreased renal function, who are receiving furosemide, or who have altered electrolyte balance are at greater risk.

Table 5.2: Dermatologic use of systemic corticosteroids	
A. Acute emergencies—definite indication, as they shorten the course of the disease and reduce discomfort.	
Acute disseminated eczema	Polyarteritis nodosa
Acute urticaria and angio-neurotic oedema	Severe erythema multiforme
Widespread drug eruption	Anaphylactoid shock
B. Chronic disorders—to be used as a last resort	
Atopic eczema	Erythroderma
Infantile eczema	Lichen planus
Psoriasis (erythrodermic and arthropathic varieties)	
C. Fatal disorders—are lifesaving.	
Pemphigus vulgaris	Systemic lupus erythematosus

To decrease the complications of oral corticosteroids, the following guidelines have been suggested by Thorn (1981).

1. Drug dosage must be reviewed frequently, and the dose reduced whenever possible.
2. Single morning/alternate-day doses should be given. This produces less suppression of the hypothalamic-pituitary-adrenal axis.
3. Steroid-sparing drugs/immunosuppressive agent (i.e., cyclophosphamide, antimalarials) should be introduced to avoid long-term high-dose corticosteroid therapy.
4. Routine chest radiographs to rule out tuberculosis, if prolonged corticosteroid therapy is contemplated.
5. Periodic urinalysis and determination of blood sugar levels to rule out diabetes.
6. If therapy is long-term, check for hypertension and cataract formation.

Depending on the acuteness of the disease, different corticosteroids with variable potency can be used, as shown in **Table 5.3**.

Table 5.3: Relative potency of corticosteroids

Steroid	*Equipotent dose (mg)*	*Half-life (Hrs)*	*Anti-inflammatory effect*	*Sodium retention and metabolic effect*
Hydrocortisone*	20–240	8–12	1	1
Prednisolone and prednisone	5–60	24–36	4	Less
Methylprednisolone	4–48	18–36	5	Half
Flucortisone	–	–	10	>100
Triamcinolone	4–12	48–48	5	0
Betamethasone	0.6–7.2	36–54	25	0
Dexamethasone	5–9	36–54	25	0
ACTH	25–300	8–12	+	+

*Hydrocortisone is taken base 1; other steroids can be compared on equivalent basis for comparing anti-inflammatory effect and metabolic upset.

Topical corticosteroids are much more frequently used in the dermatological practice.

Newer potent preparations have overshadowed the traditional triamcinolone and hydrocortisone **(Tables 5.4 and 5.5)**.

The side effects of corticosteroids should be borne in mind, namely oedema, hypertension, activation of infective process, glycosuria, osteoporosis, peptic ulcer, hyperkalemia and thrombosis. The effect on the skin is seen as acneiform eruption, hypertrichosis, hyperpigmentation, striae atrophica, impaired wound healing, ecchymosis, etc. Contraindications like hypertension, heart failure, kidney disease, diabetes and active focus of infection should be excluded before the drugs are prescribed. Further, the corticosteroids must be gradually tapered off after the disease has been brought under control.

Single dose therapy and step ladder tapering are being successfully used by many workers. Local triamcinolone and prednisone injections (intradermal infiltration with dental syringe or dermajet) are being employed in the treatment of keloids, hypertrophic scars, lichen simplex chronicus and prurigo nodules.

Antibiotics

They are very useful as bacteriostatic and bactericidal agents in bacterial and mycotic infections. Careful selection is essential according to the infection for which they are employed. Antibiotics which are employed systemically should preferably not be used topically for fear of causing sensitization. If facilities are available, sensitivity

Table 5.4: Selected topical corticosteroids and their strength

Classes	*Drug*	*%*
1.	Betamethasone dipropionate cream	0.05
2.	Dexamethasone	0.25
3.	Betamethasone valerate	0.12
4.	Fluocinolone acetonide cream	0.2
5.	Hydrocortisone butyate cream	0.15
	Triamcinolone acetonide cream, lotion	0.1
6.	Hydrocortisone	0.5
7.	Methylprednisolone acetate ointment	1

Adapted from Arndt, 1989. Class 1 is the most potent; Class 7 is least potent

Table 5.5: Indications for local use of triamcinolone and betamethasone (in the form of lotion or ointment 0.1–1.0%)

Physiological effects Extinction of inflammation Disappearance of pruritus	Protection against fibrosis Absence of sensitivity phenomena
Indications 1. Contact dermatitis 2. Infantile enzema 3. Atopic eczema 4. Nummular eczeme	5. Neurodermatitis 6. Localised pruritus (anus and vulva) 7. Prevention of fibrosis and keloidal scars 8. Insect bites

tests may help to select the most effective one. Only in serious and widespread skin infections, should antibiotics be employed systemically; it is usually sufficient to employ them locally. Because of the increasing degree of sensitivity reactions, an intradermal sensitivity test is a "must" before penicillin is administered.

The dosage and combinations of these antibiotics, if needed, are based on the principles followed in general medicine. One must familiarise oneself with cost and toxic effects before prescribing them.

There have been many improvements in the types of penicillin, e.g. synthetic penicillins like ampicillin, cloxacillin, amoxycillin and carbenicillin. They have a broad spectrum of activity. Cephaloridine, a derivative of cephalosporin C, is highly effective against gram-positive and gram-negative organisms. Gentamicin, clindamycin and kanamycin have powerful antibacterial action. Their use should be restricted to severe, fulminating infections.

The treatment schedule for the usual cutaneous infections is the same as is employed for other infections. Most skin and soft tissue infections are caused by *Streptococcus pyogenes* or *Staphylococcus aureus*. In general, systemic antibiotics such as penicillins, erythromycin, or cephalosporins are favoured for deeper infections as they are beyond the reach of topical preparations. However, the development of potent topical preparation such as mupirocin may obviate the use of systemic antibiotics in several instances. In acne vulgaris, oral tetracyclines including doxycycline or minocycline have also been used in severe cases.

Topical antibiotics are commonly used for localised impetigo contagiosa or other superficial skin infections and also in acne vulgaris. Erythromycin 2–4% topical solution or gel, clindamycin 1% solution or gel with or without benzoyl peroxide have recently got popularity in the treatment of acne.

The additional uses of systemic antibiotics apart from varieties of cutaneous bacterial infections and acne vulgaris are in several non-infectious conditions such as rosacea: exacerbations of atopic dermatitis, colonized by staphylococci, and pityriasis-lichenoides et varioliformis acuta.

Mupirocin is derived from fermentation of *Pyocyaneus fluorescens*. It is used only topically and is effective against gram-positive organisms and some gram-negative organisms by inhibiting bacterial protein synthesis. Toxicity is low. It is useful in impetigo, infective eczema and staphylococcal folliculitis.

Minocycline is a semisynthetic derivative of tetracycline, with activity against a wide range of gram-negative and gram-positive organisms, including some organisms resistant to other tetracyclines. It is effective in gonoccoccal infections, urinary tract infections, skin and soft tissue infections and acne.

Adverse reactions include anorexia, nausea, vomiting, glossitis, rashes, erythema multiforme, photosensitivity, muddy pigmentation and superadded infections. As with other tetracyclines, this drug should not be given in 3rd trimester of pregnancy and in children upto 14 years of age.

Cephalosporins

First generation	Cephalexin, cephalothin and cephazolin.
Second generation	Cefaclor, cefoxitin and cephamandole.
Third generation	Cefotaxime, cefoperazone, ceftazidime, ceftriaxone and latamoxef

The cephalosporins are broad-spectrum bactericidal agents which inhibit bacterial cell-wall synthesis. Susceptible organisms include a wide range of gram-positive and gram-negative organisms such as haemolytic streptococci, *Strep. pneumoniae*, *Staph. aureus* (both penicillin sensitive and resistant), *Neisseria gonorrhoea*, *Neisseria meningitidis*, *Proteus mirabillis* and some strains of *E. coli*, indole positive *Proteus* sp., *Enterobacter* and *Haemophilus*. Newer cephalosporins also show activity against *Pseudomonas aeruginosa*. They have been used in the treatment of respiratory tract infections, genitourinary tract infections, soft tissue infections, bone and joint infections, septicaemia and intra-abdominal infections.

Side-effects: These include false-positive reactions for glucose in the urine, positive direct Coomb tests, leucopenia, eosinophilia, granulocytopenia, transient rise in AST (SGOT), ALT (SGPT) and alkaline phosphatase levels, elevations in serum creatinine and blood urea, nausea, diarrhoea, abdominal pain, vomiting, pain and phlebitis at injection sites and hypersensitivity reactions such as maculopapular rash, urticaria and fever.

Clindamycin is semisynthetic derivative of lincomycine. It is bacteriostatic in low concentrations and bactericidal at slightly higher concentrations. It is completely absorbed from the gut and excreted in urine. Side-effects are pseudomembranous colitis, hepatotoxicity and drug eruptions. Dermatological uses are topical in acne, and systemic in acne and hidradenitis suppurativa. The dose is 150–450 mg BD.

Rifampicin is a semisynthetic antibiotic produced by *Streptomyces mediterranei*.

It is readily absorbed from the gastrointestinal tract, reaches its peak in 2–6 hours and then maintains at therapeutic levels. Presence of food delays absorption. It is a broad-spectrum bactericidal antibiotic (inhibits DNA-dependent RNA polymerase). It is effective against gram-positive and gram-negative organisms and *Mycobacterium tuberculosis* and *Mycobacterium leprae*. There is a tendency to develop drug resistance.

In leprosy, it is given in a single dose 450–600 mg daily first thing in the morning on empty stomach for 12–20 weeks. It helps to kill lepra bacilli rapidly. Morphological and bacteriological indices fall rapidly, disease comes under control and the complications of the disease especially ENL are prevented.

Side-effects

1. Increase in rate of blood coagulation, hence in heart patients increased requirement of anticoagulant coumarins.
2. Liver dysfunction.
3. Hypersensitivity reaction.
4. Abdominal discomfort, cramps, increase in sense of heat and muscular pains.

Roxithromycin

Roxithromycin is a semisynthetic macrolide. It has a better pharmacokinetics than erythromycin and can be administered twice a day. A high clinical and bacteriological cure rates have been achieved by it. The usual dose is 150 mg twice a day 15 minutes before food in adults, and 2.5–5 mg per kg body weight twice daily in children. Serious side-effects are uncommon. Usual adverse effects include anorexia, constipation, dyspepsia, dizziness, tinnitus, headache, skin rashes. Its potential for hepatotoxicity is much less than that of erythromycin.

Quinolones

Quinolones (norfloxacin, ciprofloxacin, pefloxacin ofloxacin) are bactericidal and act by inhibiting the enzyme responsible for maintaining the structure of DNA. Ciprofloxacin is active against a wide range of both gram-negative and gram-positive organisms including those that are resistant to penicillins, cephalosporins or aminoglycosides.

Ciprofloxacin is a quinoline antibacterial agent effective against gram-negative bacteria such as *E. coli*, *K. pneumoniae*, *Serratia* spp., *Proteus* spp., *P. aeroginosa* and *H. influenzae* and also gram-positive organisms such as *Staphylococcus* spp., haemolytic streptococci and enterococci. Toxicity is low and side effects few. It is very useful in gonorrhoea and urethral infection. Dose is 500 mg BD.

Ofloxacin is a synthetic 4-fluoroquinolone structurally related to nalidixic acid. It is active against a wide range of both gram-negative and gram-positive organisms found in the lower respiratory, urinary and genital tracts. Unlike other 4 quinolones, no interaction has been demonstrated between ofloxacin and warfarin. Ofloxacin as well as pefloxacin have been recommended in the multibacillary leprosy at the initiation of the therapy for 1.5–2 months. They have shown to reduce the incidence of reactions in leprosy. Dose of ofloxacin is 200–400 mg daily while that of pefloxacin is 400–800 mg daily. Lomefloxacin, the latest addition to this group has an advantage as it can be given only once a day, the dose being 400 mg daily. Their chief side-effects include GI distrubances, dizziness, headache, tremors, confusions, convulsions, rashes, blurred vision, joint pain, judgement and dexterity may be impaired. There may be transient increase in serum creatinine, haematological, hepatic and renal disturbances, vasculitis, pseudomembranous colitis, Stevens-Johnson syndrome.

Antifungal Agents

Griseofulvin is a colourless, neutral, thermostable antibiotic isolated from *Penicillum griseofulvum*. Administered orally it gets well-absorbed. On reaching the skin, it endows the epidermal cells eventually destined to produce keratin with the power to resist fungi completely.

Indications: Tinea of the skin, hair and nail caused by species of *Trichophyton*, *Epidermophyton* and *Microsporon*. It has no action on *Monilia*, *Microsporon furfur*, actinomycosis, histoplasmosis, and other deeper fungi. It should only be used if tinea is chronic, resistant and widespread.

Dose of griseofulvin FP.

Adult—250 mg 2 times a day

Children—125 mg 1–2 times a day

Duration of treatment: Improvement starts in 1–2 weeks, and it takes about 4–6 weeks to control the disease of the scalp and skin. It takes about 6–9 months to control tinea unguium. Treatment must be persisted with for at least a couple of weeks after the disease process has been completely controlled. The first symptom to disappear is itching.

In tinea unguium, it is customary to give griseofulvin FP in doses of one gram once a week. It helps to cut down cost and toxicity.

Toxicity: It has low toxicity and sensitizing capacity. The side-effects consist of headache, abdominal discomfort and occasionally, urticaria and porphyria.

Table 5.6: Fluconazole therapy

Indication	*First day*	*Daily*	*Minimum duration of therapy*
Oropharyngeal candidiasis (acute)	200 mg	50–100 mg	14 days
Oesophageal candidiasis (acute)	200 mg	50–100 mg	21 days
Systemic candidiasis	400 mg	200 mg	28 days
Cryptococcal meningitis (acute)	400 mg	200 mg	10–12 week after CSF culture becomes negative

Ketoconazole is imidazole derivative with broad-spectrum antifungal activity. When used orally, it is effective in mucocutaneous candidiasis, superficial fungal infection, onychomycosis and deep fungal infections. Dose is 100 mg twice a day.

Adverse reactions include nausea, vomiting, abdominal pain, pruritus and toxic hepatitis. Physicians intending to use ketoconazole should weigh the potential benefits of treatment against the risk of liver damage and should carefully monitor their patients both clinically and biochemically.

Fluconazole, a bis-triazole antifungal drug, is rapidly absorbed orally. Studies *in vivo* have shown that this drug is effective in infections caused by *Candida*, *Cryptococcus*, *Aspergillus*, *Blastomyces*, *Coccidioides* and *Histoplasma*.

It is indicated for vaginal, mucosal, systemic candidiasis, and cryptococcosis. It is also used as maintenance therapy to prevent relapse of cryptococcal disease in patients with AIDS. It is not recommended in children below the age of 16 years. Patients who develop abnormal liver function tests during therapy with fluconazole should be monitored for the development of more hepatic injury **(Table 5.6)**.

Acyclovir (Zovirox-P)

Acyclovir (Zovirox-P) is an acrylic analogue of deoxyguanosine. It is inactive. Unless first phosphorylated in cells by the viral genome namely, herpes virus thymidine kinase.

Acyclovir is a potent inhibitor of DNA polymerase in the virus infected cells; hence it is effective against the herpes virus (1 and 2), varicella zoster and Epstein-Barr virus only, if employed within 24 hours of onset of infection. It is useful parenterally, orally and topically. It is effective in primary and recurrent herpes progenitalis; it has being extensively tried.

Dose	Acute: 200 mg 4 hourly, 5 capsules a day × 10 days. Chronic: 200 mg TDS × 6 months.
Adverse reaction	Mutagenesis Decreased spermatogenesis Impaired fertility Emergence of less sensitive strain Teratogenic effect in pregnancy Vomiting, nausea, diarrhoea, fatigue, headache, skin rash, leg pains, adenopathy and sore throat, hair loss, depression.

Adverse reactions, seen in approximately 16% of patients are nausea, headache, skin rash, abdominal pain, vomiting and diarrhoea. It may be administered either orally or by intravenous infusion at a rate of approximately 5–10 ml/min.

Ciclopirox Olamine

Ciclopirox olamine is broad-spectrum, topical fungicide. Concentration used is 1% in cream base. It is useful in tinea pedis, tinea cruris, candidiasis and pityriasis versicolor. It can cause local irritation and sensitisation.

Treatment must be continued for at least a few weeks after clinical recovery to avoid recurrence. It should be lightly rubbed into the patches twice a day.

Antihistaminics

Antihistaminics derive their name from the fact that they inhibit various activities of histamine, an important chemical mediator in allergic reactions like urticaria, eczema and drug reactions. Besides histamine, antihistaminics may have some effect on other agents like serotonin, bradykinin, etc. By virtue of their property, it has been found out that there are 2 types of receptor organs, the H_1 and H_2 receptors. Studies have shown that skin contains both these types of receptors. According to their selectivity of inhibition, antihistaminics have been classified into two groups. (1) H_1 receptor inhibitors; (2) H_2 receptor inhibitors **(Tables 5.7 and 5.8)**.

Of these groups of inhibitors, H_1 type are the traditional antihistaminics. But if one of these groups fails the second should be chosen from a separate group. It has also been observed that histamine-mediated dermatoses such as urticaria and dermatitis might be more effectively treated with combination of the H_1 and H_2 inhibitors rather than either one alone. The traditional antihistaminics have side-effects like drowsiness, hence they should not be given when the patient has to go for work but may be beneficially used when some sedation is needed.

Newer antihistaminics show more instances of drug reaction **(Table 5.9)**.

Among the H_2 receptor inhibitors the earlier ones proved to possess renal and hepatic toxicity. Cimetidine, in this group, is free from toxicity except that it may cause mental confusion in few older people who have impaired hepatic and renal function. Antihistaminics should not be employed topically; they are not only useless but are also great sensitizers. Their adverse reactions are enumerated in **Table 5.10**.

Sex Hormones

These hormones should be used after due consideration has been given to the pros and cons of each case. Many harmful side-results have ensued from their indiscriminate use. Oestrogens are given in small doses in the first half of the menstrual cycle. In males with acne, oestrogens are employed as a last resort in order to avoid males developing feminine features. An effective herbal remedy, *Shatavari* (*Asparagus racemosus*) powder has been found to be an effective remedy for menstrual disorders regulation and melasma. The roots of this plant have nutritive, galactogogue and other digestive properties.

1. Oestrogens in acne, kraurosis vulvae, menopausal keratoderma, senile pruritus in females, hypertrichosis of females with oligomenorrhoea. It is given as tablet ethinyl oestradiol 0.01–0.1 mg daily, stilboestrol 1–5 mg daily.

Table 5.7: H_1 receptor inhibitors

Class, Name and Trade name	*Indications*	*Contraindications*	*Duration (in hours)*	*Preparation*
I. Ethanolamines Diphenhydramine (Benadryl)	Pruritus, urticaria	MAO inhibitor	4–6	Tab 25 and 50 mg and syrup
II. Alkylamines Chlorpheniramine maleate (zeet)	Pruritus, urticaria	Not to be used in elderly	4–6	Tab 2 and 8 mg and syrup
Dextrochlor-pheniramine	Pruritus, urticaria angioedema			Tab 2 and 8 mg and syrup
Triprolidine and protection	Sun sensitivity	Low sedation		Tab 2.5 mg
Pheniramine maleate	Pruritus urticaria	Low sedation		Tab 25 and 50 mg Inj 10 ml
III. Piperazines Hydroxyzine hydrochloride	Acute and chronic heat and solar urticaria	Card. Irregularity Glaucoma	6–24	Tab 10 and 25 mg
Cetrizine Dihydrochloride (Alerid)	Acute and chronic heat and solar urticaria	Benign Prostate Hypertrophy	24	Tab 10 mg
IV. Phenothizines Promethazines HCl	Dermographism phycho cutaneous diseases	Hypersensitivity, jaundice, depression		Tab 10 and 25 mg
Methdialazine	Powerful antipruritic	Photosensitivity		Tab 8 mg
V. Piperidines Cyproheptadine	Cold and mild urticaria Dermographism	Elderly person anticholinergic Photosensitivity	11	Tab 4 mg
Terfenadine	Chronic urticaria	Alopeica, insomnia palpitation		
VI. Others drugs Embramine	Antiallergic	Slight sedation	6–8	Tab 25 mg
Mebhydrolin napadisylate	Antiallergic	Slight sedation		Tab 6 mg
Dimethidine maleate	Antiallergic	Slight sedation		Tab 2.5 mg

Table 5.8: H_2 receptor inhibitor

Name: Cimetidine, Ranitidine, Famotidine, Roxatidine

1. Inhibit histamine induced gastric acid secretion.
2. H_2 receptors are also present in endothelial cells of dermal blood vessels.

Uses in dermatology:

1. When H_1 antagonists fail
2. Dermographism, chronic urticaria
3. Pruritus of renal disease, lymphoma and polycythemia
4. Immunostimulants
5. Antiandrogen effect
6. Adjuvant to H_1 antagonists

Table 5.9: Drug interactions and side effects of newer antihistaminics				
Parameters	*Cetrizine*	*Astemizole*	*Terfenadine*	*Loratidine*
Drug interaction	CNS Depressants	Diazepam Alcohol	Ketoconazole Erythromycin	No known Interactions
Side-effects	Headache Dry mouth Dizziness	Dry mouth Cardiac Arrhythmia Dizziness	Alopecia Insomnia Dysmenorrhea Tachycardia Palpitation Tremors Nightmares	Headache Fatigue

Table 5.10: Side-effects antihistaminic adverse reactions	
CVS	Hypotension, tachycardia, extra systoles
Hemat	Anemia, leucopenia, agranulocytosis, thrombocytopenia
CNS	Sedation, restlessness, confusion, diplopia, blurred vision, conv.
GIT	Epigastric distress, anorexia, constipation, vomiting
GU	Dysuria, polyuria, urinary retention, early menses, impotency
RS	Thick sputum, chest tighness, dry mouth, resp. depression
Others	Tingling, heaviness and weakness of hands, urticaria photosensitivity, shock, itching
Contraindications • Hypersensitivity, MAO therapy, nursing mothers • Phenothiazines in comatose patients/CNS depressants, Jaundice • Bone marrow depression, dehydrated children	
Warnings • Use with caution in elderly patients, pregnancy, children • Avoid in glaucoma, peptic ulcer, BPH, asthma	

2. Androgens in senile pruritus in males. It is given as testosterone propionate injections 25 mg I.M. Cyproterone acetate is an anti-androgen which has been claimed useful in the treatment of acne and hirsutism. The drug is given in a dose of 50–100 mg per day from days 5–14 of the menstrual cycle. Since cyproterone would interfere with the menstrual cycle, ethinyl oestradiol is also given from days 5–25.
3. Progesterone in herpes gestationis 5–25 mg IM.
4. Serum gonadotrophic hormone 500–1500 IU once a week in hypertrichosis and bad acne vulgaris. The author adopts the following routine for injections of serum gonadotrophic hormone, injections being given for 3–6 months depending upon the need of the patient:

Dose in IU	1000	1000	1000		1000	1000	1000
Day of menstrual cycle	0	10	20	30	10	20	30

The introduction of sex hormones in the form of birth control pills has resulted in several dermatoses, viz. chloasma, alopecia, acne. Fortunately, their incidence is still low.

Sedatives and Tranquilizers

Because of primary psychogenic stresses and secondary complicating neurotic factors in a large number of dermatoses, there may be an indication for sedatives and tranquilizers to control these factors. They are also useful in controlling intractable pruritus.

Sedatives	Phenobarbitone and other drugs of the barbiturate group. Bromides, chloral hydrate.
Tranquilizers	*Rauwolfia serpentina group*—Raudixin (P), Serpina (P), Serpasil (P) Meprobomate–Miltown (P) Chlorpromazine–Largactil (P) Chlordiazepoxide–Librium (P) Diazepam-calmpose (P) Larpose

Metals

1. ***Arsenic:*** Except in the case of syphilis, arsenic is now used only as a last resort because of the risk of toxic reactions. Even in syphilis, arsenic has been largely replaced by penicillin. The two main indications for liquor arsenicalis are dermatitis herpetiformis and lichen planus. Even in these conditions, it is seldom used now. In syphilis, the preparations employed are neoarsphenamine and mepharside.
2. ***Bismuth.*** In the form of injections—bisglucol, bismuth is useful in syphilis. Mercury and gold are not employed internally these days.
3. ***Antimony.*** Preparations like antimony tartrate and urea stibamine in kala-azar, disseminated cutaneous leishmaniasis and mycosis fungoides. Antimony as intramuscular injections in cutaneous leishmaniasis. It is a toxic drug, so should be used carefully.
4. ***Zinc.*** Daily need of zinc is 5–20 mg. Therapeutic dose is 50–150 mg daily. Sea foods and dairy products are rich sources. Wheat, green vegetables, nuts and legumes are the other good sources. It is involved in several cellular metabolic factors especially nucleic acid metabolism. Its deficiency results in disturbed cellular growth especially of the thymus, macrophages and lysozymes. Clinically, the deficiency is associated with diarrhoea, acrodermatitis enteropathica, proneness to infections, slow wound healing and mental disturbances.

Important cutaneous features are subacute dermatitis of the nose, chin, and eyebrows (somewhat like seborrhoeic dermatitis but crusts are blackish and necrotic), erosions and dermatitis in the groins and ano-vulval region, vesiculation and bullae on palms and soles, dermatitis on buttocks and upper thighs, papulo-pustules on face, psoriasiform lesions, hair loss and nail changes.

Heavy Metal Antidotes

1. Sodium thiosulphate—Ametox (P) 5–10 cc IM, or IV daily or alternate days for 5–10 days.
2. BAL (British- anti-lewisite, dimercapto-propanol) 2.5–3.0 mg per kilogram of body weight BD to OD for 7–10 days. They are employed to get rid of and neutralise the toxic effects of heavy metals—arsenic, gold, bismuth and mercury.
3. Lomodex (P) 500 cc IV drip has been successfully employed in erythrodermas due to heavy metals. It has also been found useful in lepra reaction and toxic melanosis.

Non-specific Stimulants and Desensitizing Agents

1. Calcium gluconate IV—10% 10 cc with or without vitamin C.
2. Calcium (P)—5–10 cc IV or oral tablets.
3. Collosal manganese—Injection intramuscular 0.5–1 cc 2–3 times a week.
   Tablets—one tablet 2–3 times a day.
   Syrup—one teaspoonful twice a day.
4. Tin-Stannoxyl (P)-Tablets, 1–4 times a day. Injection 0.5–1 cc IM 2–3 times a week.
5. Milk-Siolan (P)—2–6 cc IM 2–3 times a week.
6. Auto-haemotherapy—3–10 cc twice a week.
7. Indigenous preparations:
   a. *Chiraita* (*Swertia chiretta*)
   b. *Amla* (*Phyllanthus emblica*)
   c. *Trifala* (*Amla, Harar, Bahera*)—-myroblans
   d. *Neem* (*Nelia azadirachta*)

They are very useful agents without any toxic action. The authors have successfully used indigenous preparation Capyna compound (P) in reactional leprosy and *Andropogan muricatus* (*khas khas*) in urticaria, endogenous eczemas and rosacea, when associated with sense of heat (SOH).

Specific Stimulants

Vaccines

- Autogenous.
- Stock streptostaphylococcal mixed vaccine
- Acne vaccine.
- Staphylococcal toxoid.

They are useful in recurrent pyodermas—acne, folliculitis, furunculoses, infective eczemas, etc. Autogenous vaccine made by an expert is preferable to a stock vaccine.

Vitamins

They are employed for their specific action in the treatment of vitamin deficiencies. Besides, they are empirically recommended in certain dermatoses as follows:

Vitamin A (tablet or injection)	Phrynoderma
50,000–100,000 IU	Lichen spinulosum
	Acne vulgaris
	Darier's disease
	Keratoderma
	Miliaria
Vitamin A acid	Acne vulgaris
	It is keratolytic
Vitamin B_1 (thiamine hydrochloride)	Herpes zoster
	Neurodermatitis desseminatus
Vitamin B_2 (nicotinic acid)	Pellagra
	Chilblains, acrosclerosis

	Angular stomatitis
	Herpes zoster
	Seborrhoeic dermatitis
	Scurvy
Vitamin C	Bleeding dermatoses
	Chloasma
Vitamin D (calciferol tab. 50,000 IU)	Lupus vulgaris
Inj. 60.000 IU weekly	
Vitamin E (wheat germ oil	Keratoderma, epidermolysis
"Viteolin" (3–50 mg)	Collagen disease, cramps.
Vitamin K + P	Bleeding dermatoses including haemorrhagic drug eruptions

Vasodilators

Nicotinic acidamide, Duvadilan (P), Trental (P) and Priscol (P) in tablet form are employed in acrocyanosis, chilblains, Raynaud's disease and other peripheral vascular diseases. They may also be useful in early diffuse type of scleroderma especially acrosclerosis.

Miscellaneous

Chloroquine 150 mg one to three times a day is proving useful in different light-sensitivity dermatoses like lupus erythematosus, hydroa aestivale and xeroderma pigmentosum. Chloroquine can cause blood dyscrasias, corneal and retinal changes, so a careful watch must be kept. Quinine hydrochloride 5–10% in ointment form is useful as a local protective agent against light.

Isonicotinic acid hydrazide (INH) 50–300 mg daily by mouth is useful in cutaneous tuberculosis. Pellagra-like features have been seen to develop following the long-term use of INH. A combination of INH and thiosemicarbazone has been used in cutaneous and extracutaneous tuberculosis, leprosy, etc.

Thiabendazole: Useful in creeping eruption. The dose is 50 mg/kg body weight repeated after 12 hours. Such 2–3 doses. No side-effects have been reported. It is also useful in scabies and intestinal worm infestation.

Hetrazan (P): Useful in filariasis. Dose 2–6 mg/kg body weight thrice daily for 3–4 weeks.

Diamino-diphenyl-sulphone (DDS): Avlosulfone (P)/Dapsone (P) has established its place in the treatment of leprosy, dermatitis herpetiformis and pemphigoid. The dosage is 50–100 mg daily. The important side-effects are blood dyscrasias like aplastic anaemia and agranulocytosis, dapsone syndrome and skin reactions.

Nuclear toxins like radioactive phosphorus, urethane and nitrogen mustard are used in the treatment of mycosis fungoides, leukaemia cutis, etc. Aminopterin and methotrexate are used in recalcitrant cases of psoriasis.

General stimulants like liver extract, concentrated proteins, vitamins, iron, etc. are very commonly employed in the practice of dermatology; so also are autonomic nervous system drugs, purgatives, thyroids, anabolic hormones.

Retinoids are the synthetic derivatives of vitamin A. Two important retinoids are isotretinoin and etretinate. They are being tried in keratinizing disorders (like ichthyosis, pityriasis rubra pilaris and Darier's disease), cystic acne, psoriasis and skin malignancies.

Dosage: 0.5 mg/kg of body weight for 15–20 weeks. Then 8 weeks rest before recommending a second course.

Side-effects: Cheilitis, dry skin, pruritus, conjunctivitis, musculo-skeletal weakness, thinning of scalp, peeling of skin, proneness to infection, headache, diarrhoea, etc.

Blood sugar metabolism may be upset; intolerance to contact lenses and disturbed night vision are the other side-effects.

Vitamin A acid (retinoic acid) is used topically in treating acne vulgaris and chloasma. Since it is an irritant and keratolytic, it should be used with care. It has also been recommended to correct wrinkles and ageing skin. Results are controversial.

Collagen: It is an animal protein product and has been used with success in cases of chronic ulcers like nodular vasculitis, Schamberg's disease, stasis ulcers and Hansen's disease. It is used in the form of sheets or gel for local dressing. It is also under trial for local infiltration like silicone is soluble collagen in filling skin defects. The exact mode of action is unknown. It is a useful agent of promise in handling of intractable trophic and vascular ulcers.

Dextranomer-Debrisvan (P): It is a hydrophilic dextran polymer and has been tried as a 'cleansing agent' in cases of chronic ulcers, e.g. trophic ulcers of leprosy and decubitus ulcers. It is believed to exert its effects by adsorbing the wound exudate, debris and microorganisms into the dextranomer beads and thereby promotes healing.

Minoxidil is a pyrimidine derivative. It is a vasodilator used primarily in treating severe hypertension. Patients under treatment with minoxidil develop hypertrichosis. This observation has prompted the dermatologists in successfully using minoxidil in alopecia areata androgenetic alopecia and female patterm hair loss.

DNCB (2–4 dinitrochlorobenzene) immunotherapy is used to produce a locally induced cell-mediated immune response of sufficient severity to eradicate recalcitrant warts and treat alopecia areata. It may act either by immunological stimulation or simply as a non-specific inflammatory reaction.

Side-effects of treatment with DNCB are pruritus, oozing, blistering, adenopathy, auto-eczematization and urticaria.

LOCAL TREATMENT

One must be thoroughly familiar with all aspects of external topical measures, since they form the basis of curative treatment when the cause is on the surface, and can be tackled by topical measures alone; and palliative, when used to control the symptoms of the cause which lies deeper. Instructions regarding the use of local medicaments must be given in detail, and if possible, it is advisable to demonstrate the same to the patient or attendants.

CLEANSING PROCEDURES

It is common sense that before any remedial procedure is adopted, the site must be properly cleaned of the disease products like crusts, scales and previous medicaments (which may have harmed the patient). Crusts and scales not only screen the diseased part from the action of medicaments, but also favour the accumulation of disease products underneath them; the part, therefore, should be thoroughly cleaned at the first opportunity.

Poultices: A starch boric acid poultice is cumbersome to make, and is more harmful than useful if not properly made; so the authors recommends simpler and cheaper measures in underdeveloped countries, viz., first soak the crust in warm olive or coconut oil. This will soften it. The crust can then be removed by means of a soft piece of cotton dipped in a dilute potassium permanganate solution (1 in 8,000, or light pink in colour, when roughly made without the use of proper weighing scales) or diluted Savlon (P) or Cetavlon (P) liquid. In dermatitis, eczema, impetigo and other crusted lesions, this procedure is simple and easy to employ.

A kaolin poultice is useful in fomenting a boil or an abscess. Fomentation hastens the suppuration, localizes it and makes it burst. Every Asiatic country has its own indigenous local poultice, like linseed poultice, mustard poultice, etc. One must be careful not to irritate or macerate the surrounding areas.

Soaps: Medicated soaps containing tar, mercury, cetavlon or sulphur, etc. are of doubtful value in practice, for the simple reason that the active medicament in the soap is greatly diluted by the time it reaches the skin. Soap containing 3% salicylic acid and 10% sulphur is useful in scabies and pityriasis versicolor; the lather is left on the skin for at least 15 minutes before washing it off.

The use of soap is absolutely forbidden in acute inflammatory conditions particularly in those that are eczematous. Its use is restricted in chronic inflammatory dermatoses, atopic eczema and ichthyosis.

The most important indication for the use of soap is seborrhoeic dermatoses, for instance, a seborrhoeic skin, acne vulgaris and pityriasis capitis. Dry and soft soaps, particularly tincture of green soap, are very useful in such conditions to remove the grease. Particularly in acne vulgaris, the face should be cleaned by washing, and if frequent washing with soap is not possible, cleansing alcohol or eau de cologne may be employed for the same purpose. A greasy scalp should be washed more frequently, at least two to three times a week.

Superfatted soaps are very valuable for dry skins. If superfatted soap is not available, it can be prepared at home by melting finely shredded soap in hot olive or coconut oil over a water-bath, stirring it till a homogenous mixture is formed and then allowing the mixture to cool and set to form a cake.

In psoriasis, scales should be removed from the lesions with a nail brush, a roiled towel or an Indian earthen brush (Jhanwa).

Sulphonated loral is a soapless detergent. Its use is recommended when an individual is sensitive to ordinary soap. It is prepared as follows:

Sulphonated Loral
Glycerinated amylii
Lanette wax S.X
Aqua m. ft. emulsio equal parts

Baths: Bathing is contraindicated in acute inflammatory dermatoses but in chronic conditions it is not only permitted but supplemented with medicaments. Medicated baths have been in vogue in most dermatological clinics. They are useful in ameliorating symptoms, particularly itching.

Hot sulphur springs, such as the 'Sohna' spring near Delhi and other hot sulphur springs near Manali, Bombay and Kangra attract a lot of patients with skin diseases like psoriasis and seborrhoeic dermatoses. Besides the hot sulphur water, the holiday atmosphere and the mental relaxation, these resorts provide a stimulating effect on the integument. Hence, patients should be encouraged, whenever possible, to visit such places.

Because of the lack of facilities in the homes and hospitals of underdeveloped countries, the preparation of medicated baths is difficult, and so, they are seldom recommended. The different types of medicated baths are:

1. Saline bath (hypertonic)- in ichthyosis. 1–2 lbs. of table salt to 20 gallons of water.
2. Boric acid bath. 6 oz. dissolved in a jugful of water and then added to the bath. Useful in chronic pyogenic dermatoses.
3. Anti-pruritic bath (colloidal) in exfoliative dermatitis, urticaria, generalized pruritus.
   a. Boiled bran 2 lbs. to a bath. Boil bran 2 lbs. with 4 lbs. of water like porridge, put this in a muslin bag, tie securely and swish in a tubful of warm (in winter) or cool (in summer) water. An ounce of baking soda may be added to make it more alkaline to dissolve the scales. The patient relaxes in this bath for 10–15 minutes, and then pats himself dry. A colloidal bath gives the patient relief for about 12 hours.
   b. Laundry starch is also useful. It is mixed directly with the bath water.

It is preferable not to add any other medicament like potassium permanganate or chrysorabin to the bath. The good they do is doubtful; they certainly create a lot of mess in the house and bathroom; apart from this, the bath tub is stained.

Shaving: Hair interfering with treatment of affected parts should be cut. Except in the case of children, shaving of scalp is disliked by patients, and so should be avoided, unless of course the case is obstinate in responding to other remedial measures. In sycosis barbae, and filiform warts in the beard region, growing a beard should be encouraged to avoid repeated traumata and spread of infection.

Remedial Measures

With implementation of the above cleansing procedures, the patient is ready for external remedial applications. The important principles to be borne in mind when recommending them is, that applications should be cheap, easily available and not cumbersome or tedious to apply. They should not spoil or stain the clothes; if they are likely to do so, the affected parts should be kept covered.

The general rule to follow in deciding on the medicament and then decide the vehicle is as follows:

1. On dry lesions—powder or paint.
2. Oozing or vesicular lesions—lotion, as paint or wet dressing.
3. Crusted and scaly lesions—cream or paste.
4. Chronic scaly lesions—ointment.
5. Folliculitis and pustules—varnish.

Do not forget to give detailed instructions regarding dispensing and proper method of application.

Local Active Medicaments

1. *Anti-inflammatory:* Hydrocortisone (0.5–2.5%), prednisone (0.5%) or fluorocortisone (0.1%), betamethasone, fluocinolone lotion, ointment or intradermal injections.
2. *Antiseptic:* Boric acid (1%), potassium permanganate (1 in 8000 to 1 in 4000), antibiotics, quinolor derivatives like Vioform (P), Sterosan (P), Dermoquinol (P) (2–8%), Cetavlon (0.1–1%), Dequadin (P), brilliant green (1%), gentian violet (1%), hydrarg ammoniata (5%), hydrarg perchlor (1 in 1000).
3. *Anti-pruritic:* Phenol (1–2%), menthol (1–2%), camphor (1–5%), ichthammol (2–10%), corticosteroids, cocaine derivatives (procaine, benzocaine, novacaine, xylocaine etc.), chloral hydras (1–2%).
4. *Antivirals:* 5-iodo-2-deoxyuridine (5-IDU) 0.5% in vaseline base for treatment of herpes simplex, herpes progenitalis and warts. Also useful are methisazone and amantadine.
5. *Astringents:* Calamine preparata (10%), silver nitrate (0.5–1%), gentian violet (0.5–2%), brilliant green (0.5–2%), lead (liq. plumbi subacetate fortis 5%), Indian catechu (concentrated solution), bismuth subgallas (10%), amylum (20%), aluminium acetate (Burows' solution 1–5%).
6. *Bleaching:* Mono-benzyl ether of hydroquinone (MBEH in short).
7. *Caustics:* a) Mild (irritant). Cantharidin, iodine (tincture or iodex). (b) Strong phenol 95%, podophyllin 25% in spirit or vaseline or paint, trichlor-acetic acid 50–75%, acid nitrate of mercury, CO_2 snow, liquid nitrogen.
8. Cytotoxic agents-5-fluorouracil in hydrophilic ointment 1–5% for extensive keratosis; 0.5% (demecolcine) for skin cancer, podophyllin for skin cancer and warts. It is applied twice a day for 3–4 weeks; methotrexate 0.25–0.5%).
9. Fungicidal agents—Gentian violet (0.5–2%), brilliant green (0.5–2%). Quinolor derivatives: Vioform (P), Sterosan (P), Dermoquinol (P) (2–4%). Tincture iodine, Whitfield's ointment, sulphur (5%) Castellani's paint, hydrag ammon. (5%), anthralin (0.5–1%), propionic and undecylenic acids (5–20%), phenylmercuric nitrate (0.5%), salicylanilide (5%), nystatine, copper sulphate (0.5%), Hamycin (P), buclosamide, natamycin, tinactin, miconazole clotrimazole, etc.
10. *Hydrolyzing agents:* Hyaluronidase (in keloids, localized scleroderma and localized myxoedema). Corticosteroids, fibrolysin.
11. Haemostatics—Gelfoam.
12. Keratolytics—acid salicylic (2–5%), formaldehyde (2–5%), anthralin (0.5–1%), tar (1–5%), vitamin A acid.
13. Lubricants—glycerinated amyli on lips, oils (olive, coconut, arachis), eucerine (Nivea cream), butter, milk cream.
14. Parasiticides—Antimony, berberine sulphate, benzyl benzoate (25%), sulphur (5–10%), DDT (2–5%), pyrethrum, crotorax (P), gamma benzene hexachloride, tetmosol, dieldrine, etc.
15. Pigment stimulants—Ammi-majus (meladinine, P), babchi (Psoralea corylifolia), oil of bergamot; croton oil, UVR, X-rays.
16. Stimulants—Tar (Pix liquida 5–10%, liq. picis carb), anthralin 0.1–1%), chlorophyll, aloe vera, oil of cade.
17. Sun-protective agents—Para-amino-benzoic acid (5–10%), silicone (barrier cream in industry).

18. Shampoos—Selenium sulphide, Savlon (P) liquid, *ritha* shampoo, *amla* and *trifala* shampoo (last three are indigenous in India).
19. Stimulants of hair—Cantharidin, tinct K 5 (P), Ammi majus, Minoxidil.

Demulcents: They form aqueous solutions which mechanically alleviate irritation of mucous membrane and abraded integument. They are also useful vehicles to provide stable emulsions or suspensions of drugs immiscible with or insoluble in aqueous solutions. Their molecular weight is high. They swell up with water and provide protection. Common examples are acacia (gum acacia), tragacanth, agar, glycerhiza, cellulose, glycerine, propylene glycol, and polyethylene glycol.

Protectives and adsorbants: They mechanically cover the mucous membrane and skin and thus prevent contact with possible irritants. They are chemically inert and insoluble. They also adsorb toxins, bacteria and gases.

Examples:

a. Dusting powder like zinc oxide, starch, zinc stearate, magnesium stearate, bismuth subgallas, magnesium silicate (talc).
b. Collodion.
c. Activated charcoal.

Powders: They should be used only on dry lesions since oozing will change the powder into a hard mass which will irritate the inflamed skin. Powders soothe the skin, and protect it from external irritation and friction and so are useful in prickly heat and intertrigo. Ordinary powder contains talcum, starch or chalk with boric acid added to it as an antiseptic. The powder should be freely and generously used on the affected area at least 2–3 times a day. Boric acid and hexachlorophene should not be used on raw surfaces, they get absorbed and cause toxicity.

Lotions: They are usually used on oozing and vesicular lesions, though lately, lactocalamine lotion has come into fashion as an astringent make-up for women. There are four important lotions:

Lotion Silver Nitrate

Lotion silver nitrate, 0.5–1% in distilled water. It is to be dispensed in a blue bottle, and is to be kept in a dark place since the sun's rays make the lotion ineffective.

Lotion Gentian Violet

Lotion gentian violet, 0.5–1% in water. Its only drawback is the violet colour which stains the clothes and bed linen.

These two lotions are astringent as well as antiseptic; so they are very effective with infective lesions. They are used as wet dressings (strips of linen dipped in the lotion) on the affected part or as paint, 3–4 times a day. Lotion aluminium acetate 1–5% (Burrow's solution) is another popular soak for wet and oozing lesions.

Calamine Lotion

Calamine preparata	10%
Zinc oxide	5%
Glycerine	5%
Aquacalcis.	Add to 100%

Lead and Zinc Lotion

Liq. plumbi subacetate fortis	5%
Zinc oxide	10%
Glycerine	10%
Aqua	Add to 100%

These are powder suspensions which are shaken before use and dabbed on the inflamed skin with cotton wool three to four times a day. When the lotion dries up, it forms a thin scale or crust. Lotions should not be used alone for more than 2–3 days at a time. At the end of this period, crusts are removed with warm olive oil and then Condy's fluid, before the lotion is repeated. In case the scales formed are thin and dry, and the use of lotion is considered unnecessary, a paste or cream is applied over the area. These help to soothe the inflamed skin.

Pastes: They are useful in sub-acute inflammations, being soothing astringents. One effective paste is:

Bismuth subgallas	20%
Amylum	20%
Soft paraffin	to 100%

This is spread on a piece of linen or calico with a knife to form a thin layer according to the shape and size of the affected area; the linen piece is then applied to the skin and lightly bandaged. It must be strongly emphasized that no cotton wool is to be used in the dressing. The paste dressing is changed twice a day. In cases with mild infection or oozing, aqueous gentian violet is painted first, and when it has dried up completely, a paste dressing is applied. Next morning, the affected part is cleaned with warm olive oil and Condy's fluid, and the process repeated till the infection has cleared up. At this stage the gentian violet paint is stopped, and the dressing carried on with the paste only. Pastes should not be applied on hairy parts of the body unless those parts have been closely shaved.

Creams: They are cleaner, easier to apply and are aesthetically more acceptable, soothing to integument when it is affected with sub-acute and chronic inflammation. They are lightly rubbed on the skin two to three times a day. The following are examples of some useful creams:

Zinc cream	
Zinc oxide	15%
Wool fat	25%
Arachis oil	20%
Paraffin molle	20%
Aqua calcis	20%

Antiseptic creams like Vioform (P), Sterosan (P), Cetavlon (P), Dequadin (P), Nebacortril (P), Bacitracin, Soframycin (P), Tyrothricin (P) are patent creams containing quinolor derivatives, cetavlon, dequadin and the topical antibiotics, etc. Penicillin and sulphonamide creams are more harmful than useful and should be strictly avoided. Brilliant green 1% or sterosan 1 % may be added to calamine cream to make it antiseptic.

Ointments: They are used on chronic, scaly lesions, when there is absence of exudation.

Anhydrous

a. Water repellent—Paraffins. They are inert, cheap and non-sensitizing. But they are greasy, messy and non-absorbing.
b. Water absorbing—Hydrophilic paraffin.
c. Washable—Carbowax, polyethylene glycol.

Hydrous:

a. Water in oil emulsion: Eucerine
b. Oil in water emulsion: Hydrophilic ointment.

Cetomacrogols are the emulsifying agents. They are non-ionic (hence compatible) and also help to preserve by reducing microbial growth. Most commonly used agent is Lanette wax SX. Glycols are poor emulsifiers, Mono-sterin is self-emulsifying. There are others like polyoxryl stearate, cetomacrogal 4000, and derivatives.

Varnishes: They are employed in chronically thickened and pustular lesions. They are liquid preparations which are painted on the skin. On drying, a thin adherent layer is left behind. The common varnishes in use are:

a. *Gentian violet varnish:* Gentian violet 1% in 75% spirit. It is useful for chronic folliculitis.
b. Crude coal tar varnish for chronic eczema, lichenification and chronic folliculitis. It is used with tar paste as follows: The tar should be painted thinly with a firm brush. After ten minutes the area should be dusted with talcum powder and protected with cotton or linen cloth. This is left in position for 24 hours, after which, a dressing of paste on linen is applied and left for 24 hours. At the end of this period, affected part is cleaned with olive oil and then washed gently with soap and water. The process is repeated for about 15 days.

   Liq. picis carb paint is used in psoriasis-modified Goekerman's regimen and psoriasis day care centres.
c. Unna's paste

Zinc oxide	25%
Gelatin	35%
Glycerine	20%
Aqua	20%

The above formula is useful for tropical conditions. It is available in jars. When needed for use, the jar is placed in a pan of boiling water for ten minutes. This turns the paste into liquid, and when it has cooled down reasonably, it is painted on the affected parts with a firm brush or pledge of cotton wool. Within a few minutes, it dries up to form a bandageless supportive dressing. It is very useful in neurodermatitis since it is soothing and also keeps the finger nails away from the thickened skin giving it time to heal. It can be repeated as often as necessary, till the part heals completely.

Bandaging

In the olden days, dressings were unpopular, and lately, there has been a trend amongst authorities towards the same point of view, the reasons being: bandages are costly; dried-up bandages cause irritation and are difficult to remove; poorly applied bandages are troublesome to patients; open air dressing promotes healing. Only in certain cases is bandaging necessary.

1. Protective bandages to protect the affected part from the trauma of scratching and exposure to contacts, e.g. a mask in acute dermatitis of the face where the cause is not established; white cotton gloves and stockings for hands and feet. A bandage is also recommended where greasy or staining ointments have been prescribed. A mask is prepared by taking a piece of white cotton cloth or lint which has been washed clean without soap or detergents. It should be big enough to extend from one shoulder to the other, from the front of the neck to the back. Holes are cut in the mask for the eyes, nostrils and mouth to allow for seeing, breathing and eating.

   In widespread lesions, it is better to apply the medicament and keep the patient in a cotton garment at home rather than to let him go about with multiple bandages. No cotton wool should be used in the dressing, particularly in those used for eczematous patients, for the simple reason that cotton wool retains heat and will make the affected part unduly warm, and thus, aggravate the condition.
2. Occlusive bandages like elastoplast, for instance, are used to prevent trauma to diseased parts in conditions like neurodermatitis and dermatitis artefacta. They are left on for about 7 days at a time. They should not be employed in eczema. In cases of varicose ulcers, however, crepe or elastoplast bandages are supportive as well as protective. Occlusive bandages with Saran wrap or polythene paper and corticosteroid ointments are very useful in localized psoriasis and lichen simplex chronicus.
3. Restraining bandages and splints are used to prevent scratching by tying hands and feet to the sides of the bed, as for instance in conditions like infantile eczema.

SPECIAL POINTS TO REMEMBER

1. Avoid abuse and indiscriminate use of medication, both systemic and topical. As Professor Dunlop has said, a good doctor thinks and advises while a bad one rushes for the pad or the syringe. Before prescribing it is essential to ask oneself, "Is this prescription essential?" It will help to reduce the cost of scientific medicine for which the patient ultimately foots the bill.
2. Medicaments are useful, but their side-effects should never be forgotten. The untoward effects of medication are:
   a. *Systemic:* Drug eruptions; toxic reactions like fever, arthralgia, hypertension, melanosis, diabetes, metabolic changes, dyspepsia, etc.; anaphylaxis.
   b. *Local:* Irritation; sensitization and auto-sensitization; discoloration (anthralin, iodine, chrysorabin, potassium permanganate); scarring (caustics); Pigmentation (UVL, X-ray, iodine); malignant stimulation (tar, X-ray).
3. Remedies should be inexpensive, easily available and not cumbersome or tedious to use. They should not spoil or stain clothes.
4. Detailed instructions must be given regarding the use of medicine. If possible, a demonstration should be given regarding the use of topical applications by a trained nurse or dermatological assistant.
5. In allergic cases, sensitivity tests should be done- intradermal for injectants, particularly penicillin, and a patch test for local application.

6. Patients should be instructed to notify immediately any untoward effects—both local or systemic.
7. Palliatlve treatment must be preceded by the establishment of diagnosis, cause specific treatment and reassurance in every case.
8. Whenever in doubt, use a bland treatment like calamine lotion till the doubt is removed. Active medication can produce disastrous results.
9. Hospitalize all extensive, severely affected and resistant cases.
10. It is criminal to play with new drugs or formulae in general practice till the value, indications, contra-indications and untoward effects are properly established.
11. Avoid 'therapeutic panic'—changing medications every 2 or 3 days in panic.

Chapter

6

Physical Treatment and Skin Surgery

To enable the practitioner to do the maximum good to the skin patient, physical treatment and skin surgery have become an important division of modem therapeutics. They are mostly office procedures, and are done by a dermatologist to save the patient ping-ponging from doctor to doctor and also to enable the patient to receive the selected care (Sulzburger). The student of medicine should be well acquainted with the fundamentals; undoubtedly the fine essentials will be acquired with practical training and experience **(Figs 6.1 to 6.3 and Table 6.1)**.

CARBON DIOXIDE SNOW

Indications: Warts, cavernous haemangiomas, chronic lupus erythematosus, seborrhoeic warts, keratoses.

It is a convenient method of superficial destruction. CO_2 snow is prepared by letting out CO_2 liquid gas from cylinders, through a small jet, into a chamois leather bag. As the liquid gas comes out, snow forms. The snow is put into metal moulds to give it a special shape which is ordinarily like a pencil. This pencil is held in several layers of gauze and applied to the selected lesion. Firm pressure is maintained; the period of application varies from 30 seconds to 2 minutes (usually 1 minute in most cases) depending upon the amount of destruction desired. The healthy skin surrounding the lesion should be well protected from the destructive effects of CO_2 snow. The destroyed lesion forms a crust surrounded by erythema and oedema; this takes frqm one to two weeks to subside.

Mixed with acetone and sulphur, CO_2 snow has been used in the form of slush for the treatment of acne scarring. With a brush or a wooden applicator it is painted on the affected area. With the introduction of liquid N_2, CO_2 snow has fallen into disfavour.

LIQUID NITROGEN

As necrosis produces less scarring, cryosurgery by liquid nitrogen –196°C has become a good tool in the practice of dermatology. Easily available, the technique is easy to perform and postoperative wound care is simple. Useful in patients allergic to local anesthesia and people who are afraid of surgery. Less popular is cryosurgery by nitrous oxide and CO_2 snow.

Mode of action: There is cell death following cryosurgery.

- Tissue water is changed to ice which leads to cell dehydration.
- Freezing of small blood vessel leads to ischaemic changes in the tissue which ends in cell necrosis.

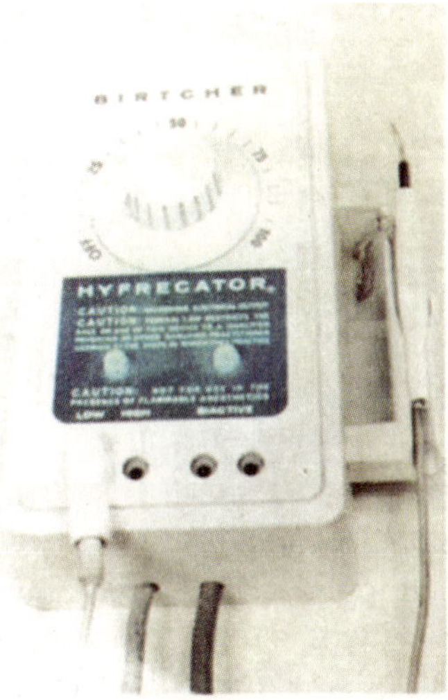

Hyfrecator

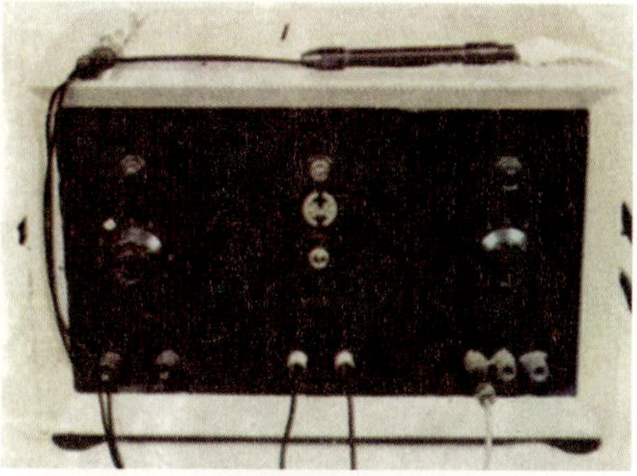

Surgical diathermy

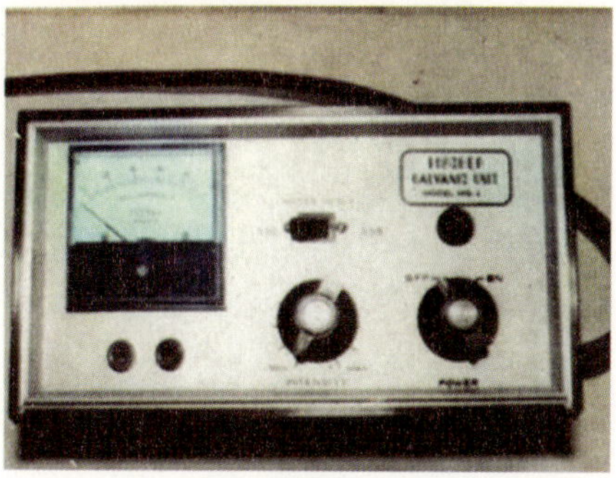

Iontophoresis unit

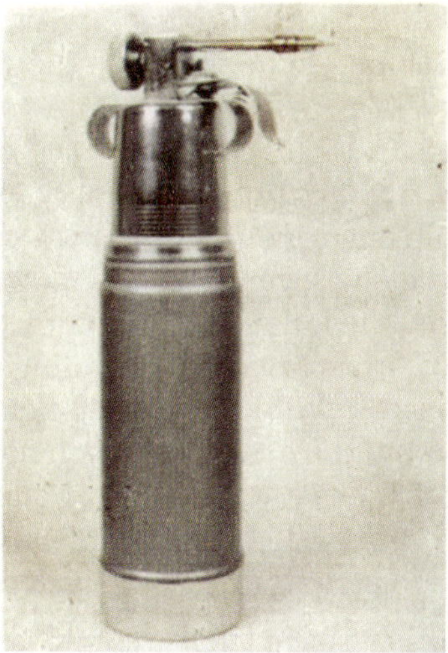

Liquid nitrogen flask

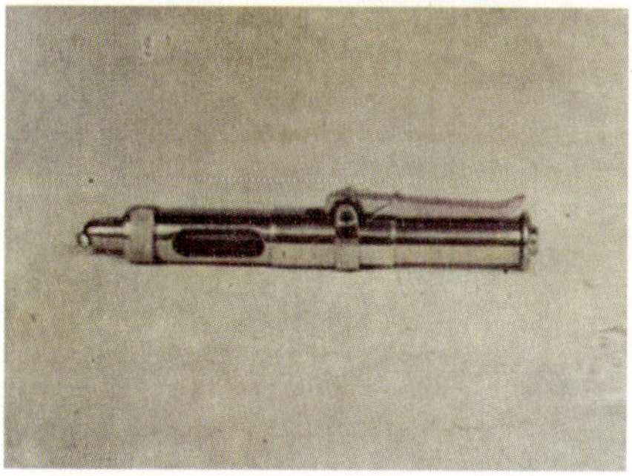

Dermajet

Fig. 6.1: Physical aids in treatment (I)

Tissue sensitivity:

More sensitive tissues	*Less sensitive tissues*
Melanocytes	Fibroblasts
Keratinocytes	Stromal structure
Hair follicle	Bone
Nerve tissue	

Depth of freeze: Controlled by rate of flow and the distance of the spray unit from the lesion and the time of contact. Development of freezing (circle) and then thawing help to decide the duration of exposure.

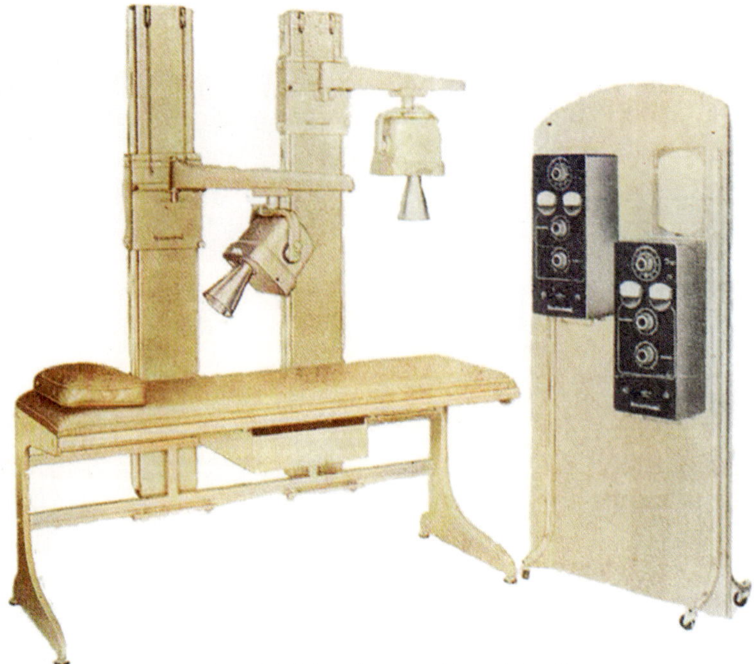

Superficial X-ray therapy with control unit

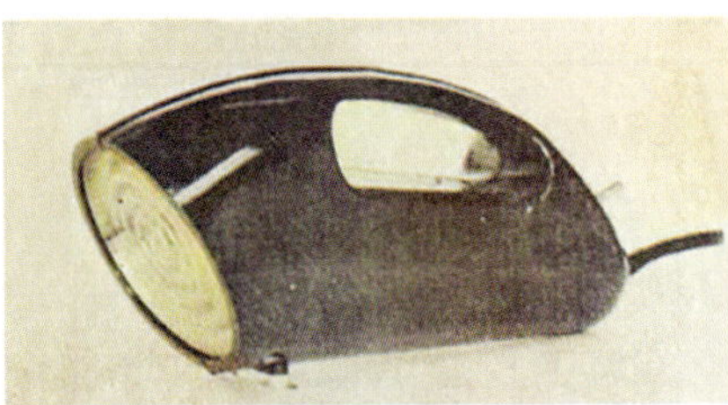

Quartz lamp

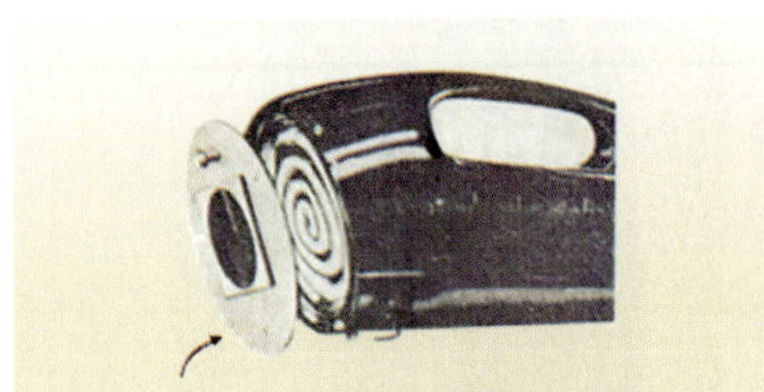

Wood's lamp

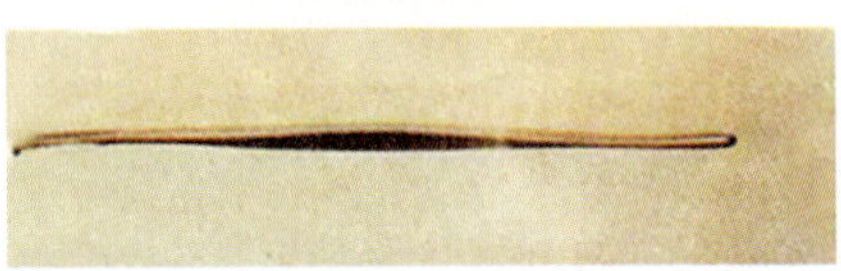

Comedone expressor

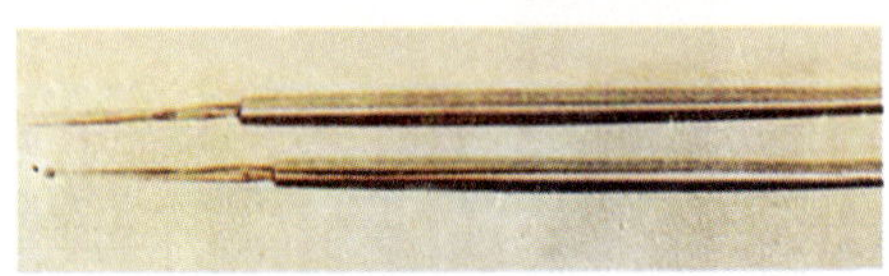

Demal curette

Fig. 6.2: Physical aids in treatment (II)

Equipments:

1. Storage tank/cylinder
2. Cotton swab
3. Cryo-probes
4. Spray unit
5. Thermocouple devices

Indication:

Actinic keratosis
Actinic cheilitis
Keloid
Keratoacanthoma
Skin tags
Syringomas

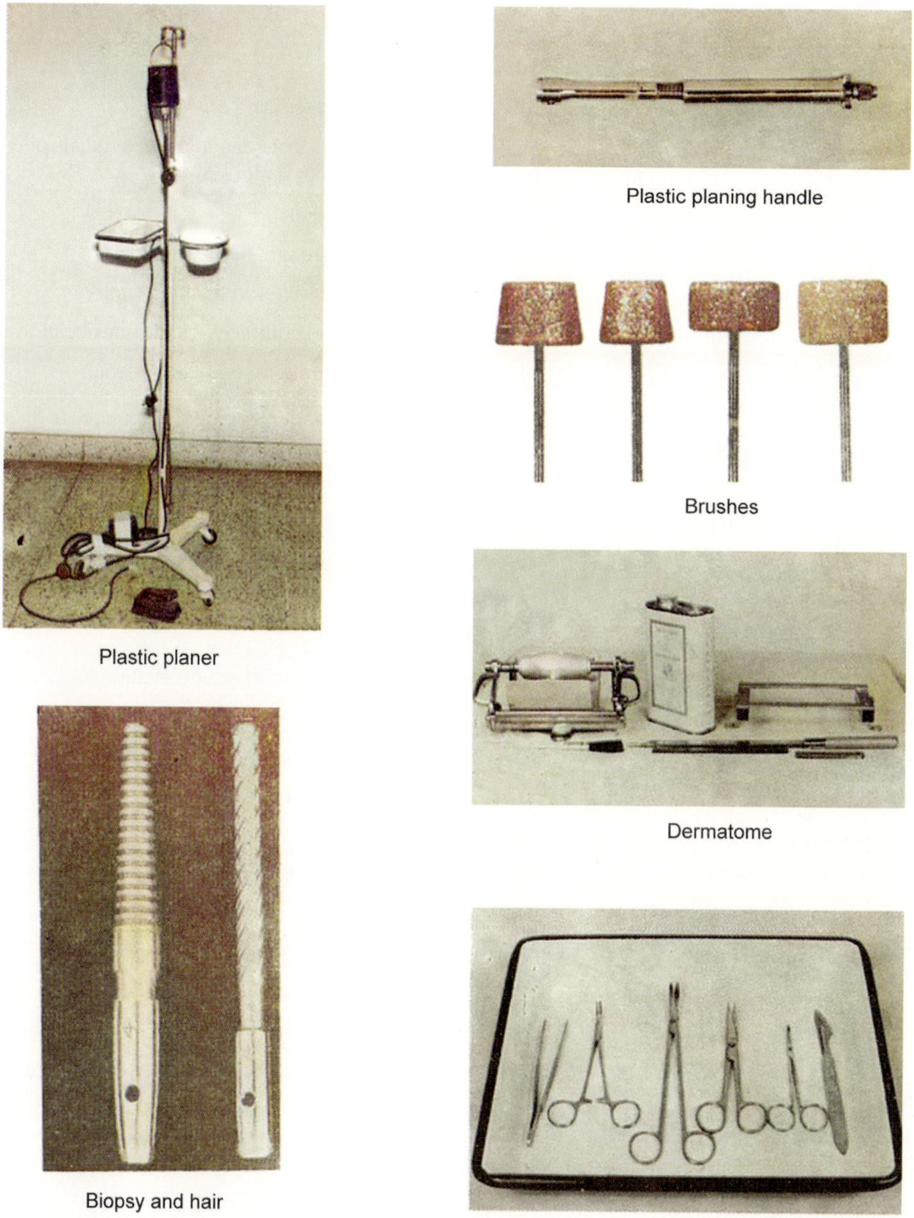

Plastic planer

Plastic planing handle

Brushes

Dermatome

Biopsy and hair transplantation punches

Surgical tray

Fig. 6.3: Cutaneous surgical instruments

Basal cell epithelioma
Condyloma accuminatum
Epidermal nevi
Leishmaniasis
Molluscum contagiosum
Trichoepithelioma
Warts

Complications: Most important is depigmentation and scar formation which is seen more frequently. Postoperative oedema, bullous formation and a throbbing sensation may be seen.

Table 6.1: Common dermatoses-needing surgery

1. Abscesses	Incision
2. Investigation and diagnosis	Biopsy (Punch, knife, excision)
3. Warts	Liq. N_2; CO_2 snow; electrocoagulation, chemicals phenol, trichloracetic acid; never scalpel surgery
4. Milia	Puncturing and expression
5. Moles	Excision, shaving and coagulation
6. Skin tags	Papilloma, pedunculated fibroma—Snip surgery
7. Keratoses (Senile, Seborrhoeic)	Dermabrasion, shaving, curettage, electro-desiccation
8. Telangiectasia and spider nevi, de-Morgan's spots	Mild electro-coagulation with epilation needle, hypertonic saline injection
9. Cysts (Sebaceous/Mucous)	Puncturing and phenol curetting of the wall
10. Xanthelasma	Trichloroacetic acid, curetting, excision
11. Lipomas and fat bulges	Excision, liposuction
12. Keloids	Laser, radiotherapy, Inj. triamcinolone
13. Freckles	Dermabrasion (DA)
14. Chloasma	Dermabrasion (DA)
15. Scars	Infiltration, scar revision, graft, scar elevation
16. Hirsutism	Electrolysis
17. Wrinkles	Face lift, DA, Chemical peel; Infiltration, belpharoplasty
18. Vitiligo	Thin Thiersch's grafts, Minigrafts
19. Acne scars	Dermabrasion (DA)
20. Baldness	Hair transplantation and scalp reduction
21. Rhinophyma	DA, Laser, knife shaving, electrocoagulation
22. Varicose veins	Vein ligation, stripping, injection, crepe bandage, elastic stocking
23. Skin cancers	Radio-therapy, excision, Laser, Moh's chemosurgery
24. Tinea nail dystrophy, ingrowing nail	Nail abrasion, avulsion, biopsy
Hyperhidrosis of axillae, hidradenitis suppu.	Sweat gland surgery

Important tips:

- Select your patient, explain the procedure to the patient and tell him/her about transient pain and possible complications.
- Select your equipment carefully (a spray unit or a cotton tip).
- Note and control your rate of flow from the spray unit, check the time of freezing and adjust the distance from the lesion. This all helps in better controlling of the depth of freeze which is seen as lateral spread of the freeze on the surface.
- Malignant lesions should be carefully monitored and a close follow-up is done to insure complete destruction. Avoid excessive freezing. Better underdo rather than overdoing and later regretting.

DIATHERMY

Surgical diathermy is a special electric unit generating a high frequency current which produces heat when passed through tissues. Depending upon the speed of the current and the resulting heat, a diathermy unit can achieve the following results:

1. Cutting with high speed or intensity.
2. Coagulation (cooking compared to burning due to heated needle in electrocautery).
   a. If weak, epilation.
   b. If strong, coagulation producing destruction.
3. Desiccation (fulgration) ensues by passing medium current through a mono-terminal electrode at a slight distance from the surface which produces sparking heat and results in drying up the tissues.

In practice, these three processes overlap each other in the same unit, depending upon the intensity and speed of the current. Before treating patients, the practitioner must familiarise himself with the basis of its working, the different regulators controlling the resistance and amperage and the electrodes—the indifferent electrode and the active, operating electrode which varies in shape and size to suit different surgical requirements. Surgical diathermy is usually bloodless and aseptic, hence its usefulness is enhanced. Unless very weak currents are used, as in epilation or mild desiccation, preliminary local anaesthesia is essential. Hyfrecator is a compact diathermy unit.

Indications

1. *Epilating current:* Epilation of superfluous hair, spider naevi, dilated capillaries as in rosacea, verruca plana on face.
2. *Electrocoagulation:* Common warts, verruca vulgaris, seborrhoeic warts, pyogenic granuloma, senile keratoses, mucous cysts, acanthomas, basal cell epithelioma.
3. *Electrocutting:* For excision of cutaneous lesions including biopsy, keloid, malignant neoplasm and plantar wart.
4. *Electrodesiccation:* This may be combined with curettage (dermal steel curettes are employed for the purpose) which precedes or follows desiccation depending upon the individual needs of the patient: warts, both plane and filiform, xanthelasma, condyloma acuminatum, adenoma sebaceum and skin tags.

Since the ultimate completeness of the cure and the cosmetic results are the important criteria for judgement, the operator must take all the facts into consideration before selecting a particular procedure for a patient.

Superficial wounds are left open and only a mild antiseptic cream or powder applied twice a day till the wound heals. In deeper lesions, particularly in the summer, an antiseptic dressing is used. These wounds heal more slowly than surgical wounds.

EPILATION

It implies methods of removal of superfluous hair. These hair are disfiguring and cause a lot of anxiety in women when present on the face, occasionally in man, when present in between the eyebrows and forehead and sometimes on the hairy naevi. When the hair are thin and few, simple bleaching with hydrogen peroxide may satisfy the patient. Epilating waxes (Wax-away) (P), Strip-tease (P), etc. help in some cases, but electrical epilation gives the best results especially when the hair is thick and dark. There are two methods in electrical epilation:

Electrolysis: It involves the use of direct galvanic current through a platinum needle which liberates hydrogen causing chemical cauterization of the hair root. It is time consuming, and needs a special instrument; hence, it is not so popular. Thermolysis is a new innovation.

Diathermy: Weak coagulation current is popular with the dermatologists. The authors find it a quick and efficient method by which we can remove 60–100 hair in one sitting of about 20–30 minutes. Wearing a magnifying (1–2 D) binocular loupe, the needle is inserted into the hair follicle and gently slid along the hair till it reaches the bulb which causes resistance to the needle. With the foot switch current is switched on and off intermittently three times for a second or so. It causes coagulation of the hair root. The current is switched off, and the needle is pulled out. If the procedure has been successful, the hair either comes out with the needle or can easily be pulled out with the epilating forceps. The hair should never be pulled out forcibly since it implies that electro-coagulation has been unsuccessful and only mechanical plucking has been performed. No bleeding or blistering should be produced; only very slight blanching may be seen around the hair follicle. After one hair has been epilated, the same procedure is repeated with another; one must make sure that at least 5 mm distance is left in between two epilated hair follicles. The least possible current that will produce epilation is employed. At the end of the sitting, the epilated area is sponged with spirit. A little inflammation or pustulation may be produced; it will subside within 4 or 5 days.

The procedure causes a little pain and discomfort. Most patients tolerate it well, except on the upper lip and neck. Very slight scarring may be evident even with expert care. Usually patients do not mind this; even so, they must be warned in advance.

Furthermore, they must be told that it is the only safe and permanent method of removing superfluous hair; but there is always a 25% chance of the hair growing back even in expert hands. Hence the procedure will have to be repeated from time to time on a maintenance basis to keep the disfiguring by hypertrichosis under control. This procedure deals only with hair which is already present and does nothing to prevent the growth of new hair or downy hair from becoming dark and thick . In every case, these facts must be explained to the patient before treatment is undertaken, and also an honest attempt must be made to correct the basic disorder responsible for the hypertrichosis.

ULTRAVIOLET RAY THERAPY

Ultraviolet lamps are useful in dermatological practice. These lamps are composed of quartz glass envelope filled up with mercury vapour and 2 electrodes. When in use electric current passes in-between these two electrodes in the form of an arc between the intervening gaseous media and UV rays are generated. Mercury atoms have the property of emitting a spectrum of 185–400 nm in the ultraviolet range.

According to the radiation energy emitted, UV rays (UVR) have been classified:

1. UVA 315–400 nm
2. UVB 280–315 nm
3. UVC 10–280 nm

UV rays have both surface and systemic actions. The former is confined to the area irradiated and consists of stimulation, killing of bacteria, peeling of the horny layer of the skin and pigmentation. Reaction to UVR appears 2–12 hours after exposure. If a strong exposure is given, the skin may be irritated or a local bum may be produced.

The systemic effect of UVR consists of stimulation of the metabolism, increasing the body's resistance and increasing also the production of vitamin D. In sunny tropical countries the cool morning sun does as much good as UVR. Photochemotherapy: UVA 315–400 nm (fluorescent black light lamp) has been employed in the treatment of vitiligo and psoriasis along with oral 8-methoxy psoralen **(Fig. 6.4)**.

Often the beneficial effects of UVR have been grossly exaggerated to the extent that it is considered a panacea by certain enthusiasts.

The contraindications to the use of UVR are: Acute eczema, acute vitiligo, spreading psoriasis; progressive alopecia, active pulmonary tubercu losis, lupus erythematosus and all light-sensitive dermatoses.

Dose schedule: After determining the minimal erythema dose (MED), exposure can be given daily or alternate days depending on the discretion of physician and convenience of the patient. Once there is improvement in the disease process, the interval time can be lengthened.

The distance of the lamp from the patient, and the time of exposure, vary with each lamp. The manufacturers' instructions must be strictly adhered to, and a log book maintained every time the lamp is used. Proper records should be maintained of the doses administered to the patient. UVR has a deleterious effect on the eyes; the patient, doctor and nurse should always wear well-fitting, coloured glasses especially meant for the purpose every time they expose themselves to the lighted lamp. When giving UVR

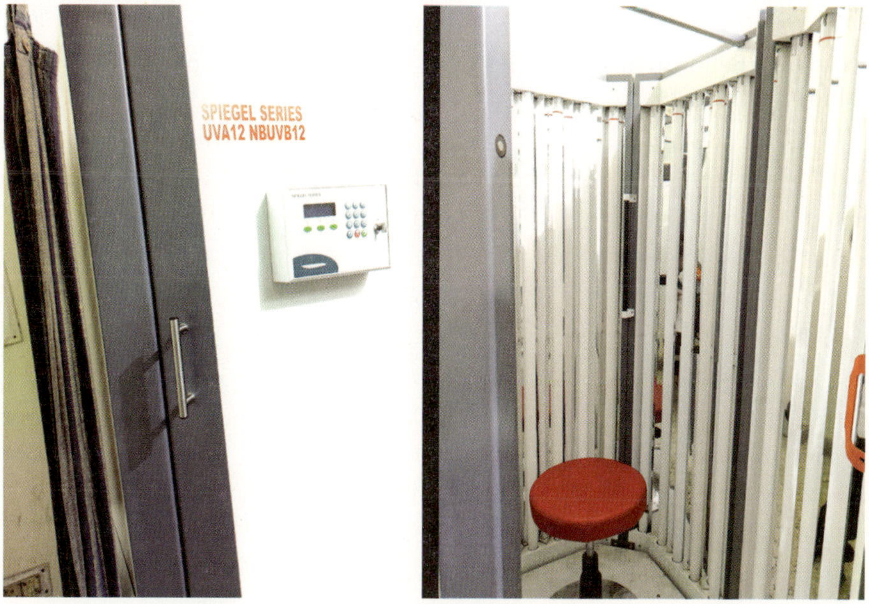

Fig. 6.4: PUVA therapy unit

to the eyelids, be sure that the patient's eyes are kept closed all the time. The lamp must be kept clean with methylated spirit. The practitioner should not carelessly expose his uncovered skin to UVR.

X-RAY THERAPY

In recent years, the use of ionisation radiation therapy has been vastly reduced due to number of factors iike easy availability of antimetabolites, cytotoxic agents and steroids, improvement in cutaneous surgical procedures, resistance of patients because of publicity in lay press, and poor training in radiotherapy to both under- and post-graduates.

Despite these developments, there is no doubt of the usefulness of radiation therapy in selected dermatoses.

X-rays or Roentgen rays are rays of very short wave-length (shorter than 100Å units). They are produced by bombardment of electrodes from a cathode filament to an anode tungsten plate at a high voltage and the resultant X-rays are emitted through a window. The present machines are shock-proof, and ensure a great deal of protection from scattered X-rays. The quantity and quality of X-rays reaching the site at different voltage (kV), milliamperes (mA) and distances are measured and charted for each machine. The unit of Roentgen ray quantity measure is called a Roentgen (r). The epilation or erythema dose is the skin toleration dose (400 r for unfiltered radiation at 90 kV). To determine the quality of radiation, we take two major factors into consideration:

1. Half value layer (HVL). This is defined as that thickness of aluminium which reduces the intensity of radiation to 50%.
2. Half value tissue depth (D½ HVD). This refers to depth of the tissue at which the absorbed dose is 50% of that at the surface. This phenomenon of penetration of X-rays should always be correlated with the depth of the pathological process **(Tables 6.2 and 6.3)**.

High voltage Betatron has been employed with success in exfoliative dermatitis and intractable erythroderma.

Table 6.2: Depth, dose data (in mm) (after Zoon and Zerry modified)

Epidermis	0.03–0.25
Hair papilla	2.5–3.5
Corium	3.0–4.0
Sweat glands (Eccrine)	2.0–4.0
Dermatitis and eczema	0.8–2.0
Psoriasis	0.7–3.0
Lichen simplex chronicus	1.0–4.0
Lichen planus	0.4–2.0
Folliculitis and acne	3.0–6.0
Basal cell epithelioma	2.0–5.0
Squamous cell epithelioma	3.0–10.0

Table 6.3: Important radiation methods

Type	*Sources*	*kV*	*TSO (cm)*	*Wavelengths*	*HVL*	*D½*
Superficial X-ray	Low voltage standard X-ray	60–100	15–30	0.5	0.7–2 mm Al	7–10 mm
Grenz ray	Ultrasoft therapy	5–20	10–15	2.0	0.03 mm Al	0.2–0.8 mm

The physio-biological effects of radiotherapy are:

1. Reduction of rate of cell division or even temporary cessation
2. Reduction of secretion.
3. Reduction of sensitivity in nerve endings.
4. Reduction of bacterial and fungal growth.
5. Permanent killing of cells.

Clinically, these physio-biological effects help to control pruritus, reduce inflammation, cure or control infections, reduce sebaceous and sweat secretion, cause falling of hair, and last of all, kill pathological tissues, as in warts and malignant radio-sensitive tumours.

Grenz rays are useful in resistant cases of pruritus ani and vulvae, dyshidrosis, psoriasis and balanoposthitis.

Definite contraindications are:

1. Light-sensitive dermatoses, lupus erythematosus, etc.
2. Acute eczema.
3. Radio-dermatitis, ulcer, atrophy and epithelioma.

Untoward effects of over-radiation. Over-radiation is the greatest danger of X-ray therapy; a better understanding of dosage will minimize this hazard. The effects of over radiation are:

1. *Acute:* Erythema, vesicles, swelling and even eczema going on to necrosis and ulceration.
2. *Chronic:* Redness, atrophy, keratoses, telangiectasia, and pigmentation; later reactions like ulcer and even epitheliomata may occur.

Chronic effects usually come up years after the X-ray treatment. In dark skinned patients, hyperpigmentation, though transient, is a great drawback when treating exposed areas. There is also risk of causing epilation in employing X-ray therapy on hairy regions and sterility when X-ray therapy is employed over the gonads.

X-ray is an invisible energy and one must always respect its destructive powers when making use of its beneficial effects. Since X-rays are cumulative in effect, erythema doses should never be repeated within 12 months. Large areas of the body should never be exposed to X-ray therapy for fear of causing depression of bone marrow and other serious systemic reactions.

The testes, uterus, ovaries and eyes must always be protected and never exposed to X-ray therapy.

Strict accuracy must be maintained regarding line voltage, kV, mA, filter, distance and there should be screening of the sensitive surrounding areas with lead rubber. Proper records must be maintained.

Last of all, the authors emphatically add, that X-ray therapy must be prescribed in properly selected cases as a last resort **(Table 6.4)**.

Table 6.4: Indications for radiotherapy

Disease	*Indications*	*Dosage*	*Total radiation*
A. Benign			
1. Acne vulgaris	Chronic pustular or keloid/cystic acne	75 r weekly	1000 r in 6 months
2. Keloid	Not hard, more vascular rather less fibrotic; less than 9–12 months duration	300 r alternate days or weekly	1500 r
3. Ch. eczema	Chronic, resistant	75 r weekly	800 r
4. Paronychia	Chronic, persistent	75 r weekly	400 r
5. Haemangioma	Strawberry/cavernous	250 r fortnightly or monthly	500–750 r
6. Warts	Periungual, subungual, plantar	750 r monthly	1500 r
7. Lichen simplex chronicus	Marked lichenification long standing, resistant to topical steroids	100 r weekly	800 r
8. Dermal leishmaniasis	One or two areas, resistant to routine therapy	600 r one dose	600 r
9. Pustular psoriasis, dyshidrosis	Resistant, recalcitrant	50-75 r weekly	500 r
10. Hypertrophic lichen planus	Recalcitrant cases	100 r weekly	800 r
11. Lymphocytoma cutis		100 r weekly	1000 r
B. Malignant			
12. Basal cell epithelioma	Avoid cartilaginous areas, scrotum and eyes	400 r alt. day	3000 r
13. Squamous cell epithelioma		500 r alt. day	4000 r
14. Kaposi's haemorrhagic sarcoma	Skin lesions	100 r weekly	800–1000 r
15. Lymphomas (esp. mycosis fungoides)		300 r alt. day	3000 r

RADIUM PLATES

Beta and gainma rays of radium are used as surface applicators in selected cases of cavernous haemangioma and epithelioma. Being a highly specialized field, a discussion of these rays is not included in this book.

THORIUM-X

The main indication is superficial capillary naevus. It emits alpha rays which hardly penetrate 1 mm depth of tissues. It has a short half-life of about 3 or 4 days. Hence it is difficult to use in practice unless employed near the source of manufacture.

IONTOPHORESIS

The term implies induction or introduction of charged medicinal ions into the tissues by electric current having like charges. To produce this ion transference effect, direct (Galvanic) current generators are used having positive and negative poles. Depending upon the different medicaments used, iontophoresis can be helpful in a number of dermatological conditions as shown in **Table 6.5**.

Table 6.5: Indications of iontophoresis

Indication	*Media*	*Electrode*	*Time (min.)*	*Current (mA)*
Hyperhidrosis	Tap water	Anode (+)	15	15–20
Oedema	Hyaluronidase	Anode (+)	20	20
Vasodilatation	Histamine	Anode (+)	3–5	2–10
Varicose ulcer	Methacholine	Anode (+)	20	5–30

LIPOSUCTION SURGERY

It is a technique for dissection and suction of body fat, without cold knife surgery, but employing a high pressure suction apparatus and long cannulas. There is no scarring. The body is contoured and sculptured to shape and mould offending bulges according to the needs of the individual patients. Hips, buttocks, abdomen, cheeks, jaws and neck are the areas normally worked on.

Equipment required are high suction vacuum apparatus, long cannulas and local/ general anaesthesia. Special bandages are worn afterwards. Body execise and massage help in preventing adhesions and dimpling of the skin. There are no long-term adverse effects . There may be temporary fluid or blood accumulation under the skin and also temporary anaesthesia.

This is no substitute for dieting and exercises in general obesity. It is recommended only in getting rid of localised bulges of fat.

DERMABRASIVE SURGERY (PLASTIC PLANING)

The following cosmetic defects may be amenable to this method:

1. Pitted scars—smallpox, acne vulgaris.
2. Pigmentation—chloasma and freckles.
3. Tattoo
4. Miscellaneous—post-traumatic scars, portwine naevus, epidermal naevus, keratoses, verrucae, enlarged pores, rhinophyma, milia, wrinkled skin due to old age, hypertrophic lichen simplex.

Procedure: The affected part is washed with soap and water and then cleansed with alcohol. Under anaesthesia, general or local, the part is peeled with a special steel or diamond brush revolving at the rate of about 12,000 revolutions per minute. This procedure requires dexterity and experience for best results. At one sitting the whole face or the affected area should be completed. Capillary bleeding is controlled with pressure gauze. It takes about 20–30 minutes to control bleeding. The affected part is dressed with a mild antiseptic cream, and a bandage is applied only for the first day and then discarded. Patients can use soap and water between the fifth and seventh day. Erythema takes about 3 or 4 weeks to disappear completely. Most patients can attend to their normal duties after 7 days or so; no hospitalization is ever necessary. A second planing is usually required; third and a fourth, only in cases with deep scars.

Sequelae are minor; only rarely are they serious. Erythema is seldom normal type, it usually disappears within 3 or 4 weeks. Bleeding can be a problem in patients with haemorrhagic disease; so when this history is available, due precautions should be taken. In susceptible individuals, hyper- or hypopigmentation may be produced, which is a great disadvantage in Indian patients; they must be warned about it. Complete healing of the operation area usually takes a short time.

No new scarring is produced in properly done cases. It does not cause loss of facial hair, an important consideration in male patients. Friction and infection are to be strictly avoided during healing of the planed area. There is an important side-consideration in acne patients; since planing tends to remove the pilo-sebaceous apparatus to a considerable extent, acne lesions usually do not develop on the planed areas. So it is a useful procedure in acne patients for therapeutic reasons.

THERAPEUTIC TATTOOING

Therapeutic tattooing with insoluble pigments and medicaments is claimed to be useful in the amelioration of certain intractable conditions. Conway has employed it to eradicate portwine marks (naevus flammeus), vitiligo and ugly tattoos. However, cosmetic results are not satisfactory. Tattooing and vibra puncture with gold and herbs has been used in vitiligo with controversial results. Newer machines (Micropigmentation) with better sterilized colours and needles are useful in vitiligo of hands, feet and lips.

SKIN GRAFTING

Homologous

Thin Thiersch grafts in vitiligo. This procedure is recommended to give normal pigmentary effect to resistant patches in properly screened quiescent cases of vitiligo. Surgery is done under local/general anaesthesia. The recipient site is abraded with a diamond brush to produce uniformly abraded area. After the bleeding has been controlled, Thiersch's graft from the matched donor site is removed with a dermatome or a blade and applied to the recipient area. Part is sealed with collodion. Pressure bandage is given. Windows are made in the collodion seal after 48 hours. Bandage is removed after 2–3 days and collodion is removed with acetone after 7–12 days. By this time, graft has taken in nicely. The margins take a couple of weeks to smoothen out. The colour takes 4–8 weeks to match. The donor site is normal or slightly discoloured on healing; occasionally there is hypertrophic scarring particularly when the graft has been deeper **(Tables 6.6 and 6.7)**. Recipient sites may have a peripheral depigmented fringe if the graft has been smaller than the recipient site. At one sitting, up to 40–50 square inches can be grafted. A slightly modified technique has also been successfully tried on the lips.

Pinch Grafts

Pinch graft is very easy to take but its use is limited. They are generally used in the treatment of chronic leg ulcers. A pinch graft is a free full thickness graft in the centre while at the periphery, it is a partial thickness graft.

Table 6.6: Split thickness grafts	
Advantages	*Disadvantages*
1. Chances of survival great	1. Vulnerable to trauma, break easily
2. Utilised to cover large areas, e.g. burns	2. Colour may not match
3. Easy to perform	3. Cosmetic look is poor
4. Thin Thiersch's grafts are useful in vitiligo	4. Cannot be applied on bare areas, e.g. bones and cartilages and tendons.

Table 6.7: Full thickness grafts	
Advantages	*Disadvantages*
1. Considerable strength; do not break easily	1. Chances of survival are less.
2. Can be used in weight bearing areas, e.g. soles of foot.	2. Large areas cannot be grafted.
3. Cosmetically more acceptable	3. Procedure is difficult
4. Functionally superior	4. Donor areas have bad residual scars.
5. Can be grafted on bare areas like tendons, cartilages, bone, etc.	

The donor site is chosen from a place where there is loose skin and the resultant scar would not show, i.e. usually from a hidden portion of the body. Pinch graft is sometimes taken from the upper eyelid to do correction on the other eyelid.

Mini Grafts

Falabella has successfully tried these grafts on post-burn leucoderma cases. A powerful suction machine is used to produce blisters on the donor area. The nozzle of the suction machine is applied on the donor skin. The vacuum created by machine produces blister on the skin. Multiple blisters are thus made according to the requirement. The blisters are then stripped off from the edges and the skin obtained from the blisters is applied on the donor area prepared by cryosurgical Liq. Nitrogen.

The grafts grow and according to Falabella, it may cover big areas or more grafts are applied at frequent intervals. The technique is slow and time-consuming. Thiersch's grafts, on the other hand, can be obtained much faster, and can cover big areas in a short time.

Vitiligo Surgery

Vitiligo is a major cosmetic disability in dark skinned patients. The introduction of autologous thin. Thiersch's grafts for the management of vitiligo has been a God-send for many of these hapless people.

Thin Thiersch's grafts in the management of resistant vitiligo patches was introduced in 1957 by Behl after experimental work in animals and human beings. By 1959, the technique was standardised. In 1964, results of this initial study were reported **(Figs 6.5 to 6.8)**.

From the clinical and treatment point of view, vitiligo has been divided into three types: V1, V2, V3 **(Table 6.8)**.

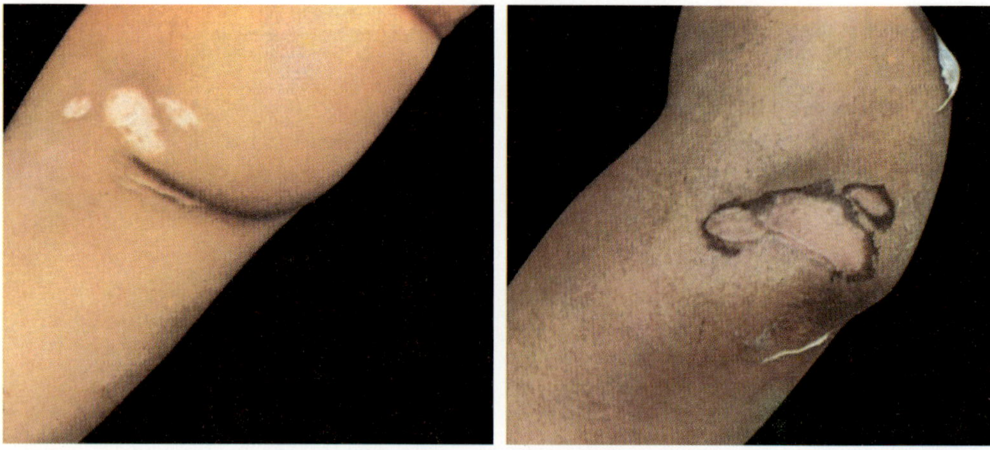

Fig. 6.5: Vitiligo surgery (pre- and postoperative)

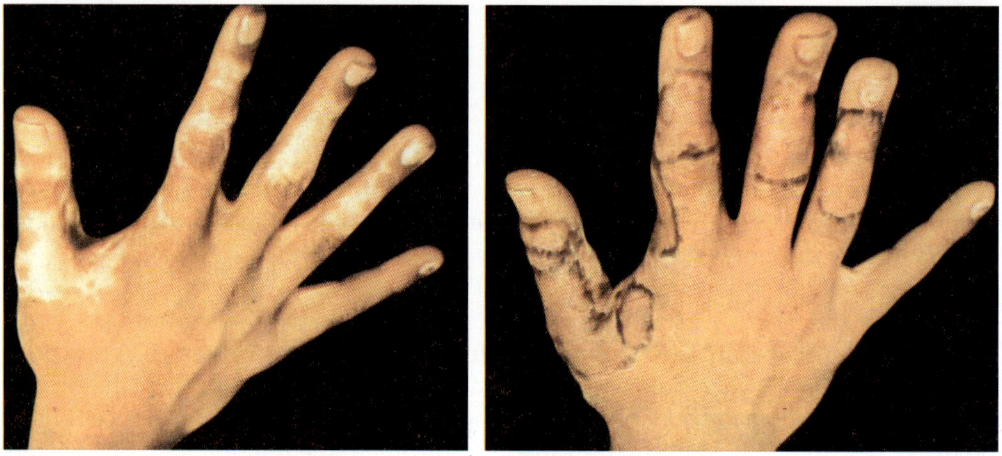

Fig. 6.6: Vitiligo surgery (pre- and postoperative)

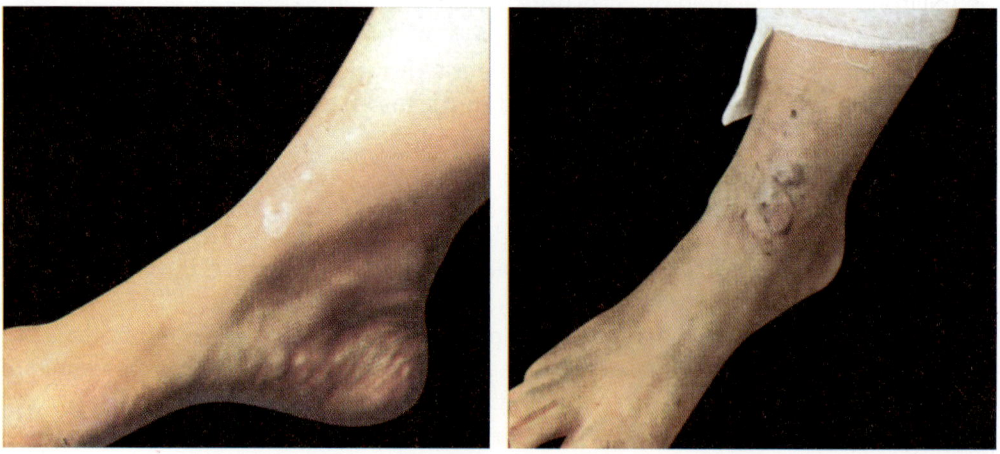

Fig. 6.7: Vitiligo surgery (pre- and postoperative)

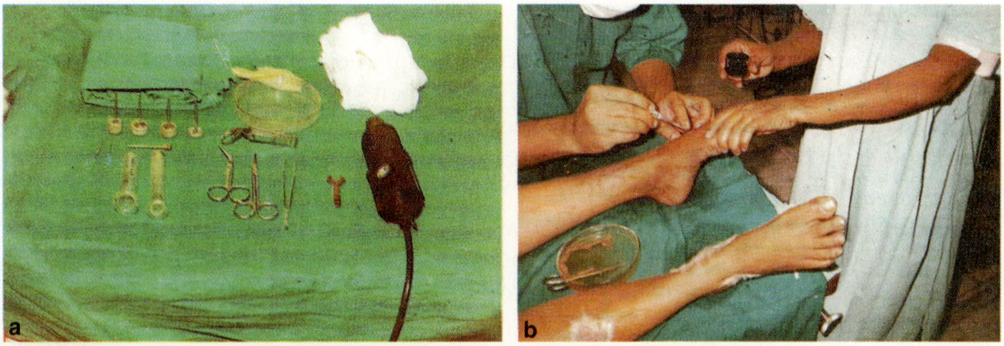

Fig. 6.8: (a) Vitiligo grafting equipment tray and hand engine; (b) The process of applying, sealing and cutting a window in vitiligo grafting. [*Courtesy:* Practice of Skin Surgery (1990). Behl PN, SISD publication]

Table 6.8: Stages of vitiligo	
Active (V1)	a. New lesions developing
	b. Lesions increasing in size
	c. Borders ill-defined
Quiescent (V2)	a. No new lesions
	b. Lesions stationary in size
	c. Borders hyperpigmenced and well-defined
Improving (V3)	a. Lesions decreasing in size
	b. No new lesions developing
	c. Presence of follicular and peripheral repigmentation.

Table 6.9: Prerequisites for doing thin Thiersch's graft	
1.	New lesions should have developed in the previous 2 years.
2.	Recipient sites should be well-defined and have hyperpigmented borders.
3.	Nutrition of the skin—both donor and recipient areas—should be good. There should be no evidence of atrophy or scarring.
4.	There should be no bleeding diathesis; general health should be good.
5.	There should be no evidence of cutaneous infection.
6.	There should be no keloidal tendency.

Normally grafting is undertaken, when the disease has progressed to the V3 stage and is not repigmenting any further with medical treatment. In other words, patients with quiescent, non-progressive, resistant, recalcitrant patches of depigmentation are recommended for grafting. This includes cases of vitiligo, leucoderma following burns, trauma, DLE, etc. Vitiligo includes both common-vulgaris and segmental varieties. In case of halo nevus, we prefer excision of the whole lesion or cauterisation of mole and later grafting when the halo nevus covers a big patch (Table 6.9). Before doing the grafting, a detailed history and thorough clinical examination are important for selection of cases.

Keloid Surgery

Keloids are a common problem in practice in Asian and African countries (Fig. 6.9). Black/brown and white ratio of incidence is 5:1. Then, there is genetic predisposition-autosomal dominant gene with variable expressibility. It is a dread of surgeons and dermatologists. Before management is discussed, it is important to understand its basic features.

Keloid means uncontrolled painful growth of scar tissue. Clinically, it is seen as a scar which has grown beyond the original dimensions, and has crab's claw appearance. Its persistence and growth are specific features.

Compared to a hypertrophic scar, it is symptomatic. Common complaints are itching, tenderness and pain. The latter can be excruciating, to the extent that it can interfere with normal activities and sleep. Common sites arc sternal and deltoid region. It is seen all over the body especially in cases of post-burn and post-traumatic scars.

Histology shows nodular collagen, broadly eosinophilic with refractile hyaline like collagen fibres. Biochemical studies reveal markedly increased collagen synthesis activity and increase in collagenase inhibitor.

Keloids increase in pregnancy and decrease during menopause. Main goal in the management of keloids should be

1. Control of symptoms—itching, pain and tenderness
2. Functional restoration
3. Aesthetic improvement
4. Prevention of recurrence, and newer lesions as produced in grafting techniques.

Surgical excision is avoided for fear of recurrence and increase in size. It occurs in over 50% of the cases. For the same reason, skin grafting is avoided in patients with keloids or keloid-prone people. Commonly used therapy include:

1. Steroid infiltration with dental syringe to provide pressure. It very useful in early scars for preventing keloid formation, and in early, soft keloids for aborting them.

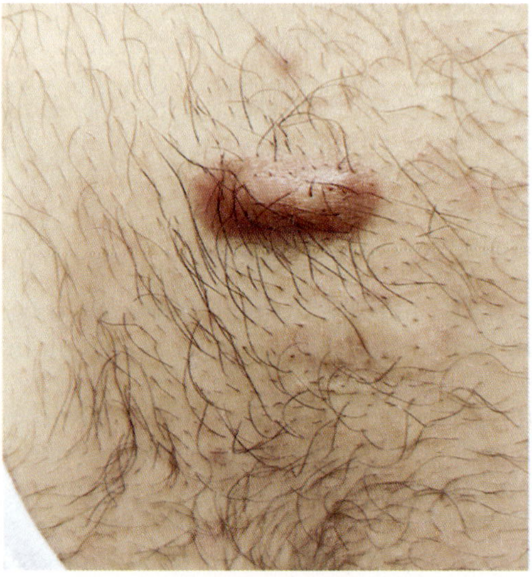

Fig. 6.9: Keloid

Properly diluted triamcinolone 10–40 mg is infiltrated at monthly intervals, all over the keloid. Long dental needles and cartridges with dental syringe are used. Proper precautions are taken to avoid its spilling in surrounding normal skin, so as not to cause epidermal atrophy and telangiectasia.

2. Radiotherapy is a useful tool in causing regression of early keloids in the first 6–24 months or so. One thousand r to 1500 r is given in 4–5 biweekly doses. Surrounding skin is well-protected with lead shield. It is probably the best treatment in preventing and treating post-burn, post-accident and acne keloids. Following radiotherapy, ultrasonic, physiotherapy exercises and pressure crepe bandage or stockinette are employed for several weeks to months.
3. Laser is now being used more and more in the management of keloids followed by grafting and/or intrarlesional triamcinolone acetonide.

Corticosteroid ointment/lotion especially clobetasol, hydrocortisone applied topically on freshly healed wounds helps to prevent keloid formation. In our experience, laser, radiotherapy and steriod injection help the most in the management of keloids.

HAIR TRANSPLANTATION

It is an accepted procedure in baldness. Initially introduced by Norman Orentreich, it is an effective means for permanent redistribution of scalp hair. There are several modifications available viz. multiple punch grafts, strip grafts, single hair transplant and scalp reduction. Autografts containing viable hair follicles are removed from the occipital area and placed in recipient areas in the frontal and vertex regions.

Scalp is properly prepared by shampooing and the patient is seated on a reclining dental chair. Donor area is trimmed along a horizontal path of 5 mm and grafts are removed with a punch 4–5 mm diameter. Spacing and angling of grafts is very important. The distance between each graft is the size of the punch. At one sitting 20–100 punch grafts can be inserted. Most transplanted hair would fall out in 3 weeks to grow again within 3 months.

Besides male baldness, quiescent resistant cases of alopecia areata, scars of trauma and lupus erythematosus and burns can also be treated by hair transplantation.

NAIL SURGERY

Surgical planing of nails with dental burrs is being employed to get rid of affected portions of the nail in cases of tinea unguium. The authors finds this technique useful in getting quick and better results in this difficult condition and also in nail dystrophies. Since the availability of griseofulvin and other newer antifungal agents, the need for nail surgery in the treatment of tinea unguium has somewhat declined. Nail resection and cauterization of lateral folds is useful in ingrowing nail. Making a hole in the nail plate with dental burr is practised to differentiate haematoma from a melanoma. Histopathological examination of nail disorders can be conducted by taking a biopsy of nail plate and underlying tissues.

Other Surgical Measures

Sweat gland surgery in cases of hyperhidrosis of axillae, venous stripping and ligation in cases of varicose veins and Z-plasty, etc. are some of the other surgical procedures employed by dermatologists.

LASERS

The term implies light amplification by stimulated emission of radiation (LASER). These are optical devices producing electromagnetic energy with their special properties viz. light output is monochromatic for each type of laser, light is coherent (complete alignment of all the waves produced and emitted) and light is highly climated (no divergence during travel- essentially directed beam without loss of intensity).

Since its first use in 1960, a lot of research has been done in this field. Not only newer lasers are being produced, but usefulness and disadvantages of each laser are also being studied extensively in different parts of the world.

A laser device has the following components:

1. Active medium—Ruby rod (solid), CO_2 (gas), liquid (fluorescent dyes).
2. Power supply—for energizing the active medium electrical, chemical, radio frequency or mechanical.
3. Optical resonator—or tube surrounding the active medium. It has a totally reflecting mirror at one end and partially transmitting one for the laser beam.

In the continuous-wave laser, shuttered pulses for certain therapeutic modalities are used like the shuttering device in a camera. Action of the laser beam on the skin depends upon the following factors:

1. Optical properties of the skin-water content, melanin, haemoglobin (red cell mass) and the presence of other colours.
2. Wavelength, power density (watts per sq cm) and energy fluence (irradiance multiplied by time of exposure expressed as joules per sq cm) of the laser.
3. Length and type of exposure.

Penetration, absorption of the laser beam by different tissues (red cells, black melanin, fibroblasts, etc.) and tissue scatter depend upon these three factors and hence the ultimate destruction of the desired diseased tissues and the saving of healthy surrounding tissues (to avoid scarring) are calculated in treatment.

It is believed that long exposures produce no specific destruction and short exposures produce specificc localised damage to desired tissues. Tissue scatter and thermal relation are the other factors to be taken into consideration while planning laser therapy.

At the present junction, six laser systems are in use. Only No. 2, 4, 6 are used in dermatology.

Their different properties are briefly tabulated in **Table 6.10**.

1. Argon laser
2. Carbon dioxide laser—for warts, keloids, lymphangiomas, etc.
3. Ruby laser
4. Helium-Neon laser—for acne vulgaris
5. Neodymium YAG laser
6. Tunable dye laser with fluorescent dyes (esp. rhodamin6G)-for haemangioma and moles.

ABSCESSES

Never lance an unripe abscess. As soon as it ripens as seen by the evidence of a yellow top, it should be incised with the point of a sharp knife. Ethyl chloride or fluoroethyl

Table 6.10: Laser systems and their properties

Properties	*Argon laser*	*Carbon dioxide*	*Ruby laser*	*Helium neon*	*Neodymium–YAG laser*	*Tunable-dye laser*
Colour of light	Visible blue green	Invisible; far infra-red	Visible red	Visible red	Invisible near infrared	Fluorescent dyes, (varying comprosition and colours)
Wave length Format-continuous pulsatory	488–514 nm Continuous	10600 nm Continuous	694 nm Pulsed high energy	– Continuous	1060 nm Continuous	400–1000 nm pulsed
Penetration (coefficient of extinction)	1–2 mm	0.1 mm Beam diameter at focal point 0.1–0.2 mm)	1–2 mm	Little energy and penetration	>3 mm	1–3 mm
Absoption	Non-selective Selective action controversal haemoglobin and melanin	Non-selective; instantaneous destruction	Selective blue or black pigment	Non-selective	High energy. No colour specifictiy	Selective dye rhodamine 6G–577 nm specific for haemoglobin
Tissue scatter	Moderate	Minimal irradiance value changable with focussing and de-focussing	Moderate	–	High	Variable

Contd...

Table 6.10: Laser systems and their properties (*Contd...*)

Properties	*Argon laser*	*Carbon dioxide*	*Ruby laser*	*Helium neon*	*Neodymium–YAG laser*	*Tunable-dye laser*
Indications	1. Vascular lesion—portwine stain • Angioma • Lymphangioma • Kaposi's sarcoma	Cutting/dessicating 1. Bloodless surgery; immediate suturing and grafts 2. Moh's histographic surgery 3. Keloid 4. Warts	1. Tattoos 2. Naevi Pigment is exploded by tissue steam and then phagocytosed Face lift	1. Mainly as laser 2. Biosumulation acceleration of wound healing 3. Non surgical cavernous 4. Controversial usefulness	1. Endoscopic coagulation of haemorr 2. Malignant tumour of GIT, bladder, bronchi	1. Vascular lesion 2. Photodynamic therapy with HPD (haemato porphyrin derivative)
	2. Pigmentary • Lentigenes • Naevus of Ota • Chloasma 3. Tattoos 4. Granuloma faciale • Lymphocytoma cutis	5. Superficial angiomas 6. Superficial angiomas 6. Superficial lymphangioma 7. Actinic cheilitis 8. Tattoos 9. Rhinophyma 10. Syringomas, trichoepitheliomas 11. Epidermial naevi lentigmes			3. Bulky and basalcell haemangiomas 4. Keloid 5. Haemangioma after putting special crystals in the beam	3. Useful in cavity tumour, malignant melonomas epithelioma
Disadvantages	Scarring Non selective action.Hence in disfavour	Nil Vergy useful	Scarring and danger of dissemination of malignant cells by shock waves	Low energy; little use in practice	Useful tool in surfical practive	Unpredictable tissue reaction levles. Undesirable photosensitivity reactions

spray helps to reduce the pain of incision. Do not allow the opening to close till the abscess has been fully drained. If abscess is big and patient is toxic, administer a systemic antibiotic according to the type of infection. Pus smear, culture and sensitivity testing facilitates the choice of antibiotic. Chronic, recurrent abscess would warrant investigation to establish the cause and causative factors, building up the general health of the patient and use of non-specific agents like *Swertia chirata*. The latter stimulates phagocytosis.

Carbuncle is an abscess with multiple openings. Diabetes may be the preceding cause. Antibiotic umbrella is essential. Indiscrete lancing can result in septicemia, a serious complication. Hidradenitis suppurativa deserves careful handling. Large area with chronic recurrent abscesses may have to be excised in toto under general anaesthesia. It is a difficult condition to treat, especially in the tropics and in hot months. Physiotherapy, proper exercises of flexures, exposure to cool fresh air and general aids are essential part of the treatment.

Chemo-surgery

Minor chemo-surgery has been in use for centuries for treatment of minor dermatoses. Only in the last five decades, phenol chemo-surgery for deep facial scars has been employed by several workers. Amongst the coloured races, because of their keloidal tendency and fear of colour changes (depigmentation or hyperpigmentation), use of chemo-surgery has to be very selective.

Indications

1. Chemical cauterisation for warts, keratoses, molluscum contagiosum, sebaceous cysts, acne scars, rhinophyma, discoid lupus erythematosus.
2. Cyto-toxic chemicals in Moh's chemo-surgery for treatment of skin cancers.
3. Chemical peel for removal of deep facial wrinkles.

Chemical Cauterisation

It has been practised from ancient times, in one form or the other. There is mention of it in *Charaka Samhita* and *Sushrut Samhita*.

Earlier, plant juices like 'Aak, Madar (*Calotropis gigantea*) juice', milkweed, euphorbia were employed. They are still being used in the remote rural areas.

Because of difficulties in procuring the correct herb and its standardisation, its use over the years has become less popular in the practice of sophisticated dermatology. Barbers used copper sulphate and lime for destruction of warts, often with disastrous results. Now with the availability of standardised chemicals, use of chemical cauterization has become well established in clinical practice.

Plantar and palmar warts: Formaldehyde soaks (10%) 5–10 minutes daily for 4–6 weeks are helpful, especially when dealing with multiple and mosaic warts.

Phenol is a good caustic agent; besides it numbs the part. In cases of plantar warts, phenol is applied, wart is scraped and then phenol reapplied. The process is repeated till the whole of the wart has been removed. Electro and cryo-surgery have over-shadowed and almost replaced this technique of phenol cauterization of warts.

Molluscum contagiosum: Squeeze the molluscum and apply 25% phenol with an ear bud just over the molluscum. After 1 minute, wipe it off with alcohol/spirit. Since it is a painful procedure, most dermatologists prefer to use a mixture of lactic acid and salicylic acid or electrodesiccation.

Chronic discoid lupus erythematosus (CDLE): After the activity of disease has been controlled with steroid infiltration/ointment, chloroquine etc, resistant patches are treated with application of 75% phenol for one minute and then wiping it off with spirit.

Sebaceous cysts: Curetting with phenol after incision and evacuation of contents is very beneficial in the management of cystic acne.

Paronychia: Phenol cauterisation and sterilization is in daily use by several workers. A pladget of cotton wool dipped in phenol is pushed into the paronychia cavity, kept for a minute and then replaced by a pladget of cotton dipped in tincture iodine. This is removed after a minute. Patient uses a tincture containing phenol 3% and tincture iodine 10% in rectified spirit 4–5 times a day, and avoids wet work.

Phenol peel has been used in the treatment of superficial acne scars. It has now been replaced by dermabrasion which is a fairly controlled method of skin peel.

Chapter

7

Aids to a Healthy Skin

The prevention of death is a fine ideal, but the prevention of disease is still finer.

A healthy skin is a source of pleasure, not only to its owner but also to the one who looks at it. To possess a nice skin is to have great social and economic advantage. Besides, the positive health of the skin is an insurance against disease, the ideal of every individual as well as every medical man.

The normal healthy skin is clear, smooth, supple, elastic, uniformly pigmented without wrinkles, and does not sag; the stratum corneum (horny layer) is thin, translucent and invisibly cast off, the pores are hardly visible, secreting an imperceptible amount of sebum and sweat (except in summer, in hot environments and when exertion takes place), and there is no evidence of active bacterial or fungal growth. This tone and glossiness is noticeably absent in the skin of the sedentary town worker.

The integument being the external covering of the human body is put to great stress and strain by the external environments involving factors like climatic changes, dust, irritants, non-pathogenic and pathogenic microorganisms, etc. Hair and nails grow constantly. Grease (sebum) of the skin is daily washed off. These agents have to be controlled. The following factors are important in keeping the skin healthy.

Diet

It should be balanced and digestible. A fair amount of animal proteins and vitamins are essential. The daily diet should contain liberal helpings of meat, fish, eggs, milk and its products, butter, green vegetables and fruits; concentrated, starchy food should be avoided. "*Sattwik*" diet is the answer. Spices, condiments, tea, coffee and alcohol should be consumed as little as possible. They produce a sense of heat, hence predisposition to allergic conditions and dermatoses. Occasional fasting is good for health. Keep your digestion healthy.

Gluttons and dyspeptics tend to be greasy, flushed, sallow, pasty and pimply. They, later, tend to develop seborrhoeic dermatoses. Besides, overeating results in obesity which predisposes to several illnesses.

Fresh Cool Air, Exercises and Mild Sun

Fresh cool air, exercise and mild sun are potent natural skin restorers. They stimulate the skin and thereby the thyroid, adrenals and sympathetic system on which are dependent the well-being and vitality of the skin and the body. Their importance is not fully realised by the medical profession. This point can be stressed with, an example: A holiday in a hill station or on the coast with a cool climate spent in loose, comfortable clothes, will tone up the skin, stimulate the musculature and improve the well-being of a person so much, that if he happens to suffer from dermatoses like chronic furunculoses, intertrigo and recurrent herpes, they will most probably disappear. This aspect of nature cure and physiotherapy has been developed on scientific lines in many countries for the prevention and cure of many diseases, both cutaneous and systemic. Intertrigo and tinea are rare in individuals who indulge in regular exercises in cool, fresh surroundings.

A moderately cold climate is the most potent natural stimulus to the integument. Exercise in fresh, cool air is very stimulating. Yogic exercises are beneficial because they exercise and relax the musculature in a scientific manner. Extreme cold is injurious, so a person should have the right clothing to protect himself from it. Several tropical conditions can be directly attributed to the scorching heat of the tropical climate causing hyperhidrosis and maceration. Due precautions, therefore, should be taken to keep the body cool. Air-conditioning, whenever possible, is the answer.

While mild sunbathing is beneficial, the strong sun produces degenerative changes and even neoplasms especially in white people. The integument must be protected from the strong sun and direct heat . An umbrella, solar hat and sun protective agents are useful aids.

Clothing

The amount of clothing worn should be very minimum, and neither the clothing nor footwear should contain sensitizers . Avoid very tight fitting and nylon clothes especially in the summer weather; only wear loose cotton clothes and soft sandals/chappals. Nylon clothes interfere with the absorption and evaporation of sweat. Furthermore , the chemicals, dissolved by unevaporated sweat can cause contact dermatitis. The same applies to footwear (especially of rubber and plastic), spectacle frames, furs, artificial jew ellery, etc.

Bathing

In tropical countries, daily bathing with clean and cool water is essential in the summer. In cold weather, one should bathe in warm water as often as possible. Clean the various body folds, genitalia and feet properly. The skin should be thoroughly dried after washing. A hot bath followed by a cold one is stimulating to the skin and the vital organs. To begin with the difference in between the two baths should not be great, but in course of time, as a person gets used to the difference he will greatly enjoy such baths with benefit.

These baths have been recommended with success in cases of chilblains, thermal urticarias and certain selected cases of atopic dermatitis.

Soap

A simple, least alkaline, soap should be. employed. People with greasy skin need more soap than those with dry skins. People with dry skins should use superfatted soaps (for method of making, refer to Chapter 5). Medicated soaps are the least useful as medication, and can be great sensitizers.

Oil

If nourishes the skin and hair; it makes them smooth. Coconut, mustard and olive oil are in common use. Medicated and perfumed oils are great sensitizers. In cold, dry weather as for example in the North Indian winter, it is a good habit to massage vaseline or lanoline or milk cream on the exposed parts of the body before retiring to bed. It helps to keep the skin smooth and fresh.

A good substitute for oil is butter, *ghee* or lanoline. In India, the first two are used abundantly to massage the skin of children. They are very useful for chapped lips, hands and feet. Butter is animal fat, rich in vitamins. In India, 'Upvatnas are popular with the fair sex for giving the required translucence, opacity and glow to the skin. They consist of milk cream, gram flour and lemon juice. Many modifications are available.

Shaving

The following points should be kept in mind when shaving:

a. Do not shave too finely by stretching the skin.
b. Shave in one direction.
c. Use clean, sterilized and sharp instruments and avoid repeated shaving on the same part.
d. The beard should be properly softened with soap or shaving cream before shaving. After shaving, rub in a little cream to lubricate the degreased skin.

Strongly alkaline or sensitizing shaving soap and cream should be avoided. The same applies to after-shave lotions.

The electric razor is a useful innovation, particularly for people with disorders on the beard region, since it avoids both trauma and the use of alkaline soap.

Cosmetics

Cosmetics contain chemicals to which individuals may be sensitive or may become sensitized to them; hence, care should be exercised while selecting them. In Europe and America, cosmetics are responsible for a great deal of contact eczema. In Asiatic countries, the incidence is fortunately still low. Chemicals in cosmetics may harm the skin, cause blockage of pores and invisible, slow degeneration; hence avoid cosmetics as much as possible.

Whenever one desires to change one brand for another in cosmetics, it is advisable to do a patch test.

Care of the Hair

It consists of: Washing with soap or shampoo. Regarding the choice of a shampoo, the same statements apply as have already been made for soaps (refer to preceding pages). Sometimes beaten egg white is employed to give glossiness to the hair. Savlon (P), Cetavlon (P) and Selsun suspension (P) are useful in controlling dandruff. In India, certain indigenous plant products like *ritha* and *amla* are used for washing the hair. They are cheap and effective. Greasy hair need frequent washing and less oil application. Dry hair requires less frequent washing and good oil massage. Frequency of washing depends upon the climate and the length of the hair, daily, alternate days or weekly. Often bland soap and water are sufficient.

Greasing or oil application is essential for effective lubrication and grooming; choice depends upon individual taste.

Combing and brushing of the hair is normally done once or twice a day. No force should be used in either combing or brushing. Combs and brushes tend to irritate the scalp; often injures and atrophies the hair.

Singeing of the hair ends is often employed by beauty parlours and hairdressers to treat splitting. It has no advantages over cutting, and is by no means curative.

Dyeing grey hair is prevalent with vegetable dyes (henna, chamomile), metallic dyes (bismuth, silver, lead) and chemical dyes (para-tolyendiamine, paraphenylenediamine, etc.). Several dye preparations are available in the market . Vegetable dyes are usually the safest, but there is limited choice of colour in them. Patch test to the dye must be applied before its use.

Permanent waving, and straightening of wavy hair (as in Negroes).

Broadly speaking, there are two methods of permanent waving:

a. ***The cold method:*** The hair is curled by means of curlers, and softened with a reducing agent like ammonium thioglycolate so that it can conform to the undulations made by the curlers; later, undulations are fixed with a neutralizer or an oxidizing agent.
b. ***The hot method:*** The hair is first softened by an alkaline sulphate solution, and then undulations are made by rods and the application of heat (electrical, steam or hemicals). The hair is shampooed before any of the two techniques of permanent waving are employed . Burning of the scalp by direct heat, or chemical irritation and sensitization are some of the risks of permanent waving. Due precautions should be taken; patch tests should precede the use of chemicals.

Hair ornaments: Pins, clips and nets. These are employed to keep the hair in a desired shape and also to enhance looks. Only rarely do such accessories cause dermatitis. Nickel and plastic materials should be used with caution to prevent irritation. Wigs are worn, particularly by women, to conceal alopecia or for improving appearance.

Part II

Diseases of the Skin

Chapter 8

Affections due to Physical Agents

The physical agents which can affect the integument vary from friction, pressure and maceration to cold, heat, sun, etc. They produce a large percentage of dermatoses seen in general practice; the majority of these dermatoses are minor problems, only a very small percentage are serious. Apart from the intensity and quality of the physical agents, the sensitivity and vitality of the individual also plays an important part in the bringing about of skin disorders.

FRICTION AND PRESSURE

Abrupt and intense friction or pressure produces erythema and sometimes, a blister. A common example is the blister produced on the heel by tight shoes. Continuous light pressure or friction produces pigmentation which is commonly seen around the waist where the sari, pyjama's string or the trouser belt is tied. If the belt or string is tightly tied over a long period, it will roughen the skin, even ulcerate it and result in depigmentation. Other examples of such irritation are the sites of the truss, corset, brassiere and the hat band.

Corn and Callus

Intermittent pressure and friction over a long period is likely to produce a callus or a corn. It represents hyperkeratosis formed by nature to protect the sensitive part of the skin and the underlying structures from such pressure and friction. A callus is a raised, uniform, painless plaque of hyperkeratosis appearing on the hands and the dorsum of feet. A corn, on the other hand, represents a conical, painful hyperkeratosis appearing on the soles and over the toe joints. Because of the body's weight and shoes, the hyperkeratosis of a corn gets pushed into the skin causing pressure on nerve endings which produces pain. Callosities are indicative of a person' s occupation and habits. Unless they are unduly uncomfortable or unsightly, they demand no treatment. On the other hand, a corn is painful, and needs attention. First of all, a corn must be differentiated from a plantar wart by the following facts: A corn is at a pressure site (over heads of the first and fifth metatarsal bones). It is painful when pressure is applied from above as well as from the sides, and there are no papillary prolongations nor any verrucous surface. Clinically, a corn is seen as a polished, flesh-coloured and circumscribed papule. Ill-fitting shoes and deformed feet are the two important causes.

The treatment of a corn consists of correcting the underlying causes. Footwear must be comfortable. Foot deformities must be corrected by exercise. The advice of an orthopaedic surgeon should be taken in cases of recurrent corns. Locally, collodion containing 10% salicylic acid is painted on the corn every night. The corn separates in about a week, but treatment must be continued till the corn area is absolutely level with the surrounding skin. Ivory horns have also been successfully employed by indigenous chiropodists.

Bunion

It is a circumscribed swelling consisting of a callus covering a fibromatous growth. A bunion is nature's protection against constant pressure and friction. Bunions commonly appear over the metatarsophalangeal joints—the first and fifth, and in deformed feet that have been confined to ill-fitting shoes. They look ugly, but are generally, painless. The treatment consists in excising the bunion, and in correcting the foot deformity by orthopaedic methods.

Cracking

It is seen mostly on the hands and feet in dry weather, particularly in the dry cold of the Indian winter which dries up the integument, roughens and cracks it because of its diminished elasticity. If the cracking is severe, fissures may be produced. The hands are further predisposed to cracking by poor general health, avitaminosis and frequent washing with soap and water. Cracking itself is uncomfortable; besides, it predisposes to secondary infection and pyoderma.

The treatment consists of:

1. Lubricating the parts with lanoline, glycerine, Nivea (P) cream, or pure fat (*ghee*). These agents soften the integument and help it to retain moisture.
2. Avoiding frequent washing with soap and water. Sodium bicarbonate soaks are useful.
3. Improving the general health.
4. Protection from dry climate by proper clothing, gloves, airconditioning, etc. Peeling the keratotic skin with a blunt knife or a common dermal abrader.

Maceration

Prolonged moisture produces two effects: (1) Maceration, (2) Paronychia. The former is seen in the flexures, like the interdigital spaces, the groins and the axillae during the monsoon when it results in intertrigo.

Interdigital maceration is common in people who wear shoes for long hours. Paronychia, due to maceration, is frequently seen in domestic servants, washermen, housewives, cooks and barmen. Macerated skin predisposes to monilia, tinea and streprococcal infection. In the case of patients confined to bed, continuous pressure and maceration results in necrosis of the tissues as is seen in bed sores.

The treatment of all these conditions consists in correcting the basic causes and keeping the affected parts dry.

AFFECTIONS DUE TO COLD

Chilblains

See Chapter 9 for details.

Acrocyanosis

It implies cold and clammy extremities of the body—hands and feet, less commonly the tip of the nose and the ears—in people with poor peripheral circulation. The parts are cold and dusky red; often accompanied by oversweating. Acrocyanotic individuals are usually young, emotionally sensitive, with rather unstable vasomotor systems. The condition becomes accentuated in the cold weather, improving as it becomes warmer.

When this circulatory disturbance affects the legs, it is called erythrocyanosis crurum. It is seen as a cold, dusky or bluish-red swelling over the outer side of the lower parts of the legs. The only subjective complaint is an ache. The condition is common in people who wear skirts and no stockings; hence, it is rather uncommon in Asiatic countries where people wear garments down to the ankles.

The treatment consists of exercising the affected parts, keeping them warm with proper clothing—gloves, thick stockings and footwear and a good, nourishing diet. Tonics, Duvadilan Retard, Complamina and nicotinic acid amide are beneficial. In some patients, good results are obtained with UVR and tab Trental (P).

Livedo Reticularis (Marbled Skin)

It implies a bluish-red reticular network enclosing islands of white skin seen usually on the legs, less so on the arms. Young girls are particularly affected in countries with a cold climate. In India, it is rare because of climate and clothing.

The reticular pattern is the result of the pattern of blood supply; the bluish network represents the anastomosis of arterial supply and the white islands are the areas getting direct blood supply from below. Slowing of the circulation due to cold is responsible for marbled skin. Application of heat results in pigmentation over the bluish network—*Ephelis ab igne*.

Frost-bite

It implies the destruction of tissues of the hands and the feet, less frequently, the ears and the tip of the nose, by exposure to extreme cold (usually below freezing point). Any part of the body being wet, strong winds and poor general health predispose to frost-bite. Cold temperatures lead to contraction of the arterioles, later, to dilatation of the capillaries and last of all, to the freezing of the parts. On thawing, necrosis of the frozen tissue and blood vessels occur; the latter results in thrombosis and gangrene. Frost-bite is uncommon in the south Asiatic countries except in the mountains.

Almost similar to frost-bite, are the effects of immersion foot, a condition brought on by immersion of the feet in cold water for long hours as in sea accidents.

Clinical features: The affected part first appears cold, and bluish-red. Then as freezing sets in, it becomes white and numb. On thawing, it becomes swollen, bluish-red and painful, and may develop bullae or ulceration due to the sloughing of the superficial tissue or frank gangrene of the digits.

Treatment:

1. Gradual warming of the parts—warm room, but no direct heat.
2. Wrapping in sterile cotton wool—no massage.
3. Antibiotics to prevent infection.

4. Anticoagulants like heparin and dicoumarin (Tromexan-P) to prevent vascular thrombosis.
5. Oxygen inhalation and anti-tetanus serum in very severe cases.
6. On recovery, gradual exercises to restore function.
7. Skin grafting or amputation in cases of frank necrosis. Epidural anaesthsia is being successfully tried.

AFFECTIONS DUE TO HEAT

Mild heat produces erythema due to the dilatation of blood vessels. Excessive dry heat produces various degrees of burns, and moist heat, scalds. They are mainly surgical conditions. Electric burns are deeper than they appear, and are generally slow in healing. Mild degree of electrical burns are occasionally seen following the use of medical diathermy in people wearing metal embroidered saris.

Frequent application of mild heat to any part of the body results in pigmentation. It is found, for instance, on the legs of cooks, and on the abdomens of Kashmiri people using the kangri*. This pigmentation is dark-brown in colour, and occurs in a network fashion dependent upon the arterial and venous circulation of the blood. This condition is called ephelis ab igne (erythema ab igne).

Exposure to heat produces profuse sweating which may give rise to different types of miliaria or prickly heat.

AFFECTION DUE TO SUNLIGHT

Sunlight when mild, stimulates the integument, but if fair skin is repeatedly exposed to it, over long periods, it will produce diffuse pigmentation or freckles (small, spotted pigmentation). Strong sunlight burns the integument; in hypersensitive individuals, certain light or sensitization dermatoses are produced.

Solar Dermatitis

Exposure to strong sunlight produces dermatitis which may be of an acute or chronic nature. The actual degree of the burns depends upon the intensity of the sunlight and the environments under which the integument is exposed. Snow and water reflect sunlight strongly especially the ultraviolet beam; hence, sunburns occur easily on the mountains and near the sea. Dark people sunburn less frequently than the white; people used to exposing themselves to the sun, can stand sunlight better than those who do not. Blondes and red heads are sensitive to sunlight. The signs of sunburn vary from redness to swelling and blistering. The eyelids may swell, if the face is affected. The eruption is usually bilateral and symmetrical. Subjectively, the patient complains of burning and itching. The signs develop several hours after exposure. A mild attack clears up within a couple of days; the inflammed epidermis peels off, leaving behind hyperpigmentation, freckles, and sometimes though rarely, depigmentation. A severe attack may be accompanied by prostration and shock, and will take weeks to subside; it may leave behind some degree of atrophy or scarring.

*It is a coke heater consisting of an earthen bowl enclosed in a cane basket.

Chronic sunburn is produced in fair people by exposure to strong sunlight over a period of years. The integument looks like that of a sailor, there being patchy and diffuse pigmentation, wrinkling, atrophy, telangiectasia and keratoses. There is a tendency to develop epitheliomata. Exposed parts like the face, neck, the dorsum of the hands and feet, are the sites chiefly affected. Cutis rhomboidalis nuchae is a form of chronic solar dermatitis of the back and neck. It is seen as thick and red skin divided into rhomboidal areas by prominent creases.

Diagnosis: It is not difficult in ordinary cases, because of the typical features, and the history of the environments under which they develop. Erysipelas and cellulitis can be eliminated by their localized nature and raised local and systemic temperature.

Treatment: It consists of:

Prophylactic: People with light skin, blondes, red heads and also those with photosensitivity, should avoid direct and prolonged exposure to the strong sun. In sun-bathing, exposure to the sun should be increased gradually, in stages. Such people should use the sun-shades, umbrellas, and apply evenly on exposed surfaces anti-actinic creams like Paraminol (P) or para-amino-benzoic acid or titanium dioxide in lactocalamine lotion (physical and chemical sunscreens).

Curative:

1. Locally, lotion calamine in mild cases, and lotion hydrocortisone in severe cases. These should be substituted by zinc cream and eucerine as the acute stage subsides.
2. Antihistaminics and corticosteroids by mouth in moderate and severe cases respectively.
3. Bed rest, plenty of fluids, salt and lime in severe cases.
4. In chronic cases, lanoline cream with vitamins may help to soften the skin, but it never returns to normal. Dermabrasive surgery may help to some extent. Keratoses and epitheliomas are treated by surgical or electrical excision etc., on the lines discussed in Chapter 6.

PHOTOSENSITIZATION DERMATOSES

It implies group of skin disorders produced by susceptibility or hypersensitivity to light—sun's rays and UVR. Refer to **Tables 8.1 to 8.3** for more detail on this topic. These disorders can be classified as follows:

Photosensitive dermatoses:

a. *Genodermatoses:* Xeroderma pigmentosum, porokeratosis, congenital porphyria.
b. *Non-specific/idiopathic:* Solar urticaria, polymorphous light eruption (PLE), hydroa aestivale (Vacciniforme), Hutchinson 's summer prurigo.
c. *Aggravation of diseases:* Discoid lupus erythematosus (DLE)—erythema multiforme (EM), herpes, lymphogranuloma venereum (LGV), pemphigus, rosacea, lichen planus (LP), psoriasis, vitiligo, lymphocytoma cutis, Darier's disease, seborrhoeic dermatitis.
d. *Nutritional and metabolic:* Porphyrias, pellagra.
e. *Foods, preservatives, chemicals and additives:* Celery, buckwheat, fish, chemicals, dyes, saccharine.
f. *Drugs:*

   I. Contact: Hexachlorophane, halogenated salicylanilide—cosmetics, deodorant

Buclosamide—antifungal
Psoralen derivatives, tar, pitch and bithional—cosmetics
Aminobenzoate—sunscreen
Furocoumarins—cosmetics and tanning agents

II. Systemic antibiotics and chemotherapeutic agents—ledermycine, terramycin, nalidixic acid, doxycyclin and cynomycin griseofulvin, sulphonamides
Antidiabetics—sulfonylureas

Table 8.1: Differences between Phototoxicity and photosensitivity

Phototoxicity	*Photosensitivity*
Associated with systemic and topical agents	Repeated exposure to photo-sensitising chemicals and medicaments
Intense light	Minute exposure
Resolution fast	Resolution slow
Burning, erythema and vesicles, scaling and depigmentation	Itching, edema, erythema and oozing
Hypopigmentation	Lichenification and discomfort

Table 8.2: Wavelength of solar and associated spectrum

Cosmic rays	5×10^{-5} nm
Gamma rays	0.0005–0.14 nm
X-rays	0.01–10 nm
UVC (Short)	10–280 nm
UVB (Medium)	280–320 nm
UVA (Long)	320–400 nm
Visible	400–720 nm
Infrared	720 nm–1000 μ
Radio waves	1000 μ–500 m

1 n.m. (Nanometre) = 10^{-9} metre
1 Angstrom (Å.) = 10^{-10} metre = 0.1 nm
1 Micron (μ) = 10 nm
Phototherapy is useful in psoriasis, vitiligo, solar urticaria and mycosis fungoides

Table 8.3: Types of skin

Type	*Characteristics*
Type I	Always burn, never tan
Type II	Always burn, sometimes tan
Type III	Sometimes burn, always tan
Type IV	Sometimes burn, tans readily
Type V	Very rarely burn, always tan
Type VI	Never burn, always tan

Diuretic—chlorthiazide
Tranquillizers and anti-depressants—phenothiazine derivatives
Vitiligo drugs and dyes—furocoumarins, psoralens
Bithionol—Cosmetics
Aminobenzoate—Sunscreen
Furocoumarins—Cosmetics and tanning agents
NSAID group—Pain killers

Xeroderma Pigmentosum

It is a rare congenital and heredo-familial disorder showing undue sensitivity to light. The disorder starts in infancy, but may begin later in childhood or adult life. The characteristic lesions are: hyperpigmentation, freckles and blotches, atrophic spots and telangiectasia. Later, warty growths, keratoses and epitheliomas may complicate the disorder. The exposed parts of the body are the sites of choice. Exposure to sunlight aggravates the condition, which may be accompanied by photophobia and keratitis. The prognosis is bad in severe cases; patients die early, but some live to adulthood (Fig. 8.1).

The treatment administered is unsatisfactory. Patients should learn to live with their skins, respecting its undue sensitivity; they should avoid sunlight, and use anti-actinic creams. Keratoses and epitheliomata need surgical intervention; radiotherapy should be avoided in these cases. Dermabrasive surgery may be helpful in mild cases.

Solar Eczema

It implies abnormal sensitivity to sunlight amounting to an allergy which results in a polymorphic type of eruption consisting of erythema, papules, vesicles, oozing, crusting, which may later on turn into pigmented freckles and blotches and even depressed scars on the parts of the body exposed to sunlight. Lesions vary from oedematous papules to frank eczema in different individuals. In others, it consists of only infiltrated, blotchy erythema of the face. The eruption is accompanied by considerable pruritus, which may result in secondary infection and even lichenification in chronic solar eczema. The etiology is unknown. The disorder usually starts in childhood, and lasts for several years. In children, it is usually seasonal and named juvenile spring eruption or summer

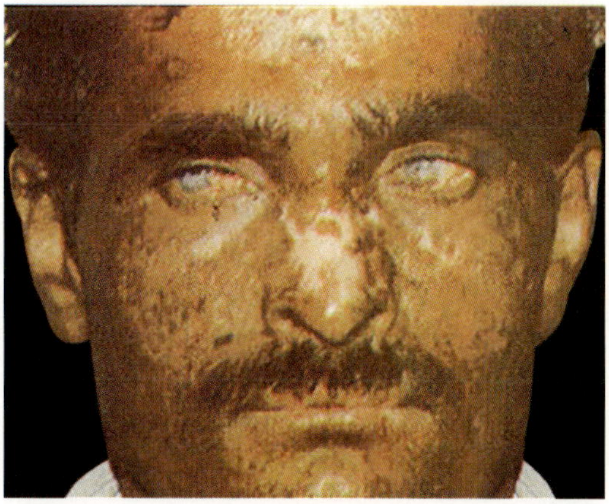

Fig. 8.1: Xeroderma pigmentosa leading to blindness

eruption or hydroa vacciniform. In young adults, the term polymorphous light eruption is used. Relation to sun exposure is the important feature.

The treatment consists of antihistaminics, and calamine or hydrocortisone lotion in active cases. Anti-actinic lotion helps to prevent the condition. Patient must avoid exposure to sun.

Solar Urticaria

It is a variety of physical urticaria, caused by sensitivity to sunlight, affecting the exposed parts of the skin. Urticarial lesions begin to develop soon after an exposure has been made to the sun. In the temperate climate, the condition is seasonal, while in the tropics, it may occur throughout the year. The condition is chronic and recurrent. The treatment consists in protecting the skin from sunlight, and the use of antihistaminics. One could try desensitizing the skin by exposing it, by degrees, to the sun.

Actinic Reticuloid

It is a feature of chronic photodermatitis causing severe itching, discomfort and emotional disability. Air-borne contact allergens like parthenium and drugs are the important causes.

Clinical features are reddish or lichenified plaques, on the exposed parts of face and hand; later they become confluent with deep furrows in between and even disfigurement. From exposed parts, the condition may spread to other parts and may even become generalised. Mycosis fungoides and malignant transformation must always be excluded **(Fig. 8.2)**.

Treatment is unsatisfactory. It consists in protection from sun, use of sunscreens, steroid creams and oral steroids.

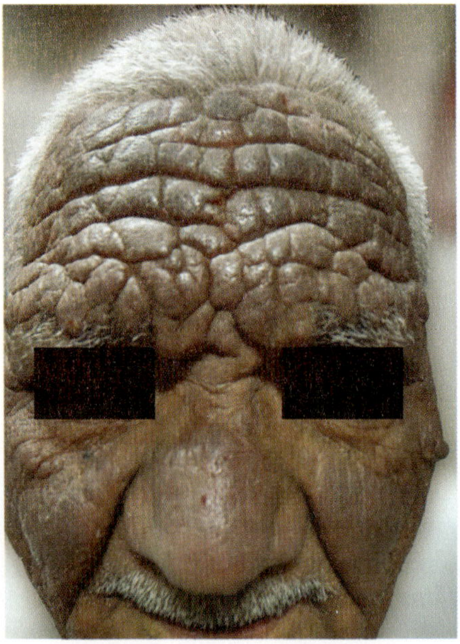

Fig. 8.2: Actinic reticuloid

Chapter

9

Erythematous, Urticarial and Purpuric Rashes

Erythema is one of the most common primary lesions of the skin. It is produced by the dilatation of the cutaneous blood vessels. If the dilatation is accompanied by increased permeability, redness and oedema of the skin are produced, features of urticarial eruption, quite familiar to everyone, as commonly seen in nettle rash. At times, the cutaneous blood vessels are so irritated and damaged, that they permit the whole blood to pass through , as in purpuras (haemorrhagic rashes). Thus, it will be seen that these three lesions, erythema, urticaria and purpura, depend upon the degree of stimulation or damage to the cutaneous vascular system. In every case, an erythematous lesion must be felt for induration or infiltration, either by palpation with gloved fingers, or with pointed dissecting forceps. Simple erythema has no resistance or infiltration of underlying tissues. Granulomas, however, like tuberculosis and leprosy, have erythema plus infiltration. Generalized erythema and infiltration of the whole integument is termed erythroderma.

ERYTHEMATOUS RASHES

The causes of erythematous rashes are as follows:

Localized erythema due to local external causes

1. Traumatic—injury, pressure, bedsores, intertrigo, napkin rash.
2. Chemical—dermatitis and eczema.
3. Heat, cold, light-burn, frost-bite, sunburn.
4. Infective—erythema in the early stages of impetigo, insect bite

Generalized erythema, usually bilateral and symmetrical, due to a systemic internal cause.

1. Specific causes, described on etiological basis:
   a. Syphilis (*see* Chapter 17)
   b. Exanthemata (*see* Chapter 26
   c. Drug eruption (*see* Chapter 21)
   d. Toxic erythema-focal sepsis, intestinal (food and its products).
2. Non-specific causes, described on morphological basis. They are definite disease entities, though the causes are indefinite.
   a. *E. nodosum* (*see* Chapter 15)
   b. *E. induratum*
   c. Lupus erythematosus (*see* Chapter 24)
   d. *E. pernio*
   e. *E. multiforme*
   f. Other rare erythemas

Erythema may take the form of localized or generalized macules or sheets. Asymmetrical, localized redness is usually due to a local, external cause. Injury produces redness; pressure may result in bedsores. Chemical and thermal burns, insect bites, bacterial infections, dermatitis and eczemas produce erythemata, at least, in the early stages. Bilateral and symmetrical widespread eruptions are usually due to an internal cause.

NAPKIN RASH

It affects infants in the areas covered by the napkin. Lesions consist mainly of simple erythema, though they may become vesicular or even ulcerative. They are situated, most frequently, on the prominences, and may occupy the inner parts of the thighs, perineum and genitalia. Usually, the flexures are not affected, contrary to what happens in intertrigo **(Fig. 9.1)**. The causes of napkin rash are: wet or soiled napkins, soap left in the napkins after washing, strong ammoniacal urine, poor general health.

Differential diagnosis: It is made from other erythematous eruptions in this area, namely, congenital syphilis (it is accompanied by other syphilitic manifestations, rash on the palms and the soles, involvement of the anal region; the lesions are erythematous or bullous); thrush (moist, red areas with peeling at the edges, also thrush lesions in the mouth); intertrigo (confined to the flexures only) and tinea (the lesions are characteristic, besides, tinea is rare in infancy).

Treatment: It consists mainly of correcting the cause or causes of the condition. Part must be kept dry and exposed to fresh air as far as possible. Rubber and nylon panties must be avoided. Napkins should be changed as soon as they become wet, and should be rinsed in clear water after being washed with soap. The general health of the patient should be improved. If the urine is strong, water should be given for drinking in between feeds. Any soothing ointment and talcum powder would do the trick, after the cause or causes have been eliminated. The authors prefer zinc and castor oil cream or eucerine for local application.

INTERTRIGO

It is a very common and annoying cutaneous affection.

Etiology: Plethoric, debilitated and over-dressed individuals with hyperhidrosis and sedentary habits are more prone to intertrigo, but in tropical heat, anyone can develop this complaint. In the authors' experience, people in good health, of normal weight, who wear comfortable clothes in the day allowing the free passage of air, and loose garments at night, and who do some exercise in cool, fresh air, usually escape intertrigo. It is an uncommon condition amongst the poor who live in the open. Friction caused by opposing surfaces or ill-fitting underclothing, heat and retention of sweat, are the important local etiological factors. The disease is most prevalent in the summer in hot tropical countries. Diabetes, obesity and gout are the three main predisposing causes.

Clinical features: The flexures are the sites of affection. In order of frequency, groin, axillae, retroauricular and inframammary regions, popliteal fossae, are the areas commonly involved. The symptoms are: an uncomfortable feeling, burning and sometimes tenderness. A clinical examination will reveal redness which leads to

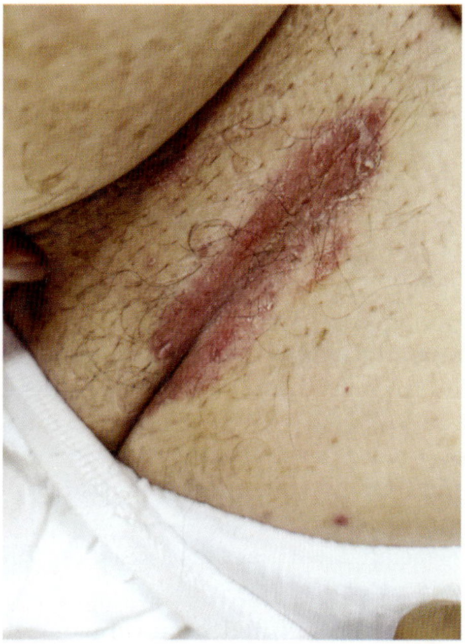

Fig. 9.1: Intertrigo in a diabetic 65-year-old man

maceration and may be to a linear superficial abrasion or fissure. The latter is found right at the angle of two opposing surfaces. There is no frank oozing of serum or crusting unless flexural infective eczema complicates intertrigo owing to secondary infection and eczematization (Fig. 9.1). Moniliasis may also secondarily complicate intertrigo. Seborrhoeic background makes it worse.

Differential diagnosis: It is made from tinea cruris. Here, the characteristic clinical features are: marked itching, sparing of the deepest angle of opposing folds, and inflammatory border of vesicles and pustules. The microscopic evidence of fungus is conclusive.

The prognosis is good if the disease is treated by an expert and the patient is co-operative, unless there is predisposing seborrhoea, obesity and diabetes.

Treatment: It must be religiously carried out for best results, otherwise this simple skin affection can become exceedingly annoying and demoralizing. The treatment consists in correcting the systemic and local factors described above.

1. The general health of the patient must be improved, and he should be instructed to lead an outdoor life, exposing the affected parts particularly to fresh, cool air for at least a couple of hours every day. If possible, he should work and live in an air-conditioned room.
2. The affected parts must be kept dry, cool and free from friction. They must be frequently oiled. Underclothing should be of cotton, and must fit properly. Tight jeans, jockey type of underwears and synthetic material should be avoided.
3. *Exercise:* Raise the legs and separate them as far as possible. Repeat it 20–30 times.
4. The affected parts must be cleaned daily with potassium permanganate lotion (1 in 8,000 dilution) and patted dry. An astringent dusting powder and/or lotion is then

usually applied. The authors prefers the use of talcum powder, lotion acid tannici or calamine lotion containing 1% chloral hydras, and 600,000 IU of nystatin (P) per 100 cc. Spirit must be avoided in the acute state; on recovery from this stage, it is beneficial, as it tends to harden the skin. Corticosteroid cream with vioform and nystatin gives dramatic results but its use should be avoided on the scrotum and groins for fear of causing atrophy.

CHILBLAINS

Synonym: Erythema pernio.

People with poor peripheral circulation, and sometimes with poor general health, are the victims. It is more common among females than males. It occurs on the fingers and toes only during the cold weather; it usually subsides completely in summer. When there is exposure to cold, itching, tenderness and burning sensation develop. The fingers and toes become dusky red and cold. Itchy swellings also develop; occasionally, these ulcerate. On healing, there is no scarring except where there has been ulceration.

Chilblains may be associated with acrocyanosis, erythrocyanosis crurum and acrosclerosis.

Differential diagnosis: It is distinguished from lupus erythematosus, which may even complicate chilblains. In lupus erythematosus of the hands, bluish-red, slightly infiltrated and scaly lesions develop on the backs of fingers, accompanied by typical lesions on the face. When one comes across chronic whitlows and erosions on the fingers or toes, the possibility of chilblains must be considered.

Treatment: It is rather unsatisfactory, the main emphasis being on proper nutrition, improvement of general health with tonics and warm clothing. The hands and feet must be kept warm with gloves and woollen stockings. Sudden changes of temperature, like exposing parts of the body to cold and then warming them near a fire, act badly on the malady. For this reason, central heating is very useful. Drug therapy includes a course of thyroid, nicotinic acid, and vitamin K—Pernavit (P), Priscol (P), Duvadilan (P) and locally UVR exposures, lead lotion and galvanic baths. All these may have to be tried one by one, since in one case, one may succeed, and in another, it may fail. There is no specific drug available for chilblains.

ERYTHEMA MULTIFORME

It is an affection uncommon in tropical countries, being a disease found mostly in the temperate climate. It occurs most often in young adults, and in the spring and autumn.

Etiology: It is considered to result from sensitization to products of infection and drugs. The infective group includes haemolytic *Streptococcus* infection of the nose and the throat. The common offending drugs are: Barbiturates, sulphonamides, phenolphthalein and salicylates. So a search for a septic focus, and an enquiry into the drugs taken, should always be made. Quite often the patient himself volunteers the history of the sore throat preceding the attack of erythema multiforme. Sometimes the disease is related to visceral disorders like allergic purpura or rheumatism or lymphogranuloma venereum or herpes simplex infection.

Clinical features: The onset is acute with mild fever, malaise and perhaps other constitutional symptoms. The lesions are multiple and polymorphic; they are distributed symmetrically on the dorsum of hands and feet, the forearms, the legs, the face and neck. Predominantly, the lesions are oedematous erythematous macules and flattened papules. Nodules, vesicles and bullae are uncommon. Bullous lesions can occur as such, generally starting on erythematous bases . Mucous membranes are usually spared, but a few lesions may be found in the mouth. The colour of the macular and papular cutaneous lesions changes from crimson-red to a purplish and even bluish colour. At times, concentric rings of various colours may be found in the lesion (erythema iris is a common annular lesion with a red centre). The cutaneous lesions are asymptomatic except for mild burning and smarting **(Fig. 9.2)**. Erythema multiforme is rarely associated with a gastrointestinal disturbance, arthritis and haemorrhages. Severe erythema multiforme with predominantly extensive bullous eruption of the skin and mucous membranes, sudden onset, high fever and prostration, is often termed as Stevens–Johnson disease or syndrome. The eyes, urethra and respiratory tract may also be involved. Bullous pemphigoid is a chronic variant of bullous erythema multiforme in elderly persons.

Pathology: The histopathological picture varies with the clinical picture. In all cases, the dermis shows dilated capillaries and infiltrate consisting mainly of lymphocytes. There may also be polymorphs and eosinophils. In bullous lesions, there is a typical subepidermal bulla while in maculopapular, epidermis shows spongiosis and intra-epidermal oedema.

Prognosis: The individual lesions last from several days to weeks. The whole attack lasts from two to four weeks. There is a tendency to recurrence, unless the causative factors are completely eliminated. Sometimes, there is a likelihood of erythema multiforme bullosa being clinically mixed up with dermatitis herpetiformis and pemphigus (*Percival*). One

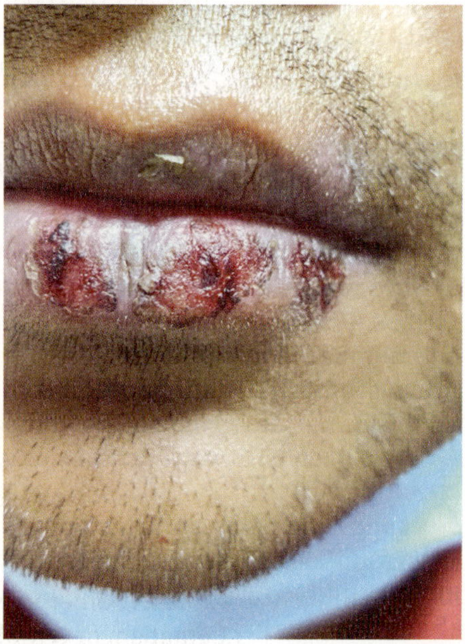

Fig. 9.2: Erythema multiforme (Steven–Johnson syndrome) lesions on the lips

can follow the other. For this reason, some authors prefer to discuss all of the three bullous conditions under the same heading.

Differential diagnosis: It is made from other erythematous and vesiculobullous lesions and occasionally from urticaria. In the latter, the diagnostic features are: asymmetrically distributed weals with whitish centres, marked itching, the short duration of the lesions and the absence of constitutional symptoms.

Main differentiation is from lupus erythematosus, dermatitis herpetiformis and pemphigus.

Lupus erythematosus shows typical butterfly lesions on the face, chronic infiltrated erythematous patches, follicular plugging and scarring. Dermatitis herpetiformis is seen as grouped polymorphic rash on forearms, scapular region and lower back, accompanied by marked itching and typical histopathology. Pemphigus bullae develop on normal skin (cf. bullae in erythema multiforme which develop on erythematous area) and there are lesions in the mouth. Nikolsky 's sign and Tzanck test are positive for acantholysis.

Treatment: The disease has usually a spontaneous resolution, subsiding within few weeks. The bullous variety, however, can be recalcitrant and can even prove fatal.

1. Immediate—for the attack:
   a. Removal of the cause—infection and drugs, the former with antibiotics, the latter by withdrawing the drug.
   b. Appropriate supportive therapy.
   c. Antihistaminics by mouth.
   d. Locally calamine lotion or cream with 1% phenol.
   e. Corticosteroids, if the attack is very severe and of the bullous variety.
2. Preventive—removal of the cause and antihistaminics.

TOXIC ERYTHEMA

It is a wide but useful term for a group of erythematous conditions, apart from exanthemata, syphilis and drug eruptions, which one comes across in practice. These erythemas are, on their own, specific, though morphologically, they present varying pictures, and have no strict association with the cause. Occasionally the term, "toxo-allergic rash" is employed. The morphological names do not convey anything to the clinician. On the contrary, they are responsible for a great deal of confusion and misunderstanding.

As the name suggests, toxins reaching the skin produce such an erythema. These toxins include products of focal sepsis in the ear, nose, throat, teeth, intestines, urinary tract etc., products of digestion and metabolism, acute illness, fever, rheumatism, drugs, injections and so forth. Clinically, lesions occur symmetrically and are usually widespread. The trunk, the upper parts of the extremities and the face are generally affected. Erythema may be morbilliform, scarlatiniforrn, roseolar or chronic, migratory variety. Erythema fades on pressure. The condition lasts from days to weeks, depending upon the cause. The eruption may be accompanied by mild constitutional disturbances like low-grade fever, headache and joint pains. Besides, there are local subjective symptoms of the causative toxic focus.

Toxic erythemas are very common. Selectively affected are children and young adults. Before the label of toxic erythema is given, pityriasis rosea, drug eruptions, secondary syphilis and infectious fever, must all be definitely ruled out.

The treatment is usually simple. All obvious causes must be removed. In idiopathic cases, the treatment consists of an opening medicine, antihistaminics and soothing, local applications, like zinc cream and calamine lotion.

URTICARIAL ERUPTIONS

1. Urticaria
2. Papular urticaria
3. Urticaria pigmentosa (*see* Chapter 27).
4. Angioneurotic oedema.

Urticarla

Synonyms: Hindustani: Chhapaki, Dhapar.

Layman's popular name: "Nettle rash".

It is a common, annoying reaction pattern affecting almost 10–15% of the population at one time or the other during their lifetime. No age is exempted, but its incidence is highest at puberty and middle age.

Clinical features: There are two varieties of urticaria: Localized and generalized, depending upon the distribution of the eruption. The nature of the lesions is identical in both varieties. Localized urticaria is confined to a small part of the body usually limbs and is caused by bites or stings of nettles, caterpillars, weaver fish, jellyfish, whiplash, on site of injection or contact with stinging plants known as 'nettles'—Urticaceae family (*Bichhu buti*). In comparison, generalized urticaria is widespread all over the body—trunk and extremities asymmetrically. Eyes, lips or hands may be swollen **(Fig. 9.3)**.

The onset is usually sudden and abrupt. The lesions resemble those produced by the sting of nettles. They start as rosy-red, erythematous macules, on which flesh or lighter colour oedematous weals soon develop. The erythema is ill-defined, and fades on pressure. The lesions are usually irregular and asymmetrical. The rash is accompanied by severe, annoying itching, burning and sense of heat. The individual lesions subside within a few hours; at the latest in a day or two. An attack of urticaria can be brought on by exposure to cold winds, baths, or by exposure to heat; also by hot, spicy food and psychogenic stress. The dermographism is usually positive, e.g. scratching the skin produces triple response.

Dermographism can occur as such without being accompanied by the spontaneous wheals and irritation of true urticaria (Fictitious urticaria) **(Fig. 9.4)**.

Pathology: Main features are capillary dilatation and accumulation of serum in the corium. Later, the serum may compress the capillaries and produce pallor, but at the edge of lesion, capillary dilatation can always be detected. Activation of mast cells and basophils by immunoglobulins IgE and IgG and complements and other stimulants results in release of mediators like histamine, serotonin and bradykinin which act on H_1 and H_2 receptors in the skin and its blood vessels.

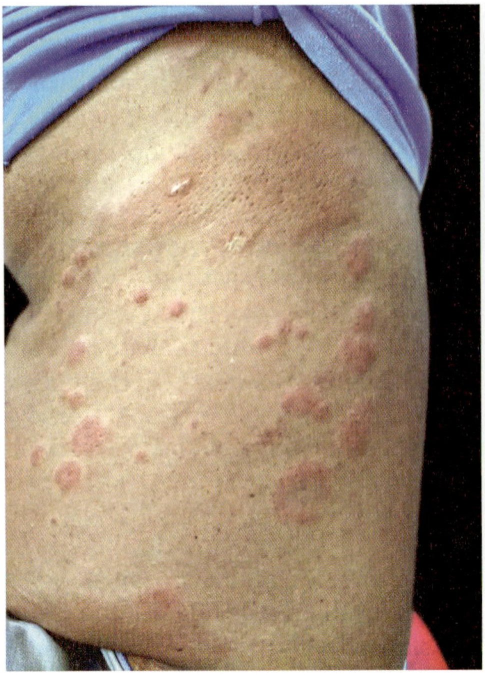

Fig. 9.3: Acute urticaria in a 27-year-old male

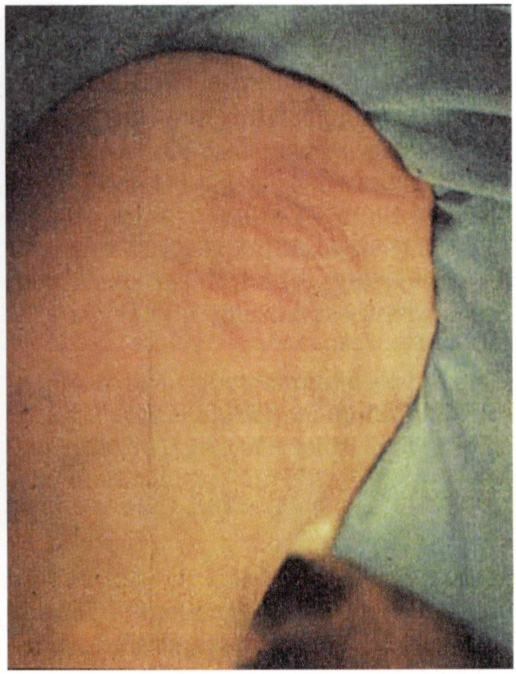

Fig. 9.4: Dermographism in a patient of urticaria and sense of heat

Etiology: In the authors' experience, besides genetic predisposition, there is increased sense of heat (*see* Chapter 3), which increases considerably at the time of attack. This is more often seen in physical urticarias and allergies to food and drugs **(Fig. 9.5)**.

Drugs: Penicillin (also penicillin in dairy products). Aspirin and other salicylates. There is cross sensitization with tartrazine and benzoic acid in areated drinks and preserved foods, and to Indomethacin.

Foods: Nuts, shell fish, oysters, prawns, eggs, milk and its products. Strawberries, Zaminkand, Mushrooms.

Food additives: Preservatives, dyes, flavouring agents—Tartrazine, benzoic acid, azo dyes, salicylates, yeast, saccharin.

Plants: The 'nettles'—Urticacae family (*Bichhu buti*).

Insect bites: Nettles, wasps, jelly fish, weaver fish, caterpillars, *trombicula irritans*.

Internal disorders: Rheumatic fever, SLE, reticulosis, hypogammaglobulinemia.

Genetic: Hereditary angioedema, familial cold urticaria.

Focal sepsis: Teeth, nose, throat, ears, sinuses, lungs, liver, intestines, kidney, bladder, vagina, etc.

Parasites: Round worms, tape worms, hookworms, thread worms, hydatid cyst, filariasis.

Psychogenic: Resentful frustration, emotional stresses, over-work, etc.

Physical factors: Pressure, vibration, heat, cold, sun, exertion.

Acute urticarias are usually due to drugs and foods. They last from a few days to a few weeks and then disappear.

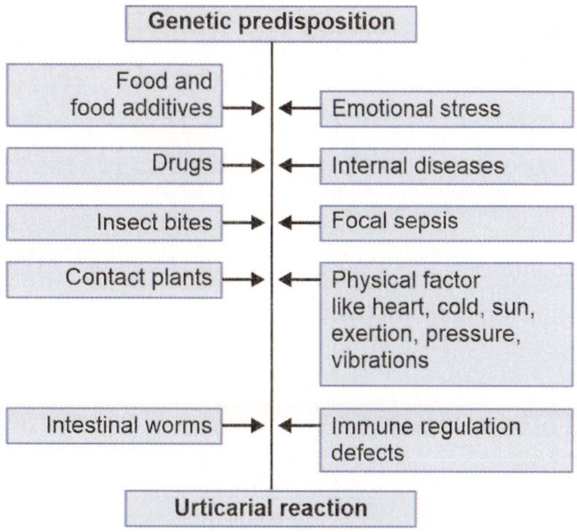

Fig. 9.5 Etiological factors in urticaria

Urticaria which is prolonged over 6 weeks is termed chronic urticaria. These pose a problem and cause considerable strain on the expertise of physician for detection of the cause. With patience, one can detect causative factors like focal sepsis, parasites, psychogenic stresses and physical factors. People consuming large quantities of hot spicy food, tea, coffee, alcohol and non-vegetarian food are more prone to urticarias. Food additives and aspirin are the two common culprits.

Cold urticaria may be familial or acquired; the former may be accompanied by fever, joint pains, and presence of cryoglobulins. Swimming or a cold bath may bring on a severe attack, hypotension and collapse. Ice cube test may be positive.

Heat, exertion and emotional stress cause cholinergic urticaria. These are more common in the Indian winter. Cycling or walking fast or standing in the sun starts a pricking sensation in the skin and an uncomfortable feeling in the body followed by urticaria. These patients complain of a sense of heat with warm clothes and bed covers. They are very uncomfortable and restless in the sun. Weals are small. Mecholyl and nicotine injection produce an attack.

Solar urticaria is confined to exposed parts and is seen on exposure to sun.

Diagnosis: In the handling of urticaria, great emphasis should be laid on history taking and physical examination. Patient's personality, food and drug habits should be thoroughly studied and a search for foci of infection made. Examination of stool for ova and cysts would help in discovering parasitic infestation, urine for kidney infection, ESR for chronic infection, and internal diseases, diet diary and single factor elimination diet for food allergies. In intractable cases intradermal testing may provide a lead to the cause. This can be supplemented by provocative administration of aspirin, tartrazine, benzoic acid and sunset yellow added one by one with a 2–3 days interval in between.

Immunology can be studied by investigative tools like cryoglobulins, ANA, skin tests, etc.

Table 9.1 would help in establishing the cause and variety of urticaria.

Differential diagnosis is from granuloma (there is infiltration, absence of itching and lesions persist while the urticarial lesions are non-infiltrated and transient typical weals accompanied by marked itching and dermographism).

Table 9.1: Differential diagnosis of causes of urticaria

Differentiating features	*Drugs*	*Foods*	*Infection, focal sepsis*	*Psychogenic*	*Physical*
1. History	Positive	Positive	Usually negative	History of emotional stresses and conflicts	Urticaria on exposure to sun, wind or exertion
2.Course-acute	Acute	Seasonal, usually acute	Chronic	Chronic	Chronic with acute exacerbations
3. Duration of individual attack	Hours to days	Few hours	Hours to days	Variable	Short duration
4. Distribution	Trunk	Generalized	Joints and pressure sites	Generalized	Cold and sun on exposed areas. Exertion on covered parts
5. Timing	Any	Any	Any	Usually evening and night	Usually day time; cold urticaria after bath
6. Features of weals	Massive large lesions, serpiginous with tendency to central clearing	Very small lesions of irregular shape	Small round lesions	Small circular lesions	Small lesions
7. Associated features	Joint pains, lymphadenopathy purpura	Abdominal pains, vomiting and burning in mouth	Run down state. Easy fatiguability	Anxious look with neurotic tendencies	Dermographism is prominent

Prognosis: Acute urticarias have a good outlook; those due to food clear up quickly within a few days, and those due to drugs, like penicillin, clear up within a few weeks. The prognosis is good when the specific cause has been established and eliminated. Chronic urticarias, without a traceable cause, have a bad prognosis, because in such cases treatment can only be symptomatic. In severe acute urticarias with swelling of the face, there is always danger of laryngeal obstruction.

Treatment: It consists in the following:

1. *Eliminating the cause:* Food allergy by an eliminative diet, drug allergy by the withdrawal of the causative drug, parasitic infection and focal sepsis by a treatment that will eliminate them, psychogenic urticaria by the removal of psychogenic causes, physical urticaria by the correction of the existing physical stress.
2. Reassurance.

3. Symptomatic treatment:
   a. Patient is advised simple bland diet and rest in acute urticarias. A saline purgative is often useful. Alcohol and tea/coffee are preferably avoided.
   b. *Main line of treatment consists in use of antihistaminics:* H_1 blockers: Benadryl (P), Phenergan (P), Practin (P), Dilosyn (P), Incidal (P); H_2 blockers cimetidine.
   With experience, most of the workers are inclined to use a combination of antihistaminics. Since they help to block the effect of released histamine at the receptors and there are two—H_1 and H_2-types of receptors, the combination is useful. In case of failure to get good response with usual antihistaminics, cimetidine should be recommended. Side effects of each antihistaminic should be properly studied. Patients should avoid driving especially when taking antihistaminics which cause drowsiness.
   c. Steroids should be used discretely in acute, severe attacks of urticaria. Their routine use is to be discouraged. In acute angioneurotic oedema with tendency to suffocation, tracheotomy is to be considered in emergency to keep the air-way open.
   d. Terbutaline and cromoglycate help to prevent release of mediators; thereby curbing the urticarial reaction right at the point of onset. Epsilon-amino-caproic acid (EACA) is useful in hereditary angioedema. Tranexamic acid and danozol have also been used. Locally, calamine lotion or Fuller's earth or diluted vinegar water is soothing to the integument. Tranquilisers, IV calcium, milk injections, autohaemotherapy, adrenaline and ephedrine have their own supporters. A quiet holiday in a quiet place with moderate climate and congenial environment may do the trick in a chronic case when other measures have failed. Authors have reported good results with *Andropogan muricatus* (*khas khas*) syrup particularly in cholinergic urticaria and patients with complaint of sense of heat.

PAPULAR URTICARIA

It affects infants and children between the age of 3 months and 6 years. It is usually seen during the summer months. It is a common condition in tropical countries.

Clinically, the lesions are erythematous macules or whitish weals, surmounted by a central papule or sometimes papulovesicle. The weal usually disappears in an hour or two, but the papulovesicle may last a few days. Lesions are accompanied by itching and scratch marks. The limbs and trunk are the sites of choice; the course is chronic with seasonal variations (Fig. 9.6).

According to some authorities, papular urticaria is due to infestation with animal parasite, *Trombicula irritans*. Lesions are arranged in lines, and may show puncture in the early stages. If an animal parasite is the cause, Crotorax (P) will cure the condition. Papular urticaria may also be caused by sensitivity to food or its digestive products, certain metabolites or focal sepsis. The treatment is on the same lines as for urticaria.

ANGIONEUROTIC OEDEMA

Synonym: Quincke's disease.

It is an acute giant variety of urticaria, characterized by the sudden development of circumscribed swellings of the skin and subcutaneous tissue, the mucous membrane

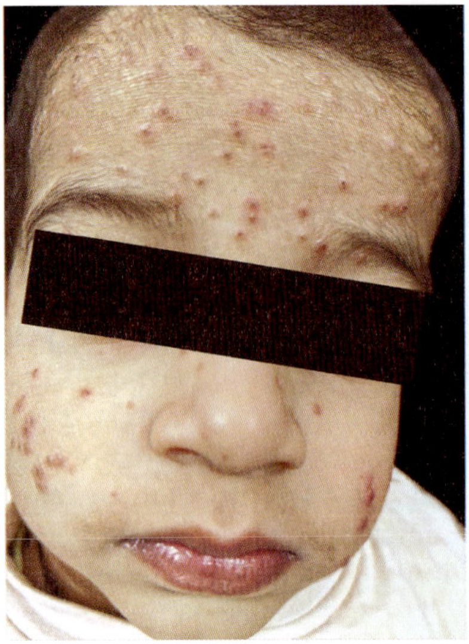

Fig. 9.6: Papular urticaria in a 2-year-old child

and submucous tissue. The swellings are reddish or skin-coloured; the local temperature may be raised. The consistency is firm. The swellings are single or multiple, usually arranged asymmetrically. The common sites involved are: the eyelids, the tongue, the lips, the glottis, the hands, the trunk, the feet and the genitalia. Angioneurotic oedema of the glottis is a serious condition because it interferes with the respiration and if not controlled in time can prove fatal.

Swellings appear suddenly, and last from a few hours to a few days, leaving neither atrophy, scars or stains when they subside. The swellings recur from time to time or in quick succession.

Angioneurotic oedema may be accompanied by urticarial lesions. There are no constitutional symptoms except for local tension, heat, pain, moderate itching and tenderness. If the gastrointestinal tract is involved, there may be a concomitant attack of colic. Involvement of the glottis, however, produces difficulty in breathing, hoarseness and even death.

Etiology: Young adults are most frequently affected, females more often than males. Heredity is an important predisposing factor. The exciting causes are: psychogenic stresses and allergic offenders, similar to urticaria.

Diagnosis: It is based upon the acute, transient and recurrent nature of these tense, circumscribed swellings. The other local causes of oedema, like insect bites, cellulitis, erysipelas, venous thrombosis, also gravitational oedema and the kind produced by lymphatic obstruction as in filariasis, should first be excluded.

Prognosis: It is favourable in the acute, cutaneous varieties . Death can occur when the glottis is involved. Recurrent cases are rather resistant to treatment.

Treatment: It is almost on the same lines as in urticaria. The patient must be reassured. The cause must be established, and an attempt made to remove it. Psychogenic cases with chronic emotional problems should be referred to a psychiatrist and/or social worker for help.

Acute cases: Treat with antihistaminics, adrenaline or corticosteroids. If the glottis is involved, and there is difficulty in breathing, a tracheotomy should be done as an emergency measure.

Chronic cases: Treat with antihistaminics, a simple diet, non-specific stimulants, sedatives and a holiday.

PURPURA

Purpura implies a haemorrhagic eruption. If it is punctate, it is called a petechial haemorrhage; if it is large in size, it is called ecchymoses. To begin with, the eruption is bright-red; however, it differs from erythema in that the redness does not disappear on pressure. It changes colour like a bruise, becomes dark-red, bluish, and then disappears in a couple of weeks. Localized purpura is due to localized injuries, sprains, blows, insect bites, needle punctures, etc. Generalized or widespread purpura signifies severe damage to the blood vessels by internal toxins, allergens or disturbance of the platelet or coagulatory mechanism **(Fig. 9.7)**. It should be viewed with concern, and the opinion of a medical expert should at once be sought.

Causes of Purpuric and Haemorrhagic Conditions

1. *Hereditary:* Haemophilia, hereditary haemorrhagic thromboasthenia. Hereditary haemorrhagic telangiectasia.
2. *Fevers:* Typhus, smallpox, scarlet fever, rheumatic fever, meningitis.
3. *Toxic:* Nephritis, septic focus, snake venom.
4. *Drugs:* Phosphorus, arsenic and anaesthetics (liver damage). Benzol, NAB, sulphones (bone marrow depression). Salicylates, penicillin, Irgapyrin (P), sedormid, sulphonamides, sera (vascular damage).

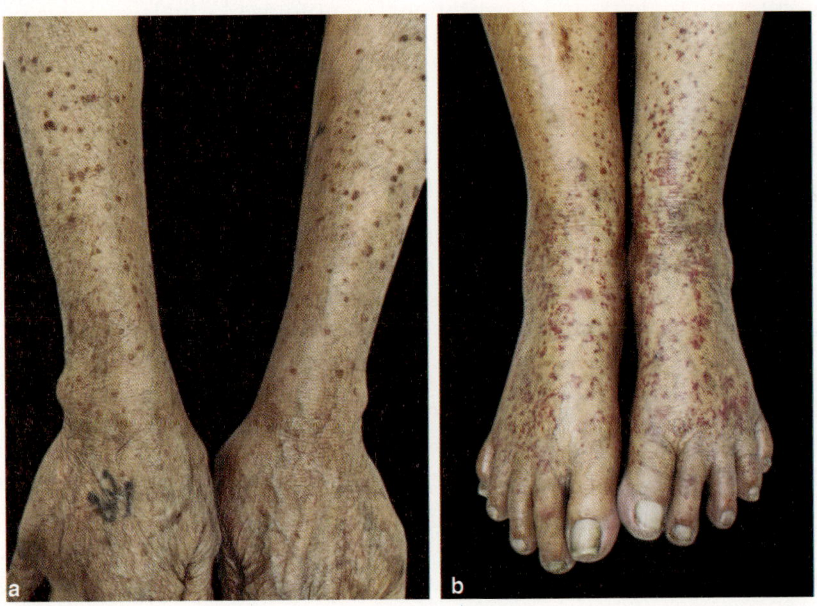

Fig. 9.7: (a) Henoch–Schönlein purpura over hands; (b) Henoch–Schönlein purpura over legs and feet

5. *Allergic and anaphy-lactoid:* Henoch–Schoenlein purpura (drugs and toxins)
6. *Liver disease (jaundice):* Acute yellow atrophy (including drugs, cirrhosis of the liver).
7. *Splenic disease:* Felty's, Banti's, Gaucher's syndromes.
8. *Bone marrow:* Thrombocytopenia-essential and idiopathic and symptomatic, aplastic anaemia, carcinomatosis, pernicious anaemia, drugs.
9. *Nutrition:* Scurvy, cachexia, vitamin K and P deficiency.
10. *Mechanical:* Hypertension, polycythemia vera, venous thrombosis and convulsions.

Only occasionally do people with purpuric and haemorrhagic conditions seek the help of a dermatologist, because these diseases come under the department of internal medicine. Hence, they are only mentioned here, with the exception of allergic and anaphylactoid purpura. A case of purpura calls for a detailed history and examination. Laboratory aids are usually resorted to for the following: The tourniquet test (Hess's), platelet count, coagulation time, bleeding time, clot retraction, prothrombin time, fibrinogen content of the blood, and a complete blood and bone marrow examination. These tests are ordered according to the provisional diagnosis.

Purpuric haemorrhages are common in thrombocytopenia (both idiopathic and symptomatic), allergy and anaphylaxis, hereditary haemorrhagic thromboasthenia and telangiectasia, liver diseases and scurvy. In others, there is only a tendency to increased bleeding.

ALLERGIC AND ANAPHYLACTOID PURPURA

Synonym: Henoch–Schönlein purpura.

The common symptoms are: purpuric spots usually on the lower limbs and buttocks, less so on the other parts of the body; urticaria, joint pains, visceral haemorrhage causing intestinal colic and malena, and constitutional symptoms like malaise, fever, headache, etc. The onset is sudden, and relapses are common. Occasionally, nephritis occurs. The blood count shows eosinophilia.

Causes

1. Streptococcal infection- tonsillitis, pharyngitis, etc.
2. Drugs like penicillin, sera, salicylates, Irgapyrin (P), sulphonamides, etc.
3. Rarely, food allergy.

Prognosis: It is good in an average case. In the severe, fulminating variety with kidney involvement, the prognosis is bad, and death may occur. In cases with recurrent causes, relapses occur.

Treatment

1. Rest in bed, light food and reassurance.
2. Treat the cause, eradicating streptococcal infection with broad-spectrum antibiotics, and by withdrawing drugs that have produced toxic effects (for details, refer to Chapter 21 on drug eruptions).
3. Symptomatic
   a. For allergy—antihistaminics, adrenaline, calcium gluconate IV, corticosteroids in severe cases.
   b. For bleeding—Vitamin C and P [Styptobion (P) tablets or injection].

Chapter

10

Dermatitis and Eczema

INTRODUCTION

Dermatitis and eczema are a common problem all over the world. Their incidence is 2–3% of all medical problems seen in practice (about 30% of all the dermatoses). Because of the jungle of terminology, definition and classification of the subject are often controversial. Despite this confusion, the two terms 'dermatitis' and 'eczema' are being used synonymously by most dermatologists. Hence, they are being lumped together.

In the practice of dermatology, the first step is to establish the clinical diagnosis of dermatitis and eczema. Then decide the clinico-morphological pattern, viz., contact, atopic, neuro-dermatitis, gravitational, endogenous or seborrhoeic. The final and most important step is to make an etiological diagnosis, i.e. establishing the role of the different cause or causes responsible for the dermatitis.

Definition: Dermatitis and eczema is non-contagious inflammation of the skin, characterized by erythema, scaling, oedema, vesiculation and oozing. Hebra says, "Eczema is what looks like eczema". Dermatitis literally means inflammation of the skin and as such can include all inflammations of the skin except by specific infections. The term 'Eczema' is a Greek word (*Ec* means out, and *Zeo* means boil). The whole word implies 'boil out'. The Hindustani name for eczema is Chambal. Eczema is a specific type of allergic cutaneous manifestation of antigen-antibody reaction. It is characterized by superficial inflammatory oedema of the epidermis associated with vesicle formation. Itching varies from mild to severe: paroxysms which may even interfere with work and sleep.

The natural history of eczema is diagrammatically represented as follows:

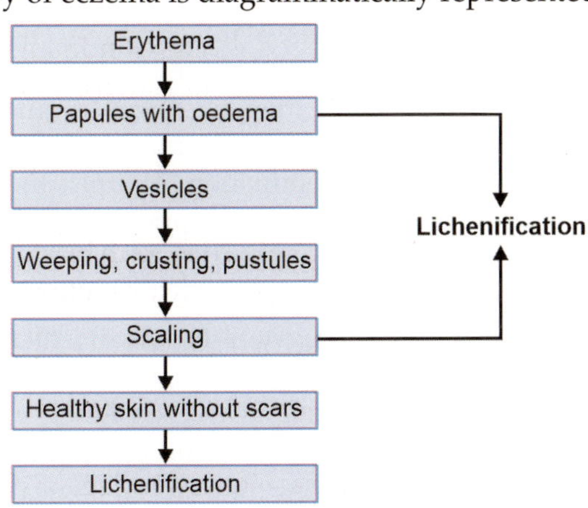

The morpho-clinical classification into acute, sub-acute and chronic stages, helps us to decide about the prognosis and the line of symptomatic treatment. The acute stage is characterized by itchy erythema followed by oedema, papules, vesicles, oozing and crusting. Most of the typical eczemas of moderate intensity start with these morphological features. This stage does not last long. In about a couple of weeks, the lesions start to heal. If the cause persists, and the eczema lasts over months or years, it becomes chronic. In such cases, the integument appears thickened and pigmented with prominent criss-cross markings (Lichenification). This is the end result of all types of long-standing eczemas. The thick, dark, Asiatic skin, has a tendency to early lichenification if not properly handled. In between the acute and chronic stages, is the sub-acute stage, characterized by papules and scaling with moderate oedema and erythema. Acute eczema may pass through this stage before it heals completely or becomes chronic.

Histopathology: Characteristic features are intercellular oedema (spongiosis) and vesicle formation. There may be mild-to-moderate dermal reaction. In chronic cases, hyperkeratosis, acanthosis and infiltration of upper dermis with lymphocytes are seen.

Etiology: Basically, two factors cause dermatitis and eczema: Firstly, an allergic or a sensitive skin, and secondly, exposure to an irritant. Darier has correctly said that, "there is no eczema but an eczematous patient."

The general predisposing causes are: age, familial predisposition, allergy, debility, climate and psychological factors. Eczema sometimes occurs in infancy, at puberty and at the time of menopause. Familial sensitiveness is an important factor. There is usually a personal or family history of allergy, viz., asthma, eczema, hay fever, etc. Genetic predisposition is responsible for the preponderance of eczemas in certain families and their absence in others. General physical debility predisposes to eczemas by lowering the resistance of the individual and hence, the threshold. Climatic extremes like heat, dampness and severe cold and also psychological stresses, promote the development of eczema. Besides the above mentioned conditions, local factors like xeroderma or ichthyosis, a greasy skin, hyperhidrosis, varicose veins causing congestion and focus of lowered resistance, hypostasis or chilblains predispose to eczema development. In the dry winters of Northern India, cracking of the integument of exposed parts may result in eczematization—"eczema crackle".

Exciting causes are varied, viz. chemicals, plants, clothing, cosmetics, medicaments, infections, drugs, diet, focal sepsis, etc. Once the skin has been irritated and sensitized, it becomes prone to further insults. Scratching, chemical trauma, climatic strains and psychogenic stresses keep the process going with the result that dermatitis becomes chronic. Auto-sensitization results in dissemination. At times, the integument becomes so sensitive that it reacts unfavourably to all applications—'status eczematicus'.

There is no eczema but an eczematous patient. Establish the cause/causative factors. While managing eczema, treat the patient and respect the skin.

It is still controversial whether the endogenous factors like diet, emotional strain and stress, focal sepsis, state of digestion, nutrition and metabolism, etc. are more important than exogenous factors like infections, irritants and sensitizers or vice versa.

In practice, mixed eczemas are much more common than pure entities. History and clinical observation are helpful in establishing the exact etiological diagnosis. The case of an eczematous patient, therefore, must be studied from all angles, attention being given to multiple precipitating, exciting and aggravating factors which may be summarized as follows:

1. Irritants—physical, chemical or electrical.
2. Sensitizers—plants, cosmetics, clothing, medicaments and occupational hazards.
3. External infections—streptococci, staphylococci, fungus, etc.
4. Mental and emotional conflicts, strains and stresses.
5. Internal septic focus shedding toxins or causing bacteraemia.
6. Diet and state of digestion.
7. Diathesis—allergic, xerodermic, hyperhidrotic or seborrhoeic.
8. Drugs—given for the disease, or otherwise.
9. State of local or general nutrition.
10. Climate—temperature and humidity.

Eczemas which appear resistant to treatment and do not correspond to the known picture, must make one suspect conditions like reticuloses and drug eruptions.

Immunology

According to Kubba (1980), what is intriguing is individual susceptibility to contact allergens. Is it genetic? However, a more important factor determining the susceptibility may be a transient or sustained malfunction in immune regulation. Sensitization develops when a different clone of T-lymphocytes is activated. The sensitized T-lymphocytes yield two sub-populations of lymphocytes, viz. memory cells that are responsible for the persistence of contact allergy, and the effector cells that initiate the allergic response when appropriately challenged.

Reaction time is the time taken by a sensitized individual to manifest a clinical reaction following contact with a known sensitizer. It is usually 12–24 hours but may vary from 1 hour to 120 hours. The reaction time is inversely proportional to the severity of the allergy.

Dissemination reaction is a fleeting, erythematous, macular reaction, involving the face and flexures, seen in some cases of contact dermatitis. There are some evidence that dissemination reaction is caused by the escape of lymphokines in the circulation resulting in vasodilatation at a distant site.

Flare reaction, another clinical feature of contact dermatitis reaction or a positive patch test reaction following renewed challenge or exposure to the same allergen at another site. This is because of persistence of sensitized lymphocytes at the site of earlier reaction, which react to minute amounts of antigen that sometimes escape in the circulation from the new site and find its way to the old site.

Langerhans cell, at long last, has been given a role. There is evidence that it may be responsible for antigen processing in contact allergy.

Studies of HLA antigens in contact allergy have so far been negative, i.e. no specific associations have been observed.

According to Baer (1981), there is possible role of systemically administered contact allergens (in the food additives, drugs, metals in prostheses, intrauterine devices, dental fillings, nickel in water and chocolates, etc.) in causing unidentifiable drug eruptions like skin lesions, flare up of old lesions and vesicular eruptions of the hands and feet.

Common example is propylene glycol used in industry as substitute for glycerine and in topical preparations.

PHOTODERMATITIS

Dermatitis in this condition, is confined to the exposed parts of the body viz., face, neck, 'V' of the chest, hands and external surfaces of the forearms and dorsa of feet and the adjoining parts of legs. Because of different clothing patterns prevalent in India, different parts of the body may be exposed producing different pictures. The integument is sensitive to sunlight and ultraviolet rays. Eruption develops, or becomes aggravated on exposure to light. Seasonal variations are an important consideration, particularly, more so, in countries with extremes of climate (Fig. 10.1). (Photosensitization dermatoses have been discussed in detail in Chapter 8)

The common causes of photodermatitis are: (i) Drugs like sulphonamides, chlorpromazine, promethazine, declamycin, terramycin, chlorthiazide diuretic, different hypo tensive and antidiabetic drugs, quindexin in animal feeding stuff. (ii) Foods like figs, buckwheat. (iii) External application of bithionol, tetrachlorsalicylanilide etc. (iv) Plants and their products-like parsnips, cow parsnips, meadow grass, mustards, lime oil, psoralea, celery, bur clover, bergamot oil, etc. Vitamin B complex deficiency, porphyrinuria, seborrhoeic diathesis and liver disorders predispose to photodermatitis.

Phytophotodermatitis means photosensitization of the skin after contact with plants which have either phototoxic or photoallergic action. The same condition has been described as Berloque dermatitis. Clinically, the lesions consist of a linear erythematous, bullous rash which heals in a week or two. On healing, pigmentation is left behind which takes several months to disappear. The rash develops after contact with the plant during, or followed by, exposure to sunlight.

Photodermatitis must be differentiated from contact dermatitis due to pollens particularly congress grass. Both occur on the exposed parts. While the former is seen in winter, the latter is seen at least to begin with, in the pollinating season, in parthenium growing areas. Both get aggravated by exposure to sun, the former more than the latter. In some cases, it is difficult to distinguish the two.

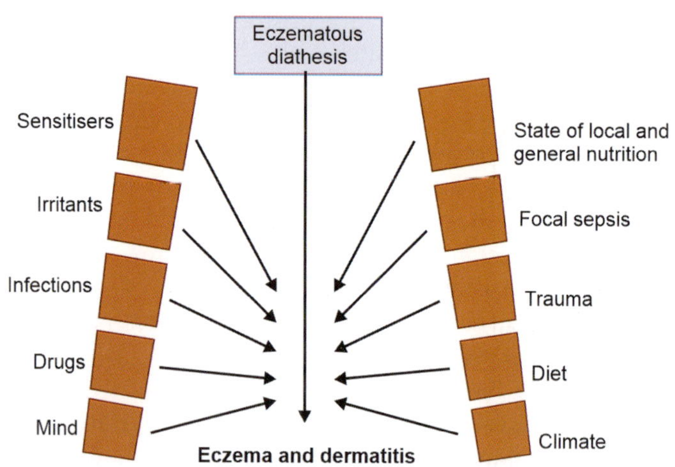

Fig. 10.1: Factors responsible for causation of dermatitis and eczema

CONTACT DERMATITIS

Synonym: Chemical eczema.

With industrialization and increasing use of chemicals and synthetics, the incidence of contact dermatitis is on the increase everywhere. Contact dermatitis develops within a few hours after contact with the offending agent (allergen to which the patient is potential ly hypersensitive). The eruption develops briskly, spreading far beyond the original point of contact. It has an ill-defined margin, fading at the periphery. Brisk oedema and uniform vesiculation are the features that dominate the eruption. Distribution depends upon the offending agent. Hence the localization of dermatitis helps in establishing the cause.

An unprejudiced history and patch tests are of considerable help in finding out the exact allergen. Failure to discover the cause results in chronic eczema and lichenification. It has been appropriately said that, especially in the diagnosis of contact dermatitis and eczema, the dermatologist should be a good "detective", with powers of observation and deduction almost like those of Sherlock Holmes. Patch tests may be done to confirm the diagnosis.

Causes of contact dermatitis:

1. Plants
2. Clothing and footwears
3. Cosmetics
4. Occupational chemicals
5. Medicaments

1. Plants: Phytodermatitis is fairly common in practice. Irritant and sensitizing properties of plants have long been known to Indian physicians. Mechanical, chemical and physical irritants should be separated from true sensitizers. Primary irritants on contact, set up dermatitis in the form of redness, blisters or even ulcers. Common examples are marking nut, cashew nut, euphorbias, buttercups, anemones, delpheniums, mustards, radish, lobelia and podophyllum. Turpentine is also a primary chemical irritant. In allergic contact dermatitis the skin reaction consists of typical eczematous lesions varying from erythema to violent vesiculation, pustulation, oozing and crusting accompanied by marked itching. The sticky sap of plants containing phenolic oily resins or like substances is usually responsible. Handling of bulbs (tulips and hyacinths) causes dryness and fissuring of fingertips.

The plants responsible for sensitization dermatitis are many and the etiological diagnosis can be difficult indeed unless this fact is borne in mind. Contact dermatitis usually occurs on the exposed parts, particularly the face and hands. Well-known examples of such plants are: Anacardiaceae (marking nut, cashew nut, mango, rhus, holigarna); Euphorbiaceae (blinding tree, castor oil plant, purging nut, euphorbias); Asclipiadaceae (Ak); compositae, (ragweed, chrysanthemums); Primulaceae (primulas); Liliaceae (tulip); Amaryllidaceae (daffodil, narcissus); celery, hops, peel of oranges and lemons; garlic and onions; chewing of plants like buttercup stalks causes severe cheilitis.

Cutting of vegetables especially garlic, onion, tomatoes, ladyfingers produces dermatitis on the tips of thumb and index fingers of left hand and right thumb. Peeling of oranges affects the thumb and index finger of right hand. The eruption develops briskly, spreading far beyond the original point of contact. It has an ill-defined margin, fading at the periphery.

Sometimes, allergic dermatitis is produced by inhalant allergies from pollens and moulds. Acute recurrences of dermatitis are observed on the head, neck, limbs, and hands which do not correspond to direct external contact; even parts covered by clothes may be affected by inhalant allergies. Occasionally, generalized erythroderma-like picture may be produced. Common example is congress grass (Air-borne contact dermatitis).

Dermatitis due apparently to plants, but really due to adventitious factors associated with plants are conveniently labelled pseudo-phyto-dermatitis (Wood). These adventitious factors are parasites, smuts and rusts, insecticides, fertilizers, fungicides (particularly those containing thiuram). Latter is also used in rubber industry and is related to disulfiram—antabuse.

The diagnosis of contact dermatitis due to plants is based on the following criteria: (i) Seasonal incidence, (ii) distribution on exposed parts, (iii) eruption, (iv) marked itching and burning sensation after exposure to contact, (v) history of previous attacks of sensitization. Diagnosis is confirmed by patch testing.

2. ***Clothing and footwears:*** The common offending substances are: Rubber chappals and footwear, spectacle frames, watch straps, furs, suspenders, artificial jewellery, clothes. The basic substances commonly responsible for contact dermatitis are rubber, nickel, dyes, synthetic finishing chemicals, resins etc. The distribution of eczema produced by clothing is typical; a knowledge of regional dermatology is very helpful.

Rubber contact dermatitis is a common problem in practice. Distribution of footwear dermatitis is typical; dorsa of the feet are more involved than the soles. It is not the natural rubber but the additives like TMT, MBEH, resins, oil, etc. which are responsible for sensitization. Dermatitis is more common in summer than in winter because of increased sweating and the leaching effect of sweat. Rubber is used in footwear particularly Hawaii chappals, also in rubber suspenders, condoms, gloves, etc.

Incidence of nickel dermatitis is markedly on the increase. Nickel in earrings, artificial jewellery, suspenders, corsets and brassiere hooks causes nickel sensitization **(Fig. 10.2)**. It takes a long time before dermatitis develops; it may extend beyond the site of contact. Car ignition key is another culprit.

Nylon dermatitis is not so common as tinea and dyshidrosis produced in individuals who wear nylon. Synthetic dyes and resins are potent sensitizers. Nylon hairnets cause dermatitis on the scalp margins, ears and back of the head.

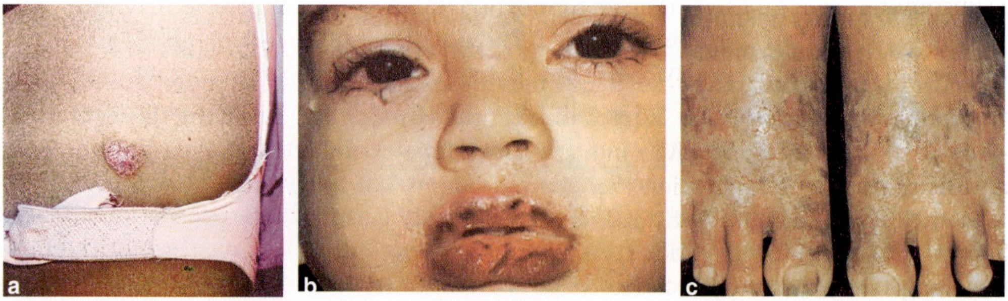

Fig. 10.2: (a) Contact dermatitis to nickel hook in the brassiere; (b) Contact dermatitis due to latex nipple; (c) Contact dermatitis due to rubber chappal

Textile dermatitis is characterized by severe itching and purpuric dermatitis on the body. The trunk is involved in *khaki* uniform dermatitis and the legs in trouser or pyjama dermatitis. Children who sleep wearing polyester clothes and wet the bed, can sometimes develop dermatitis. Urine helps to liberate formaldehyde from formaldehyde-resins used in the finish of terrycot. Most buttons are formaldehyde resins; so are tissue papers, magazine covers and sanitary napkins. Epoxy resins are also common sensitizers.

Laundry mark dermatitis (due to the juice of *Semecarpus anacardium*) is fairly common in individuals visiting India for the first time, particularly those who are sensitive to poison ivy. It causes contact dermatitis on the back of the neck (shirt), back (brassiere) and small of the back (underwear).

3. Cosmetics: Incidence of contact dermatitis due to cosmetics is on the increase all over the world, particularly in urban areas. Hair dyes, particularly the derivatives of paraphenylenediamine and *'kumkum'* are the common culprits; less so are lipstick, red sandal paste, eau de cologne, powders (particularly medicated or perfumed), face cream, nail polish and remover, eyebrow pencil, perfumes, depilatories, deodorants and hair oil. Selective distribution of dermatitis is very typical. Common ingredients in cosmetics responsible for dermatitis are the perfumes, parabens, dyes and anti-microbial agents.

Lipstick dermatitis is confined to the vermilion of the lips, the lower lip more than the upper. The presenting features are swelling and oozing or dryness and cracking . The cause is mainly the eosin dye. Such patients should be recommended a hypo-allergenic lipstick containing some other colouring agent.

Nail polish dermatitis is usually seen on the cheeks, eyelids and neck because of accidental contact depending upon the individual's habits.

Hair dye and hair oil dermatitis are common problems. Mustard and Brahmi oil (an indigenous herbal preparation) contact dermatitis should be distinguished from oil acne produced by it on the face and scalp. Dermatitis due to oil and dyes is usually severe; it affects the forehead, eyes and ears more than the scalp. A prior patch testing is essential in the prevention of hair dye dermatitis. Dermatitis of the scalp and face may also be seen following the use of shampoos, hair sprays and "wave lotions".

Deodorants and depilatories cause dermatitis in the axillae. *Bindi* (*kumkum*) is a symbolic mark Hindu women make on their foreheads with red powder, paste or liquid; Modern girls make this mark with lipstick or synthetic dyes, coloured or adhesive strips. So, the dermatitis is seen on the forehead. Similarly, *Sindhur* (mercuric sulphide) causes dermatitis on the scalp when applied at the site of parting of the hair. Henna dermatitis is uncommon, if it is pure. Perfumes commonly produce dermatitis behind the ears and upper part of breast. After-shave lotions and eau de cologne cause dermatitis on the face, neck and hands. Feminine hygiene sprays produce eczematous reaction in the vulval region and groins.

4. Occupational chemicals: With industrialization, technological advances in agriculture and increasing use of chemicals in different vocations, there is a definite rise in the incidence of contact dermatitis due to industrial and occupational agents. According to Schwartz, 80% of all occupational dermatoses are caused by primary skin irritants and not allergens. Green workers are more susceptible; with the natural process of hardening the incidence goes down, increasing again in the older age group of workers due to the ageing of the skin and lowered resistance. Besides contact dermatitis and eczema, other industrial dermatoses like warts, acne (oil acne in persons handling cutting oils), infections (folliculitis, anthrax, erysipeloid, glanders, fungus infection), dyschromias (leucoderma of tannery workers, melanodermatitis toxica, argyria, Collier's stripes), keratoses (solar, pressure and toxic), livedo reticularis (steel workers exposed to blast furnaces) and cancers (caused to persons handling tar, radium, and to chimney sweeps, etc.) may be encountered and so have to be differentiated from true dermatitis. A good physician systematically puts the condition under the right category and establishes its definite causation (Table 10.1). Important examples of dermatoses due to industrial and occupational agents are as follows:

Diagnosis is based upon the following criteria:

i. History of exposure to known offending agents.
ii. Examination shows lesions and their distribution with known pattern.

Table 10.1: Causative agents of occupational dermatitis

Occupation	*Causative agents and dermatitis*
Agriculturists and gardeners	Plants, weeds, insecticides, fertilizers and oils—mechanical injuries and contact dermatitis
Automobile	Oils, petrol, solvents, grease, paints, thinner—acne and dermatitis.
Building workers	Cement, lime, insecticides, fungicides, wood, paints, kerosene oil, turpentine oil, etc.
Chemical and pharmaceutical industries	Different dyes, chemicals, pharmaceuticals, explosives, solvents, oils, disinfectants, detergents, etc.—contact dermatitis
Coal miners	Mechanical injuries
Dentists	Cocaine and its derivatives—contact dermatitis
Engineering industries	Cutting oils, solvents, detergents, etc.—oil acne and dermatitis
Housewives	Soaps and detergents, vegetables and fruits, nickel polishes, paraphenylene diamine, keys, kerosene oil, wooden cutlery, flowers, rubber gloves and sensitisers added to foods like sodium bisulphide in salads, artificial flavours, parabens, dyes, fluorescent whitening agents in laundry products
Nurses and doctors	Iodine, streptomycin, chlorpromazine, sulphonamide, tinct. benzoin, cocaine derivatives—contact dermatitis
Painters	Turpentine, paints, detergents—contact dermatitis
Photographers	Metal, bichromate—contact dermatitis
Plastic factory workers	Resins, hardeners, solvents, glues, cellulose esters, etc.—contact dermatitis
Printers	Dyes, acrylic plates and inks causing dermatitis; rarely lichenoid rash
Rubber workers	MBEH, TMT, MBT, dyes, glues, oils, etc. contact dermatitis and depigmentation
Tannery workers	Chromate, formaldehyde, dyes, arsenic, alkalies, acids, etc. dermatitis and depigmentation
Tar workers	Dermatitis and tar acne
Textile workers	Formaldehyde, solvents, dyes, bleaches, etc. contact dermatitis

iii. More than one case of similar dermatitis in an industrial plant should cause suspicion, bearing in mind the new techniques and chemical processes added to industry from time to time.
iv. Confirmation by patch testing.

Do specific patch test with suspected agents in clinically obvious cases of contact dermatitis. In chronic, resistant cases and also atopic ones it is worth- while to test with a standard battery of common allergens.

It has to be stressed that contributory factors like environment, trauma, infections, constitutional and genetic factors (diathesis), psychogenic stresses, previous sensitization, pre-existing diseases and the cleaning agents used to clean up at the end of the day's work must be taken into consideration in proper evaluation of the patient.

A good industrial dermatologist helps to educate the workers on how to prevent industrial disease and dermatoses, use proper garments, boots and gloves, avoid direct contact and provide proper environment. Barrier cream and silicone cream also help in preventing contact dermatitis. For further information, reference should be made to detailed books on the subject (*see* "List of Reference Books" at the end of the book).

As a general rule, dyes, synthetic chemicals, plastics and resins are the basic offenders. Substances and materials containing these should arouse suspicion. Patients and their relatives have a tendency to distort facts when giving history. There is absolutely no place for prejudice and haste in history taking. Quite often the patient is allergic to more than one thing; besides, he may have used a certain agent all his life, and suddenly one fine day finds himself sensitive to it. A history of familial sensitiveness to such agents is also helpful.

Contact dermatitis sometimes fails to respond to treatment because of certain complicating factors like super-added infections, emotional stresses, focal sepsis, additional sensitizations arising from the patient's hobbies, friction, scratching, etc. An attempt must be made to eliminate these complicating causes too, in addition to the basic offending agent (Refer to **Table 10.2** for more detail).

5. Medicaments: Almost every medicament may cause reaction occasionally but common examples are the sulphonamides, penicillin, Furacin (P), streptomycin, cocaine derivatives (local anaesthetics), tincture benzoin, neomycin, formalin, Phenargan (P) cream and sticking plaster. Savlon (P), Cetavlon (P), and Dettol (P) are primary irritants.

During the use of these medicaments, any untoward reaction should be noted and investigated. Amongst doctors, nurses, and dentists, dermatitis is occupational and is usually seen on the dorsa of hands. In the patient, site of contact or application is affected.

Anaesthetic and antipruritic ointments are common culprits. Antihistaminic creams are also allergenic **(Table 10.3)**.

INFECTIOUS ECZEMATOID DERMATITIS

Synonym: Infective eczema.

This results from sensitization to certain organisms like streptococci, staphylococci, dermatophytes and yeast organisms. Infective eczemas are very common in tropical countries; about three-fourths of hospital eczema cases fit into this category . Clinically, they are characterized by their slow development; so no vesiculation is usually evident, a crust

Table 10.2: A list of common regional contactants

Face	• Those directly applied like cosmetics—face powder, cream, bindi, vermilion (*sindhur*), eyebrow pencil, perfume, soap, oil (Brahmi, Loma and Cantharidine etc.), shampoos, dyes (Inecto, Crest and paraphenylenedixmine (PARA), etc.), spectacle frames, hat-bands. The distribution is typical in all these contactants. • Volatile-dust, pollens (Airborne contact dermatitis), fumes, paints. • Those conveyed by the patient's fingers—almost any irritant or sensitizer may get onto the face, since it is natural for any person to touch the face with the fingers from time to time. Nail varnish is a common example.
Lips	Lipstick, toothpaste, cigarette holders, pipes and balloons.
Neck	Scarf, dyed fur, collar, collar buttons, marking ink, jewellery (particularly chrome or nickel), hat strap, perfume.
Body	Clothing, buttons, marking ink (*dhobi*'s mark).
Axillae	Dress, armpit pads, dyes, depilatories, deodorants, astringents.
Genitals and Anal region	Contraceptives (rubber, quinine and other chemicals), toilet paper, medicaments used by Women in douches, anti-pruritics (particularly cocaine derivatives), feminine hygiene sprays, nylon/plastic underwear.
Buttock	Toilet paper, lavatory seat (varnish), jute and straw mattresses, toy horses.
Hands	Occupational—primary irritants and sensitisers. Hobbies—gardening, photography, painting, etc. Cutting vegetables like garlic, onions, tomatoes, ladyfingers, drivers steering wheel, ignition key; detergents, cigarette paper, etc.
Wrist	Watch and its strap, bracelet and bangles.
Thighs	Clothing, things in pockets particularly matchboxes, and suspenders (rubber or nickel).
Feet	Footwear, shoes (chrome dyes and rubber). The dorsum and sides of the feet are selectively involved, interdigital spaces are spared (comparison: tinea pedis). Coloured socks (dyes and nylon), elastic shoe strap.

Table 10.3: Ten common allergens come across in practice

1. Paraphenylene diamine	6. Neomycin sulphate
2 Nickel sulphate	7. Formaldehyde
3. Potassium dichromate	8. Turpentine
4. Parthenium hysterophorus	9. Garlic
5. Nitrofurazon ointment	10. Epoxy resin

is formed instead. The patch or patches are sharply defined, and there is no erythematous halo; they take the form of circles which by union become polycyclic . The lesions spread not only by direct contiguity but also to the other body folds, parts and hair follicles **(Fig. 10.3)**. These eczemas respond to mild antiseptic astringents. They become notoriously recurrent in some cases. A trivial itch is sufficient to reproduce it; the genetic susceptibility for sensitization seems operative. Infectious eczematoid dermatitis is commoner in the monsoon and summer than in the winter.

Infective eczemas can be divided further into three sub-types according to their distribution:

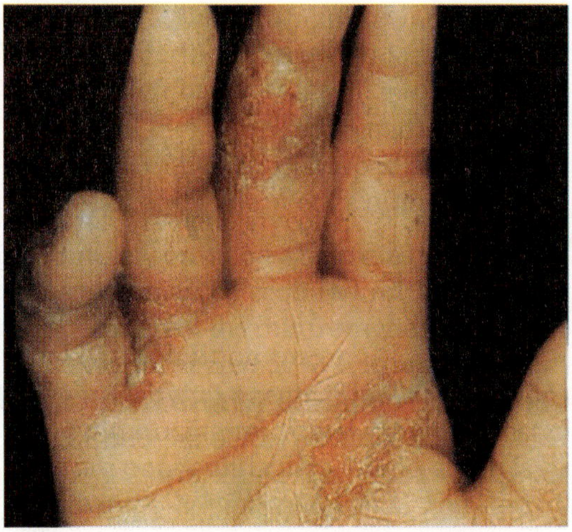

Fig. 10.3: IED secondary to scabies

Post-traumatic infective eczema: The history is usually very typical. It starts with a crack in the integrity of the skin brought on by an injury, a blister, an insect bite or exposure to a severe cold wind, etc. This gets infected; sensitization results in eczematization and a well-defined circular or oval patch of eczema consisting of erythema, oozing and crusting is formed. If there are several patches, the intervening skin is completely clear. Similarly, prickly heat can become eczematized.

Eczematization, secondary to acute tinea, particularly tinea pedis, is frequently seen. It starts from the interdigital spaces and spreads to the dorsum of the feet or the soles. Treatment has to be skilful; the condition must first be treated like eczema. Only when the eczematization process has been controlled completely, must fungicidal agents be employed .

Follicular infective eczema: It involves hairy regions, like the scalp, beard and legs. When it occurs on the scalp, it is often labelled as seborrhoeic dermatitis. It starts usually with pityriasis capitis which gets complicated by one or several itchy patches of oozing, pits and crusting. These patches become confluent. The eczema spreads to the forehead, retroauricular folds and cheeks. Streptococci, staphylococci and, less so, pityrosporon species are the causative organisms. If accompanied by seborrhoeic diathesis, both the infective eczema and seborrhoeic background should be treated at the same time. Infective eczematides may develop later, on the back, sternal region, pubic region, arms and legs, if the disease is not properly controlled. On the beard region, it must always be differentiated from ordinary folliculitis. The latter is a chronic disease, spreads slowly, and there is no oozing or itching in contrast with infective eczema. In infants, cradle cap may get complicated by infective or seborrhoeic dermatitis. True constitutional infantile eczema should be excluded in such cases.

Flexural infective eczema: The flexures (body folds) are the sites of predilection. Common examples are: the retroauricular folds, the eyelids, the neck folds, the axillae, the cubital fossae, the groins and the popliteal fossae. It starts with a crack in the depth of the fold, and the two opposing surfaces are equally' affected like the leaves of a book. The inner part looks moist and red; only at the periphery is crusting clearly evident. In the groins, it usually complicates simple intertrigo; oozing and crusting are added to the redness and maceration of intertrigo. Tinea cruris can be eliminated by the fact that it affects the inner surfaces of the thighs, but spares the inguinal fold; the peripheral border is most inflamed consisting of vesicles and pustules; the scraping for fungus is positive.

ENDOGENOUS ECZEMAS

There is no evidence of external irritants or allergens in endogenous eczema; parts of the body become sensitized to internal body products-toxins from focal sepsis, metabolites, i.e. products of digestion or elements of diet and drugs—with or without familial predisposition. To this list should be added psychosomatic influences. ln most cases, the cause is hypothetical; big names often boil down to nothing in practical dermatology. For this reason, the treatment of endogenous eczemas is rather unsatisfactory, and will remain so, till more light is shed on their exact etiology and pathogenesis.

There are three common patterns produced according to their distribution: (1) Atopic—involving the eyelids, the sides of neck, the cubital fossae and the popliteal fossae. (2) Nummular pattern—affecting the dorsum of fingers and hands, the feet, the arms and the thighs; in short, the extremities. (3) Centripetal pattern—affecting the trunk, particularly, the upper chest, the scapular and gluteal regions. Then, there is the sympathetic variety in which the corresponding site on the other extremity is affected through endogenous distribution from a patch of eczema on one extremity. This sympathetic dennatitis is comparable with sympathetic ophthalmia seen in eye lesions. Occasionally, unilateral dissemination of eczema from the right foot to the right hand, and the left foot to the left hand is seen. How nature brings about these selective affections and disseminations is difficult to explain. The common sub-varieties of endogenous eczemas are infantile eczema, atopic eczema, nummular eczema, disseminated eczema and cheiropompholyx.

INFANTILE ECZEMA

This occurs in children between the ages of three months and two years. It usually starts on the cheeks, spreading slowly to the forehead, chin, scalp, arms, trunk and legs. On the buttocks and in the groins, napkin rash-like dermatitis may develop. The dermatitis are characterized by erythema, vesicles, exudation and crusting. Pruritus is a prominent symptom; it comes in spasms. The progress is marked by spontaneous remissions and exacerbations. Teething, digestive upsets, change of season, dietetic indiscretions and tantrums affect lhe condition adversely, and may even cause flare-ups. To start with, the infants are 'usually plump. They soon go off food, have restless days and nights resulting in debility, misery and fretfulness. The general belief is that there are two types of infantile eczemas:

1. With high famílial predisposition to an allergic disease—the atopic variety. These are rather resistant to treatment. The infant becomes restless, fatigued, very irritable and pruritic. The condition develops later into typical atopic dermatitis.
2. Without familial predisposition—the simple variety. The infants are plump and good natured. Itching is moderate. These do well with treatment, and the child recovers completely by the age of two.

Table 10.4: Distinguishing features of true infantile and seborrhoeic eczema

Infantile eczema	*Seborrhoeic eczema*
Disease develops at 3–6 months after birth, sometimes earlier.	'Cradle cap' at the time of birth, seborrhoeic dermatitis afterwards.
Child is irritable and weak.	Child is usually healthy and happy otherwise.
Starts from cheeks and extends to forearms and legs.	Starts from scalp. posterior auricular folds, and involves neck and trunk. On the trunk flat macular erythematous or hypopigmented and scaly rash. In some cases, it manifests as diaper dermatitis.
Oozing more. Areas look clean.	Crusting more and the areas have a dirty appearance.
Family history of atopic disorders except in simple variety.	Family history of seborrhoeic disorders.
Itching is severe and spasmodic.	Itching, mild to moderate.
Recurrences frequent and usually independent of season	Recurrences mostly seasonal, i.e. summer and monsoon; at times in winter also.
On the whole, poor response to treatment.	Comparatively better response.

Parents must be told that infantile eczemas are not infectious, and they heal completely without scarring unless a secondary infection occurs. Contact eczemas are rare in infancy for two reasons: Firstly, sensitivity is extremely uncommon before puberty, and secondly, chemical contacts are few. But one does see infective or seborrhoeic eczema in infancy **(Table 10.4)**. This type of eczema starts as scruff or cradle cap on the scalp which develops into slight exudation and thick crusting; eczema spreads from the scalp to the auricular region, the periphery of the face and neck, sparing the centre of the face in comparison with true constitutional infantile eczema. Similarly, infective eczema in infancy may develop as a complication of suppurative otitis media, conjunctivitis, rhinitis or neglected boils and impetigo. The response to mild antiseptics is good in this infective variety.

Etiology: The exact causation of infantile eczema is not well-established but the following factors must be kept in mind. Dietetic allergies may play an important role in the causation. Infants who are overfed, and are too rapidly introduced to adult foodstuffs, frequently suffer from infantile eczema. In the authors' experience infantile eczema is rather uncommon amongst Indian infants who are fed the conservative way, namely they are given mainly milk only for the first year; eggs, bread, fruit and vegetables being added slowly in second year.

Treatment

1. The diet must be corrected, breast-feeding stopped, and powdered milk substituted; the type of powdered milk depends on what suits the patient. Other foodstuffs should not be added too quickly.
2. Physical restraint, to prevent scratching, with the help of splints and bandages.
3. Palliative treatment on the lines discussed at the end of the chapter. Use of steroids should be restricted.
4. The general state of nutrition must be maintained; sedatives are useful as a standby.

General Instructions for Infantile Eczema Patients

1. The child should be bathed in 1 in 8,000 warm Condy's solution, or bran bath, and then, blotted dry with a smooth towel. If water is not tolerated, the tender skin may be cleansed with a little boiled milk. Following this, a simple talcum powder may be used, or a lotion or cream prescribed. Any soothing preparation is suitable for eczema, but strong ointments often do more harm than good.
2. Cardboard splints may be necessary to prevent the child from scratching and damaging the skin. If these are not used, the hands should be restrained by bandages at nights. Mittens should also be used on the hands.
3. A mixture, if prescribed, ensures sleep and prevents the child from scratching himself.
4. The normal diet may be given; but if certain foodstuffs constantly aggravate the skin condition, they should be omitted. Diet diary or single foodstuff eliminative diet is useful.
5. Healthy play should be encouraged, because if the child's attention is diverted from his skin, there will be better chances for a quick recovery. The child should not be allowed to play with fluffy toys, grass, flowers and weeds without the permission of the specialist in charge.
6. Fresh air and the mild sun are usually beneficial, but sunburns should be avoided.
7. Woollen garments should not be worn next to the irritated skin.

ATOPIC ECZEMA

Synonym: Besnier's prurigo. It is also called asthma–eczema syndrome.

There is a strong familial predisposition to allergic diseases like asthma, eczema and hay fever; frequently, a personal history of collateral allergies is present. The eczema is characterized by a selective flexural distribution, extreme chronicity with acute exacerbations from time to time, a familial and personal allergic predisposition and a very sensitive emotional nature. The eczematous process is usually the result of endogenous sensitization, but exogenous allergies may also play a part. The latter can be proved by patch tests, and the former, by scratch tests, which show allergy to multiple agents. There is more than normal susceptibility to develop passive transfer antibodies in the blood serum (Prausnitz Kustner reaction). Besides allergens, emotional stresses and parental attitudes can also cause this condition. The parents are usually the anxious type, and the patient is usually very sensitive and highly strung but often very intelligent. The atopic patient is also very sensitive to physical stresses like heat, cold and humidity and also infectons. There is also vasomotor sensitivity.

Clinical features are rather characteristic **(Fig. 10.4)**. The integument is generally dry and rough with a definite tendency to dermographism. The eyelids, the sides of the neck, the popliteal and cubital fossae are the sites predominantly affected. Itching is a predominant symptom; it usually occurs in spasms. Clinically, there are three stages of atopic eczema: (1) Infantile stage, described above. (2) Childhood type, in which the main lesions are lichenoid and succulent, polyhedral papules. The eczema may become generalized on the face, trunk and upper part of the extremities. It starts at about the age of five, either as such, or as a continuation of infantile eczema; this goes on till the age of about twelve (3) Adult type is marked by ill-defined, lichenoid patches, scratch marks and blood crusts with exacerbations of acute eczema from time to time.

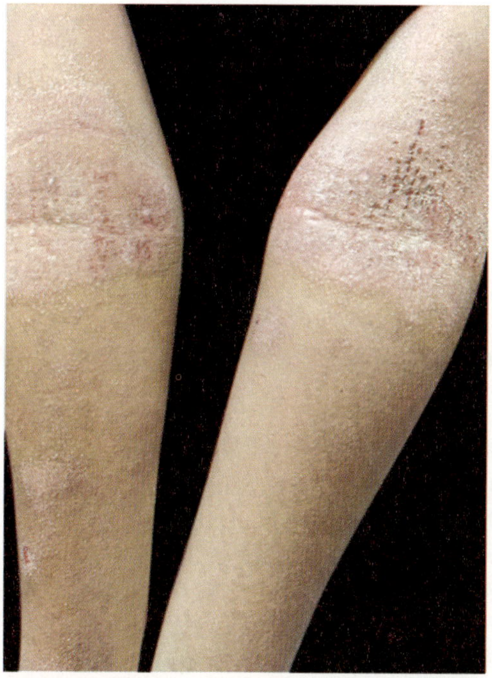

Fig. 10.4: Atopic dermatitis in a 12-year-old boy

The skin is dry and injures easily. This stage is most marked till the age of 25, and may last through life.

There may be associated cataract. Intolerance to high temperatures and humidity is fairly common.

Diagnosis is not difficult in a typical case. In an atypical case, differentiation is from lichen simplex chronicus, endogenous dermatitis, seborrhoeic dermatitis and prurigo. In every case, an attempt should be made to establish the specific etiology and assess the personality of the individual.

Prognosis: The course of atopic eczema through all stages is marked by spontaneous cures, remissions and exacerbations. Seasonal variation is autumn and spring, by pollens; summer and monsoon, by heat and high humidity. Besides eczema, asthma, hay fever and other allergies may be present at the same time or may alternate with eczema. Lately attention has been drawn to ophthalmic changes in connection with atopic dermatitis; they are conjunctivitis, keratitis, and juvenile cataracts. The pathogenesis of these is not understood. It may also be associated with other ectodermal defects. There is a constitutional susceptibility to different stresses. The blood count shows eosinophilia.

Etiology: In every case, an attempt should be made to discover the cause or causes: (1) Emotional—by psychiatric evaluation of the patient's home, parents' occupation and other environments. (2) Allergic—by a search into his diet, external contacts and inhalants, if any.

A detailed history will help considerably; also the patient's own ideas as to the cause, an eliminative diet or diet diary, along with scratch and patch tests. As a general rule, it should be impressed upon the patient that he has an inborn weakness of the skin, and an unstable, emotionally sensitive nature, and that he should learn to live with these weaknesses, avoiding stresses as far as possible.

Treatment: It consists in:

1. Impressing upon the patient the etiological factors—the allergic, psychogenic and inborn weakness of his skin.
2. Advice about climate and occupation.
3. Corticosteroids—locally and systemically should be used discriminately.
4. General palliative treatment.
5. X-ray therapy in chronic cases.

Extensive cases try the patience and ingenuity of the attending doctor. Extensive and resistant cases, therefore, should be treated in hospitals, and an attempt made to change the patient's environment after his discharge.

General Instructions for Atopic Eczema Patients

1. The patient should have a warm starch bath in winter and a cold Condy' s bath in summer. After the bath, he should blot himself with a smooth towel and avoid rubbing. Olive oil or lanoline cream may be applied on the dry, thickened skin after the bath. In generalized dermatitis, or dryness of the skin, an oil, butter or ghee massage for about an hour before a bath, helps lubricate and soften the skin. 10% urea ointment is also beneficial.
2. Moderate temperature suits these patients best, and so they should avoid extremes of climate. Where it is not possible to change the place of residence, air-conditioning is the answer.
3. The patient should not scratch and keep his nails short. In resistant cases, particularly in children, measures for physical restraint by splints should be employed, and sedatives given at night.
4. The diet should be light. The exact composition of the diet depends upon the history of the patient, the diet diary and the results of the allergy tests. Allergenic food-stuffs should be avoided.
5. The patient should be told not to fatigue himself either physically or mentally.
6. Healthy hobbies and play should be encouraged. They help to divert attention and speed up recovery. Play with fluffy toys, grass, flowers and chemicals should be forbidden.
7. Any side-effect while taking medication should be reported to the physician. Local medicaments should be properly employed .
8. Relatives must be advised to respect the patient's weakness of the skin and his sensitivities.
9. The patient should learn to live within the limits of his mental and physical strength, knowing his inborn weakness. It is a chronic but not a serious disease and, therefore, should not depress him. He should avoid anger, resentment and frustration.

NUMMULAR ECZEMA

Synonym: Discoid eczema.

It is characterized by circular coin-shaped plaques of papules, vesicles and crusting, distributed bilaterally and symmetrically on the dorsum of fingers, the hands, the

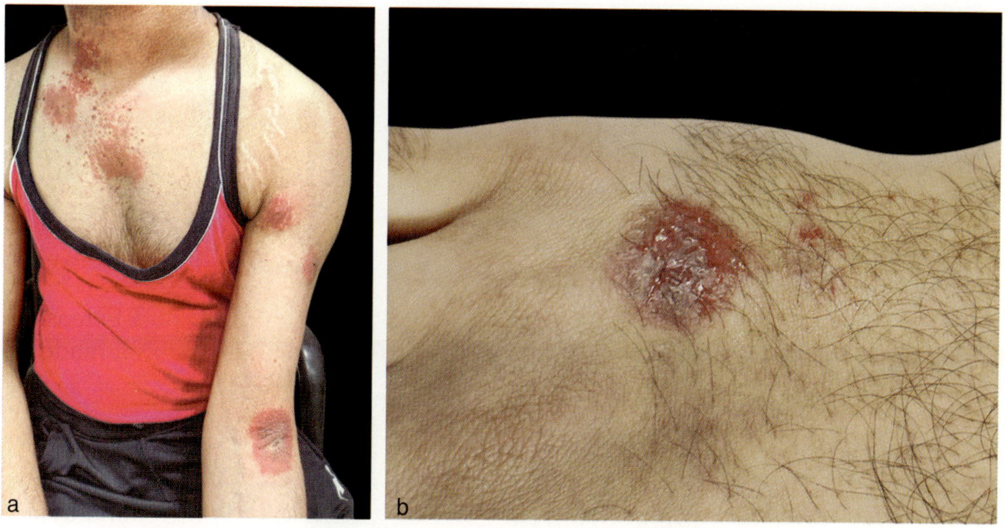

Fig. 10.5: (a) Nummular eczema; (b) Coin-shaped lesions of nummular eczema

forearms, the arms, the legs and the thighs. These plaques may enlarge slowly with a tendency to clear at the centre. The condition is chronic and recurrent (Fig. 10.5).

Etiology and pathogenesis: These are not definitely established; psychogenic stresses, focal sepsis, food allergies, alcohol, debility and drugs are usually held responsible. A dry skin and cold weather may be associated with it.

Nummular eczema should be distinguished from circular patches of infective eczema and tinea circinata. Both of these are asymmetrical, acute and non-recurring conditions. Focal sepsis may produce bilaterally symmetrical patches of infective eczematoid dermatitis resembling discoid dermatitis; these do well with administration of appropriate antibiotics, with the surgical removal of the septic focus, and the local use of mild antiseptics.

Dermatitis papulosa alba (Sugarthan) and miliarial dermatitis (Behl) are seen in the hot summer, on forearms; sweat retention may be the exciting cause. Sometimes, discoid dermatitis may be associated with dyshidrosis of palms and soles, and discoid patches of keratoderma.

Treatment: This consists in reassuring the patient, correcting the known etiological factors, administering antihistaminics and according to the morphological appearance, in resistant cases, steroid application and pix liquida prove helpful. Dry skins are massaged with oil and the nutritional status of the patient must be improved.

DISSEMINATED ECZEMA

Synonym: Eczematides.

It is characterized by tiny papular, vesicular and occasionally, bullous crusted lesions occurring singly or in small patches resulting from sensitization to the products of primary active eczema being conveyed by the bloodstream to distant sites producing dissemination of the eczematous process. This process is called auto-sensitization, brought on particularly by the use of strong medicaments (irritants or sensitizers, or

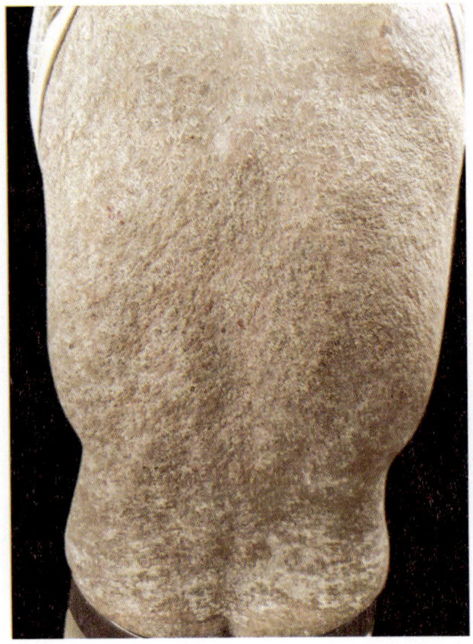

Fig. 10.6: Disseminated eczema

both) applied to the primary eczematous site. When primary eczema is infective, the eczematides are termed infective eczematides (Fig. 10.6).

Sympathetic dermatitis from one foot to another, and unilateral eczematides from one foot to the hand on the same side, are further examples of dissemination. Primary active eczemas on the feet usually disseminate to the palms, producing an eruption resembling cheiropompholyx; primary eczemas on the hands disseminate to the ears, face and trunk. If the process is wide-spread, bilaterally symmetrical and generalized eczema may develop, which may involve even the face, accompanied by swelling of the eyelids.

Constitutional symptoms like fever, headache, pains and malaise, are produced by toxaemia during dissemination. The patient looks ill and weak. Disseminated eczemas should not be treated lightly. Firstly, they take a long time to heal, and even after the condition clears up, the integument is left in a weak and hypersensitive state, and is, for some time, prone to pyoderma. Secondly, patients suffering from this kind of eczema are very sensitive to local medication, therefore, the medication employed should be as simple as possible. In underdeveloped Asiatic countries, disseminated eczemas are a common problem because of the ill-treatment of primary eczemas by the laity and the presence of quacks. If scientific treatment is delayed, recurrences are common and eczema becomes chronic.

Eczematides must be distinguished from other ide-eruptions, namely:

1. Dermatophytides. Ide-eruption from a primary active fungus infection. When it is due to trichophyton, it is called trichophytide; when due to epidermophyton, it is called epidermophytide.
2. Seborrhoeides from seborrhoeic dermatitis of the scalp.
3. Bacterides from a primary bacterial septic focus. They are found on the soles and palms when there is a septic focus in the nose, throat, lungs and abdomen.
4. Tuberculides from a primary active tuberculous focus.

VARICOSE DERMATITIS OR ECZEMA

This is simply traumatic, chemical or infective eczema, complicating varicose veins or ulcers of the legs. The predisposing factors are chronic congestion and stasis which lower the local resistance. A similar situation is created by hypostasis following white leg in pregnancy, and fracture in the lower extremities. The dorsum of the foot and lower part of the leg show telangiectases, oedema and pigmentation produced by varicose veins. Itching in varicose legs may start eczema by excoriation, secondary infection and by the use of medicaments. The eczema has the features of the exciting cause which may be traumatic, chemical or infective (Fig. 10.7).

Varicose eczema may become disseminated due to auto-sensitization. Because of the indolent nature of the basic condition, varicose veins and hypostasis–varicose dermatitis is a very chronic and persistent condition. Secondary complications like thrombophlebitis are common.

Treatment: It consists in (1) Controlling the congestion and stasis by avoiding 'long hours of standing, elevating the legs while resting, foot exercises. (2) Crepe bandages or elastic stockings. (3) Injections or surgery for the varicose veins. (4) Symptomatic treatment of eczema.

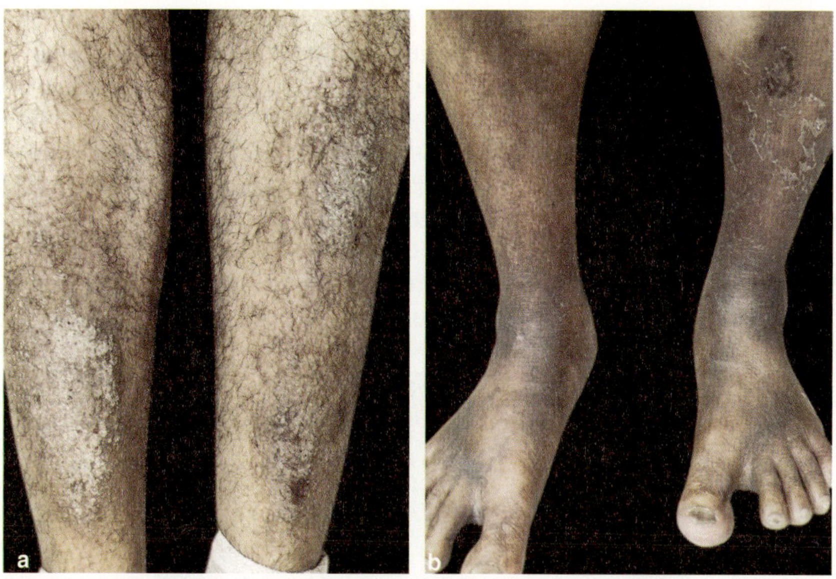

Fig. 10.7: (a) Stasis dermatitis with lichenification; (b) Stasis dermatitis with nail dystrophy

NEURODERMATITIS

Synonym: Lichen simplex chronicus.

Affecting more commonly neurotic people, this condition may be defined as the lichenification process resulting from chronic scratching and rubbing of the skin under stress and anxiety. The condition is common amongst young people and menopausal women. These patients tend to tear off their skin when they cannot get at others for social reasons. Any emotional conflicts particularly those arising from sex, financial

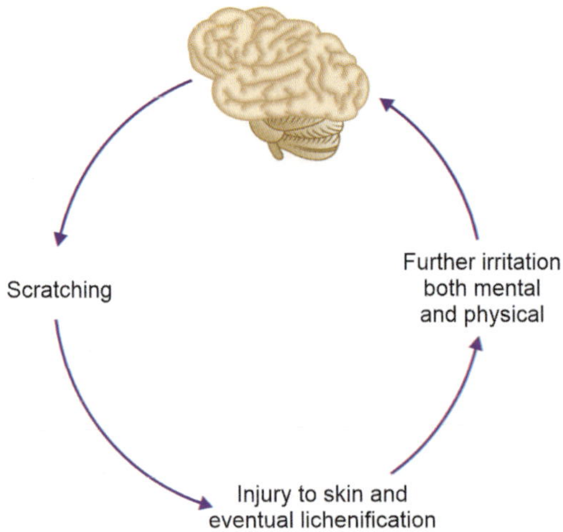

Fig. 10.8: Vicious cycle in neurodermatitis

and social problems, may initiate itching; scratching produces further irritation, and a vicious cycle is established resulting in lichenification (Fig. 10.8).

The integument becomes thickened, infiltrated and pigmented; the criss-cross markings become more prominent. Margins are irregular but usually well-defined. There may be one or several localized patches. Occasionally, an extensive disseminated variety of neurodermatitis may be seen with multiple disseminated lesions of lichenified integument. The sites commonly affected are: the nape of the neck, arms, ano-genital area, scrotum, back of knees, legs and ankles (Fig. 10.9).

Chronic eczemas may become lichenified through constant scratching. Lichenification is a prominent feature of atopic eczema. In the dark Indian skin, lichenification occurs early. Neurodermatitis should be distinguished from lichenified eczemas, atopic dermatitis and lichen planus hypertrophicus.

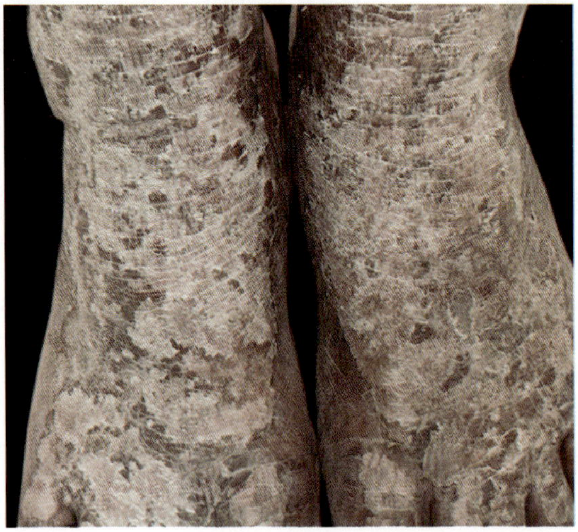

Fig. 10.9: Neurodermatitis showing chronic lichenification

Prognosis: This is good if the primary emotional conflict can be resolved satisfactorily.

Treatment consists of psychotherapy, tranquillizers and locally, crude tar, hydrocortisone ointment and Grenz-ray therapy. In practice, satisfactory response is obtained with occlusive dressing of steroid ointments especially betamethasone valerate and triamcinolone acetonide. Dermabrasion helps in bringing the skin appearance to normal.

RADIODERMATITIS

It implies dermatitis produced by excessive doses of X-rays received by the skin. This was common in the past when X-ray machines were crude and people, inexperienced. Acute radiodermatitis is rarely seen; what one usually comes across in practice is the chronic type. The features of acute radiodermatitis depend upon the degree of burn, and hence, vary from erythema, scaling, vesicular or bullous reaction to ulceration; in chronic cases, there is a long latent period of months and years, followed by redness, telangiectasia, pigmentation and atrophy. In severe cases, however, ulceration and even epitheliomas may develop. Hydrocortisone lotion is helpful , and so also is the juice of the '*Aloe vera*' (Hindustani name: *gwar ka patha*). Plastic surgery gives the best results in chronic localized X-ray burns with ulcers and a tendency to neoplasms. Epitheliomas caused by X-ray burns, should, under no circumstances, be treated with further X-ray therapy. Complete excision and Z-plasty/skin flap are the answer.

DERMATITIS MEDICAMENTOSA

It comprises all cutaneous eruptions resulting from the internal (by mouth or injections) use of drugs. These have been discussed in detail in Chapter 21.

DERMATITIS AUTOPHYTICA

Synonym: Dermatitis artefacta.

It implies self-produced dermatitis brought on with strong physical agents or acids by hysterical individuals. Young single girls are the usual victims; sympathy is the motive. The sites of affection are the commonly accesible regions. Lesions have the features of dermatitis, but are usually bizarre and do not conform to any known picture. The use of liquid irritants by the patient produces trickle lines.

DYSHIDROSIS

Synonym: Cheiropompholyx.

It consists of bilaterally symmetrical eruption affecting the palms of hands, and less frequently, the sides and soles of feet. Lesions consist of deeply-set vesicles, looking like embedded sago grains, accompanied by tingling, burning and itching. The interdigital spaces, the sides of fingers and the palms are the typical sites **(Fig. 10.10)**. The dorsum of the hands is rarely affected. The vesicles dry up in 10–14 days, leaving behind slight scaling. Sometimes they become infected with pyogenic organisms, or complicated by infective eczema. To begin with, the condition is acute and occurs in attacks. If the attacks become frequent, and the condition becomes chronic, the clinical picture shows a thick hyperkeratotic skin accompanied by deeply-set vesicles. At times, it takes a dry and hyperkeratotic form from the very beginning, then it is called dyshidrosis sicca.

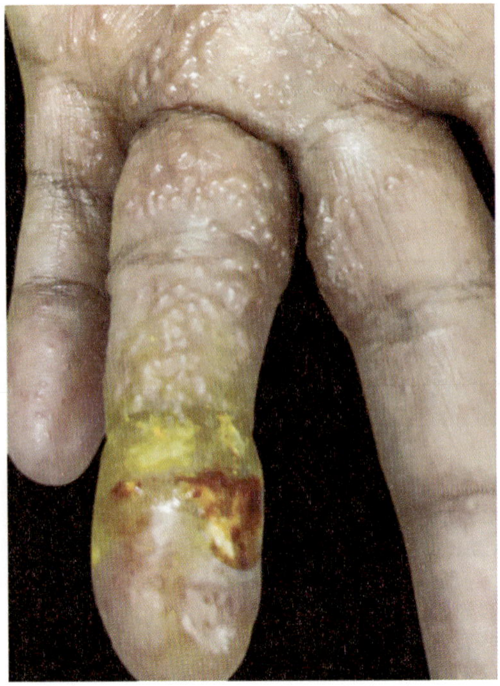

Fig. 10.10: Dyshidrotic eczema (Pompholyx)

Etiology: The disease usually affects neurotic individuals with hyperhidrosis of the hands. Psychogenic stresses and active focal sepsis are the important causes. The disease usually occurs at the change of seasons, particularly in spring and summer, and may develop every year at the same time.

Differential diagnosis: Cheiropompholyx has nothing to do with the obstruction of the sweat glands. It must be distinguished from ide-eruption, in which a similar clinical picture is produced by active fungus infection in the feet; eczematides; contact dermatitis and drug eruptions. History and physical examination help in establishing the diagnosis. In contact dermatitis, lesions are confined to specific fingers—thumb and index fingers due to cutting vegetables and flower bulbs, middle and ring fingers to cigarette paper and dorsum of fingers due to soaps and detergents. Condition is usually asymmetrical. If the primary lesion is pustular from the beginning, pustular bacteride should be suspected, and a search made for a septic focus. The hyperkeratotic form should be distinguished from other types of keratoderma.

Treatment: It consists of (1) Correcting the causative psychological factors and focal sepsis. (2) Local palliative treatment in the form of Condy's soaks, 1 in 4,000 solution, for 15–30 minutes every morning, or Burrow's solution soaks or alum or hydrocortisone lotion application. (3) Sedatives and antihistaminics. (4) In resistant cases, X-ray therapy in small doses.

PERIORAL DERMATITIS

Dermatitis is seen on the lower part of the face, mainly chin and around the mouth. Erythema is more evident and is accompanied by slight crusting or scaling and

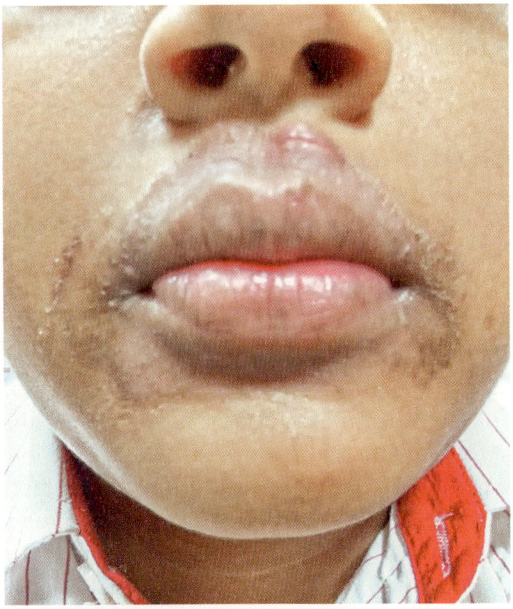

Fig. 10.11: Perioral dermatitis

itching; oozing is little (Fig. 10.11). Presumable causes are seborrhoea, emotional stress, gastrointestinal disturbances, photosensitivity, hormonal contraceptives and use of fluorinated steroids. Course is chronic, slow and insidious with occasional exacerbations. Treatment consists of correction of the underlying causes, local use of calamine lotion and a course of tetracycline 1 g daily till the disease is controlled and then maintained on 250 mg biweekly for 6–8 weeks or so. *Andropogan muricatus* infusion is very beneficial.

Prognosis in Dermatitis and Eczema

The outlook rests mainly on correct elicitation and the complete eradication of the cause or causes. It is regrettable that potential sensitizers are sold so freely in the market and advertised as panaceas in the lay press. The skin is a superficial subject and so it is easily accessible to over-treatment and ill-treatment.

Dermatitis and eczema are, as a rule, curable conditions. Eczemas are non-infective except when they are impetiginized and of the infective variety. They do not leave scars. The patient needs reassurance of these points.

It must be remembered that epidermis is an ectodermal structure, and so, takes time to heal. Patience must be the watchword; energetic treatment is to be strongly discouraged. Once warned, the patient will readily cooperate.

Acute eczemas heal readily, in about 1–4 weeks, with treatment. Chronic eczemas, in which anatomical and functional changes set in, take time to disappear. Disseminated and generalized eczemas are not only slow to heal, but are accompanied by ill-health. Infantile and atopic eczema as are troublesome and uncomfortable. The former lasts till the age of two unless it develops into atopic eczema which may continue till the age of 25 or even through life. Its course is marked by spontaneous remissions and exacerbations. Climatic extremes, psychogenic stresses and poor health, aggravate dermatitis and eczema. The cure of these conditions is retarded in tropical countries, by heat, humidity and the prevalent unhygienic conditions.

Treatment

It consists of:

1. Reasuring the patient and his relatives about the disease being curable, non-infectious and non-scarring. A patient with chronic eczema naturally worries about the chronic nature of his illness, the expense of treatment and the loss of income because of his inability to work. Hence reassurance on all these accounts is very important in winning his confidence, and thus his cooperation in treatment. Tactful bed-side psychotherapy pays dividends in all cases.
2. Elimination of predisposing, exciting and complicating causes. In one individual, more than a single cause' may be at play. Where it is impossible to remove a known cause from a patient's environment, attempts should be made to desensitize or hyposensitize him. To prevent recurrence, advice should be given to the patient regarding exposure to causes. Anyone suffering from contact eczema, for instance, should be advised against exposure to the possible sources of the causative allergens and allergo immunologically related substances. Patients with infective eczemas should be advised regarding the sources of infection, the building up of resistance against infection with specific autogenous and stock vaccines, etc. Improving the general state of nutrition is also important.
3. Palliative treatment must be properly carried out to effect a complete cure. Half-hearted measures carried out in an inefficient manner, far from being helpful, are demoralizing.

Principles of Symptomatic Treatment

Correction of Environment

a. Moderate atmospheric temperature and humidity help recovery, whereas heat, sweating, high humidity (particularly in the monsoon), dust and unhygienic surroundings, have an untoward influence. Poverty and backwardness of the people are great obstacles especially when the climate is extreme. A change to a moderate climate should be recommended to a patient suffering from chronic eczema.
b. Rest to the affected part may be recommended; bed rest becomes necessary in generalized eczemas. With rest, healing is accelerated; that is why hospitalization is so beneficial for chronic, resistant cases.
c. Diet should be simple; salt and fluids should be cut down. Sattvik (vegetarian food without spices and beverages like tea, coffee, alcohol) is helpful in bad cases. In acute disseminated eczemas, it is advisable to put the patient on light food for a few days to help the body to get rid of toxic substances. In allergic eczemas, eliminative diets may be tried.
d. The protection of the affected part is desirable; more so, in exogenous eczemas where a cotton bandage or a glove or a mask ensures complete protection from offending agents. Cotton wool must never be employed in bandaging, it retains heat, thereby worsening the eczema.
e. Patient should be asked to refrain from scratching as far as possible. In difficult cases, particularly in infantile and atopic cases, physical restraint with splints and bandages may be necessary.

Internal or Systemic Therapy

There are no panaceas. No specific medicines or injections can cure eczemas. The few drugs which are available, are for symptomatic relief only. Their indiscriminate use is criminal.

a. *ACTH and corticosteroids:* They are undoubtedly helpful, but by no means curative. Their use is recommended for generalized and disseminated eczemas. They may also be employed to control troublesome complaints temporarily in conditions where the cause is in the process of being eliminated. Prednisolone (orally) is used in doses of 5 mg QDS or so; it cuts down the period of morbidity in disseminated and atopic eczemas.
b. *Antihistaminics:* They help to control itching, and to a certain extent, acute sensitization.
c. Calcium gluconate [Calcibromate (P)] and strontium bromide [Ekzebrol (P)]: Some workers recommend gamma allergen therapy.
d. *Antibiotics in acute extensive infective eczemas:* They are also useful whenever there is a secondary pyogenic infection. In chronic cases of infective eczemas, auto-vaccine, stock vaccine, staphylococcal toxoid, are useful. Sulphapyridine is sometimes useful in resistant sub-acute extensive eczemas.
e. *Sedatives and hypnotics:* Chloral hydrate and barbiturates are exceedingly helpful in controlling restlessness and insomnia. Infants tolerate chloral hydrate very well. Tranquilizers are useful for psychogenic upsets. Discretion, however, should be exercised in their use.
f. General tonics like multivitamins, iron and liver extract for debility.

Local Treatment

Its nature depends upon the morphological appearance. Sensitizing and strong medicaments should not be used locally, as they act like petrol on fire instead of sand on water and so produce therapeutic panic! The local medicaments employed should be free from smell and should not produce stinging sensation. They should be inexpensive and easy to apply. A doctor must choose his medicament, vehicles and mode of their use carefully.

Weeping eczemas react well to astringents (wet soaks and lotions). Examples of some good ones employed are: lotion silver nitrate 0.5–1% in aqueous solution, lotio calamine and lotio aluminium subacetate 1–5%. They should be applied every 2–4 hours in most cases. In infective eczemas, crusts are removed with Condy's fluid and then silver nitrate lotion or lotio gentian violet 0.5–1% in aqueous solution is applied. A potasium permanganate soak, 1 in 4,000 is also useful. The use of lotions should not ordinarily be continued for more than 48 hours or so. If a crust tends to form, it should be removed, and treatment re-started. Bismuth subgallate and amylum paste or zinc cream are recommended for eczema that is scaly and papular. The paste/cream is changed twice a day.

In infective eczema, the affected part is painted with gentian violet, and when this dries, is covered with a medicated paste. As the infection clears up, gentian violet is gradually discontinued. Antibacterial creams like Vio-form (P) cream, Cetavlax (P), neomycin, bacitracin, soframycin (P) may also be employed, but cautiously, and with discretion. Simple, conservative measures give the best results in the long run. Local antihistaminic ointments are to be definitely avoided for fear of producing sensitivity.

In chronic eczemas, steroid and other allied local preparations, crude tar, tar paste and superficial X-ray therapy may be tried. The last of these falls in the sphere of the specialist. Steroid cream/lotion gives good results in infantile, atopic and endogenous eczemas; occlusive dressings with steroids and intralesional infiltration with prednisolone/triamcinolone have been successfully used in resistant lichenified eczemas. X-ray therapy helps to control the lichenification process, and to bring the skin to normal. So it is very useful in localized cases of chronic eczemas, lichenification, resistant cases of nummular eczemas and dyshidrosis. The authors have used dermabrasion in recalcitrant patches of lichen simplex chronicus with success.

Chapter 11

Superficial Bacterial and Tropical Infections

PYODERMA

Pyoderma is a group name for pyococcal dermatoses which are generally purulent. In tropical countries, pyoderma is a common problem, particularly in the summer and the monsoon.

The two important pyogenic organisms are the *Staphylococcus aureus* and the *Streptococcus pyogenes*. The former is more important in skin infections than the latter. Follicular infections are mainly due to staphylococci; while erysipelas and cellulitis are caused by streptococci. Besides these, other organisms which occasionally come across in pyodermas are *Bacillus, Proteus, Pseudomonas* and coliform bacilli.

The following are, broadly speaking, the different conditions produced by them depending upon the causative organisms and the location of the lesions:

1. Epidermal	Impetigo pityroides.
	Streptococcal intertrigo.
	Impetigo contagiosa, pustular bacteride, granuloma pyogenicum, pyoderma gangrenosum, infectious eczematoid dermatitis, otitis externa.
2. Subepidermal	Erysipelas.
3. Follicular	Bockhart's impetigo, sycosis, furunculoses, carbuncle, stye, marginal blepharitis.
4. Sweat glands	Eccrine—Sudoripora suppurativa.
	Apocrine—Hidradenitis suppurativa.
5. Dermis	Cellulitis.
6. Subcutaneous fat	Panniculitis.
7. Blood vessels	Arteritis, capillaritis, vasculitis, phlebitis.

In the handling of pyoderma, the following principles should be borne in mind:

1. In every non-typical case of acute and chronic infection, a smear must be made, stained and examined for causative organisms.
2. In chronic cases, when the use of an antibiotic is called for, a sensitivity test should first be undertaken. Proper selection of antibiotics can help considerably to reduce the incidence of resistant strains and also incidental misuse of antibiotics.
3. In cases of superficial and localized infection, only local antiseptics should be employed. In cases where the infection is deeper or extensive, the systemic use of chemotherapeutic agents and antibiotics is indicated. Those antibiotics which are

used systemically, should not be used topically. Several antibiotics exclusive for local use are now available, viz. soframycin, bacitracin, neomycin, gramicidin, tyrothricin, fusidin, mupirocin, polymyxin, etc.

4. The treatment should be continued for at least three to seven days after the disease has been apparently controlled, to prevent recurrence.
5. In cases of recurrent pyoderma, try to establish the cause or causes, improve general health of the patient and give non-specific stimulants.

IMPETIGO CONTAGIOSA

The causative organisms are mainly pyogenic staphylococci, less so *streptococcus pyogenes*; diminished local resistance leads to the development of this disease. Impetigo contagiosa can occur primarily as such, or secondarily, as a complicating factor in scabies, pediculoses, eczemas, seborrhoeic dermatitis and herpes simplex. To this second process we give the name, impetiginization.

Impetigo contagiosa has a world-wide distribution. Though it can occur at any age, it is commonly a disease of childhood. Patients are usually undernourished or run down. Infection is transmitted by contact with any individual carrying pyogenic organisms, directly or through towels, handkerchieves, etc. The sites of predilection are the exposed regions of the body, especially the face and scalp; though it can occur on any part of the body. The incubation period is two to three days.

Clinical features: It starts as a superficial bulla containing seropurulent matter. The contents soon coagulate producing a thick, stuck-on, honey-coloured crust. This characteristic crust is the most important diagnostic feature of impetigo. At the periphery of the crust may be seen the epidermal tags or the edge of the bulla. The removal of the crust reveals moist, glistening surface with copious serous secretion which is infectious to contiguous areas and to other persons. One or several lesions may be seen in one individual; usually, however, the lesions are multiple. Infection may spread to hair follicles in the scalp or beard region and set up folliculitis. In the tropics, bullous impetigo may even be seen in adults **(Fig. 11.1)**.

The intervening skin is completely normal. Usually no pain or itching accompanies the condition. The regional glands are only slightly enlarged. Constitutional symptoms are noticeably absent, except in children and in extensive impetigo. There is no scarring. Sometimes impetigo lesions heal in the centre and spread at the periphery producing circinate lesions.

In cachectic and debilitated individuals, the impetigo lesions are rather deep, giving rise to epidermal necrosis, thereby producing shallow ulcers with dirty brown crusts and pus underneath. This condition is called ecthyma; the legs are the sites of predilection. The lesions heal slowly; on healing they leave permanent scars. Streptococci may produce streptococcal gangrene and fuso-spirochaetal infection may spread from the gingiva to produce extensive necrosis of the lips, mouth and face (Cancrum Oris—noma).

Pyoderma gangrenosum is a hypersensitive reaction necrosis of the skin associated with trauma, coccal infection, ulcerative colitis, rheumatoid arthritis and drug addiction. Ulceration, deep necrosis, boggy violaceus, undermined edge, surrounding red areola and rapid evolution are characteristic. Outlook is serious but has improved with steroids (systemic and local injections into the rim), antibiotics, rifampicin and better topical management. Precipitating causes must be properly managed.

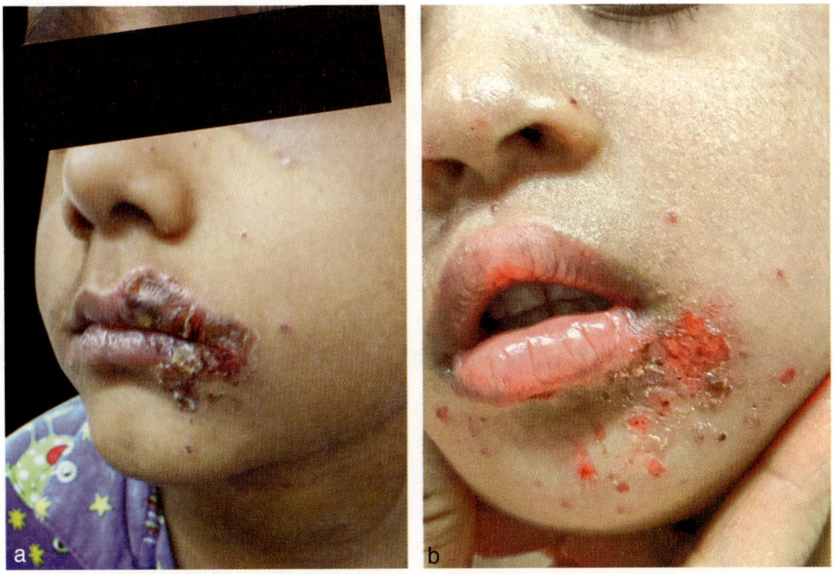

Fig. 11.1: Impetigo contagiosa in: (a) A 5-year-old boy; (b) A 3-year-old girl

Histopathology: The impetigo lesion is a superficial bulla, the roof of which is formed by the stratum corneum. The contents are seropurulent; later a crust is seen. The underlying epidermis remains intact. The upper corium shows dilated capillaries and polymorphonuclear infiltration.

Impetigo neonatorum implies impetigo contagiosa of the newborn. The eruption is extensive and involves the limbs, trunk, face and neck. Palms and soles are spared. The bullae are tense, and contain clear fluid; rupture produces a superficial, raw surface with overlying epidermal tags. Crusting is not prominent. Toxaemia is marked by fever, emaciation and collapse. Infection is conveyed by an infected genital passage, infected nipple, attendants with infected wounds or throats, or from other impetigo cases in a maternity ward. The condition used to be dreaded in maternity hospitals because of its easy communicability and high mortality rate. Prophylactic measures are important in controlling the spread of disease.

Diagnosis: The diagnosis of impetigo is not difficult if the disease and its features are remembered. In persistent impetigo of the scalp, pediculoses must be suspected, and a search should be made for nits and parasites. Persistent, impetigo-like lesions on the body may be due to scabies and dermatitis herpetiformis. The former is characterized by intense nocturnal pruritus, burrows, a typical distribution of lesions and by a history which reveals that several members of the patient's family have been affected. Acarus and ova can also be demonstrated in skin shavings. Dermatitis herpetiformis is distinguished by the presence of chronic, symmetrical polymorphous lesions on the arms, scapula and lower back accompanied by itching. Annular lesions need to be differentiated from tinea.

In the latter, there are no bullae or honey-coloured crusts. On the other hand, it shows an inflammatory border of papulovesicles, accompanied by itching.

Impetigo is usually an acute condition. In chronic, crusted lesions, infective granulomas like syphilis, tuberculosis and leishmaniasis must be borne in mind. A chronic history, underlying infiltration and associated accompanying features, a biopsy and bacteriological examination, help to distinguish them. Impetigo neonatorum is differentiated from syphilitic pemphigus by the presence in the latter of symmetrically distributed bullae on the hands, feet and face. The child is poorly developed and has a waxen appearance. Lesions develop within a few days of birth, and there is no history of a septic source of infection . Serological tests for syphilis are positive, both in the mother and the infant.

Prognosis: The disease usually lasts for 3–4 weeks. In some cases, particularly when it complicates other skin conditions, it may last for months. An average case can be cured in 6–10 days leaving behind no scars. Being a contagious disease, it can spread to other parts of the body and to other people.

Treatment: It has improved considerably with revolution in the field of antiseptics and antibiotics. Due precautions should be taken to prevent spreading of the infection. The affected parts must be kept dry, clean and covered. In children with extensive affection of the scalp, the hair must be shaved off. This procedure is rarely necessary in adults.

To begin with, crusts are removed with warm Condy's lotion, and an antiseptic lotion or cream is applied. Quinolor derivatives, Cetavlon (P), bacitracin, and soframycin (P) creams give good results. They are cosmetically acceptable to the patient. The ointment should be applied 2–3 times a day. Gentamicin, fusidin and mupirocin are the other useful topical agents.

In adults, local measures are usually enough, except in extensive cases and ecthyma.

Septran (P) or broad-spectrum antibiotics by mouth should be given in such cases.

In infants, penicillin injections, or broad-spectrum antibiotics by mouth are given as a routine. This procedure has reduced the mortality rate considerably. As for local measures, blisters are aspirated aseptically, the flaccid roofs clipped away, and the raw surface sprayed with Vioform (P) powder or painted with 1% silver nitrate lotion followed by soframycin (P) cream.

The treatment must be continued until all the lesions have healed up completely, and have stayed so, for at least a week.

BOCKHART'S IMPETIGO

Synonym: Follicular impetigo.

It is characterized by staphylococcal infection of the superficial part of the hair follicles and the perifollicular area giving rise to the formation of follicular pustules covered by tiny yellowish crusts. Infection spreads from one hair follicle to another, producing, multiple but discrete lesions which are usually found on the legs, thighs, forearms and the pubic area **(Fig. 11.2)**. There is no scarring, and the hair is not shed after the lesions have healed, unless the infection has descended into the hair follicles and produced furunculoses.

Occasionally, follicular impetigo follows the local application of irritant mercurial and tar preparations or croton oil on hairy regions.

Treatment is similar to that employed for impetigo contagiosa.

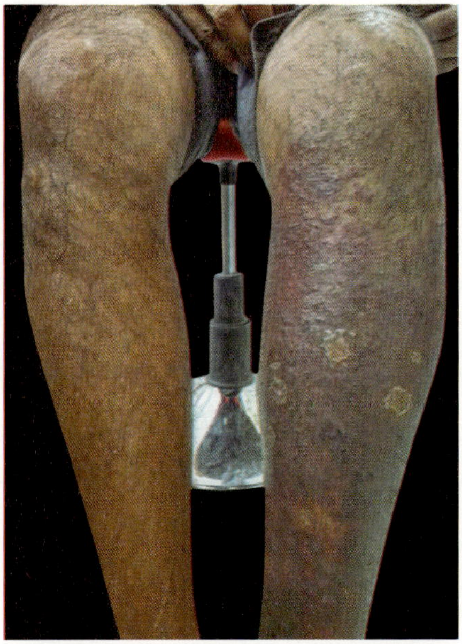

Fig. 11.2: Bockhart impetigo

PITYRIASIS ALBA

Synonym: Impetigo pityroides. Hindustani Synonym 'Thim'.

It is a common problem in practice. It is characterized by ill or well-defined, chronic patches of mild erythema, hypopigmentation and furfuraceous scaling. Size of patch is about that of a rupee; lesion is solitary or there may be 2–3 patches. The condition mainly affects the forehead, cheeks and chin of children, to a less extent, that of adults. It can occur at any time of the year, but is more common in cold winter and dry hot summer. Though the exact cause has not been well established, the disease is usually attributed to a low grade streptococal infection in a run-down individual. It can also follow an attack of gastroenteritis, dysentery or the use of broad-spectrum antibiotics. According to some authorities, lack of sunlight and avitaminosis are responsible for the condition. In India, people blame the dry weather and hence call it *Kushki ke dag* **(Fig. 11.3)**.

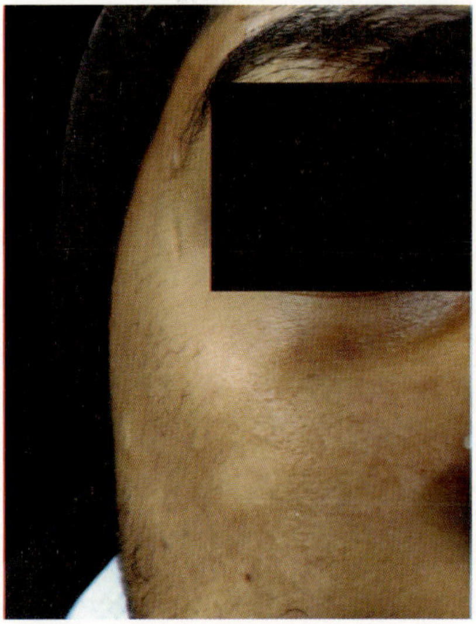

Fig. 11.3: Pityriasis alba

It is a harmless, non-scarring and usually non-infectious affection, which responds slowly to treatment. The treatment consists of a nourishing diet, mild sunbathing, tonics, particularly vitamins, and the application of mild antiseptics like ammoniated mercury (5%) ointment, Bradex-vioform (P), bacitracin ointment etc. Integument must be properly lubricated. Children should not play in the hot sun and cold winds.

STREPTOCOCCAL INTERTRIGO

It is seen as a crack or a fissure covered by a honey-coloured, stuck-on crust at the skin flexures, viz., behind the ear (retroauricular), below the ear (infraauricular), angles of the mouth (perleche), the naso-labial junction and, less commonly, the groins, the junction of the penis with the scrotum and the inframammary region. The removal of the crust reveals the crack and produces slight bleeding. It is usually a chronic condition. It may be associated with seborrhoeic dermatitis, avitaminosis and focal sepsis. Streptococcal intertrigo should be differentiated from monilial intertrigo. In the latter, there is more maceration than in streptococcal intertrigo, in which there is more crusting. Gram's stain and potassium hydroxide preparations help to confirm the diagnosis.

The treatment is on the same lines as for angular stomatitis.

ANGULAR STOMATITIS

Synonym: Perleche.

It implies bilateral linear cracks at the angles of the mouth . It is a clinical entity which can be brought about by several causes, viz., malnutrition particularly deficiency of riboflavin, monilial infection, as a feature of seborrhoeic dermatitis, or as a complication brought on by an ill-fitting or sensitizing denture, or by pipe smoking. It is rarely seen as an evidence of secondary syphilis.

Clinically, it is seen as erythema and as a crack covered by a yellowish crust.

Perleche is usually a chronic condition. The prognosis depends upon the cause; unless the cause is corrected , the patient cannot be helped very much. So, in every case of angular stomatitis, instead of relying on vitamins, the attending physician should examine the patient thoroughly.

The treatment consists in correcting the underlying cause, removing the crust with potassium permanganate lotion, and painting with 1% aqueous silver nitrate lotion, 1% gentian violet in 25% spirit. Vitamins should be prescribed only when considered necessary.

OTITIS EXTERNA

Inflammation of the external auditory meatus is a common and annoying condition. Itching is troublesome and scratching aggravates it by causing secondary infection and even infective eczematoid dermatitis. Clinical features are redness, slight crusting and occasional discharge. Common causes are seborrhoeic dermatitis, streptococcal infection and neuroderm atitis. Occasionally, it is secondary to suppurative otitis media.

Treatmeut consists of cleaning with spirit and application of corticosteroid and bacitracin cream. The underlying causes must be tackled at the same time. Nystatin and polymyxin are useful in monilial and pseudomonas infections respectively. Grenz ray therapy is useful in chronic resistant cases.

ERYSIPELAS

It is a haemolytic streptococcal infection of the skin produced by the entrance of micro-organisms through small abrasions or already established wounds. The patient is ill, and has a raised temperature and pulse rate. The face is the site of predilection. The affected part has an angry red colour; it feels hot and firm." The margins are raised, and well defined. The blood count shows polymorphonuclear leucocytosis. Like all streptococcal infections, erysipelas is most prevalent in temperate climates, occurring usually in the winter and spring months. Chronic and recurrent erysipelas produces swelling of the affected part .

The differential diagnosis is made from dermatitis, eczema and erysipeloid. The features mentioned above are absent in these conditions.

Treatment: Treatment consists of a course of a broad-spectrum antibiotic like erythromycin and tetracycline. There is no need for antitoxic sera and local medicament any more. Recurrent erysipelas requires complete eradication of the septic focus from the sinuses, ears, gums, etc.

SYCOSIS

It simply means chronic folliculitis due to staphylococci affecting the hairy regions of the body. In order of frequency, the beard region, neck, scalp, legs, arms and pubic region are most often involved. Characteristically, this condition is seen as small, superficial, follicular pustules; some rupture to discharge beads of pus, the rest dry up to form crusts. Folliculitis develops rapidly, involving more and more follicles. Soon the infection becomes chronic; the skin looks congested, swollen and infiltrated . Usually no pain is present; itching and burning are the only symptoms. The eruption looks unsightly and is annoying. In the beard region (Sycosis barbae), the chin and upper lip are most affected; the eruption later spreads to other parts. There is no oozing and weeping at any stage; this feature helps in differentiating the disease from follicular infective eczema in which the whole of the beard region is rapidly involved and oozing is a dominant feature.

Sycosis nuchae: On the back of the neck, sycosis has a tendency to produce small, keloidal papules and nodules (Acne keloides nuchae) which are chronic and relapsing. It starts as discrete, follicular papules, some of which turn into pustules, others develop into firm nodules or plaques of thick; scar-like tissue by coalescence. The hair appear twisted and tangled. It is accompanied by marked itching and occasionally pain.

Sycosis lupoides: It is a rare, chronic and progressive folliculitis of the beard region and scalp. It is seen as a small, smooth, atrophic patch of alopecia, surrounded at the periphery by small follicular papules. It is presumably caused by *Staphylococcus* or virus. The prognosis is bad. X-ray therapy, local hydrocortisone injections and broad-spectrum antibiotics (systemically or locally) are worth trying.

Folliculitis decalvans: It is comparatively an acute and severe skin disease involving the scalp. Furunculoses, abscesses and cicatricial alopecia are the important clinical features.

Etiology: The most common causative organism of sycosis is *Staphylococcus aureus*; less commonly, other staphylococci. Discharges from the nose, throat and teeth are the source of these organisms . They may enter the skin through slight injuries or abrasions caused by shaving. Use of unhygienic shaving kit, blunt razors, fine shaving by stretching the skin and shaving against the grain of hair tend to cause sycosis. Folliculitis has a tendency to occur amongst people working in dusty and dirty environments, e.g. miners, building workers and sweepers. Workers handling or coming in contact with oil tend to develop oil acne which must be distinguished from primary sycosis. Predisposing causes are many. Seborrhoeic diathesis is a common feature. Sedentary habits, under-nutrition or obesity, diabetes, unhygienic living, neurotic temperament and emotional strain are the common predisposing factors.

Differential diagnosis: Tinea barbae can be distinguished from this condition by the presence of deep-seated, indurated, boggy swellings, and microscopic examination for fungus. Secondary eczematization and follicular infective eczema, on the other hand, can be distinguished by the features described above. Impetigo has special features like interfollicular epidermal involvement, tense bullae and stuck-on honey-coloured crusts, etc. In etiological diagnosis, seborrhoeic diathesis and/or acute seborrhoeic dermatitis must be seriously considered.

Prognosis: The course of sycosis is chronic; it is marked by exacerbations and remissions. The disease can continue for years. The prognosis is good if proper treatment is given and the patient cooperates. Only a very small percentage of cases are intractable.

Treatment: It consists of:

1. Removing the causes, viz., eliminating the septic focus from the nose, throat, teeth etc.; change from dusty environments; improving the general health with tonics and exercises.
2. Avoiding trauma to the affected parts, viz., by shaving in one direction; by keeping away from the use of strong soaps and irritating oils like mustard oil ; by using sharp razor blades to prevent repeated shavings; by keeping the hair short, and by refraining from fine shaving which would necessitate stretching of the skin. In resistant cases, shaving should be avoided.
3. Medicaments. The ones usually employed are: Vioform cream (P), Cetavlex cream (P), topical antibiotic ointments like bacitracin, and soframycin (P), etc. These are applied three times a day. Gentian violet 1%, ammoniated mercury paste and 5–10% tannic acid lotion are useful for resistant patients. The latter is very useful in tanning (hardening) the integument and increasing its resistance to infection and trauma.
4. In resistant cases, a course of fractional X-ray therapy is recommended: Only occasionally are epilating doses of X-ray therapy indicated. X-ray therapy retards the growth of hair, reduces the bacteria present, and disperses chronic dermal infiltration. Keloidal acne on the back of the neck is best treated with fractional X-ray therapy, with or without excision of the keloid or dermabrasion.
5. Autogenous or stock staphylococcal vaccines and toxoids are effective in chronic cases.

FURUNCULOSIS

It is a condition familiar to every one. A furnucle or boil is a deep-seated septic affection of the hair follicle in which the hair root is completely destroyed and comes out as the core of the boil (Fig. 11.4). Multiple boils are given the name of furunculoses. A carbuncle is a big conglomeration of boils, the inflammation spreading from one follicle to another under the epidermis. The intervening corium is destroyed, and pus is discharged through multiple holes.

Etiology: The causative organism in these conditions is *Staphylococcus aureus*, less frequently other staphylococci. Furunculosis is a common skin problem, very prevalent in the tropics. It is more common in the summer, especially the monsoon season.

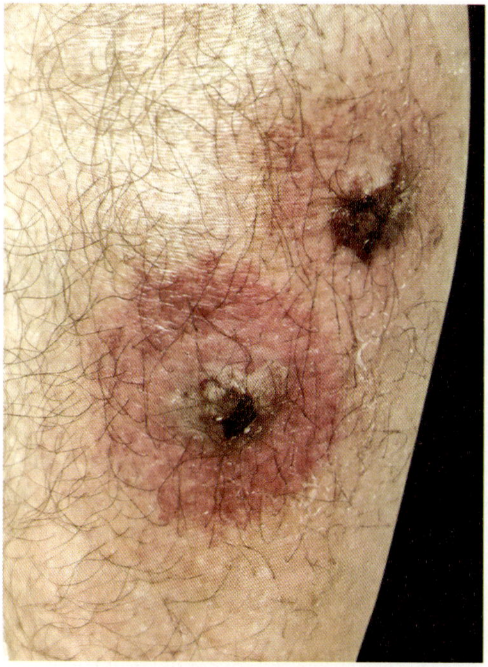

Fig. 11.4: Furunculosis

Maceration of the skin, dusty and dirty environments, and the ingestion of too many carbohydrates, predispose to furunculoses. The eating of too many mangoes has a similar effect (mango boils). A stye is a boil around an eyelash. When one deals with chronic furunculoses, the following predisposing causes must always be kept in mind:

Constitutional

1. Diabetes mellitus.
2. Chronic nephritis.
3. Poor general health—malnutrition, worries, anxieties, etc.
4. Seborrhoeic diathesis.
5. Ichthyosis.

Environmental

1. Oily occupations or dusty jobs.
2. Friction or chafing at work or by rough garments.
3. Scabies, pediculoses, etc.

In acute furunculoses, the pain is intense, replaced by uncomfortable itching when the condition becomes chronic.

Treatment: It consists of:

a. *In acute cases:*
   1. Surgical incision only when the boil is ripe.
   2. Course of Septran (P) or penicillin or broad-spectrum antibiotics.
   3. Removal or correction of the pred isposing cause.

4. Applying an antiseptic locally and dressing the affected part. Kaolin poultice helps to ripen the boil.

b. *In chronic cases:*

1. Chemotherapy is unnecessary. Locally, gentian violet or brilliant green 1% in 75% spirit, or lotio acid tannici may be used.

Tannic acid	5 g
Spt. methylated indust.	60 cc. Liquor hydrarg perchlor 1 in 1000 to 100 cc.

These tend to harden the skin. Magnesium sulphate pastes and hot fomentation are strongly contraindicated.

2. Diet—Carbohydrates and fats should be cut down, and extra proteins, fresh fruits and vegetables added.
3. Autogenous or stock vaccines or staphylococcal toxoid.
4. Course of Stannoxyl (P) or collosal manganese (P). These tend to increase the resistance against infections by increasing the phagocytic coefficient. Septilin (P) has similar effect. In India, bitter chirata* and neem** are used with benefit.
5. Improvement of general health: A holiday by the seashore has cleared up many an intractable case. Sunbathing, tonics, UVR exposures and sulphur spring baths are also beneficial.
6. Course of fractional X-ray therapy in case of localized chronic furunculoses. For more information of chemotherapeutic agents and antibiotics, refer to Chapter 5.

HIDRADENITIS SUPPURATIVA

It is a chronic pyogenic infection of the apocrine sweat glands of the axillae, less so, of the breast, genitalia or peri-anal region. Hyperhidrosis, obesity, lack of fresh air, irritation by clothing, shaving, use of depilatories or the presence of intertrigo, are the predisposing causes; *Staphylococcus aureus* is presumably the causative organism.

Clinically, it is seen as small, chronic, painful and tender nodules and discharging abscesses. The hairy cores of the boils are absent in the discharge (Fig. 11.5). There is slight itching. Treatment is unsatisfactory; but if due care is taken, every patient can be helped considerably.

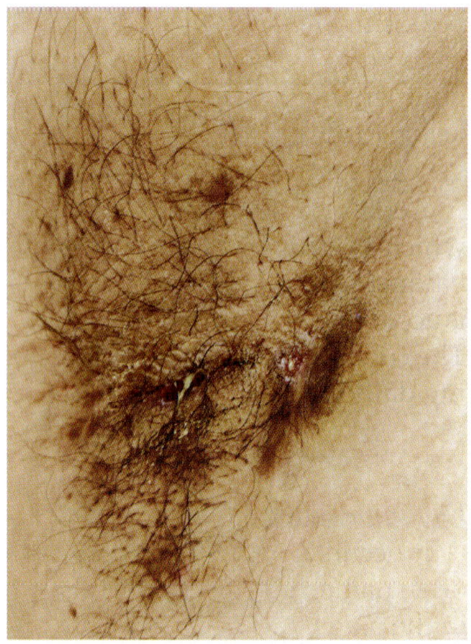

Fig. 11.5: Hidradenitis suppurativa in armpit

(*) *Swertia chirata:* The dried herb (whole plant) is used to make a bitter infusion useful as a tonic. In India, it is extensively used by indigenous practitioners to treat and prevent skin infections.

(**) *Neem-Azadirachta indica:* The leaves and the dried barks of the stems and roots are used for making a bitter tonic. Local actions are antiseptic and astringent. A poultice is made out of the leaves to treat boils and a decoction to treat bacterial infection.

The treatment consists in keeping the hair short and the affected part dry, bathing with potassium permanganate lotion, local application of gentian violet or tannic acid spiritous lotion, or Burrow's solution soaks, and the systemic use of penicillin or other antibiotics. In chronic cases, X-ray therapy may benefit, and in intractable cases, surgical excision and skin grafting may be necessary.

ACRODERMATITIS CONTINUA

Synonym: Dermatitis repens.

It is a chronic, slowly progressive and persistent pyogenic dermatitis occurring on the hands, less so, on the feet and other parts of the body. It usually complicates suppurative *paronychia* or an injury on a finger. It starts as a bulla or a pustule, which spreads peripherally by extension of an undermined epidermal border. New lesions arise by contiguity, or at some distance from the initial lesion. Rarely does it become disseminated or generalized. This condition differs from pustular bacteride which is characterized by bilaterally symmetrical pustular eruption on the palms and the soles accompanying an active pyogenic focus.

The course is chronic with acute exacerbations from time to time. It is regarded as being caused by *Staphylococcus aureus*. Underlying monilial and tinea infections must be excluded. In every case, a thorough search should be made for an active focal sepsis. The treatment is unsatisfactory. It consists in cleaning up and exposing the peripheral edge, potassium permanganate soaks, and painting the lesions with 5% aqueous silver nitrate once only. This is followed by the local application of bacitracin and hydrocortisone ointment twice a day. The ointment should be rubbed meticulously into the edges of the lesion to obtain good results. In resistant cases, superficial X-ray therapy and autogenous vaccine may be tried.

Acrodermatitis continua must be distinguished from acrodermatitis enteropathica which is characterized by persistent eczematoid skin lesions on the hands and feet, baldness, a dull, inelastic skin, a stunted growth coupled with a sallow complexion; it is accompained by chronic intestinal infection. It commonly affects infants and children. The condition responds specifically to di-iodoquin (2 TDS), and zinc sulphate (100–150 mg daily).

TROPICAL ULCER

Synonym: Ulcus phagedenicum tropicum.

It occurs in tropical countries, particularly in those with a hot, damp climate. It is often named after the region where it is specifically prevalent e.g., Naga sore occurring in the Naga hills of Assam. Occasionally it takes an epidemic form. It is uncommon in north India, most probably because of the dry, hot climate. It is by no means an easily communicable disease.

Etiology: A run-down condition and diminished vitality of the skin predispose the body to the disease. Soldiers and labourers are affected more often than others. The causative organisms are fusiform bacilli and Vincent's spirochaetes which enter the skin of the feet and legs through abrasions.

Clinical features: The tropical ulcer starts as an abrasion, bite or a wound, on which develops a bulla containing sero-sanguineous material. Rupture of the bulla produces a dirty, stinking slough; destruction of the skin and superficial tissues gives rise to an ulcer which is superficial, 2–5 cm in diameter, and has a granulomatous base. Pain is present. The diagnosis is established by the exclusion of other causes of ulceration like cutaneous leishmaniasis, veldt sore, syphilis, pyoderma, tuberculosis, etc.

Treatment

1. Course of penicillin or erythromycin (P) or cephalosporin.
2. Clean the part with Condy's fluid or Dettol (P).
3. Bacitracin dressing twice a day.
4. Improvement of general health.

In resistant cases, the ulcer may have to be excised or curetted and caustics applied.

VELDT SORE

It is called desert sore. It occurs under desert conditions in tropical and subtropical countries. It is caused by excessive dryness of the skin; the causative organisms are not definitely known, but diphtheria bacilli and streptococci are supposed to cause the condition.

Clinical features: The sites of predilection are the exposed parts of the body, particularly the backs of the hands. It starts as a painful herpetiform vesicular eruption . The vesicles rupture, discharging a straw-coloured fluid and leave behind a shallow ulcer which continues to spread and becomes chronic. The chronic ulcer is circular, and has a diameter of about one and a half inches. The margins are thick and the edges undermined or straight. The base contains greyish debris but no pus. An adherent membrane may be seen. The ulcer is usually chronic and indolent. Healing produces a papery scar. Only in the early stages can the diphtheria bacilli be demonstrated in the veldt ore.

Treatment: It consists of:

1. A course of penicillin injections—4 lac of procaine penicillin intramuscularly daily for about 12 days, or till complete recovery.
2. Anti-diphtheritic serum 20,000 IU.
3. Bacitracin ointment (locally). The affected part must be kept covered.
4. A course of broad-spectrum antibiotics in resistant cases.

ERYSIPELOID

This rarely seen entity is an acute infection caused by *Erysipelothrix rhusiopathiae* and *Bacillus erysipiletus sui*. It is a disease mostly found in fishermen, butchers, meat handlers and pathologists. Clinically it consists of painful, tender, raised erythema with a characteristic purplish red tinge. The sharply demarcated lesion spreads peripherally. Due to a clearing in the centre, it may take an annular form. Mild-to-severe constitutional symptoms may accompany it. At times it may also become generalized. Treatment with penicillin and broad-spectrum antibiotics is curative.

CUTANEOUS ANTHRAX

The incubation period of anthrax is from 2 to 5 days. Anthrax bacillus is the causative organism. The sources of infection are: wool, hides, infected animals and shaving brushes. For these reasons, wool sorters, hide porters and butchers are often affected. The commonest clinical feature is a malignant pustule. It starts as an itchy, red spot which looks like an insect bite. Soon a vesicle is formed which dries to form a reddish black slough. Typically, a malignant pustule consists of a central slough with surrounding induration, with or without vesicles. Further towards the periphery, there is oedema and redness: If the disease is not controlled at this stage, fulminating septicaemia with intestinal and pulmonary symptoms develop. The common sites are the hands, shoulders and face depending upon the source of infection. Anthrax oedema and erysipelas are uncommon; they are caused by deeper inoculation by the causative organisms.

Bacillus anthracis can be demonstrated infrequently in cutaneous anthrax. The diagnosis should be made on clinical grounds. The prognosis is good in the early stages when the disease is localized. Once dissemination occurs, the outlook becomes grave, and the mortality rate becomes high.

Treatment

1. Scalvo's anti-anthrax serum. 100 units immediately (intramuscularly), and 60 units daily, till the disease disappears.
2. Crystalline penicillin injections intramuscularly, 4 lac four times a day, till the pustule subsides. Broad-spectrum antibiotics are also useful.
3. Local dressing with bacitracin ointment.

GLANDERS

It is an occupational disease conveyed by horses to their attendants. The causative organism is the *Bacillus mallei*. The hands and face are the sites of choice. Clinically, it is an ulcer, looking like a syphilitic ulcer, but developing rather rapidly, accompanied by constitutional symptoms like fever and an increased pulse rate. Infrequently, pustules and pustular swellings are seen.

Diagnosis: It is made by the clinical exclusion of other conditions; from the occupational history; by a microscopic demonstration of the causative organisms and by guinea-pig inoculation.

Treatment: It consists in the radical destruction of the ulcer. Mallin vaccine has been tried with success. Septran (P) and antibiotics are usually recommended.

CUTANEOUS AMOEBIASIS

It is rather rare compared to the high incidence of intestinal amoebiasis in tropical countries. It is seen as a chronic, granulomatous ulcer in the perianal area or buttocks. A scraping may show amoeba or cysts of *Entamoeba histolytica*. Intestinal amoebiasis is usually present. Treatment is with emetine injections and local management with silver nitrate lotion and condy's soaks.

Chapter

12

Affections Caused by Vegetable Parasites (Fungi)

INTRODUCTION

Vegetable parasites are a group name for fungi which are pathogenic both to human beings and animals. Fungal diseases are very common. Like most infections, they are prevalent in tropical and subtropical countries. Unless properly treated, they become chronic.

Baer and Sulzburger's work has established that fungus diseases occur only in certain susceptible persons and on certain susceptible areas. Furthermore, the present feeling is that these fungi are only facultative pathogens. Only in the presence of certain adjuvant factors like trauma, maceration, warmth, lack of fresh air and sunlight to a part, previous infection, sensitization and debility, are these fungi facilitated to develop pathogenic lesions. A better understanding of these adjuvant factors will help us to understand why some people develop fungus diseases, and others do not despite living in intimate contact with infectious patients. Hence, importance of the body's basic resistance (in other words "condition of the soil") must be appreciated in comparison with the causative organisms and fungi, on which, undue stress has been laid in the past.

Fungi usually attack keratinized structures like the skin, hair or nails **(Fig. 12.1)**. Only in deep mycoses, deeper living structures are invaded. Fungi from animal sources (zoophilic), particularly horses and cattle, usually cause severe inflammatory ringworm and kerions. In conditions like pityriasis versicolor, invasion of the stratum corneum is very superficial, indeed.

Immunology: Body ringworm particularly caused by zoophilic fungi induces delayed sensitivity. It can be demonstrated by intradermal reaction to trichophytin.

Diagnosis: Fungus affections is usually confirmed by demonstration of fungus in potassium hydroxide preparation and/or culture on Sabouraud's medium.

Histopathology: It is seldom helpful.

Treatment of fungus disease has been revolutionized in recent years. It consists in:

i. Correction of the underlying facilitating factors enumerated above and increasing the local resistance of the parts by keeping them properly dry; exposure to fresh air, exercise, etc.
ii. Topical fungicidal agents like Natamycin (P), tolnaftate, miconazole, buclosamide [Jadit (P)], quinolor derivatives, econazole, Whitfields' ointment, tincture iodine, tinct. merthiolate, ciclopirox olamine (Laprox-P), gentian violet, Castellani's paint, salicylanilide and copper sulphate; nystatin topically in monilial infections.
iii. Systemic griseofulvin in tinea. It has no action on monilial or deeper fungi or pityriasis versicolor. Ketoconazole, fluconazole and itraconazole in superficial and deep

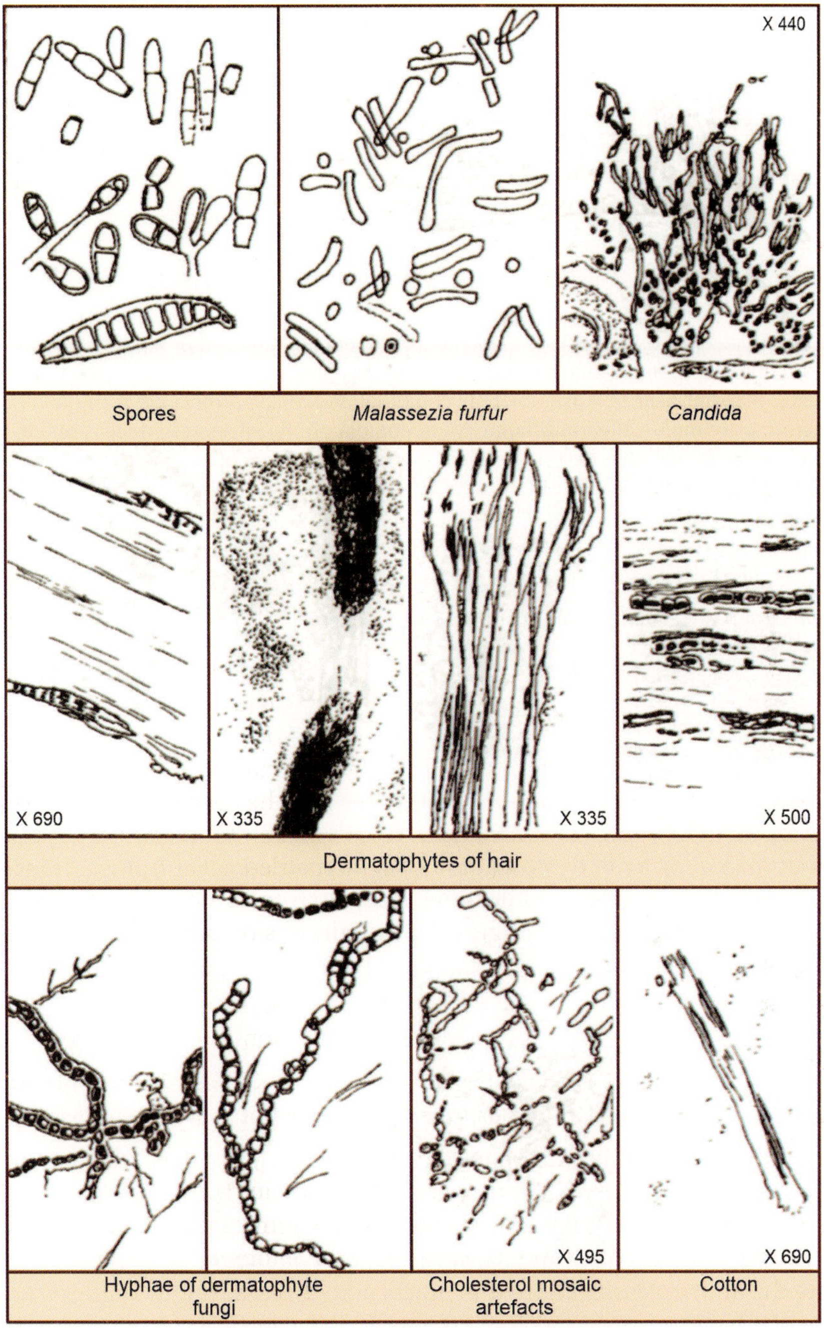

Fig. 12.1: Fungi (*Courtesy:* Mr P Chaturvedi)

mycosis. It is also useful in pityriasis versicolor-topically and systemically. Nystatin is effective in systemic moniliasis. Amphotericin-B is effective in disseminated moniliasis and deeper fungus affections like blastomycosis. Stilbamidine is useful in blastomycosis.

Also useful are sulphonamides and penicillin in some cases of actinomycosis.

Flucytosine is useful in *Cryptococcus*, *Candida*, *Torula* and *Cladosporium* spp.

The prognosis has improved. Tinea has become curable though deeper fungus affections are still troublesome.

Mycologlcal Terminology

Fungus: Lower member of the plant or vegetable kingdom without chlorophyll and without differentiation into root, leaves or stem.

a. When a daughter cell is formed by budding from a spore, it is called a blastospore, e.g., *Monilia* (*Candida*).

b. When a spore is borne on a specialized filament, and remains attached or separated on maturation by constriction at its point of attachment, it is known as conidiospore (or simply conidium), and the specialized filament bearing it is known as conidiophore. Macroconidia are those conidiospores which are mostly multi-celled and large. Microconidia are those spores which are single-celled and small. Spore formation is best studied in cultures. The division of fungi into various genera and species is based on the characteristics of these spores.

Hypha: A single filament of the fungus. It may be septate, e.g. divided by means of transverse walls or septa into a chain of cells, or non-septate, when not so divided.

Mycelium: A mass of hyphae produced by elongation and branching.

Dermatomycoses: All fungus infections of the skin; both superficial and deep, e.g. tinea, actinomycosis, blastomycosis, etc.

Dermatophytoses: Superficial infections of the skin, e.g. tinea.

Epidermophytosis: Infection with *Epidermophyton*

Trichophytosis: Infection with *Trichophyton*.

TINEA OR RINGWORM

It is a group name for a highly contagious, segmented mycelial fungus. It is the most common, single fungus group of infections found in tropical countries. There are three distinct genera in this group (distinguished by cultural characteristics):

Epidermophyton: It affects only the human skin. There is only one important species—*E. floccosum*.

Trichophyton: It is more virulent than the others. It affects the hair, the glabrous skin, as well as the nails, Ii includes both the human and animal species. The important species are: *T. rubrum*, *T. mentagrophyte*, *T. violaceum*, *T. verrucosum* and *T. schoenleini*.

Microsporum: Septa on mycelia are very close producing small segments which look like spores but are not so-in reality; therefore, the name is a misnomer. It affects mainly the hair, and less commonly, the glabrous skin. The important species are: *M. audounii* (human variety), and *M. canis* and *M. lanosum* (animal varieties).

Despite the above classification, it is practical to discuss fungus diseases according to the site of affection.

TINEA CAPITIS

It is rather uncommon in India and the other Asiatic countries except in Kashmir. The causative fungi are the different species of microsporum and trichophyton. Infection takes place from both affected human beings and animals. It is more frequent in boys than girls, because boys have shorter hair, visit barbers more often and play about with each other's caps. The occipital and temporal regions are the sites of choice **(Fig. 12.2)**.

Clinical features: There are three varieties: The scaly variety is the most common. It is caused by microsporum. The salient features are: a circular patch or patches of partial alopecia with thin greyish scales; broken lustreless stumps of hair, with, may be, a greyish film around them; a greenish fluorescence seen under Wood's light and a positive scraping for fungus. The fungus grows in the Stratum corneum of the epidermis, entering the hair follicles through their openings. Penetrating the cuticle and cortex of the hair, it grows inside the hair as well. Consequently, the hair weakens and breaks, producing alopecia, which is usually partial, and broken stumps can be seen. A microscopic examination will show the irregular broken end of the hair, the disturbed hair structure and the mosaic pattern of the mycelia of fungus, both inside the hair and also in the scales. It is not just a coincidence that tinea capitis (particularly the scaly variety caused by *Microsporum*) does not affect individuals after puberty. There is a scientific explanation for it, namely, there is an alteration in the function of sebaceous glands at puberty. Specific fatty acids like undecylenic and propionic acid, etc. (Rothman) are produced. These have definite fungicidal properties, with the result that fungi, particularly microsporum, cannot get a hold on the scalp.

The kerion variety is caused more often by trichophyton than by the microsporon of cats and dogs. Kerion is produced either by penetration of the mycelia into the dermis or virulent strains and/or due to sensitivity to the fungus. In the beginning, there are small boil-like lesions with little oozing and no pus. Later red, painless, boggy swellings are produced . These, likewise, have no pus. These lesions are irregularly distributed on the scalp along with the areas of partial alopecia. A greyish sheath is visible on the hair

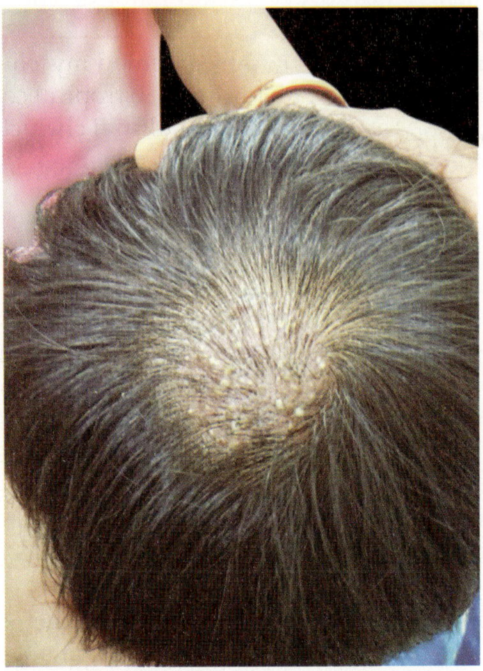

Fig. 12.2: Tinea capitis

when the latter is pulled out of the kerion; this pulling out of the hair is easy because the hair is only loosely attached. It should be distinguished from folliculitis decalvans and pyoderma.

The black-dot variety is caused by a species of trichophyton (endothrix) in which the mycelia of the fungus grow inside the hair; the hair breaks off flush with the surface of the skin, thereby producing the appearance of black dots. The alopecia may look almost complete, but tile black dots can always be detected at the periphery of the lesion. Wood's lamp examination may not show any fluorescence in the black-dot variety of tinea capitis.

Differential diagnosis: In tinea capitis, the differential diagnosis is made from other causes of patchy alopecia such as syphilis and alopecia areata. The features of ringworm of the scalp are typical; Wood's lamp and microscopic examinations will help further to establish the diagnosis.

Syphilitic alopecia has an irregular, moth-eaten appearance. Usually affecting the occipetal and temporal regions, it is accompanied by other features of secondary syphilis. Alopecia areata is characterized by well-defined patches of complete alopecia, absence of dull, broken hair and greyish scales, and the presence of "exclamation mark" hair.

Treatment: Griseofulvin (fine particle) in doses of 125 mg two to four times a day for 6–8 weeks is very effective. Fungicide lotions like miconazole, tinaderm (P), and econazole are useful topically.

Patients are instructed to keep a linen or paper cap on their head day and night; to wash the scalp every morning with soap and hot water, to scrub the affected part with a soft nail brush all over the scalp; to report any undue irritation and to come for a check-up with the ointment removed, every fortnight. The ointment usually prescribed is tolnaftate or miconazole.

Treatment is continued till shining, smooth hair has regrown to the length of about half inch and the Wood's lamp shows no fluorescence.

In kerion, the hair is clipped short. To begin with, hot compresses of 1 in 2,000 liquor hydrarg perchloride, or Condy's lotion are used. When the acute inflammation subsides, miconazole cream is advised.

The prognosis is fair in good hands. There is usually no scarring except in the kerion variety. In resistant cases, course of itraconazole/ketoconazole is prescribed. It is a useful standby.

TINEA BARBAE

There are two clinical varieties: Tinea circinata is characterized by a patch or patches of scaling or vesiculopustules with inflammation most marked at the periphery and accompanied by itching (described in detail under the heading of "Tinea Corporis").

The kerion type affects the scalp. This variety is common amongst farm workers; it is caused by the trichophyton species, and is conveyed by infected cattle.

Tinea barbae should be distinguished from sycosis barbae, actinomycosis and other granulomas. If the clinical features described above are remembered, the diagnosis is not difficult; it can be confirmed by a microscopic examination. In sycosis barbae there is chronic congestion of the skin of the beard region with superficial, follicular pustules.

Actinomycosis produces a hard, indurated, lumpy swelling below the angle of the jaw, chronic suppuration, sinuses and sulphur granules.

Treatment: It is on the same lines as for tinea capitis. The prognosis is good as regards to complete cure. Scarring and alopecia, however, are the end results of the kerion variety.

TINEA CORPORIS

In practice, this is a very common fungus affection. It is caused by *Trichophyton* in the majority of cases; infrequently, microsporon and epidermophyton have been known to cause it. The latter two produce a milder reaction.

Clinical features: They are typical. Marked itching is a characteristic symptom. There may be one or more lesions which are more or less circular, sharply demarcated from the surrounding skin; their sizes vary, say, from that of a one rupee coin to the palm of the hand (or bigger). Confluent patches produce figurate areas. The affected area or areas show vesicles, pustules or scaling; these vary from case to case depending upon the virulence of the fungus and sensitivity of the individual. Inflammation in the form of vesicles and pustules is most marked at the periphery of the lesion. There is a tendency to clearing at the centre; if the central clearing is complete, ringed lesions are formed due to centrifugal spread. The exposed parts of the skin particularly the non-hairy (glabrous) skin, are the sites of choice **(Fig. 12.3)**. Frequently, tinea corporis develops from tinea cruris; under such circumstances, big areas of the trunk are affected. The disease is usually chronic, and the course extends over months to years. Eczematization and lichenification may become the complicating features of chronic cases. Ringworm infection can almost always be confirmed by scraping the active periphery of the lesion, by the demonstration of mycelia under the microscope and by culture. The sources of infection are infected human beings or animals, particularly cattle. Infection is conveyed by direct contact, less frequently, by fomites like clothing.

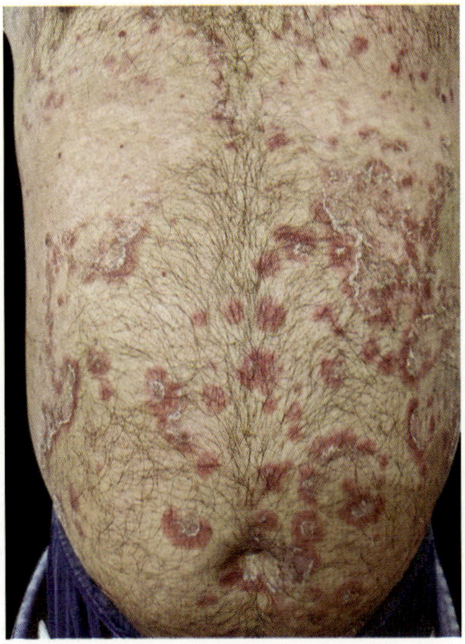

Fig. 12.3: Tinea corporis

Differential diagnosis is from nummular eczema (no active inflammatory borders, bilaterally symmetrical patches, usually on limbs, in winter), psoriasis (silvery scales, candle grease sign, distribution), erythematous rashes and lupus.

Prognosis: It has improved and tinea has become curable, if the source of infection is eliminated completely, and the right treatment is given persistently. Half-hearted treatment is demoralizing and results in chronicity. The superficial varieties of this disease do not leave any atrophy or scarring.

Treatment: It consists in: (1) applying fungicidal agents, (2) removing the sources of infection in infected nails, fomites, animals, etc. and (3) treating complications like eczema and lichenification along the usual lines.

When inflammation is marked, silver nitrate 1% in distilled water, is used. Energetic treatment is risky at this stage. It may bring about acute eczematization and a troublesome ide eruption.

The fungicides commonly advised are Tinactin (P), econazole, miconazole. Whitfield's ointment, tincture Merthiolate (P), Vioform cream (P}, and preparations of undecylenic and propionic acids like Tineafax ointment (P). Ciclopirox olamine (Laprox-P) also give good results.

Any of these fungicidal agents can be used with benefit. They are applied twice a day after the affected part has been cleaned. The part must be kept covered with a thin bandage all the time. Griseofulvin is very useful in extensive and chronic cases of tinea corporis. It should not be indiscriminately used in every case of tinea; topical agents should be employed in localized cases.

TINEA CRURIS (DHOBI'S ITCH)

It is most prevalent in the summer months. It is commonly caused by the *Epidermophyton* and *Trichophyton* from infected toes or nails; fungus may also be conveyed by infected lavatory seats (most commonly in public lavatories) and by laundry clothes. Infection can also be transmitted during sexual intercourse.

Affection occurs on the inner sides of the upper part of the thighs, spreading to adjoining parts of the scrotum, penis, vulva, perineum and later to the buttocks and trunk. Intense itching is the characteristic symptom. It starts as small circinate lesions. Typically, it is seen as well-defined patch or patches of scaling, vesicles and pustules with inflammation most marked at the periphery of the lesions **(Fig. 12.4)**.

Differential diagnosis: It is made from intertrigo, infective eczema and flexural psoriasis. The first two always start at the inguinal cleft which is usually cracked. Inflammation is more marked towards the centre than the periphery. Moreover, the demonstration of fungus clinches the diagnosis of tinea cruris. Flexural psoriasis has no real resemblance to tinea cruris, except that it occurs on the same site; lesions of psoriasis are present on other areas of the body as well.

Prognosis: It is good if the treatment is persisted with the newer fungicidal agents and the predisposing causes are corrected.

Treatment: It is the same as in tinea corporis. Under-clothing must be washed daily. Toes and nails, if infected, must be treated at the same time. Patients should be advised against the use of public lavatories. The infected part must be kept cool and dry. Griseofulvin should only be used as a last resort in extensive and resistant cases.

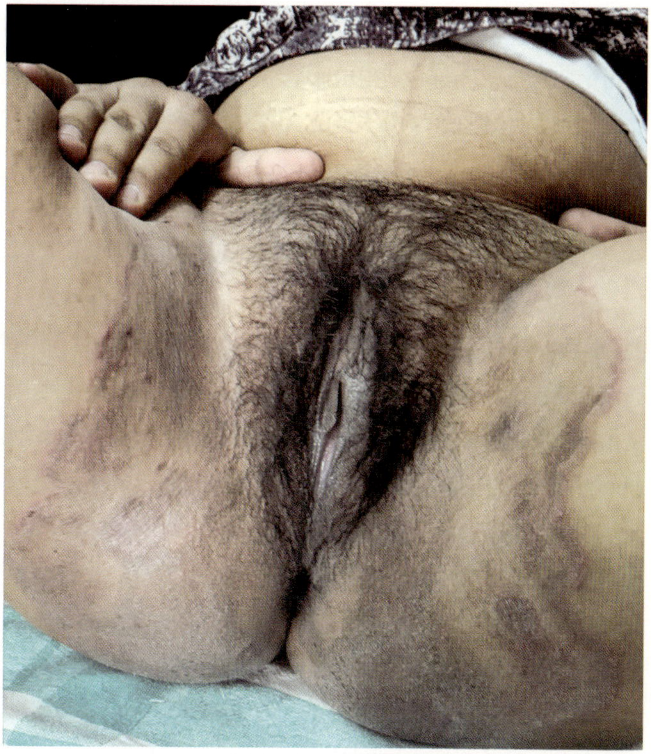

Fig. 12.4: Tinea cruris

TINEA OF FEET AND HANDS

It is very common in tropical and subtropical countries; common in the summer and the monsoon than in the winter. Men are more frequently affected than women. The incidence is directly related to the spread of civilization (Western). Heavy, closed and ill-fitting shoes worn for long hours predispose the individual to infection. The fungus is conveyed from one individual to another through bath mats, tubs and swimming pools. Europeans are very sensitive to it; they pick up the infection quickly and suffer from it more severely than the native population. The fungus grows in the stratum corneum of the epidermis in warm and moist areas; for this reason the fourth interdigital spaces of the feet are selectively affected. Here it is seen as a sodden, white membrane covering a red, glazed, fissured skin. Vesicles may be seen at the periphery. This is the chronic interdigital form. There are no symptoms except slight itching. From the fourth interdigital space, the disease may spread to the sole, to the adjoining toes and even to the dorsum of the feet. Lesions may appear as isolated vesiculopustules, or bullae, or as patches of erythema and oedema with a scattering of vesicles and pustules, the vesicles may develop into ulcers. Oozing is slight. It is accompanied by intense itching and burning. Secondary infection results in pain, lymphangitis and regional lymphadenitis. This variety has the appearance of an eczematoid or pompholyx eruption. Autosensitization produces an ide eruption (which resembles dyshidrosis from which it must be differentiated) on the palms of hands, and, may be, the, other parts of the body as well.

In the chronic hyperkeratotic variety, well-defined patches of hyperkeratotic, powdery scaling on erythematous-thickened bases are seen on the soles and sides of the feet and the palms of the hands. This condition is asymptomatic except for an annoying roughness. It must be differentiated from other causes of hyperkeratosis like syphilis, psoriasis, menopausal keratoderma, eczema, congenital keratoderma, arsenic drug eruption, etc. The fungus is rather difficult to demonstrate in this variety.

The interdigital variety of tinea of the feet is the most common variety found in practice. A search must be made for this chronic focus in patients presenting dyshidrosis; keratoderma, tinea cruris and tinea unguium.

Diagnosis: If the, characteristics. described above are borne in mind the diagnosis of tinea of the hands and the feet is not difficult. It should always be confirmed by a microscopic demonstration of the fungus.

Prognosis: The outlook as to complete cure is fair if the disease is treated by an expert, and the patient is cooperative.

Treatment: The acute stage must be treated like acute eczemas with potassium permanganate soaks and silver nitrate or gentian violet paint. Only when the acute inflammation has subsided should active fungicidal agents be gradually introduced on the lines recommended in the treatment of tinea corporis. Tinactin (P), econazole lotion or cream and Whitfield's ointment are effective in the hyperkeratotic variety. Castellani's paint or tincture Merthiolate (P) is often employed to treat the chronic interdigital variety. Paints containing spirit tend to harden the skin. It is better to use the paint in the morning and a fungicidal ointment like Vioform (P), Sagatrun (P), in the night. The best results have been reported with tolnaftate/econazole.

Shoes and socks must be sterilized; the former, with formalin vapours by putting cupful of commercial formaldehyde in a closed box containing the shoes, for 48 hours. The shoes must be exposed to the mild sun and fresh air for atleast two days before being worn, so that the feet are not irritated by the formalin. Socks are sterilized by boiling. Fungicidal dusting powders like Nycil (P), Mycozol (P), Teoquil (P) and Tineafax (P), etc. help to keep the feet dry and so discourage the growth of fungus. Topical corticosteroids are very useful in acute cases of tinea for controlling acute inflammation till the necessary fungicidal agents can be safely employed by themselves or in combination with them. Griseofulvin is useful in chronic, extensive and resistant cases.

Prophylaxis: It consists of wearing open-type shoes or sandles, drying the feet properly after bathing and the use of fungicidal dusting powder.

TINEA UNGUIUM

Synonym: Onychomycosis.

Ringworm of the nails is caused by a species of *Trichophyton* and *Microsporon*. Saprophytes like *Scopularia* and *Aspergillus* have also been incriminated. In contrast to *monilial* infection, *Tinea* affects first the free edges of the nail. One or more nails may be involved but only rarely, all of them. The history usually reveals that the infection has been present for years. Tinea unguium is characterized by opaque, brittle and deformed nail or nails and hyperkeratotic debris under the free edges **(Fig. 12.5)**.

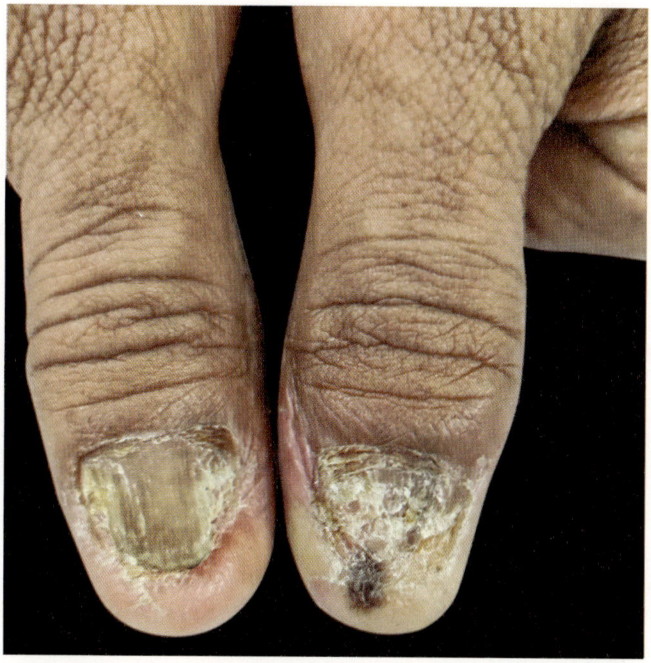

Fig. 12.5: Tinea unguium

There is no pain or itching. The condition is very rarely bilateral and symmetrical. The diagnosis is confirmed by the demonstration of fungus in the hyperkeratotic debris and nail cuttings. The differential diagnosis is arrived at from conditions like psoriasis, moniliasis, eczema, syphilis and dystrophy of the nails (for details, refer to Chapter 33: Diseases of the Nails).

According to Bendek and Sagher, there is a strong feeling that primary tinea unguium is a rare condition and what we usually take for tinea unguium is pompholyx of the nail due to an internal septic focus, metabolic upset, a run-down condition or emotional stress causing dystrophy of the nail, which acts as suitable debris for the growth of fungus, which according to them, is a secondary contaminant.

Prognosis: Because of primary pompholyx, and because the fungus grows inside the hard nail plate which cannot be penetrated by fungicidal agents, the outlook is poor. It has, however, improved.

Treatment: It consists in:

1. Griseofulvin FP, terbinafine, fluconazole or itraconazole as oral antifungal agents
2 Filing the affected nail regularly with broken glass, a nail file or a dentist's burr till the healthy nail begins to grow.
3. Local application of fungicidal agents like tincture iodine, betadine or econazole liquid/cream or glutaraldehyde.
4. Correcting the internal, physical, metabolic and emotional factors and building up the general health.

Persistent treatment on these lines gives good results. The occult focus of ringworm in the toes and groins must be treated at the same time.

Ide Eruption

It implies a distant, localized or generalized reaction due to sensitization to the products of an active, primary, fungus infection. According to some authorities, actual dissemination of the fungus is responsible for the ide eruption. An example of a localized ide reaction is the vesicular, cheiropompholyx-like eruption on the palms of the hands caused by ringworm of the toes. A deep-seated, inflammatory, *Trichophyton* infection produces follicular, papular lesions on the trunk and limbs. These lesions are rarely vesicular and erythematous. Ide eruption tends to subside spontaneously when the primary focus is cured. In practical therapeutics, it is a red signal against energetic treatment of acute tinea.

Treatment

It consists in:

1. Treatment of the primary focus with lotion silver nitrate during the day and miconazole with prednisolone cream in the evening.
2. A course of griseofulvin FP/ketoconazole/fluconazole.
3. A short course of systemic prednisolone and antihistaminic.

FAVUS

It is an uncommon affection these days. *Trichophyton schoenleini* is the causative fungus. Favus occurs where there is overcrowding and in unhygienic environments, particularly when these conditions are accompanied by rat infestation. The scalp is most frequently affected, the glabrous skin of the neck and trunk and the nails, only rarely. The salient features are: yellowish cup-shaped crusts embedded in the depressions on the skin (Scutula), mousey odour, and secondary cicatricial alopecia. Scutulum is composed of densely-knitted mycelia. The diagnosis is confirmed by microscopic demonstration and culture of the fungus, and a Wood's lamp examination. The prognosis is rather *unsatisfatory*; scarring and alopecia are the end results. Treatment is by the use of fungicidal agents and griseofulvin FP as in tinea capitis.

PITYRIASIS VERSICOLOR

Synonym: Tinea Versicolor.

It is caused by *Malassezia* which is seen as short, fine, straight or curved mycelial filaments and masses of small spores. It is most prevalent in countries with warm and humid climates. The affection occurs most often in the monsoon and affects people who sweat profusely. The sites of choice are the upper part of the trunk, the upper parts of arms, the neck, and less frequently, the forehead and cheeks. It is characterized by light-brown macules, plaques or sheets with furfuraceous scaling, which is most evident when the affected part is scraped. The exact colour varies from race to race. In dark races, it appears lighter, almost white, like leucoderma; in white races, the colour of tinea versicolor macules is like cafe-au-lait. Pathological lesions have convex borders; hence they can be easily picked up **(Fig. 12.6)**. The malady is asymptomatic except for slight itching and cosmetic discoloration. The diagnosis can be confirmed by a microscopic demonstration of the fungus. The prognosis is good; a cure is possible if re-infection is prevented, and treatment is continued on the following lines:

1. Underclothing must be washed daily in hot water.

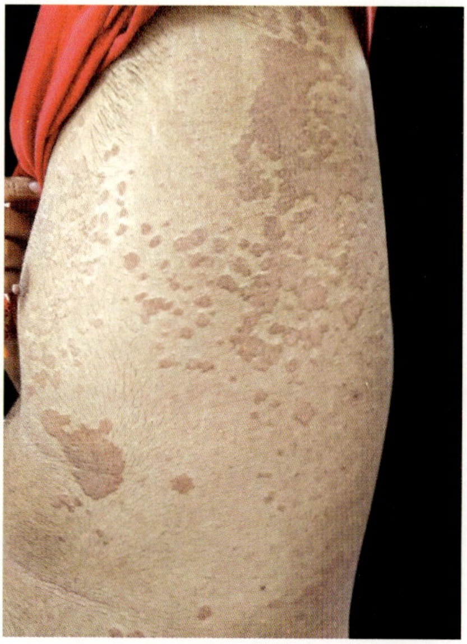

Fig. 12.6: Pityriasis versicolor

2. The affected part must be cleaned with fresh lemon or vinegar; following it, the patient must sit in the sun for 15–20 minutes. During bath, apply a little oil on the skin. After the bath, the affected parts must be dried thoroughly.
3. At night, paint sodium thiosulphate 25% in aqueous solution. Tincture merthiolate, or 3% acid salicylic and 3% acid benzoic in spirit, or miconazole or econazole, tincture iodine and UVR are other useful agents in treatment. Some workers have claimed good results with selenium sulphide suspension-Selsun (P) Ketoconazole orally is useful in resistant cases.

Patients must refrain from swimming in public pools. Sunbathing, proper washing with special soap containing sulphur and acid salicylic, oil lubrication, and thorough drying of the skin after washing, help to prevent the recurrence of tinea versicolor.

CANDIDIASIS/MONILIASIS

It is a yeast-like fungus (*Candida albicans*), which by nature is a saprophyte. Only under favourable conditions like moisture, warmth, lowered resistance due to the presence of sugar and lowered immune resistance, does it become pathogenic. In adults, diabetes may be a predisposing cause of cutaneous monilial affection; a good principle is to get the urine examined in such cases. Even if the urine is negative for sugar, efforts must be pursued to unearth pre-diabetes by elaborate blood tests. Moniliasis is also very common in obese individuals who suffer from hyperhidrosis and hence chronic maceration in the folds of the body (Fig. 12.7). Lack of exercise and fresh air and the wearing of tight clothes for long hours also predispose the skin to this infection .

In recent years, increasing incidence of candidiasis has been brought about by increasing use of antibiotics, trichomonicidal drugs, corticosteroids, contraceptives and immuno-suppressants. Morbidity due to *Candida* is definitely on the increase. Besides *Candida albicans*, other yeast fungi like *C. krusei* and *C. tropicalis* may be seen.

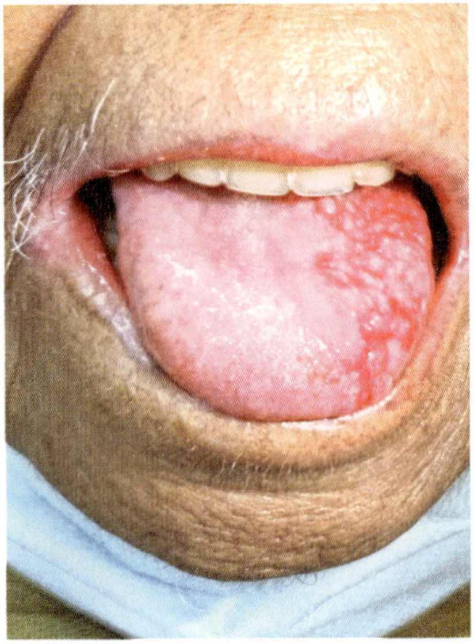

Fig. 12.7: Oral candidiasis with involvement of angles of the mouth

It is estimated that *Candida* may be present in the mouth and genitalia of 20–40% of individuals.

In adults, the common monilial affections observed are: Paronychia, erosio interdigitalis and a variety of intertrigo affecting flexures and toes; in infants, *Monilia* produces thrush and napkin eruption.

THRUSH

It is seen as easily scrapable, dry whitish patches on the tongue and buccal mucosa produced by growth of monilia in the superficial layers of the mucous membrane. Bottle-fed babies are most commonly affected, the fungus being conveyed by unclean milk bottles and teats. Proper sterilization prevents the disease. Thrush must be distinguished from curdled mlk which lie loosely on the surface of the mucous membrane. Thrush must also be distinguished from diphtheria and syphilitic mucous patches. In both these conditions, the membrane cannot be scraped easily without causing bleeding since it is firmly adherent. Besides, there are other stigmata, and the bacteriology is decisive.

In the napkin area, red, moist macules or areas, are produced with sodden epidermal edges. This is usually accompanied by monilial gastroenteritis and thrush . Diaper rash like dermatitis may also be seen.

Superinfection of seborrhoeic and infective eczema by candidiasis, may also be seen. Granuloma gluteale infantum is diaper dermatitis complicated by fluorinated steroid creams promoting the proliferation of *Candida*, more so because of plastic panties.

Lesions appear in the form of pea-sized violet nodules, firm and elastic, may be covered by fine scales. Lesions improve on removing the causes. Eczema like weeping or dry plaques of erythema with scaling may also be seen on the face and trunk.

Treatment is with 1% gentian violet in aqueous solution or nystatin cream or imidazole derivatives. Gastrointestinal lesions should be treated with oral Nystatin (P) tablets. Amphotericin-B lozenges are also useful.

PARONYCHIA

It implies chronic inflammation of the posterior nail folds of one or several fingers, and less so, of the toes. The malady affects housewives, servants, waiters and bar attendants whose hands are constantly in water. Injury to the eponychium by careless manicuring can also cause the disease. Clinically, the nail fold becomes red, swollen and boggy. There is separation of the posterior nail fold from the nail plate, leading to the formation of a space full of cheese-like material **(Fig. 12.8)**. The only symptom is slight irritation or pain. Paronychia is a very chronic condition. The nail is secondarily deformed and atrophied; atrophy starts from the proximal end and slowly extends forwards. To begin with, one finger is affected but soon the other fingers may be involved . Streptococci of low virulence may produce a similar picture. The outlook, in properly treated cases, is good.

Treatment: The authors adopt the following regimen (Brain's modification): The space between the posterior fold and nail plate is cauterized with 95% phenol. A small pledget of cotton wool dipped in carbolic acid is pushed under the nail fold with the aid of a dissecting forceps or a sharpened matchstick, and kept there, for one minute. The excess of phenol is then neutralized with tincture iodi mitis; another pledget of cotton wool soaked in tincture iodine being pushed under the nail fold as before, and kept there for one minute. This is only done once or twice in the beginning. The patient is advised to keep his hands out of water, and is told to apply tincture Merthiolate (P) 1 in 1,000 twice a day or a special lotion containing 3% phenol and 6% tincture iodi fortis in rectified spirit. The nail fold is massaged from above downwards before the paint is applied. In resistant cases, a course of superficial X-ray therapy is very beneficial. Treatment must be carried on until there is complete recovery and the eponychium is formed. Surgery and antibiotics are not necessary. The patient must avoid too much contact with water and use cotton gloves covered by rubber gloves for doing the essential wet work. The general health of the patient must be improved. Accompanying diabetes, if present, must be treated.

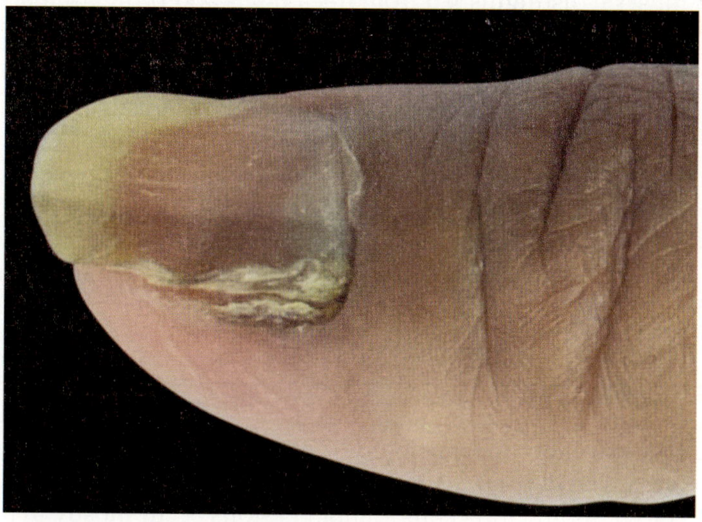

Fig. 12.8: Chronic paronychia

EROSIO INTERDIGITALIS

It occurs as chronic, moist, red erosions with sodden epidermis at the periphery, or as white, macerated skin on the interdigital webs and neighbouring areas of skin. Classically, it involves the space between 3rd and 4th fingers.

MONILIAL INTERTRIGO

It affects flexures, particularly under breasts, the perineum, the groins, the natal cleft and the axillae. The typical lesions consist of moist, smooth, red patches with overhanging edges of white, sodden epidermis.

There may be vesiculation, pustulation or squamous lesions. Exudation is mild. Base is macerated and densely covered with a whitish coat. Sometimes cracks or fissures may be seen. Lesions spread peripherally either as erythematous spots or patches. Differential diagnosis is from flexural eczema, tinea, intertrigo, erythrasma and Hailey Hailey disease.

VULVOVAGINAL CANDIDIASIS

It is seen in young women. There is severe vulvovaginitis, severe pain/itching and erythematous surface covered by whitish coat. On removal, small erosions are seen which may bleed. Vagina and cervix may be affected. Discharge is whitish or caseous like. Differential diagnosis is from gonorrhoea, trichomoniasis and syphilis. Similar picture is seen in balanoposthitis. Diagnosis is confirmed by smear and culture examination. Acute and subacute urethritis has also been described. It is characterized by whitish green discharge, painful micturition and red inflamed urethral orifice.

MONILIAL TOES

The area in between and under the toes may be infected. The lesions show as moist, red, peeling areas with white, sodden epidermis which looks like wet blotting paper. This infection must be distinguished from tinea pedis and ordinary macerated skin.

Treatment: All these conditions are treated with 1–3% aqueous or spiritious solution (in 25–75% spirit methylated) of gentian violet or tincture Merthiolate (P) or nystatin ointment or imidizole derivatives like chlormidazole, miconazole, econazole lotion or cream.

They must be applied twice a day, and the treatment must be persisted with, till all evidence of infection has cleared up. Reports indicate the usefulness of amphotericin-B topically in superficial moniliasis and intravenously in systemic *Candida* infections. Candicidin spray and powder are also very useful. The affected parts must be kept constantly dry. Underlying predisposing causes like obesity and diabetes must be corrected.

ERYTHRASMA

A *Corynebacterium* infection, morphologically looking like a fungus disease, is found all over the world . The clinical features are: well-demarcated areas of varying sizes, brownish-red colour and furfuraceous scaling. Lesions occur mostly in the axillae and groins. The centre is not pigmented and the margin not inflamed **(Fig. 12.9)**. Itching is

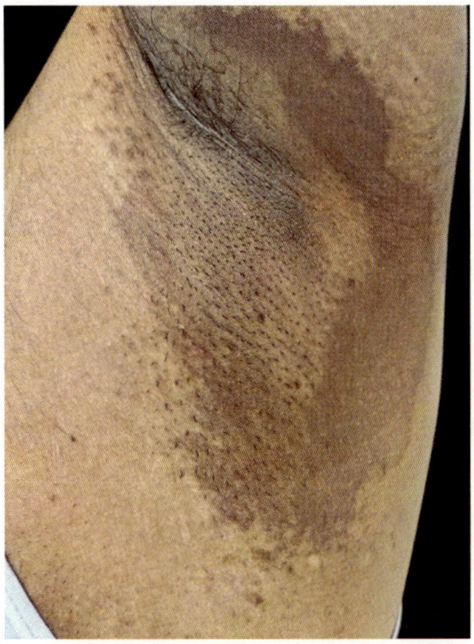

Fig. 12.9: Erythrasma

minimal. Treatment consists of Erythromycin (P) 250 mg four times a day for about a week and topically clotrimazole lotion.

TRICHOMYCOSIS AXILLARIS

It is a very common condition in the tropics and subtropics, and is caused by *Nocardia tenuis* or *Corynebacterium*. Since it is asymptomatic, very few persons consult a physician. It involves the axillary and pubic hair. The infection is seen as yellowish or greyish (rarely reddish) nodules along the hair distributed in a discrete manner, or as a continuous sheath which is firmly adherent to the hair. The hair is brittle and without lustre. The skin is never involved.

Treatment consists in shaving the hair, followed by the use of mild antiseptics on the same lines as in pityriasis versicolor.

TINEA IMBRICATA

This infrequently seen fungal infection is caused by *T. concentricum*. In India, its incidence is comparatively more in Nagaland and the adjacent Eastern States. It is characterized by intensely itchy concentric rings of scales which affect extensive areas of the body. Hairy regions are mostly spared. The infection is not contracted by children below six years. It should be distinguished from ichthyosis and at times erythroderma. Diagnosis is confirmed by demonstration of fungus. Treatment is the same as for other varieties but recurrences are more frequent in tinea imbricata.

ACTINOMYCOSIS

It is the most common of the systemic fungus affections. There are two important varieties depending upon the nature of the causative fungus: *Actinomycosis bovis* is an anaerobic fungus with world-wide distribution. The fungus is present around carious teeth and cryptic tonsils. The infection is endogenous. It affects the cervical lymph glands, lungs, and intestines. The skin is only secondarily affected. The jaw is the site most commonly affected, the infection producing a lumpy jaw. It is characterized by a chronic, solid, indurated granulomatous swelling, and abscess formation and sinuses discharging sanguineous material containing sulphur granules of ray fungus. On healing, there is fibrotic scarring.

Penicillin is the drug of choice in the treatment; it may have to be supported with sulphonamides, iodides and surgical drainage.

Nocardiosis is an aerobic actinomycosis, prevalent mostly in the tropics and subtropics. *Nocardia* is present in the soil; so the infection is exogenous since it is introduced into the tissues from the outside of the body by injury. *N. brasiliensis* is one of the causative agents of mycetoma of the foot.

Mycetoma or Madura Foot: More often seen in surgical than in dermatological practice. It is usually a unilateral affection of limbs, mostly feet. Patient gives history of piercing trauma, like thorn or splinter prick, etc. followed by development of multiple, painless, indurated and chronic sinuses discharging coloured granules on sole/dorsum of foot. The part is globoid, swollen and smells offensive. Changes usually affect deeper tissues and bones . Its etiological agents are *Madurella mycetomi, Nocardia brasiliensis* and *A. boyddi,* and imperfect fungus.

Treatment: In early and uncomplicated cases opening and drainage of sinuses and a course of Septran (P) may be useful. A course of Dapsone (P), new generation fungicide and antibiotic may be tried before radical measures are taken.

CHROMOBLASTOMYCOSIS

A few cases of this previously less known mycotic infection have been described in India. It is caused by *Hormodendrum pedrosoi, Hormodendrum compactum* and *Philialophora verrucosa.* Patients are usually those prone to trauma and contact with dirt—the sons of the soil! Sites of affection are most commonly the feet and legs, less so the hands and only rarely the other parts of the body.

Lesions start as indurated, dirty-looking, papulonodules which slowly increase and take verrucous cauliflower-like appearance in a period of years. The condition is practically asymptomatic. In due course, secondary symptoms like lymphoedema due to extensive fibrosis, ulceration and secondary infection may develop. Regional lymphadenopathy is seen only after secondary infection. At times, the clinical picture may be confused with lichenoid eruptions and lupus vulgaris.

Diagnosis is established by culture or demonstration of spores in biopsy material.

Treatment is unsatisfactory. Depending upon the clinical state electrocoagulation, iodides, cryosurgery and newer fungicides, local infiltration of amphotericin-B, etc. can be tried. Amputation of the limb is considered only as a last resort since the progress is slow, the condition is benign and the usefulness of the limb can be retained for a long time.

RHINOSPORIDIOSIS

This very rare condition affecting mucous membranes of the nose, eyes, ears and larynx is caused by *Rhinosporidium seeberi,* presumably fungal by nature. Other areas of the skin esp. genitalia may also be involved at times.

It is characterized by papillomatous, polypoid and tumor-like masses hanging (may be sessile too) from the anterior part of nasal mucosa and profuse mucoid discharge. The growths are benign and cause concern only by obstructing air and food passages.

Treatment is by desiccation and surgery. Pentavalent antimony may sometimes be helpful.

The other deeper fungi like sporotrichosis, histoplasmosis, coccidiodomycosis, cryptococcosis, North and South American blastomycosis, etc. are very rare in India. Their cutaneous manifestations, except sporotrichosis, are minor as compared to systemic ones. A detailed account of these entities is beyond the scope of this book and the interested reader should refer to detailed books on mycology.

Chapter 13

Cutaneous Disorders by Animal Organisms

INTRODUCTION

Animal organisms produce cutaneous affections all over the world, more so in the tropical and subtropical countries of Africa, South America and South East Asia. The term animal organisms includes animal parasites found on human beings, but it is not necessarily restricted to them, since non-parasitic organisms can also produce cutaneous disorders by simple trauma and the resultant irritation, etc. as a transient phase. The latter group covers a large percentage of cutaneous disorders met with in practice. These disorders are usually the product of unhygienic environment, and so occur mainly in areas and communities where crowding, filth and poverty prevail.

Classification

Medical parasitology has three main sub-divisions:

1. Protozoology—disturbance caused by single-celled animal organisms.
2. Entomology—disorders principally due to insects and mites belonging to phyllum Arthropoda: (a) Arachnida—Acarus (Scabies), ticks, mites, harvest itch, cheese itch, demodex, etc. (b) Insects—Lice, bugs, mosquitoes, etc.
3. Helminthology—diseases due to worms—flukes, leeches, ankylostoma (creeping eruption), filaria, onchocerca, schistosoma, guinea worm, threadworm.

Higher animal organisms like adders, fish, anemones and bees may sometimes cause cutaneous disorders as well. The dermatologic protozoology includes diseases caused by protozoans like *Entamoeba histolytica, Trichomonas vaginalis*, various species of genus Leishmania, etc. These have been described in Chapters 11 and 16. In this chapter we shall confine ourselves to affections mainly due to important members of entomology and helminthology.

Mode of Action

These organisms produce disorders in different ways:

Trauma in the process of burrowing into the skin in search of food, sucking blood or laying eggs. Most of the arthropods fall into this group. Common examples would be pediculosis, *acarus scabiei*, bed bugs, flies, and mosquitoes. Trauma produces irritation and pruritus; the traumas themselves are often visible on the skin.

Secondary infection: The traumas may become secondarily infected with ordinary pyogenic organisms giving rise to different types of pyodermas viz., impetigo, folliculitis, erysipelas, etc.

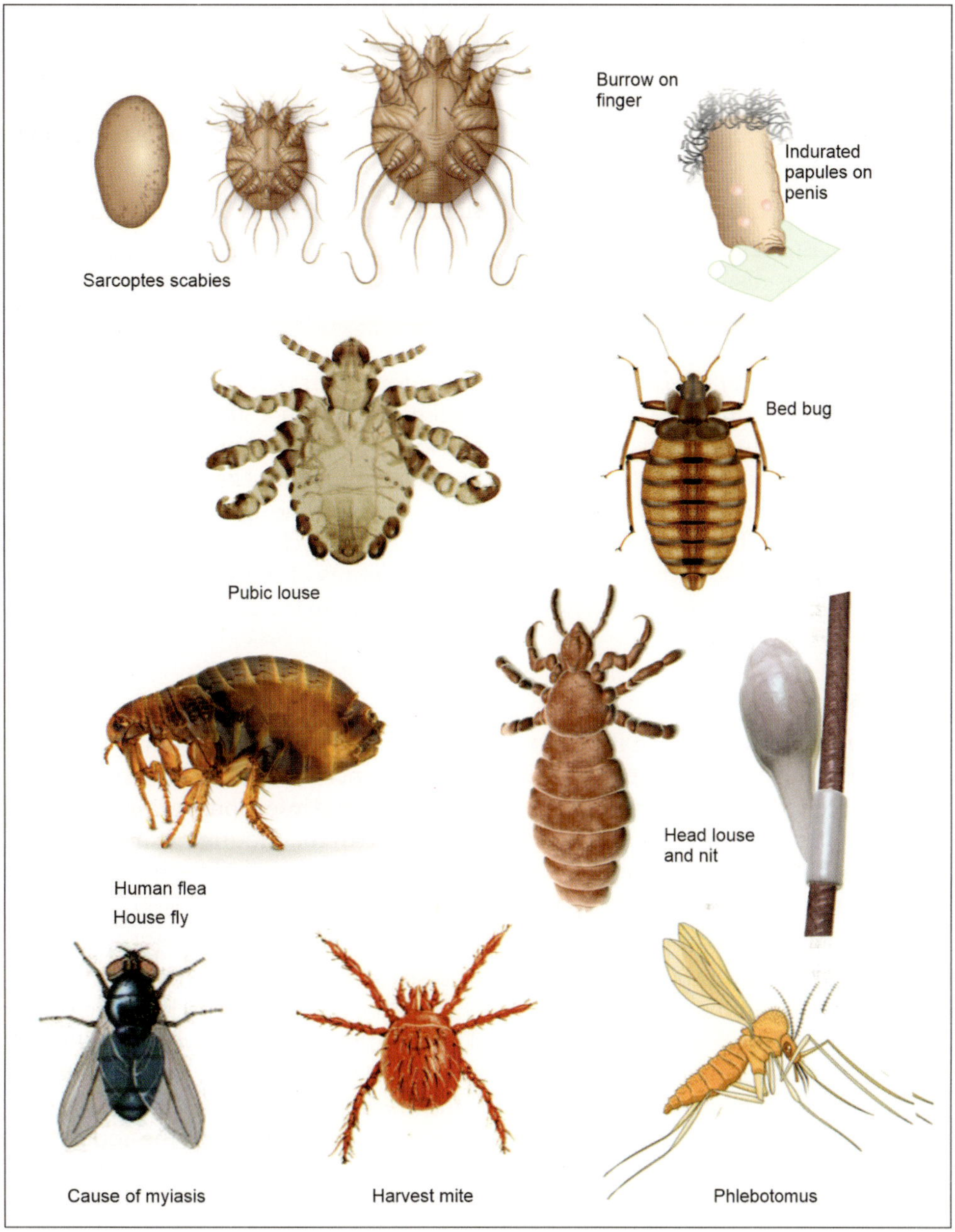

Fig. 13.1: Animal parasites

Transmission of specific infectious diseases: From the public health point of view this feature deserves the utmost attention, and hence, the eradication of the causative animal vectors should form an important part of any public health programme (**Fig. 13.1**). A brief summary is given below:

a. Mosquitoes—Malaria (Anopheles), dengue fever, yellow fever, filariasis (Culex).
b. Lice—Epidemic typhus, relapsing fever.

c. Fleas—Tularaemia, plague, typhus, leptospirosis.
d. Ticks—Typhus, tularaemia.
e. Flies—Typhoid, cholera.

Sensitization reaction: Bees, wasps, sea-fish. Local and systemic allergic reactions ensue, resulting occasionally in collapse, shock and even death.

SCABIES

It is a contagious disease caused by a parasitic mite called *Sarcoptes scabiei*. The disease is contracted by intimate contact with infected individuals, or through infected bed linen or clothing.

The parasite, *Sarcoptes scabiei*, is a mite having four pairs of legs unlike bugs, lice and fleas, which have only three pairs of legs. The female is 400 μ × 300 μ in size, and grey in colour. This parasite is just visible to the naked eye. The male is smaller than the female, and has a very brief span of life; it dies shortly after copulation. The impregnated female acarus, having burrowed her way into the horny layer of the epidermis, lives there for about two months. In these burrows, she lays her eggs which develop into larvae. They pierce the roofs of the burrows, find shelter in the pores of the skin, and develop into adult mites. The life cycle of the acarus, from the ovum to the adult stage, is from 13 to 21 days.

Clinical Features

1. *Nocturnal pruritus:* Intense itching which is worse at night. The young acari pierce the roof of the burrows in the warmth of the bed and try to reach the pores. Usually there is no itching in the first 4 weeks of contracting the infection, because the itching is due to the development of sensitization to some of the products (saliva-scabin) of the mite, and about this much time is required for it. In case of re-infection, itching starts early.
2. History of exposure or multiple cases in the family.
3. Burrows are a very important feature of the disease. They represent the path traversed by the parasite in the horny layer of the skin. They are tortuous. Their lengths vary from a quarter of an inch to half an inch. They are flesh coloured, with dark dots here and there. If the roof is lifted with a fine needle, the mite can be demonstrated. The common sites of burrows are: The fingers, the interdigital webs, the palms, the wrists, the points of elbows, the anterior axillary folds, around the nipples, the abdomen, the buttocks, the genitalia, the legs and the feet. The neck and the face are not involved, except in children. By scratching and secondary infection the burrows are deformed or mutilated and hence, are often difficult to demonstrate. For this reason, they are not absolutely essential for diagnosis.
4. Fine, pin-head sized, follicular papules. Besides, papulopustules on erythematous bases (studs) are commonly seen. They are helpful in diagnosis. Scabetic dermatitis and dyshidrosis-like eruption, following an attack of scabies have often been reported. Occasional individual dermal nodules may develop due to deeper penetration by the acarus or a severe dermal reaction to the toxins of the acarus **(Fig. 13.2)**.
5. Excoriations and scratch marks.

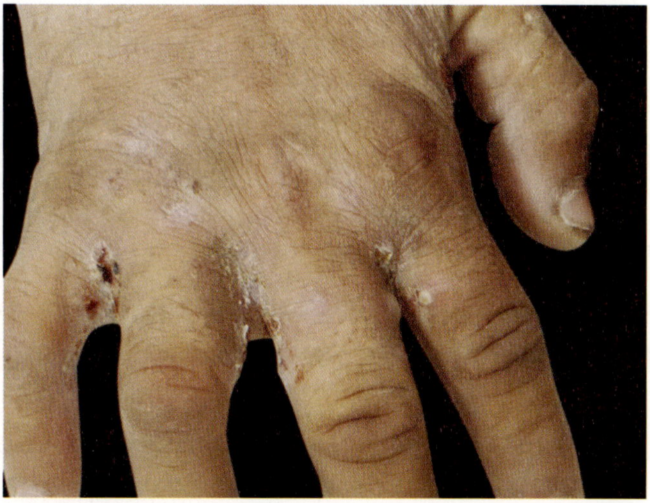

Fig. 13.2: Classical scabies involving interdigital web of the hands

Complications

a. Impetiginization
b. Eczematization
c. Secondary lymphadenitis.

If untreated, the disease may last for months. Ultimately natural desensitization may develop.

Norwegian Scabies

The lesions are so severe that the whole body and limbs including face, scalp and nails may be enveloped in crusts and scales in which large number of parasites are present. It is mainly seen in mental and geriatric patients and persists for years.

Animal Scabies

The acarus from cats and dogs rarely attack the human skin, as man is not a suitable host.

The affection in such cases is more inflammatory and usually transient.

Differential diagnosis: It is made from other causes of pruritus, eczematization and impetiginization. In cases of intractable impetigo on the body, and multiple cases of pruritus in family, particularly in an endemic area, one must suspect scabies. The features described above are characteristic of the parasitic affection. Skin shavings can confirm the diagnosis by demonstration of ova/acarus. Pediculosis, insect bites (bugs) and dermatitis herpetiformis should be specially excluded.

Treatment: It consists of:

Preventive: Personal hygiene and daily bath; separate clothes, bed linen and towels; use of medicated soap containing 3% acid salicylic and 10% sulphur.

Curative: The aims are: Specific destruction of parasites with use of special medication like benzyl benzoate emulsion (25% in adults, half strength in children), sulphur ointment 5–10%, Crotorax, the gamma benzene hexachloride and permethrin. Few cases may need oral Thiabendazole or Ivermectin in a single dose according to body weight. Strict adherence to instructions is enforced as follows:

a. First thoroughly scrub with soap and water.
b. After drying, thoroughly rub the ointment/emulsion for at least 15 minutes all over the body. The affected areas are given special attention. Since the acarus is in burrows, unless the application is thoroughly rubbed it will not reach the depth of the burrow. Emulsion is not applied over the face, scalp and neck except in children.
c. Medication must be kept on the body for at least 36 hours before taking the next hot bath.
d. Hot bath and thorough scrubbing followed by new clothes. Old clothes should be disinfected.
e. Re-application of the ointment in the same manner after 7 days. Itching will take at least 3–4 weeks to subside even after proper treatment.
f. Treat all contacts—conjugal, family members, school friends, etc. whether they have symptoms or not. This is most important to prevent ping-ponging of the disease.

For mass treatment sulphur ointment or benzyl benzoate emulsion is useful. So also is special medicated soap.

Day care centre can shorten the course of treatment in endemic areas. Urban day care centre gives initial scrubbing followed by sauna bath, rubbing of ointment for 1/2 hr and then another scrub with medicated soap and hot water. In the rural areas, instead of sauna bath, patients are asked to stand in the hot sun for 10–20 minutes. Water is heated by putting it in the sun in steel tubs. Whole procedure takes an hour and the whole family is treated at the same time. Cure rate is about 95%. Boiling of clothes and interference with night life are avoided by giving day care centre treatment.

Management of cutaneous lesions and complications: The specific remedy alone may be enough to control pruritus. If not, an antihistaminic may have to be administered and a soothing ointment prescribed. The authors prefer to use Phenergan (P) tablets, 10 mg at bed time, and zinc cream containing 1% boric acid rubbed on all itchy parts twice a day.

The management of complications like eczema, impetigo, etc. along the usual lines. In severe cases, the complications are treated first, and then the specific treatment is started; in mild cases, the reverse is the rule. In wide-spread pyoderma, a course of sulphonamides–Madribon (P), septran or penicillin is indicated.

It must be remembered that pruritus may persist for a few weeks even after the acari have been got rid of by specific treatment. Half-hearted, inadequate application of medicament without proper preparation of the patient (scrubbing and hot path), ineffective treatment of contacts and inadequate disinfection of clothing are responsible for failure to cure and eradicate scabies.

PEDICULOSES OR LICE

The Indian name is *juan*. There are three varieties of lice classified—head, body and pubis—according to affected area.

Pediculosis Capitis

It is caused by the head louse. The female louse is about 2 mm long and half as broad; the male is slightly smaller. These parasites are greyish in colour; the females are much more numerous than the males. The female and male copulate and produce ova which attach themselves in sacs (nits) to the hair by collagenous bands. Ova mature in about 2 weeks. Pediculi have three pairs of legs.

Children, particularly girls, are usually affected. The occipital regions are the sites of choice. Infection is transmitted through combs and head-dresses. Pediculosis affection, as a rule, is an index of poor personal hygiene.

Lice traumatize the skin in search of food. The trauma produces irritation which results in scratching, scratch marks and may be secondary pyoderma, impetigo and infective eczema. Persistent secondary infection brings about regional lymphadenitis. Examination reveals living lice and nits. The latter are firmly attached to the hair, but can be moved along it towards the free end **(Fig. 13.3)**. Persistent impetigo of the scalp usually indicates the presence of pediculi. It may even cause cicatricial alopecia.

Treatment: There are several methods and drugs recommended but the ones commonly used are:

DDT—Application 2–5% in an emulsifying base. About a tablespoonful of it is applied all over the scalp by parting the hair, and is rubbed thoroughly into the scalp. The hair is washed and combed after 24 hours. This can be repeated 2–3 times till the infection is completely eradicated. Synthetic pyretroid (Mediker-P) is safe and effective.

Lorexane (P)—Only one tablespoonful is required. It is applied in the same way as the DDT application with the following difference: the hair is washed at the end of 7 days, and the application is not repeated before the lapse of a week. Biweekly washing of the scalp with medicated soap containing 3% salicylic acid and 10% sulphur is also useful. Lather must be left on the scalp for 15 minutes before washing it off.

Bed clothes, head-dress and combs must be sterilized to prevent re-infection and transmission of infection to others. Secondary complications are treated in the usual way.

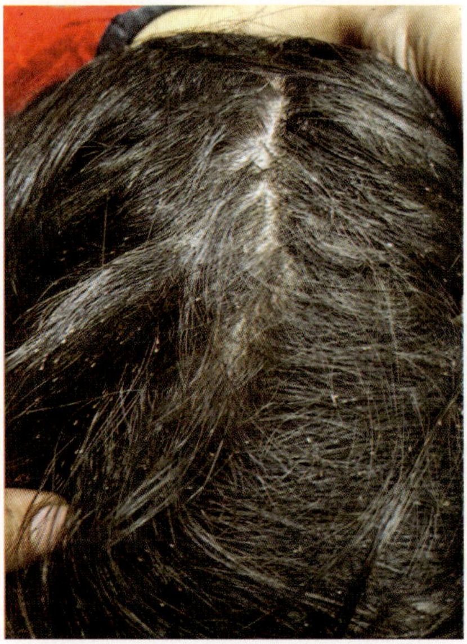

Fig. 13.3: Pediculosis capitis

Pediculosis Corporis

It is caused by body louse which is longer (about 3 mm in length) than the head louse. The life cycle of the former is about the same as that of the latter. Pediculi shelter themselves in the seams of underclothing, usually vests. They prefer to lay their ova on the clothing rather than on the hair or the skin. In their search for food, the lice produce minute haemorrhages, crusted papules and resultant scratch marks. In chronic cases, parasitic affection may be complicated by pyoderma, eczematization and pigmentation. Persistent impetigo and itching of the trunk usually indicate pediculoses (Vagabond's disease). The scapular regions and the shoulders are the sites of choice.

Young adults and old people are most commonly affected by the parasite. The body louse multiplies rapidly in conditions of mass migration of people, over-crowding and unhygienic environment. Under such circumstances, pediculoses may start epidemics of typhus and relapsing fever.

Treatment: It consists in sterilizing clothes with a hot iron, by boiling or steaming. DDT 5% solution or powder may also be employed. Secondary complications may be treated in the usual manner. Benzyl benzoate emulsion, Crotorax (P) and 0.5% gamma benzene hexachloride are also useful.

If these preparations are used, the sterilization of clothes by heat may not be necessary. If dermatitis ensues with DDT the application must be washed off and a soothing preparation applied.

Pediculosis Pubis

It is caused by stout, pubic lice which, besides affecting the pubic region, may also affect the eyebrows, axillae, and the hairy sternal region. The life cycle of this parasite is about the same as that of the head louse. Infection is transmitted through sexual intercourse, or the use of common bathing costumes and lavatories. The clinical features are intense itching, scratch marks, nits and the lice. The latter are firmly attached to the hair and skin. They appear as dark dots on the skin. On touching they move.

The treatment consists in shaving the pubic hair, rubbing in DDT powder or ointment and in the after-use of a mild soothing ammoniated mercury ointment. Underclothing must be disinfected with DDT, or by boiling. Hot tub bath with medicated soap is beneficial.

OTHER COMMON PARASITES

Bed Bugs

Synonym: *Climex lectularius*. The Hindustani name is *Khatmal*.

Bed bugs hide themselves in the crevices of beds, old furniture, and dark comers. They are reddish-brown in colour, and usually emerge from their hiding places at night to feed on human skin by sucking blood. There is marked itching. The lesions are urticarial weals, pruritic papules or haemorrhagic vesicles occurring in groups of two or three. The common sites are the back (which is attacked in bed), ankles, wrists and neck.

Fleas

There are two distinct varieties—the human or common flea (*Pulex irritans*), and the animal flea which lodges itself in the hairy coats of cats, dogs and rats. Both varieties can bite man. The common flea breeds in floor cracks, and bites man usually on the legs. The lesions are urticarial weals with central haemorrhagic puncta. Since they are carriers of serious infectious diseases like plague and typhus, eradication of the parasites is important.

Ticks

Synonym: Ixodes.

They live on pine trees or animals, and suck blood and stick to the skin looking like cysts: they may fall off when gorged with blood. Tick bites produce marked itching, urticarial weals and bleeding points. Their larvae also produce itching. Dogs are common culprits. The latter should be thoroughly washed and treated with Ticol (P).

Harvest Mites

Synonym: Trombicula irritans.

The affection caused by harvest mites usually occurs in the harvest season, and is picked up by people who walk through vegetation. The parasites attack the legs producing irregular weals and papules.

A severe burning sensation is characteristic, beginning a few hours after the attack by the parasite.

Demodex Folliculorum

It is found in young adults. It produces itchy folliculitis, mostly on the face due to the hair follicles being penetrated by the mite. Lesions may later on become secondarily infected. This affection must be considered in differential diagnosis of troublesome, itching folliculitis of the face. It is picked up from vegetation mainly siting under trees.

Tungiasis

This is an affection which occurs mostly in South America, in the West Indies and Africa.

During the Second World War, Indian troops stationed in Africa were affected. The condition is caused by the sandflea (*Tunga penetrans*), the female of which, penetrates the skin of the feet, less often, the hands and buttocks, producing itchy, indurated papules with central black dots. Secondary infection produces suppuration. Multiple lesions produce honey-combed solid patches.

Grain Itch

It is caused by a mite, *Pediculoides ventricosus*, which infests grain or straw. It affects workers, porters and people sleeping on new straw mattresses. The whole body, including the face and neck, may be involved in severe infestations. The main lesions are papules, vesicles and weals.

Copra Itch and Cheese Itch

They are caused by a mite, *Tyroglyhus langior*, infesting copra and cheese. The lesions on the skin consist of urticarial} papules with blood crusts.

Water Itch

It is caused by a particular mite found in tea plantations in the rainy season. Lesions are usually on the legs in the form of scratch marks and papular urticaria. Wearing of long trousers and long boots helps to prevent the affection. Crotorox (P) is both prophylactic and curative.

Bees, Wasps, Hornets, Ants and Insects

These insects are common in India, particularly in the summer and monsoon. On being bitten or stung there is little or no reaction in a majority of people. Simple home remedies are beneficial and no doctor is consulted except in cases of reaction which occurs in a few sensitive individuals.

Locally the sting produces an urticarial weal with a central punctum or an immediate eczematous reaction and occasionally indurated papules which take time to subside. In sensitive individuals the unpleasant consequences are due to protein-like substances, kinins. There is immediate or delayed generalized allergic reaction in the form of urticaria, swollen lips, sinking feeling, paralysis, and shock. Death has been reported to occur in severe cases.

Mosquitoes

Both Anopheles and Culex are responsible for the transmission of infectious diseases. In the monsoon mosquitoes breed in stagnant pools of water, dark corners and abundant vegetation. They are attracted by artificial light. Their bites produce papules and urticarial weals accompanied by stinging and itching.

Sea-side Stings

Swimmers and fishermen get stung by rice-fish, jelly-fish, sand-hoppers, etc. Local papular urticaria or generalized urticaria may be seen. Acute painful inflammation is sometimes come across. Rarely a generalized reaction, as after bee-stings, may develop in sensitive individuals.

Treatment of Insect Bites

Prophylaxis is most important. It is primarily a public health problem. Environmental hygiene must be improved since the animal organisms usually breed in unhygienic environment.

Insecticides: Some good ones are: DDT in powder or solution form, gamma benzene hexachloride—Gammexane (P), Dieldrin (P) and pyrethrum. The toxic symptoms are few; sometimes one comes across sensitization dermatitis. In the use of these insecticides, the manufacturer's instructions must be strictly followed to prevent serious side-effects.

Insect Repellents

1. The use of protective clothing and nets.
2. The use of wire netting all around the house-doors, windows, and verandahs.
3. Medicaments over the exposed areas. Common examples are:
   a. Rx
      Oil of citronella 16 ml

Oil of cedri 8 ml
Spt. camphor 8 ml
Paraffin molle to 100 g

b. Dimethyl-phthalate—30–50% in a vanishing cream base.

It acts by burning the feet of insects. It tends to dissolve certain synthetics like plastics and fibres; hence during use, it should not be allowed to come in contact with artificial synthetic plastic.

Curative treatment: It varies with the nature of the lesions, complications and causative organisms.

The specific treatment has been described above, along with the discussion of different organisms. Hydrocortisone ointment, ammonia or dilute tincture iodine helps to control the local reaction of an insect bite; in severe cases where there is a wide-spread, dangerous allergic reaction, corticosteroids may have to be used systemically. Antihistaminics help to control pruritus. Secondary infection is checked with local antiseptics; in extensive cases, course of Septran (P) or Doxycycline is useful.

MYIASIS

It is of two distinct varieties:

1. *Myiasis linearis,* creeping disease of Larva migrans. It is caused by the larvae of Bot files (Oestradia) or Helminths (*Ankylostoma brasiliense, A. canunum,* the common nematodes of cats and dogs). It is rather rare in this country. The incubation period is about one month. Lesions are found mostly on the legs and buttocks but may also be seen elsewhere. A lesion consists of an itchy, reddish or flesh-coloured creeping stripe; the advancing point consists of a bulla or a weal which advances by 1–3 cm every day. The treatment consists in applying CO_2 snow or freezing the advancing point with ethyl chloride. Thiabendazole by mouth (50 mg per kg in single dose) has been found very effective.
2. *Constant myiasis* (Maggots). It occurs mostly in summer months when flies are common due to heat and unhygienic environments. Flies lay eggs in open wounds; the eggs grow into maggots which penetrate the tissues causing necrosis. This condition can be prevented by dressing all open wounds, and keeping flies away from the patient by hygienic measures and the use of mosquito nets.

The treatment consists in thoroughly cleaning the infested wounds, extracting all visible maggots and applying maggot oil containing chloroform and turpentine oil in water.

CYSTICERCUS CELLULOSAE CUTIS

The cysticercae of *Taenia solium* and other tapeworms reach the subcutaneous tissues and produce multiple tumours. In cysticercosis, man is the intermediate host, acquiring the infection by the ingestion of pork or drink contaminated with eggs. The subcutaneous lumps are, at first, rounded and elastic and vary in size from a pea to a walnut and are asymptomatic; The old cysts dry up and may calcify. Diagnosis usually comes as a surprise, when biopsy specimen reveals the parasite. Treatment consists of surgical excision and a course of Praziquental. An anthelmintic should be administered to clear the tapeworms from the intestines.

SCHISTOSOMIASIS

Synonym: Bilharziasis.

Schistosomal affections are rather rare in India. There are two clinical varieties: Cercarial dermatitis (Swimmer's itch) caused by cercaria of non-human schisto somiasis of birds and mammals, has been recorded in Mysore (India), though it is commonly seen in other parts of South-East Asia. In summer and the monsoon, the cercaria penetrate the skin of swimmers producing prickly sensation; later, erythematous macules and urticaria develop due to sensitization.

Systemic Bilharziasis is rare in India, hence its allergic manifestations, and later, cutaneous features like vulval warty masses and indolent nodules in the skin, have not been found in this country. This condition is fairly common in Egypt (Zawahry, Mofty). Antimony is employed in the treatment.

DRACUNCULOSIS

Synonym: Guinea-worm infestation.

It is a very uncommon affection. Man is the main host of the parasite, *Dracunculus medinensis*, and the water flea (Cyclops) is the intermediate host. Man is infected by water contaminated by the parasite; hence the infection occurs amongst people who drink water from the tanks in which they bathe. Cyclops are digested in the stomach. The mature larvae penetrate the stomach wall and lie in retroperitoneal connective tissue, spaces or in the subcutaneous tissues; here it grows into adult worms and mates. No signs or symptoms are produced. The male dies after copulation, and the female migrates under the skin to a part of the body which comes in contact with water, usually the feet, but sometimes the buttock. The whole process takes from 10 to 14 months. The adult female worm measures about 30–50 inches. On reaching the foot it produces a blister which bursts, producing an ulcer. It may be preceded by urticaria, fever, severe itching and other anaphylactoid symptoms. From this ulcer, protrudes the worm discharging larvae when the ulcer comes in contact with water. On discharge, these larvae find their way into the cyclops.

Clinical Features

i. During the long incubation period of about a year, there are no symptoms, until the gravid female undertakes her journey usually towards the legs and feet. As the worm carrying the distended gravid uterus nears the surface, under the stimulus of water, pronounced prodromal symptoms, e.g. erythema, generalized itching, dysponea and asthma-like symptoms may appear.

ii. Soon a blister forms which ruptures giving rise to an ulcer on the malleolus of a foot, less so, the buttocks and back (in water carriers). All toxic symptoms subside when the blister ruptures.

iii. A protruding worm which can be rolled around a stick. Complications develop if the worm dies under the skin, or the track becomes secondarily infected producing cellulitis, gangrene or septicaemia.

Treatment: The oriental treatment consists in gently making the worm protrude out by douching with water. The worm is then pulled out slightly and rolled around a sterilized stick; in this way it is pulled out gradually, bit by bit every day. If proper care is not taken the worm will tear, producing disastrous complications, which can nowadays, be controlled with antibiotics and surgery.

Phenothiazine is recommended by Manson Bahr. This is injected intramuscularly into the leg. The worm dies within 7–10 days, and can then be pulled out.

The prophylaxis consists of filtered water supply to the people. In villages drinking water wells should be kept separate from tanks where people bathe and wash.

FILARIASIS

It is caused by *Wuchereria bancrofti* deposited in the lymphatic vessels and glands. The male is about 4 cm × 0.1 mm and the female 6 cm × 0.2 mm. They copulate, the female becomes gravid, discharging microfilariae (living embryos) into lymphatics; these enter into the blood stream unless the lymphatics have become occluded by inflammation due to primary irritation and secondary infection . Microfilariae are found in the peripheral blood at night time in the early stages of infection. Mosquitoes (Culex) are the intermediate hosts in whom microfilariae, sucked during biting, mature into infective larval filariae. They are transferred to human beings through bites by infected mosquitoes; larval filariae enter the lymphatic system, maturing in about 3 months.

Filariasis is common in Central and Eastern India. It also occurs in other countries of South-East Asia and throughout the Pacific region.

Clinical features: During the stage of invasion, the symptoms are mainly allergic, taking the form of painful swelling of the scrotum, arms and legs (like erythema nodosum), urticarial lesions, lymphadenitis, lymphangitis and filarial fever.

After the adult worms have lodged themselves in lymphatic vessels and glands, the microfilariae are liberated. Only at this stage can they be demonstrated in the peripheral blood. Filarial abscesses, enlarged groin glands, lymph scrotum, lymph hydrocele and chyluria, arthritis, etc. are the usual symptoms at this stage. Inguinal and femoral glands are hard and fibrous; when punctured with a syringe, microfilaria can be demonstrated in the lymph. Indurated lymphatics are also seen. In lymph scrotum, the scrotum is enlarged, bulky and itchy. Surface shows lymph varices which on rupture keep on discharging continuously straw coloured fluid.

The most common infestation one comes across is elephantiasis of the legs and scrotum produced by the obstruction of the lymphatic vessels and glands. There is tense solid oedema (which does not pit on pressure) with furrowed skin **(Fig. 13.4)**. This is usually preceded or accompanied by repeated attacks of lymphangitis, and eosinophilia. Elephantiasis is a very distressing symptom; it often cripples the patient. The lymphatic glands in the groin are often enlarged. Microfilariae are absent from the blood at this stage. Surgical measures may have to be undertaken to relieve this distressing and crippling symptom. Filariasis should be distinguished from streptococcal elephantiasis and lymphogranuloma inguinale.

Diagnosis: It is confirmed by the demonstration of microfilariae in the night blood, eosinophilia, complement fixation and skin tests.

Treatment: It consists of administration of hetrazan in doses of 150 mg daily for 20 days (2 mg per kg. of the bodyweight). The course can be repeated after about a month. Course of penicillin or other antibiotics is also indicated. Pressure bandages and surgery help the bad case of elephantiasis. The prevention of filariasis consists of mass treatment of all infected individuals in an area and the eradication of mosquitoes by the use of insecticides in the breeding places.

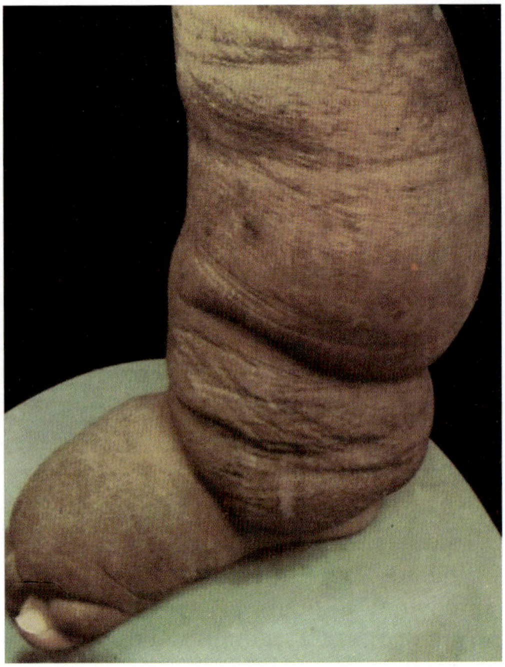

Fig. 13.4: Elephantiasis

LOIASIS

It is a common filarial infection found in tropical Africa. The microfilariae are found in the blood stream during the day. The characteristic clinical feature is the presence of Calabar swellings which are transient, itchy, oedematous swellings, occurring periodically on the extremities and the face. The diagnosis is confirmed by the demonstration of eosinophilia, microfilariae in the day blood, complement fixation and skin tests. The treatment is with hetrazan.

ONCHOCERCIASIS

It is confined to tropical Africa, being a filarial infection caused by *Onchocerca volvulus*. Clinically, it is characterized by intense pruritus, cutaneous nodules, thickening of the skin, elephantiasis and blindness. The diagnosis is established by the demonstration of microfilariae in the skin shavings particularly from the neighbourhood of nodules, eosinophilia, by complement fixation and skin tests. The treatment is with hetrazan and Suramin (P).

OXYURIASIS

Oxyuriasis is caused by threadworms. These parasites are responsible for peri-anal, and less often, vulval pruritus. Itching is worst at night. Children are most commonly affected. The adult worm comes out of the anus to lay eggs in the peri-anal skin; in the process it produces irritation.

The diagnosis, once suspected, is confirmed by the examination of stools which show ova. The treatment consists of administering an antihelmintic like mebendazole or single dose of albendazole. The hands must be tied in mittens or gloves at night to prevent reinfection by the transfer of the ova from the anal region to the mouth.

Chapter

14

Diseases due to Viral Infection

INTRODUCTION

Viruses are the smallest infectious agents (18–300 nm in diameter: one nm = one millionth part of a millimetre) whose genome is an element of either deoxyribonucleic acid (DNA) or ribonucleic acid (RNA) but never both, enclosed within an outer shell of protein, capsid. Viruses can reproduce only inside living cells and utilise the synthetic machinery of the host cell for synthesis of specialized particles, the 'virions', which contain the viral genome and serve as a vehicle to carry the genome to other cells. When a virion enters its host cell the capsid is stripped off and its nucleic acid is liberated within the host cells entering into an eclipse phase in their reproductive cycle, a characteristic of all true viruses. The surface proteins of the virion have special affinity for specific receptor sites on the host cell. Proteins also contain the viral antigens that stimulate the host's immune responses during infection. Viruses possess the property of haemagglutination.

Interferon, a protein produced by the cell after infection with a virus interferes with the replication of the other viruses. Inactivated virus and also a few other substances (foreign nucleic acids and other synthetic polynucleotides) also induce synthesis of interferon.

Any of the following events may occur following presence of virus within a cell:

1. Destruction, e.g. primary herpes hominis virus infection.
2. Stimulation and multiplication first forming a papule which then undergoes destruction associated with inflammatory exudate forming vesicle, which subsequently evolves into a pustule and finally drying up to form scab, e.g. variola, varicella, monkeypox virus.
3. Stimulation of the cells to proliferate indefinitely forming papillomata, e.g. warts. Skin is one of the principal target organs for viral attack. Rashes (exanthemata) are characteristic of many acute systemic viral infections where virions in the blood invade the endothelium of the capillaries and venules of the dermis. Viral rash may also be related to antigen–antibody reaction and the circulation of immune complexes. The rash may be an outward sign of the neutralization of circulating virus by antibody. Haemorrhagic rashes may be due to disseminated intravascular coagulation precipitated by the circulating virus antibodies and immune complexes.

In some instances where the primary process of invasion is in the epidermis, the skin lesions are characterized by intracellular inclusions and the formation of multinucleate giant cells.

Skin probably offers a peculiarly sensitive situation for some viral growth because of its lower temperature.

In dermatologic practice the following group of viruses appear important:

DNA viruses (Deoxyriboviruses)

1. *Herpes viruses*
   Herpes simplex, varicella zoster
   Epstein-Barr virus
   AIDS virus-HIV-I
2. *Pox viruses*
   Variola,
   Vaccinia
   Monkeypox
   Molluscum contagiosum
   Orf. Milker's nodes
3. *Papova viruses*
   Warts

RNA viruses (Riboviruses)

1. Picoma viruses
   Coxsackie:
   Herpengina, rubella
2. Echo viruses
   Hand-foot-mouth disease (HFMD)
3. SARS CoV19

The term 'Herpes' signifies a group of vesicles on an inflammatory base like a bunch of grapes. Clinically, herpetic lesions are typical and are seen in two main herpetic conditions—simplex and zoster.

HERPES SIMPLEX

It occurs after stress, for instance, a psychogenic stress, injury, fever, particularly malaria, pneumonia, meningitis, general illness, debility, etc. The virus of herpes is ubiquitous; it is more prevalent in the temperate climate and the cold season. This accounts for the layman's name of 'Cold spots'.

There are two distinct antigenic types of herpes simplex viruses: HSV-1 and HSV-2. While HSV-2 is responsible for genital herpes simplex, all other clinical varieties are due to HSV-1. Development of carcinoma may be related to HSV-2 infection of the cervix.

Clinical features: Herpes starts with a sensation of burning or itching after there has been an exposure to the cold wind, sun, etc. Erythematous macules appear, on which grouped, pinhead sized, superficial vesicles rapidly develop; their contents soon become opaque. They may rupture and become crusted, or dry up to leave faint, reddish stains (Fig. 14.1). There are usually negligible constitutional symptoms. The course of herpes is about 7–14 days. There is usually no scarring except when secondary infection occurs. Occasionally, hyperpigmentation or depigmentation may follow.

Besides the common herpes simplex affection, primary infection may manifest in the following three ways:

1. Gingivostomatitis or vulvo-vaginitis or keratoconjunctivitis associated with fever, malaise, regional lymphadenopathy.
2. Herpetic whitlow-painful vesiculopustular eruption around the nailfold, often associated with regional lymphadenopathy.
3. Eczema herpeticum type or Kaposi's varicelliform eruption.

Recurrent herpes implies relapsing type of herpes simplex occurring on the same site-usually perioral and genitalia. Local resistance is low; emotional stress, fever, exposure to cold and lack of personal hygiene tend to bring on an attack.

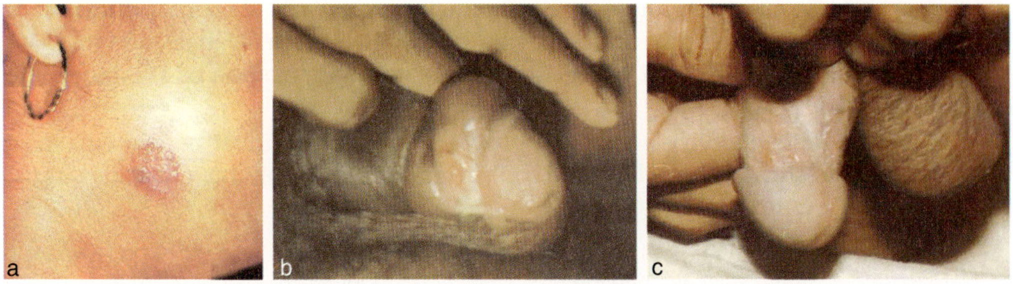

Fig. 14.1: (a) Herpes simplex; (b and c) Herpes progenitalis

Erythema multiforme may be a complication at times.

Herpes progenitalis implies herpes simplex lesions on the genitalia. It is transmitted sexually. In the male, the lesions are on the glans, prepuce or body of the penis; in the female, on the labia, vaginal wall and cervix. The eruption on the genitalia is painful, and may cause a constitutional upset. Genital herpetic lesions rupture early producing erosions, which at times, are in a circinate pattern. The common predisposing causes of recurrent genital herpes are phimosis, lack of personal hygiene, discharge per vaginum and sexual neurosis. Furthermore, recurrent herpes progenitalis is responsible for syphilophobia in some cases.

Buccal herpes is rare in adults but common in infants as aphthous stomatitis which involves the mucous membrane of the palate, cheeks and tongue. Because of moisture and friction, the vesicles get rapidly eroded producing painful, superficial erosions on erythematous bases accompanied by constitutional upset.

Diagnosis: Herpes simplex of the face is so characteristic that it can be diagnosed without any difficulty. Herpes zoster is unilateral; the lesions appear along the nerve distribution; they are painful and non-recurrent.

Herpes progenitalis should be differentiated from syphilitic chancre by the presence of multiple, superficial lesions and the absence of induration, shotty regional lymph glands and spirochaetes in the dark-field examination. Moreover, herpes develops within a few days of exposure while syphilitic chancre develops much later (about 4 weeks).

Chancroid is characterized by painful ulcers which are deeper than the superficial erosions of herpes; suppurating bubo, and the presence of *Haemophilus ducreyi* in the smear (for details, refer to **Table 18.1**).

Very rarely can scabies of the penis, monilial balanitis, lichen planus and fixed drug eruption be confused. If their respective features are remembered, there will be no difficulty at all.

Prognosis: In an individual attack of herpes the prognosis is good, in the sense that lesions heal up nicely and no scarring results. Only in recurrent herpes is the treatment rather unsatisfactory, and the malady can become a nuisance especially in herpes progenitalis.

Treatment: Locally, any antiseptic and astringent application is sufficient; the lesions soon dry up, secondary infection is prevented. Authors prefer the use of lotion silver nitrate 1% and savlon cream (P) or dequadin paint (P), spirit camphor or pure alum applied repeatedly has been found to abort attacks in the early stages. Application of anaesthetic ether has been also advocated by pressing a cotton swab soaked in anaesthetic ether for 5 minutes on 2 consecutive days. Prior application of 1% lignocaine will minimise the pain.

In recurrent herpes which is a knotty problem, an attempt must be made to raise the general resistance and to eliminate the precipitating causes like chronic rhinitis, phimosis, debility, anxiety, stress, etc.

Other measures recommended are as follows:

A. Topical chemicals	Ether Glutaraldehyde 2%
B. Topical systemic anti-viral	Idoxuridine Acyclovir
C. Photo-dynamic	Proflavine and UVR
D. Immunological stimulants	Auto-vaccination Levamisole
E. Grenz-ray therapy	

Antiviral therapy is useful if started early on the first day of eruption. Multiplicity of modalities available is a fair indication of their inadequacy. Lotio silver nitrate 0.5% usually gives the best results. Circumcision is very useful in resistant and recurrent herpes progenitalis. Superficial epidermal surgical removal and applying 25% phenol for 30 seconds is also beneficial.

In intractable cases, a relaxing holiday, preferably at a spa or sulphur spring, may do the trick and cure the patient when every other therapeutic measure has failed.

HERPES ZOSTER

Synonym: Shingles.

Varicella-zoster virus (VZV) is the causative organism, and the site of its pathology is the posterior root ganglion; the skin is only secondarily affected. One or several posterior root ganglia may be involved. The inflammation, sometimes, though rarely, spreads to the posterior horn and then to the anterior horn and even the meninges. Physical injuries, mental trauma, febrile illnesses and drugs are also known to act as triggers as well as predisposing factors.

Shingles may occur at any age, though of course, adults are more often affected.

Occasionally, herpes zoster may take an epidemic form.

Herpes zoster is closely related to chickenpox on microbiological, serological and epidemiological basis. Patients are infectious; in the first week, virus can be isolated from the vesicles.

Clinical features: An attack starts with neuralgic pain, local increased sensitivity of the skin (hyperaesthesia) and fever with a range of 102–103°F. Cutaneous lesions develop three days after the onset of the attack. Sometimes, the rash may develop suddenly without any premonitory symptom. The rash develops in the segmental dstribution of the affected nerve roots, and consists of typical herpetic lesions, e.g. groups of vesicles on inflammatory base in several patches with intervening areas of normal skin.

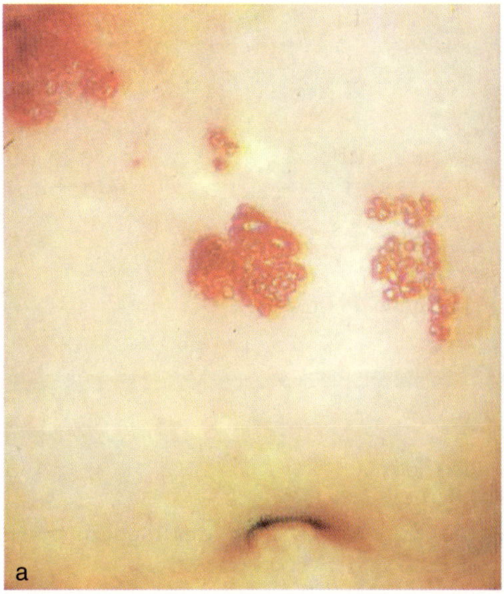

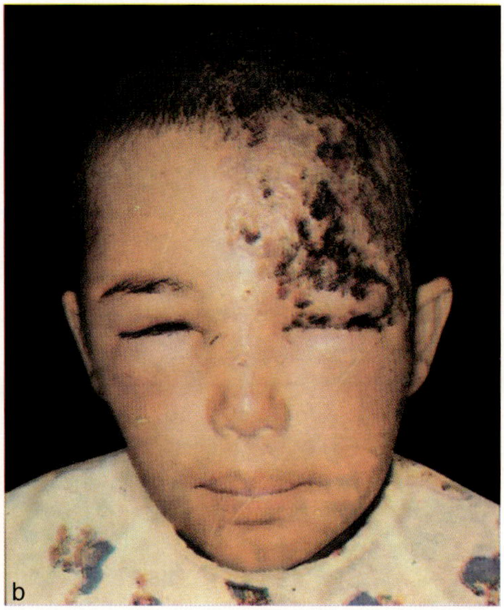

Fig. 14.2: (a) Herpes zoster; (b) Herpes zoster ophthalmicus—grouped vesicles distributed unilaterally along the ophthalmic division of Vth nerve and also eye involvement

The contents of the vesicles soon turn opaque. The vesicles may become confluent to form flat bullae. The lesions develop in several crops, each crop lasting a week or so **(Fig. 14.2)**. Towards the end of this period, the lesions rupture or dry up to form crusts. When the crust separates in about a week's time, there is temporary pigmentation and faint scarring. The latter is marked when there is secondary infection and ulceration. The regional glands may be enlarged and painful. An attack lasts for 2–3 weeks. The sites of predilection are the trunk (intercostal nerves), neck (cervical) and the face (trigeminal distribution). Involvement of the first root of the trigeminal nerve gives rise to lesions on the eye herpes ophthalmicus. The rash is mainly unilateral; very rarely it affects both sides. Immunity in herpes is lifelong; second attack is rare. Important sequelae are the post-herpetic neuralgia and rarely muscular paralysis. The former is seen in middle age and old persons having severe attack of the disease. Pain is along the course of nerve; it can be very severe and excruciating. It may interfere with work and sleep. Neuralgic pain lasts for months to years.

Diagnosis: It is based upon the sudden onset of a unilateral, herpetic eruption along the distribution of one or more nerve roots accompanied by pain and hyperaesthesia. In the initial stage of sudden pain, before the rash develops, confusion may occur with other local causes of pain like mastoiditis, pleurisy, appendicitis, cholecystitis, pyelitis, etc.

Prognosis: It is good as far as the cutaneous lesions are concerned. An individual attack subsides nicely, leaving faint scars. The troublesome sequelae may be the annoying post-herpetic neuralgia and muscular paralysis due to extension of inflammation to anterior horn of the spinal cord. Viremia and meningoencephalitis may rarely occur in susceptible patients or in patients under immunosuppressive drugs.

Treatment

Mild cases and young persons:

1. Lotio calamine with 1% phenol topically.
2. Savlon or Cetavlon cream.
3. Aspirin, if painful.

Severe cases and older person past 40 years of age:

A. Topical
   1. Vesicular stage: Silver nitrate 1% or 1% Gentian violet
   2. Crusting and scaling: Neosporin (P) or Bacitracin or Savlon (P) Cream

B. Systemic:
   1. Prednisolone—15 mg daily for 3 days.
      —10 mg daily for 3 days and
      —5 mg daily for 3 days (if suspecting PHN)
   2. Septran (P) or tetracycline, short course, if secondary infection
   3. Crocin (P) or Proxyvon (P) for pain.
   4. A course of Acyclovir/Famcyclovir/Valacyclovir for a week, or longer insevere cases and immuno-depressed individuals and AIDS. Useful only if started within 24 hours of onset.

Post-herpetic neuralgia

1. Analgesics-cum-tranquillizers
2. Infiltration of affected nerves with xylocaine in oil or infiltrate with triamcinolone if keloids have developed on the scars.

Herpes ophthalmicus

1. Opinion of ophthalmologist
2. Cleaning with boric acid solution l%.
3. Acyclovir drops 5–6 times a day.

VERRUCAE

Synonym: Warts (Hindustani equivalent is 'Masse').

These are benign epithelial growths developing as a result of infection of the skin with a filterable virus. The infection is autoinoculable and transmissible. Warts are a very common problem in practice, particularly amongst children. The virus is ubiquitous, so the infection is worldwide. The incubation period is about 90 days. It can affect any part of the body. The age of the patient and the part affected, tend to produce different varieties of warts, e.g. plane, vulgaris, filiform, plantar, mosaic and condyloma acuminatum.

Verruca plana: The face and back of hands are the sites of choice. Children are most commonly affected. That is why the name verrucae juvenilis is sometimes given to this condition. But not infrequently they are seen on the face of young adults particularly women. Verruca plana appear as small, smooth papules with flat tops. These papules are flesh coloured (or, a shade darker), about the size of pinhead or a little bigger. They are multiple; usually several dozen warts, many of them in lines, occur in one individual.

Differential diagnosis is from molluscum contagiosum and early lichen planus. The latter occurs in older people and the characteristic lesions are symmetrically distributed violaceous, itchy, polyhedral, shiny papules; the lesions appear in the mouth as well. The lesions in molluscum contagiosum are pearly in colour, look like solid vesicles, and when squeezed cheese-like material is demonstrated.

Verruca vulgaris: These can occur on any part of the body, but the areas usually affected are the exposed parts. The sites of choice are the hands and feet, around and under the nails, the arms, legs and less so, the face and scalp. Paronychial warts frequently occur in nail biters and cuticle pickers. These warts may occur singly or in groups. The lesions are flesh coloured or somewhat darker, rounded or oval papules or nodules. The size of these varies from that of lentil seeds to split peas (sometimes bigger). Their verrucous surface is very typical; once seen, it is seldom missed. On the scalp, the wart may have a cauliflower-like appearance. The warts do not itch but subungual warts may be painful. Koebner's phenomenon represented by linear groups of warts following inoculation of virus into scratch marks may be seen. In the beard region, they may take the form of finger-like processes; hence are called filiform warts **(Fig. 14.3)**. These spread by shaving by way of implantation.

A single common wart should be distinguished from Butcher's or postmortem wart (tuberculosis cutis verrucosus) which is marked by induration around the periphery of the lesion. Verruca vulgaris should be distinguished from seborrhoeic warts which are multiple circumscribed, flat elevations, covered with dark, greasy scales. They occur mainly on the trunk, forehead and temples.

Plantar warts: As the name suggests, they occur mainly on the soles of the feet; they can sometimes be found on the palms of the hands. They are deeply set in the skin, lying in flask-shaped cavities, being wider at the bottom than at the top. The important symptoms are pain and tenderness. Plantar warts occur singly at pressure sites of the feet and the heel; daughter warts are found in the contiguous areas. Clinically, a plantar wart appears as a painful, tender, hyperkeratotic, circular plaque, with a diameter of about one to one-and-a-half centimetres **(Fig. 14.4)**. Scraping the surface of the wart with a blade reveals papillae with punctate capillary bleeding; papillae can be seen more clearly when silver nitrate paint is applied on them. An agglomeration of these warts on the sole with a polygonal outline and a roughened surface is called mosaic wart. It is usually superficial and painless. The infection is contracted in swimming pools: Public bath rooms and less commonly, on the beaches.

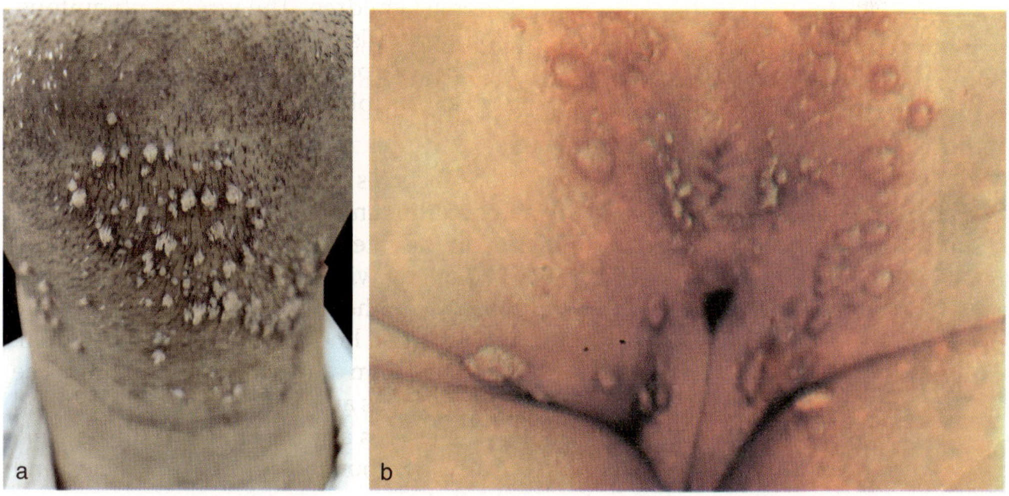

Fig. 14.3: (a) Verruca vulgaris on the beard area and neck; (b) Perianal warts

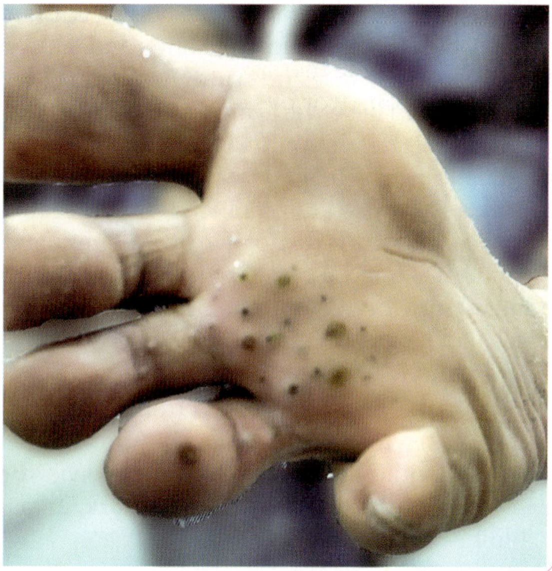

Fig. 14.4: Mosaic/plantar wart

A plantar wart must be differentiated from a corn. The latter is at a pressure site and has a smooth surface and when its surface is scraped, found absent is the papillomatous surface typical of the plantar wart. The greatest amount of pain is felt when the corn is pressed from the top, the pain increases towards the evening; in contrast with a plantar wart, in which pain is felt when the wart is pressed from the sides as well as from the top, it being the greatest in the morning, on first putting the weight of the body on the feet.

Epidermodysplasia verruciformis is considered by many to be caused by invasion of the virus warts in genetically predisposed persons, manifested by profuse coalescent eruptions of verruca plana type lesions, usually on the limbs.

Condyloma acuminatum: It is simply an hypertrophic common wart occurring on the genitalia and the peri-anal region, very frequently in the sexually promiscuous young adults. The papillomatous or vegetating verrucous lesion, pedunculated as a rule is typical. Secondary infection may produce a little purulent discharge; the base is not infiltrated. Infection is contracted during sexual intercourse or accidentally through the fingers.

The differential diagnosis is made from condylomata lata (*see* Chapter 18). In long standing cases. giant condyloma acuminatum of Buschke and squamous cell carcinoma must be excluded by microscopic examination. Genital warts are often acquired along with other venereal infections and as such tests for syphilis and gonorrhoea should also be carried out.

Histology: All warts are papillomatous, epidermal hypertrophies, seen as hyperkeratosis and acanthosis with finger-like processes in the corium. Vacuolation of the prickle cells is characteristic of viral affections. Only in the plantar warts and condyloma acuminatum slight or moderate lymphocytic infiltration is present in the upper corium. Inclusion bodies can be well demonstrated only in plantar warts.

Treatment of warts: It consists mainly in destroying the warts chemically, electrically or surgically; the exact mode of treatment depends upon the site, nature and number of lesions. There is no specific systemic therapy available. The warts especially the plane warts may disappear spontaneously or by psychotherapy.

Management of Warts

Plane wart vulgaris	Psychotherapy
	Levamisole 150 mg weekly
	Cryosurgery—liquid nitrogen (N_2 oxide)
	Podophyllin
	Wart paint
	CO_2 Laser—electrocoagulation
Plantar	Podowart occlusive dressing
Formalin soaks	
	40% salicylic acid
	Cryosurgery
	CO_2 laser
	Bleomycin infiltration
Condylomata	Cryosurgery
	CO_2 laser
	Infiltration with interferons
Subungual	Podophyllin
	CO_2 laser electrocoagulation

The chemicals usually employed are phenol 25–95%, trichloracetic acid 25%, CO_2 snow, liquid nitrogen and podophyllin paint.

Podophyllin Paint

Podophyllin	20% (1 part)
Acid salicylic	20% (1 part)
Acetone	20% (1 part)
Collodion flexible/tincture benzoin	40% (2 parts)

Simple Wart Paint

Acid salicylic	16.6% (1, part)
Acid lactic	16.6% (1 part)
Collodion flexible or Tincture benzoin	66.2% (4 parts)

Wart paints are most effective in condyloma acuminatum and also may be effective in plantar warts, filiform warts on the scalp and beard region: Podophyllin paint should not be applied more than once a week. After application, the plantar wart is covered with polythene and then elastoplast bandage. It is left like this for 5–7 days. At the end of this period, the elastoplast is removed and the wart curetted. If the wart has not been completely destroyed, the application is repeated.

In case of pain, the bandage is removed earlier. A simple wart paint can also be tried in all types of warts. Glutaraldehyde solution also gives good results. Pregnant women should not be treated with podophyllin since its absorption may cause foetal abnormalities. Formaldehyde 10% soaks are very helpful in treating multiple plantar warts or mosaic warts. Soles are soaked daily for 30 minutes for 4–6 weeks. CO_2 snow is useful in destroying warts, by freezing. It is applied in the form of a pencil, under firm pressure for 30–60 seconds. Cryosurgery with liquid nitrogen is helpful and so is CO_2 Laser.

Electrocoagulation with surgical diathermy or infrared coagulation and electro-cauterization carried out under local anaesthesia gives the best results, because the amount of destruction is under direct control, scarring is minimal, and the recurrence rate low. It is the treatment of choice for filiform warts in young adults. Levamisol therapy (150 mg per day on 2 consecutive days in each week for 12 weeks) may be worth trial specially in verruca plana. Surgical excision and X-ray therapy may be employed as the last resort for plantar warts. The destruction of the normal skin should be avoided at all costs, whatever be the mode of treatment. Infiltration with Interferon or bleomycin helps some cases.

Subungual warts can be treated with podophyllin painted twice daily on the wart, the latter is scraped before application. X-ray therapy or liquid nitrogen has also given good results. Good results have been claimed with ultrasonic therapy, intralesional smallpox vaccination or bleomycin infiltration (0.1% solution, 0.01–1 c.c.) into the wart. The latter is painful. Only one injection is enough.

A recurrence is possible so long as even one infected cell remains. If the virus has been transplanted in the neighbouring area, new lesions will develop even after the primary lesions have been removed. These facts should be explained to the patient and his attendants before treatment is undertaken.

MOLLUSCUM CONTAGIOSUM

It is more common in the summer than in the winter though one may come across cases throughout the year. The trunk, arms, neck and face are the usual sites of affection. Infection is picked up at gymnasia, swimming pools, play grounds, etc. It is contagious; school children are selectively affected.

Clinical features: The lesions are usually multiple. They are seen as multiple, pearly or flesh-coloured, smooth, shiny, globular papules. The size of a papule varies from that of a pin-head to split pea. A molluscum contagiosum looks like a vesicle, but is solid and firm. The top may be flat but more commonly umbilicated **(Fig. 14.5)**. When squeezed, cheesy material is ejected. There is usually no pain except when secondary infection sets in.

Histology: Molluscum cantagiosum is seen as an acanthotic mass with a well-developed basal cell layer. The prickle cells become round and show eosinophilic masses (inclusion bodies) with nuclei pushed to the periphery. The process becomes more and more marked as the epidermal cells reach the surface. There is slight round cell infiltration in the upper corium.

Diagnosis: Molluscum contagiosuin is not difficult to diagnose if the above features are remembered. Vesicles, bullae, lymphangiomas and warts can all be easily excluded.

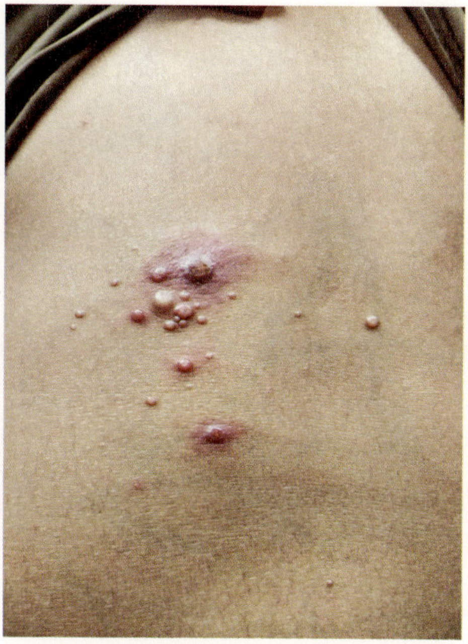

Fig. 14.5: Molluscum contagiosum

Treatment: There is no specific treatment. Lesions disappear spontaneously in few cases. In children, wart paint containing 1 part salicylic acid, 1 part lactic acid in 4 parts collodion flexible is beneficial. It is painless and gives good results. It should not be applied for more than 5–7 days. 10% podophyllin paint applied for 12–24 hours is useful; avoid irritation at all costs.

Electrocoagulation is very useful in selected cases particularly adults with limited number of mollusca. Phenol application has been discarded as it is painful and children resist the application.

OTHER VIRUS INFECTIONS

Vaccinia: Primary vaccination with calf lymph, and also accidental inoculation produce typical vaccinia. In primary vaccinia, a papule appears after three-day incubation period. The papule develops into an umbilicated vesicle on the sixth day, and a pustule on the eighth day; the latter dries up to form a crust and then leaves a depressed scar. A secondary vaccination produces an accelerated reaction subsiding within three to seven days, or no reaction at all, depending upon the immunity developed by the person concerned. The only complications that can occur are impetigo and pyoderma at the site of the inoculation, regional lymphadenitis, and rarely encephalitis. Sometimes a generalized vaccinia which is characterized by a sparse vesiculo-pustular rash, may be seen at the height of the local vaccinia reaction, i.e. 10th day after vaccination; the rash involutes quickly without leaving any scar. In eczematous patients, the vaccinia tends to cause eczema vaccinatum (Kaposi's varicelliform eruption). So the vaccination shout be given with caution to such individuals. Acute pemphigus is a very rare complication of vaccinia.

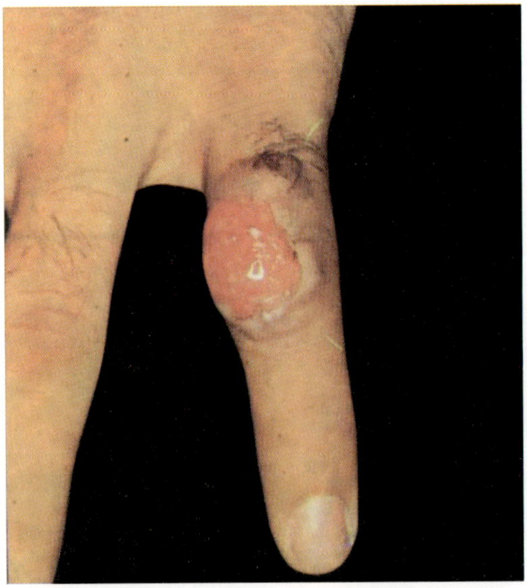

Fig. 14.6: Orf—typical lesion

ORF

Synonym: Ecthyma contagiosum; contagious pustular dermatitis of sheep (Peterkin). It is common in sheep from whom man occasionally becomes infected by contact. The initial lesion is single dark-red, painless, indurated papule, appearing on an exposed part of the body, usually the hands, It slowly enlarges into a pustule with haemorrhage and surrounding inflammation (Fig. 14.6).

Spontaneous recovery takes place in 3–6 weeks, hence no treatment is required except to control secondary infection, if it occurs. Erythema multiforme may occur 1–2 weeks after orf.

Milker's Nodes (Paravaccinia)

The lesions consisting of multiple, purple, elevated, non-umbilicated, slightly tender nodules on the fingers; may appear in persons who are engaged in the act of milking (cows and sheep). The lesions start disappearing in about 2 weeks time.

Kaposi's Varicelliform Eruption

This may manifest as either Eczema herpeticum or as eczema vaccinatum. The former is caused by herpes simplex hominis virus (HSV-1) in primary infection and the latter by vaccinia virus. Both are complications of atopic dermatitis. Eczema herpeticum is a serious, sometimes fatal complication of atopic eczema manifested by sudden widespread papulo-vesicular eruption often umbilicated, chiefly on the areas usually affected in atopic dermatitis with associated fever and lymphadenopathy. It can occur even in patients whose atopic dermatitis is quiescent.

Eczema vaccinatum occurs usually in a child who has recently been inadvertently vaccinated against smallpox with live vaccinia virus or has come into contact with an individual with an active vaccinia lesion. Profuse clusters of umbilicated vaccinal vesicles and pustules arise on the affected skin.

Clinical picture usually consists of:

1. Pre-existing eczema.
2. A constitutional upset in the form of fever and malaise.
3. A sudden onset of rapidly developing vesiculo-pustules on the face, neck and extremities, less so, on the trunk. Sometimes, the lesions may be umbilicated, or impetiginized.
4. The regional, cervical and axillary lymph glands are enlarged.

Cytological examination of the smears demonstrates intranuclear inclusion bodies in herpes and intracytoplasmic in vaccinia and also typical ballooning degeneration with multinucleate giant cells in herpes simplex. Relatively milder constitutional symptoms and adenopathy and associated oral lesions will suggest herpes infection.

Treatment: Consists in isolation from susceptible subjects, managing the preexisting eczema and secondary infection. Broad-spectrum antibiotics may give good results. Hyperimmune vaccinal gammaglobulin should be given in eczema vaccinatum. It may be a useful standby in eczema herpeticum. Acyclovir is worth using in cases with fresh lesions.

Chapter

15

Tuberculosis of the Skin

INTRODUCTION

It is an uncommon skin affection found all over the world. Its incidence is directly proportional to the incidence of pulmonary tuberculosis. In advanced countries where the incidence of pulmonary tuberculosis is on the decline because of improved hygienic conditions, good public health and better general nutrition, the incidence of cutaneous tuberculosis has followed suit and declined as well. However, in the developing third world, its incidence is still high. Moreover, tuberculosis cutis is diagnosed late and is therefore, often seen at an advanced stage when the cosmetic result is very poor, and the prognosis is not so favourable.

Several different pictures are produced in tuberculosis of the skin. These depend upon: the mode of local infecction, affection by bacilli or toxins, the degree of patient's immunity and/or sensitivity, age and the site of affection. Among Asian and African people, verrucous lesions are more common than other varieties because of the tendency of their skin to lichenify early and due to climatic conditions. Secondly, in debilitated persons, liquefaction occurs earlier, hence scrofuloderma.

Mode of Infection. Tubercle bacilli reach the skin by the following routes:

1. Exogenous inoculation into the skin either from an autopsy, infected animals, or sputum or contact with infected lesions, e.g. primary tuberculous chancre, postmortem wart.
2. Spread from neighbouring areas either by contiguity or by lymphatics, e.g. scrofuloderma.
3. Blood stream bringing the tubercle bacilli to the skin from a distant focus in the lungs, bones or glands.

Classification of tuberculosis cutis based on type of infection and morphology of lesion (Table 15.1): Prognostically, acute generalized miliary tuberculosis and tuberculosis cutis orificialis are lethal conditions; lupus vulgaris, tuberculosis cutis verrucosus and scrofuloderma are stable conditions with a fairly good prognosis, while the tuberculide group is unstable, and has an indefinite outlook. Prognosis has improved impressively with the availability of many antitubercular drtigs.

In primary infection, the tuberculin test is negative, and in the remaining conditions, it is positive, though the degree of reactivity is variable.

Laboratory Investigations

1. Demonstration of tubercle bacilli
   a. Direct smear-stained with Ziehl–Neelsen stain.

Table 15.1: Classification of cutaneous tuberculosis

Mode of infection	Localized	Disseminated
A. Primary infection	Primary tuberculous complex	Acute generalized miliary tuberculosis
B. Reinfection	1. Lupus vulgaris	Tuberculids allergic or toxic reaction
	2. Tuberculosis cutis verrucosus	1. Lichen scrofulosorum
	3. Scrofuloderma	2. Papulo-necrotic tuberculides
	4. Tuberculosis cutis orificialis	3. Erythema induratum
		4. Erythema nodosum
		5. Acne agminata
		6. Rosaceous tuberculides

b. Culture.
c. Guinea-pig inoculation.
d. Demonstration in the biopsy sections.

2. Tuberculin test.
3. Existence of tubercular focus in lungs, glands, bones, intestines, etc.
4. Histopathological features of dermal miliary tubercles are characteristic. They consist of epithelioid cells, lymphocytes and a few giant cells. Caseation is usually absent. A few tubercle bacilli may rarely be seen in the centre of the tubercle. It must be emphatically stressed, that the tuberculoid histological picture does not necessarily indicate tuberculosis since other granulomas can produce an identical picture.

Tuberculosis of the skin manifests itself in several clinical forms. Non-tubercular, atypical mycobacteria **(Table 15.2)** produce infective granulomas like swimming pool granulomas (*M. marinum*), ulcerating granuloma and chronic subcutaneous abscesses (*M chelonei* or *M. fortuitum*).

According to several workers, the term 'tuberculides' is questionable for the reasons that there is no obvious active tuberculous focus in the body, tuberculin test is negative, AFB have never been isolated, cultured or produced in animal inoculation, tuberculoid histological picture is found in other non-tuberculous conditions and clinical features resemble other diseases like pityriasis lichenoides et varioliformis and other dermatoses. Further, these conditions do not respond to anti-tuberculous drugs, but may respond to steroids.

Primary tuberculosis complex: It is a rare, cutaneous complex like Ghon's focus in the lungs. It occurs most frequently in children. It starts as a nodule which breaks down to form an ulcer. It is accompanied by regional adenitis. The face is the site of choice. Tubercle bacilli can be demonstrated from the ulcer. The tuberculin test is negative. There is a tendency for the ulcer to heal and leave a scar. It rarely disseminates or develops into lupus vulgaris. It is occasionally seen in adults following trauma.

Miliary tuberculosis: In fulminating pulmonary or meningeal tuberculosis in children, miliary tuberculosis may be seen in the skin and other organs. The cutaneous lesions are usually maculo-papular. It is usually a fatal condition. In subacute and less severe cases, the papules may undergo necrosis producing ulcers.

Table 15.2: Differential diagnosis of different mycobacterial infections

	M. tuberculosis	*M. marinum*	*M. ulcerans*	*M. chelonei and M. fortuitum*
Incubation period source of disease	Lupus vulgaris-years; external as well as endogenous-blood, lymph glands, joints, bones	Three weeks, Trauma and bathing in sea or pools	Two months or so, external inoculation from vegetations	Two months or more, injection, inoculation and surgical incision
Clinical features	Typical features of lupus vulgaris-reddish brown patch, apple jelly nodules, tissue paper scarring, destruction of cartilages	Dermal granulomas and nodules along the lymphatics. Lymphadenitis rare	Necrosis spreading Closed swellings	Subcutaneous abscess intermittent discharge, chronic granulomas
Lab. investigations	1. Tuberculin-positive 2. Histopath–Tuberculoid	1. Culture-positive 2. Histopath–granuloma	1. Culture-positive 2. Histopath—Liquefaction necrosis especially in fatty layers of skin	1. Smear and culture 2. Histopath—Tubercles and suppuration
Natural course Treatment	Years and decades: Streptomycin, INH, ethambutol, rifampicin	6–12 months: Cotrimoxazole and tetracycline	Arrest after 1 year: Rifampicin, clofazimine and co-trimoxazole	Many months: Doxycycline, tetracycline and other antibiotics.

Lupus vulgaris: It affects the face primarily; children and young adults are usually affected, though no age is exempt. One or several patches may be seen. The disease is usually asymetrically distributed. Lupus vulgaris starts as a reddish-brown macule, the size and shape of a freckle from which may be difficult to differentiate at this stage except by histological examination. It enlarges slowly over months and years to form a big patch with a well-defined but irregular margin (Fig. 15.1). The colour is reddish-brown. In dark-skinned people, colour changes are difficult to demonstrate. On healing, a tissue paper-like scarring is produced, a feature very characteristic of lupus vulgaris. This is seen at the healing centre or edge. Adjoining mucosa of nose, eyes and mouth may be involved by lupus vulgaris.

On the hands, feet, knees and the buttocks in people living in tropical climates, the lesions may show thickening of the overlying epidermis which takes on a rough and

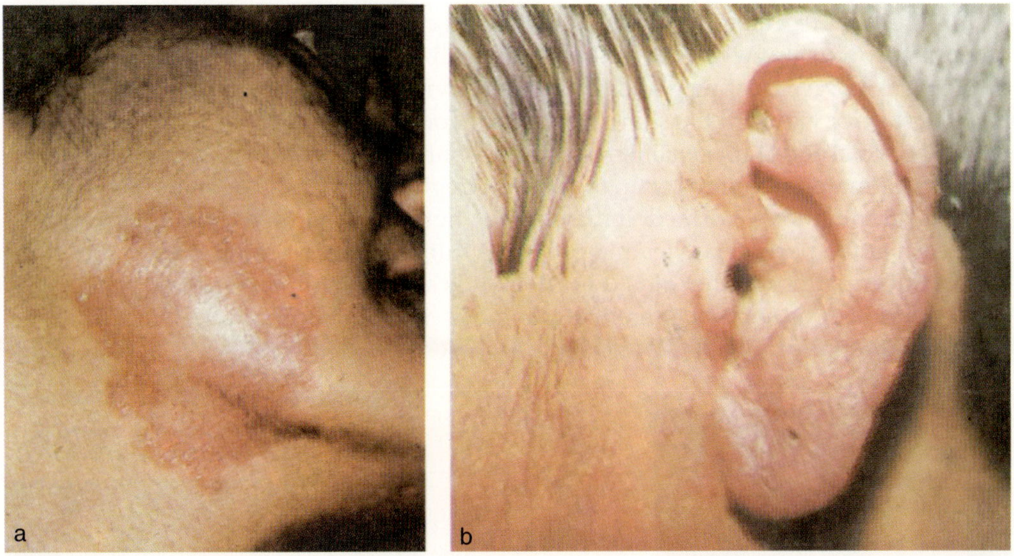

Fig. 15.1: (a) Lupus vulgaris—typical reddish brown plaque with tissue paper wrinkling; (b) Lupus vulgaris

verrucous appearance, very much resembling tuberculosis cutis verrucosus. Ulceration complicates lupus vulgaris in a small proportion of cases. Tuberculosis cutis can also develop as a complication of BCG vaccination. Rarely, squamous cell carcinoma may complicate.

The diagnostic features are:

1. Persistent, brownish-red, well-defined patch with dermal infiltration.
2. The presence of apple-jelly nodules.
3. Match-stick test positive. An apple-jelly nodule has no resistance to pressure by a sharp match-stick.
4. Tissue paper wrinkled scars.
5. Long history extending over years.
6. Tuberculin test positive.
7. Miliary tubercles in a biopsy specimen.

Differential diagnosis is made mainly from lupus erythematosus. It is differentiated by the presence of the lesions on the face, usually in a butterfly pattern; the affection of persons past puberty; well-defined lesions with adherent scales, follicular plugging and cayenne-pepper appearance on diascopy. The biopsy is characteristic. Dermal leishmaniasis affects persons who have lived or are living in endemic areas. Typical lesion is noduloulcerative; nodules are bluish red and indolent; LT bodies can be demonstrated in smear preparation. In the authors' experience, dermal leishmaniasis recidivans can easily be confused with lupus vulgaris in the endemic areas; the only distinguishing features are the presence of papules at the periphery of a healed erythematous patch and negative tuberculin test.

Syphilitic and leprotic lesions are characteristic and can easily be distinguished clinically and also by positive serology in the former and sensory changes in the latter.

Scrofuloderma: It is relatively frequent in India. It commonly affects the neck and groins but it may occur anywhere. The tubercle bacilli reach the skin from an underlying active focus like a caseating gland, joint bone or viscera. The history and sign of such a focus may be obvious. In the skin, it starts as a non-specific, chronic inflammation or a painless dermal nodule or swelling which softens and ruptures to discharge purulent and sanguinous material. A sinus or an ulcer with irregular borders, pale undermined edges and pale granulation is formed. It may or may not be surrounded by a lupus vulgaris-like patch at the periphery. Healing produces thin atrophic or retracted scars. Lesions have a linear pattern in the folds **(Fig. 15.2)**. It is a chronic disease, developing slowly over a period of months. Differential diagnosis is from suppurative lymphadenitis, hidradenitis suppurativa, LGV and deep mycoses.

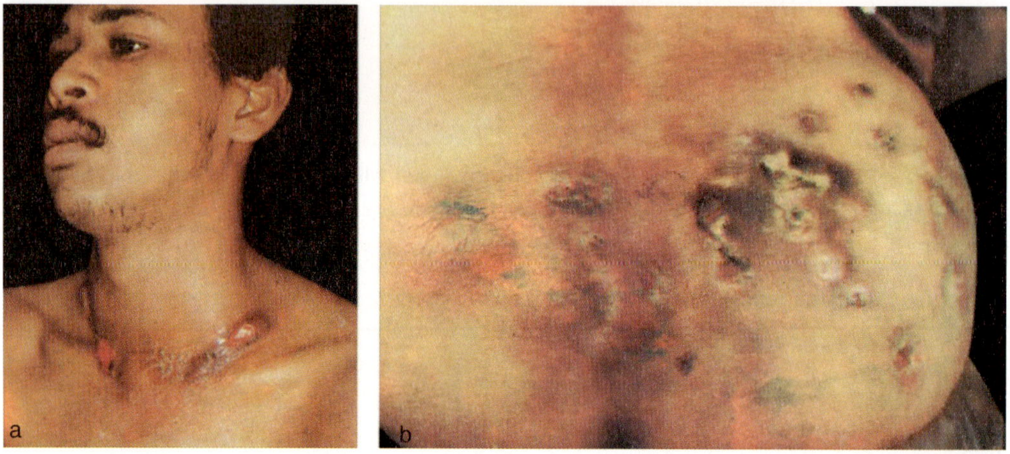

Fig. 15.2: (a) Scrofuloderma—discharging sinuses in destructive tuberculosis cutis; (b) Scrofuloderma

Tuberculosis cutis orificialis: It is seen occasionally in patients with laryngo-pulmonary or gastrointestinal tuberculosis. Lesions are around the mouth in the former and around the anus in the latter. Typical lesions are chronic shallow ulcers with pale granulations as ischiorectal abscesses.

Verruca necrogenica: Synonym: Tuberculosis cutis verrucosus. It is seen in pathologists, butchers, veterinary surgeons and patients with pulmonary tuberculosis. Tubercle bacilli are accidentally inoculated into the integument. Common sites are the hands and feet. Clinically, the condition starts as a reddish-brown, firm, indurated papule. The surface becomes crusted and later verrucous. At this state, it can look like a common wart with the difference that at the periphery, a bluish indurated tuberculous nodule can always be detected. Deep mycosis and orf are the two other conditions to be considered in the differential diagnosis **(Fig. 15.3)**. Cases of disseminated verruca necrogenica and tubercular pseudoelephantiasis have also been seen. Spontaneous healing may occur, but it is usually a slow and chronic process.

Papulo-necrotic tuberculides: It is not so common a condition in the tropics. It is supposed to be due to sensitivity to tubercle bacilli or other toxins. It occurs more commonly in females than males. The sites of choice are the face, arms and legs.

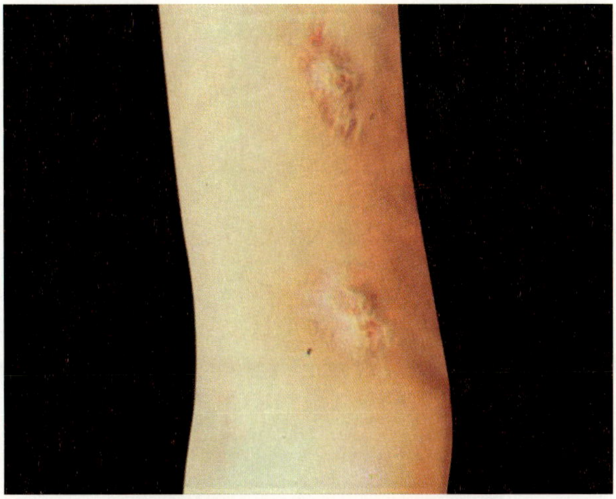

Fig. 15.3: Tuberculosis verrucosa cutis

The lesions are symmetrical and develop in crops over several months. Clinically, the lesions consist of discrete, indolent, red, deep-seated papules or nodules, the centres of which slowly undergo necrosis to form pustules. A small ulcer covered by a crust is formed when the necrotic material of the pustule is discharged. The lesions heal spontaneously leaving behind pitted, achromic scars with hyperpigmented periphery. The tuberculin test is strongly positive. On the face, the papulo-necrotic tuberculides take two forms, acne agminata and rosaceous tuberculide. In acne agminata, the papules are distributed around the eyes, nose and upper lip. The papules necrose to form crusts, and on healing leave behind pitted scars. In rosaceous tuberculide, yellowish tuberculous papules and telangiectasia are distributed on the periphery rather than on the centre of the face in contrast with rosacea. Tubercle bacilli have not been demonstrated in these two conditions.

Being an unstable condition, prognosis is indefinite and usually not good. The treatment is not very satisfactory, hence the condition tends to be chronic and recurrent.

Lichen scrofulosorum: It is an uncommon questionable tuberculide. It affects children with or without systemic tuberculosis. The shoulders and trunk are the sites involved. Clinically, the lesions consist of patches of grouped, firm, follicular, bluish-red, indolent papules with central spines **(Fig. 15.4)**. It itches slightly. Histopathology is tuberculoid. Tuberculin test is negative.

Bazin's disease: Synonym: Erythema induratum. Young women are selectively affected. Sites of choice are the backs of lower part of legs. Typical clinical features are symmetrical, bluish-red, infiltrated and indurated plaques. There may be nodules under the surface. The centre of nodules may soften and result in ulceration. The patients usually suffer from acrocyanosis in the form of cold feet and legs. The disease is marked by the absence of pain.

Onset is usually in the cold weather; lesions tend to heal spontaneously with the advent of the warm weather, recurring again in next winter. The exact cause of erythema induratum is not established. Acrocyanosis is the basic, predisposing factor; hence the seasonal recurrence. Sensitivity to tubercle bacilli or its toxins and sarcoid are the two

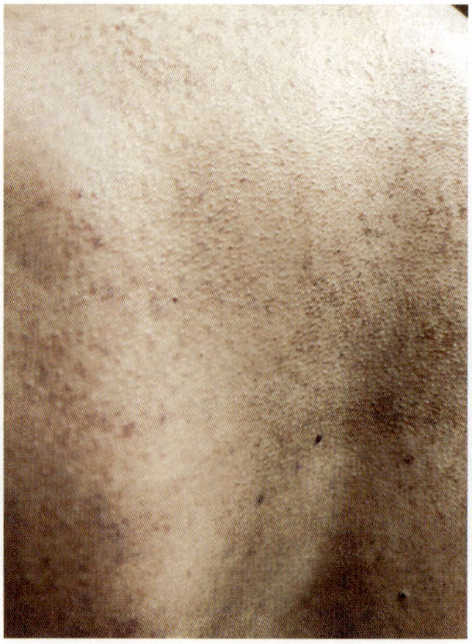

Fig. 15.4: Lichen scrofulosorum lesions on the back

supposed causes. Differential diagnosis is from erythema nodosum, nodular vasculitis, gumma and panniculitis.

Histologically, necrosis of the subcutaneous fat and granulomatous infiltration are the two dominant features.

Treatment

A. ***Prophylaxis:*** It consists of correcting the causative factors. The milk supply must be from non-tuberculous animals. Open cases of tuberculosis must be treated early till full recovery, and proper follow-up must ensue.

B. ***Curative:*** Due to recent advances in anti-tubercular therapy more stress is laid on systemic therapy. Good, nourishing diet is routinely recommended.

Medicinal treatment has become fairly standardized. First line of therapy consists of streptomycin intramuscularly, Para-amino-salicylic acid (in short, PAS) and Isonicotinic acid hydrazide (in short, INH) preparations, particularly thiosemicarbazone with isonicotinic acid hydrazide orally in established standard doses. Streptomycin and INH are given together in advanced and extensive cases, while the latter is given alone or in combination with PAS in ordinary cases of tuberculosis cutis. Improvement starts within a month; within six months or so, small lesions disappear. In extensive cases, treatment is continued for 12–18 months or even longer. It must be emphasized that treatment must be continued for at least 2–3 months after complete clinical recovery.

Alternative drugs like ethionamide (ETH), rifampicin (RM), ethambutol, pyrizinamide (PZM) and cycloserine are used in resistant cases. These are the second line of therapy. They are expensive and toxic; hence discretion must be employed in their use. Pefloxacin 400 mg BD or ofloxacin 200 mg OD are the new useful drugs. They may replace rifampicin because of drug resistance to it.

Vitamin D (Calciferol) is now rarely employed since the cure rate is low.

TB vaccine (Polysaccharide extract of pure culture of human-type tubercle bacilli) has been successfully used by Maruyama (1964) in the treatment of skin tuberculosis. This vaccine acts by producing an antigen-antibody reaction in the lesions; this is antibacterial in cases of genuine skin tuberculosis and as a desensitizer in cases of tuberculides. Further confirmation about its effectiveness is still awaited.

Verruca necrogenica may require excision (surgical or with diathermy) in resistant cases. In scrofuloderma, underlying tuberculosis in glands, etc. may also require surgical intervention.

Management of tuberculides is unsatisfactory. Anti-tubercular drugs are not generally helpful. Antihistamines and steroids may be beneficially employed in resistant cases. Many cases improve on their own in course of time. Ulcers need dressing with acriflavin or bacitracin; on dry lesions steroid ointment may be used with care.

In Bazin' s disease, treatment consists in improving the circulation by keeping the affected part warm with woollen stockings or an elastoplast bandage. The patches are dressed with 1% ichthamol paste. In cases of ulceration, acriflavin in cod liver oil is recommended. Good nourishing diet and regulated leg exercises are essential. Systemic treatment is usually unsatisfactory. Anti-tubercular drugs and steroids may be used in resistant cases.

ERYTHEMA NODOSUM

It is quite a common cutaneous condition seen as frequently by a general physician as by a dermatologist. One usually comes across these cases in the autumn and winter. Usually affected are the young people. It is more common in females than males.

Clinical features: The disease starts with a constitutional upset, e.g. malaise, moderate pyrexia, headaches and joint pains. The eruption is usually confined to the pretibial surface of the legs, but may occur on the elbows, face and trunk. The mucous membranes are usually spared. Lesions are bilaterally symmetrical and consist of red, painful, tender nodular swellings, the sizes of which vary from 1–2 cm. The lesions last for about 6–8 weeks. As they involute, they take on the bluish hue of a bruise. The eruption usually appears in crops.

Etiology: The exact pathogenesis is not definite, but the reaction, presumably, is due to the patient's sensitivity to the toxins of tubercle bacilli and streptococci, often brought about by the use of drugs like sulphonamides, particularly sulphathiazole (may be a biotropic action). It is also associated with rheumatic fever which, itself, is supposed to be caused by a person's sensitivity to streptococci. An erythema nodosum-like eruption can also develop during an attack of meningitis, lymphogranuloma inguinale, leprosy, sarcoid and coccidiodomycosis.

Prognosis: It depends upon the causative factor or factors. With the control of the latter, the eruption slowly disappears without leaving any scar. Usually there are no relapses.

Diagnosis: It is usually not difficult. The differential diagnosis is made from nodular vasculitis; syphilitic gumma and erythema induratum; all these have characteristic features of their own. So, if the features are remembered, these diseases can be easily differentiated. Once the diagnosis has been arrived at, an attempt should be made to establish the cause.

Cases of chronic erythema nodosum are usually caused by nodular vasculitis, erythema nodosum leprosum, and panniculitis.

Treatment: Very important is the general management of the patient. He should be put to bed till his temperature comes down to normal and the causative factors are controlled. There is no specific therapy for erythema nodosum as such; the main treatment consists of management of the cause. Sedatives and analgesics may be needed to control the symptoms. The local use of corticosteroids, in ointment or lotion form, may help to reduce pain. Systemically, both corticosteroids and ACTH are contraindicated. Ichthammol Belladonna in glycerine is popularly advised as a local paint.

SARCOID

It is a rare, benign and non-infectious skin disease with a doubtful etiology, often occurring with systemic involvement. Cases are infrequently reported in India. The exact causation is not definite, but the two causes usually put forward are tuberculosis and reticuloses. The histology is characteristic; no tubercle bacilli have ever been satisfactorily demonstrated. The tuberculin test is characteristically negative and may be due to a state of anergy. Sarcoid usually affects the young, and middle-aged women.

Clinical features: The cutaneous lesions consist of papules, nodules and plaques, single or multiple. They vary in size, being anywhere between the size of a pea and the palm of a hand. The face, ears, arms and toes are the areas usually involved. The lesions show definite infiltration, and their colour varies from bright-red, purple, brown to a bluish-hue; the bluish hue is commonly seen in the centres of old lesions. There is no itching or burning or any other symptom.

The cutaneous lesions may occur by themselves or in association with systemic affection of the lymph glands, bones, particularly of the fingers, uveal tract, parotid (uveo-parotid disease), lungs, spleen, liver and even the brain. In such cases, there are signs and symptoms referable to the tissues or organs involved.

Investigations

1. An intradermal test using the saline extract from the sarcoid tissue (Kveim test). It is not as specific for sarcoidosis as was generally believed. It has, however, some degree of prognostic value.
2. The plasma globulins are often increased.
3. The negative tuberculin test.
4. Typical histology. It is characterized by the presence of epithelioid cell tubercles surrounded by lymphocytes. There is never any caseation. The characteristic lesions may later be replaced by fibrosis, hyalinization or both.
5. X-ray of the small bones of the hands shows rarefied areas.

Prognosis: It is rather unsatisfactory. The clinical course is chronic with no constitutional disturbances; however, there may be acute phases characterized by a general reaction with malaise and fever. Sometimes the lesions involute spontaneously; at other times, they are resistant to every form of therapy.

Treatment: There is no specific treatment. Calciferol (vitamin B_{12}) has brought about occasional cures. Lately, corticosteroids and ACTH have given some degree of success. The general health must be looked after in every case, and the cause, if specifically found, must be eradicated.

Chapter 16

Dermal Leishmaniasis, Yaws and Rhinoscleroma

DERMAL LEISHMANIASIS

Synonyms: Oriental sore, Delhi sore, Baghdad sore, etc.

Etiology: Leishmaniasis cutis is a specific cutaneous granuloma caused by a parasite, *Leishmania tropica*. Though widespread, it is most prevalent in countries where there are dry, hot summers and short winters. It exists endemically in West Asia, Pakistan and North India. It also occurs in North Africa, parts of China and Russia. In India; systemic leishmaniasis (Kala-azar) exists in the eastern provinces of Bengal, Bihar, Assam and Orissa, but cutaneous leishmaniasis is non-existent in these regions.

Leishmania tropica has two forms: Leishmanial form (LT bodies) in mammalian hosts, and flagellates in the culture, and an insect vector, for instance, the sandfly (*Phlebotomus papatasii*).

LT bodies exist intracellularly in the reticuloendothelial cell where they multiply. The typical LT body is 2–4 µ in diameter, is elliptical in shape, and contains a prominent nucleus and a rod-like parabasal body or kinetoplast. LT bodies lie singly or in groups in vacuolated spaces inside the cells, but may occasionally be found extracellularly on rupture of cells.

Grown on NNN medium (Novy, MacNeal, Nicolle) or Noguchi's medium, the parasite develops into a flagellate (*Leptomonas* form) measuring 15–20 µ by 0.2–0.6 µ and develops a 15–20 µ long single flagellum; the nucleus and the kinetoplast are retained.

Insect vector: The sandfly (phlebotomus) is responsible for transmission of *L tropica*. Inside the insects, LT bodies develop into flagellates which transform into parasitic form after inoculation into the mammalian host. The fly breeds in unhygienic conditions, in the cracks of buildings, open drains, tunnels, and dungheaps.

Host: Apart from human beings, one comes across cutaneous leishmaniasis in dogs, cats and circus bears; lesions are seen on the exposed parts of the bodies of these animals. In several regions, rodents have also been found to harbour infections; breeding on them transmit the disease to man.

L tropica is related to other leishmaniasis: *L. infantum* and *L. braziliensis*. They can be distinguished from each other by electophoretic enzyme analysis of culture isolates.

Immunity: Infection with *L. tropica* evokes an integrated cellular and humoral immune response with elimination of the infection and subsequent permanent immunity against that particular strain of the organism. The notable feature of the *L. tropica* infection is the tropism it displays, i.e. following inoculation at the site of insect bite the organism is incapable of moving away to distant sites except in diffuse cutaneous leishmaniasis.

The severity of the infection, i.e. the number of skin lesions relates to host susceptibility. In the endemic area the residents enjoy a certain measure of protective immunity as evidenced by cryptic infection or a mild infection (often a solitary lesion). In comparison, immigrants or long stay visitors to the endemic area develop more severe infections with multiple lesions.

Clinical features: The incubation period is variable and has not been definitely established. Ordinarily, it varies from 1 to 3 months.

The lesions appear generally on exposed parts like the cheeks, nose, ears, lips, neck, elbows, arms and hands. The lesions may be single or multiple. In endemic areas, several clinical forms of cutaneous leishmaniasis have been described. The most common variety is the oriental sore- nodulo-ulceration. It starts as a papule which develops into a firm, solid nodule which undergoes necrosis to produce ulceration. The chief characteristics of an oriental sore are its indolence, bluish-red infiltration and erosion covered by a crust. Untreated lesions last from 6 to 12 months, even longer. The size of an oriental sore varies from a quarter to 4 inches in diameter. When the sore heals, it leaves a depressed pigmented and deforming scar which is a great cosmetic blemish.

The other clinical varieties one comes across are: furunculoid, rhinophyma, nodular, extensive infiltrative plaques, verrucous and vegetating varieties. When the latter variety occurs on the nose, it produces a picture of rhinophyma- rhinophyma variety of dermal leishmaniasis. There is relapsing form of dermal leishmaniasis which is a sequelae of ordinary leishmaniasis; pin-head-sized bluish papules develop at the periphery of the apparently healed primary scar, usually sparing the centre, it resembles lupus vulgaris; apple-jelly coloured spots may also be seen **(Figs 16.1 to 16.3)**. It lasts for years. The smear is usually negative for LT bodies in the specific relapsing variety—leishmaniasis recidivans.

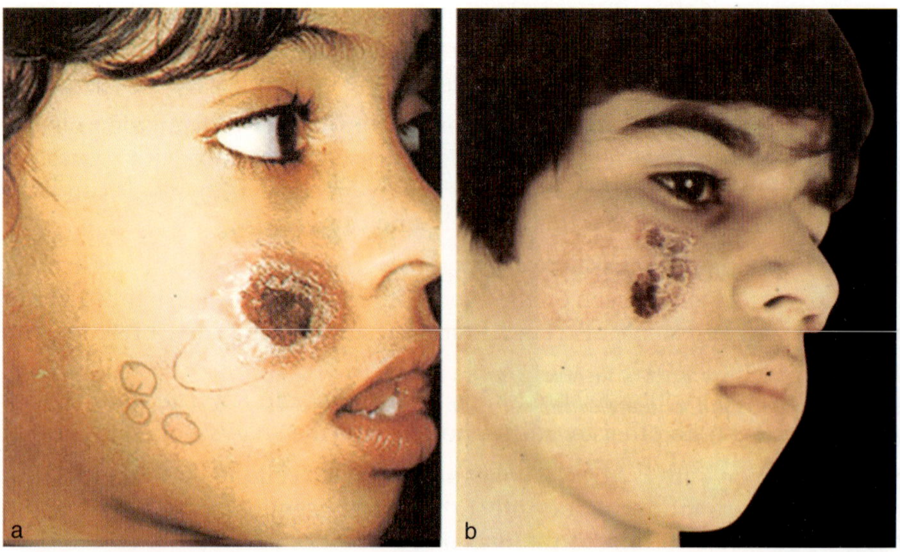

Fig. 16.1: (a) Cutaneous leishmaniasis; (b) Dermal leishmaniasis

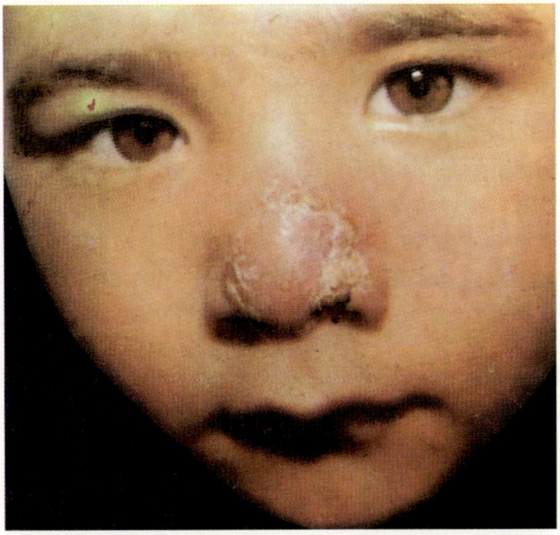

Fig. 16.2: Leishmaniasis—typical indolent bluish red nodule

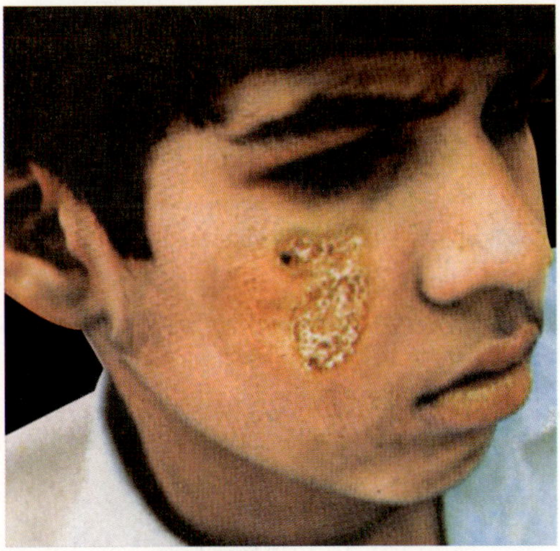

Fig. 16.3: Dry type cutaneous leishmaniasis showing closely adherent crust

The mucous membranes of the nose and throat may be affected. This is most commonly seen in American leishmaniasis caused by *L. braziliensis*. Destruction is marked. Condition is seen in South America and is called Espundia.

Dermal Leishmanoid

Synonym: Post-kala-azar dermal leishmaniasis. It is a skin eruption due to generalized infection with *Leishmania donovani* as sequelae to an attack of kala-azar. It is sometimes related to inadequate therapy. The cutaneous lesions appear in 1–2 years after recovery from kala-azar. The face is the site of choice, less commonly, the limbs and the trunk. The rash varies from maculo-papular to nodulo-verrucous. Butterfly erythema is usually seen on the face. There are no constitutional or subjective symptoms. The eruption heals after passing through a stage of depigmentation. The parasite can easily be demonstrated in smears taken from the nodular and erythematous cutaneous lesions, but it is absent in the blood and spleen. People suffering from this condition are the carriers of the disease. Rarely do kala-azar and dermal leishmanoid occur together.

Pathology: The essential feature is the proliferation of the reticuloendothelial cells which may show LT bodies when stained with Leishman's stain. Secondarily, there is round cell and plasma cell infiltration. In the early stages, there is marked inflammation consisting of mixed infiltrate and plenty of LT bodies. In the late stages, the histology resembles that of tuberculous granuloma and may be completely indistinguishable from it.

Investigations

1. Demonstration of LT bodies in a smear made from the serum sucked with a pipette from the periphery of a lesion. The smear is stained with Leishman's stain. The LT bodies can also be demonstrated in a biopsy section. Stained with Leishman's stain, the protoplasm of the LT body becomes darker in colour.
2. Culture on NNN medium or Noguchi's medium.
3. Histology of the biopsy material.
4. Skin test. 0.1 cc. of antigen containing 1,00,000 parasites in a phenolized saline emulsion is injected intradermally into the skin. At the end of 24 hours, a reddish papule is formed which develops fully in 2–3 days time. The strongest reaction is seen in cases of leishmaniasis recidivans.

Differential diagnosis: It is made from other infective granulomas, chiefly tuberculosis, leprosy, syphilis and deeper fungi, e.g. sporotrichosis, blastomycosis and chromoblastomycosis. Occasionally, chronic pyogenic ulcer, tropical sore and epithelioma have to be excluded. In endemic areas, leishmaniasis should be suspected before any other disease, and confirmed by the demonstration of LT bodies. At times, this is really difficult to do, but if the essential features are remembered, and the necessary investigations conducted, there is little likelihood of confusion.

Prognosis: It is favourable except for the disfiguring scar. Dermal leishmanoid is somewhat resistant to treatment. Depigmented lesions take a long time before they disappear.

Treatment

Prophylactic: This consists in eradicating sand flies and infected rodents, dogs and cats. There should be no open drains or tunnels burrowed in the ground by animals and dump heaps near residential areas.

A vaccine made from a leishmania culture has a certain degree of prophylactic value in endemic areas.

Curative: It consists of local or systemic measures, depending upon the number of lesions, the site and the age of the patient. When only 1–3 small lesions occur on the easily accessible parts of the patient's body, the treatment is local viz:

1. Infiltration of the lesion with 1% mepacrine solution, or 1% emetine hydrochloride solution, or berberine sulphate solution—Orisol (P). 1–2 cc of any of these solutions is usually required for one injection. The needle is entered just outside the periphery and directed towards the centre of the lesion. Generally, there is an inflammatory reaction for two or three days. When it subsides, another infiltration is done at a small distance from the first one. In this manner, usually between 3–12 local injections are

given to bring about complete healing. It is a somewhat painful procedure, especially in lesions near the eyes, ears and lips. Glucantime (N-methyl glucamin antimonate) has also been used with success.

2. Cauterization with CO_2 snow, liquid nitrogen, or electro-cautery.
3. X-ray therapy, 600–800 r in one to two doses, gives very good results. It is a painless procedure, and if carried out by an expert, the cosmetic results are indeed very good.

When there are multiple lesions, systemic measures are preferable. Anthiomaline (P) intramuscularly, sodium antimony tartrate 10–50 mg intravenously, and neostibosan (organic pentavalent antimony) intravenously, are the usual preparations employed in cutaneous leishmaniasis as well as dermal leishmanoid. Glucantime 50–60 mg per kg intramuscular daily for 12 days and also intralesionally appears to give the best results. It is also used in PKDL. Course can be repeated after 15 days interval. Intravenous antimony preparations are very toxic to the kidneys, lungs, heart and gastrointestinal tract; so they should be given very carefully and only in selected cases. Rifampicin (600 mg once daily for 10 days), metronidazole (Flagyl), trimethoprim sulpha-methoxazole (Septran), dapsone and amphotericin-B are also useful in resistant cases.

YAWS

Synonyms: Framboesia (German), Pian (French)

It is a spirochaetal, non-venereal, contagious and communicable disease, rampant in warm and humid tropical areas. In India, it is most prevalent in the south; the rest of the country is almost free from the disease. It is endemic in certain regions of Asia, Africa and South America.

Etiology: *Treponema pertenue* is the causative spirochaete which resembles *Treponema pallida* of syphilis morphologically. Even serologically, it is difficult to separate the two organisms. Their behaviour in the human body is the only differentiating feature, the former attacks the skin and bones primarily, while the latter affects all organs including the heart, brain and eyes (Hassellman) and is transmitted by sexual intercourse.

Yaws is transmitted through intimate bodily contact between an infected person with an open wound and an uninfected person with abraded or excoriated skin. *T pertenue* cannot penetrate the intact skin, from one individual to another; though flies have been demonstrated to convey the infection mechanically. Hence the primary lesion usually appears on an exposed part of the body, particularly the legs. The incubation period is about 3–4 weeks.

Clinical features: Yaws starts with a primary sore (mother yaws) at the site of the inoculation of the spirochaetes. After about a month or so, a secondary eruption (polypapillomata) appears in the neighbourhood of the primary lesion by lymphogenous spread. The tertiary stage develops after a latent period of several years; it consists of destructive skin and bone lesions. The central nervous system, the heart and other viscera are never involved.

Primary Stage

It starts as a small papule which is solid and well-defined. It soon grows into a papilloma with a coarsely granular, raw and pinkish surface (raspberry—framboise in German) covered by a crust. It is about one inch in diameter. The crust is shed from time to time;

the serous discharge is replete with spirochaetes. The lesion is painless and non-itchy. Regional glands are enlarged and painless. Primary lesion may persist for months and then heal with an atrophic scar.

Secondary Stage

1. Rudimentary papillomata, around the primary lesion (daughter yaws) which resemble the latter clinically and histologically. These are produced by a regional lymphatic spread or direct contact. These regional metastatic lesions are separated from the primary lesion (mother yaws) by healthy-looking skin.
2. Papillomata on the face, limbs or chest are multiple; they may number any where upto a couple of hundred. Their clinical features are identical with those of the primary lesion—the same granular, pinkish surface covered by a crust. They vary in size from one to two inches in diameter. The scalp and trunk are less involved than the exposed parts of the body. The lesions of yaws are frequently itchy. They may occur on mucocutaneous junctions like the lips, peri-anal region, etc. but the mucous membranes are not directly involved.
3. The lesions on the palms and soles are uniform, well-defined, discrete, wet papules, with or without fungation. They are very unlike the hyperkeratotic lesions found in the tertiary stage.
4. One kind of lesion which occurs less commonly in yaws, being quite atypical, is the acuminate follicular papule: It appears in groups or singly. Infiltrative alopecia is uncommon in yaws.

   Cutaneous lesions are frequently accompanied by rheumatic pains, discomfort and malaise. Secondary lesions are short-lived and non-destructive, but there is a definite tendency to relapses for two to three years. Healing leaves behind faint, wrinkled scars. Desquamation may be found only on the glabrous skin.
5. Bony lesions which occur in the secondary stage are characterized by cortical rarefaction and periosteitis. They are accompanied by considerable pain and tenderness. Swelling of the fingers (polydactylitis) and hypertrophic osteitis of the para-nasal bones, unilateral or bilateral (Goundou) are typical. Either one of the two bony lesions—erosions in the cortex of bones or hyperplastic periosteitis—may predominate over the other in different bones. As a rule, destruction is not so pronounced in the secondary stage as it is in the tertiary.

Tertiary Stage

It is characterized by hyperkeratotic and ulcerative lesions of the integument, and bony deformities.

1. Lesions on the palms and soles are very characteristic. The main feature is the hyperkeratotic thickening of the skin which desquamates, becomes fissured, or erodes, leaving behind pitting (moth-eaten appearance) or cribriform erosion (sieve-like appearance).
2. Late ulcers can occur with papillomata of the secondary stage. They may be single or multiple and localised or extensive. The ulcers are painful, indolent, and have infiltrated borders. They may be destructive; they may therefore result in mutilations. which when occurring in the region of the nose and throat are characteristic of yaws

(Gangosa- rhinopharyngitis mutilans). Tertiary cutaneous lesions heal slowly, leaving flat, pigmented atrophic scars.

3. Tertiary lesions of the bones are more destructive. One or more bones, anywhere in the body, may be involved. The skull may show nodes; the palate, perforation : nasopharynx, mutilating destruction of the bones; the hand, destruction of phalanges; the tibia, a sabre-like deformity and so forth.
4. Hard fibromatous nodules in the proximity of the joints (juxta-articular nodes) especially close to the elbows, knees and ankles are frequently found in yaws. After some years, the disease tends to become latent, or dies out, leaving deformities of the integument and bones, which would make any person exceedingly miserable.

Laboratory Investigations

1. ***Blood serology:*** Flocculation and precipitation reactions (Wassermann and Kahn) or VDRL become positive within eight weeks of contacting the infection. It stays positive throughout the secondary, latent and tertiary stages.
2. The presence of spirochaetes in the primary and secondary lesions by dark field examination.

Histopathology: At the microscopic level also, yaws is similar to syphilis, except that in yaws endarteritis is not a feature. Primary and secondary stages are similar and show acanthosis, papillomatosis, spongiosis, neutrophil exocytosis and intra-epidermal microabscesses. In the dermis there is a diffuse mixed inflammatory infiltrate with predominance of plasma cells. Treponemas are readily visualized lying in between the epidermal cells. The microscopic appearance of tertiary stage is non-diagnostic and does not show the organisms.

Diagnosis: It is based on the presence of typical cutaneous and bony lesions in children and young adults in endemic areas. It is confirmed by dark field examination of the smear, and positive blood serology. Early lesions require differentiation from pyodermas, tuberculosis, sporotrichosis, leishmaniasis, etc. and late lesions from syphilis, leprosy, and muco-cutaneous leishmaniasis.

Prognosis: Since penicillin has come into use, the outlook in yaws has changed for the better. There are bright prospects of exterminating the disease from endemic areas by mass treatment of all infected individuals by making them non-infectious.

Regarding the individual sufferer, he can be cured, but nothing can be done to alleviate the misery produced by the scars, mutilations and deformities left by the disease, once it has been allowed to become advanced. Therefore, if good results are to be achieved. Every case must be diagnosed at an early stage.

Treatment: This consists in educating the slum dwellers and the poor illiterate classes, improving sanitation, mass diagnosis and treatment. Penicillin is very effective. The recommended dosage is benzathene penicillin 2.4 mega units (1.2 mega units to each buttock) IM in one visit or PAM 600,000 units IM daily for 8–10 days. Penicillin sensitive patients may be treated with tetracycline as for syphilis. Open wounds should be dressed with an antiseptic cream.

Aim of the treatment should be: (1) To make all the lesions disappear. (2) No new lesions should develop. (3) The serology should become negative or to a low titre. (4) Cases must be followed up to detect early clinical relapses.

RHINOSCLEROMA

Synonym: Scleroma.

It is a rare, contagious, chronic, granulomatous disease of the upper respiratory tract. particularly the nose and the adjoining part of the skin. It occurs endemically in certain parts of Asia, Africa, America and Eastern Europe. The disease is spread by close and intimate contact; it usually affects people living in crowded and unhygienic environments.

Etiology: *Klebsiella rhinoscleromatis* is the causative organism, though this fact is disputed by several authorities. The bacillus is typically seen as Gram negative diplococcus inside vacuolated histiocytes called Mikulicz cells which are typical of rhinoscleroma pathology. Young adults are most commonly affected. Transmission is by droplet infection. Incubation period is unknown but probably very long.

Clinical picture: It mostly affects adults and shows no sex predilection. Three distinct stages are recognized. In the first, 'rhinitic' stage, the symptoms are rhinorrhoea with foetid odour, headaches, progressive difficulty in breathing and occasional epistaxis. The clinical findings are non-specific at this time, showing hypertrophy of the nasal mucosa. In the second, 'infiltrative' stage, painless, reddish induration of the mucosa, and sometimes adjacent areas of the skin of the upper lip, develop **(Fig. 16.4)**. The obstructive symptoms may become more pronounced with possible extension of the disease to larynx or palate. In the final, 'nodular stage', the clinical appearance is more amenable to recognition. Nodular swellings of mucosa and the adjacent skin are apparent, the sense of smell is lost, and complete nasal obstruction develops. The disease progresses relentlessly, ending in asphyxia, and possible death if tracheotomy is not performed. There is no metastatic spread or systemic symptoms.

The course is slow and usually extends over years.

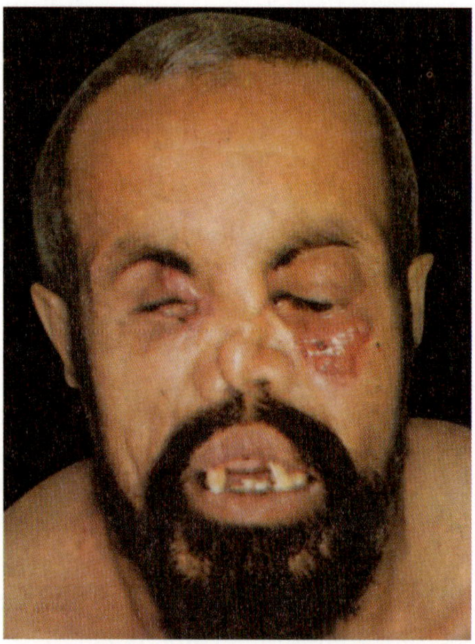

Fig. 16.4: Rhinoscleroma—typical site and lesion

Diagnosis: It is based upon: (1) The clinical picture. (2) Biopsy. The diagnostic features are abundant foamy histiocytes, many containing the klebsiella bacilli (Mikulicz cells), and Russel bodies. These are round or ovoid non-nucleated eosinophilic, refractile structures (20–40 nm diameter). The overall picture is that of a histiocytic granuloma. In late lesions, the number of Mikulicz cells diminishes and fibrosis becomes more evident. (3) Demonstration of bacillus rhinoscleromatis.

Differential diagnosis is mainly from dermal leishmaniasis, leprosy, rhinosporidiosis and syphilis.

Treatment: It is unsatisfactory. Deformities cause disfigurement and misery. Tracheotomy may have to be done to relieve respiratory embarrassment in laryngeal stenosis. The treatment consists mainly of: (1) Streptomycin—Long course of 1/2–1 g daily. Chloramphenicol, tetracycline, cephalosporodine and oleandomycin are also useful. (2) Antiseptic cream or spray locally. (3) Surgery may be required in late case to correct deformities and to restore function.

Chapter

17

Leprosy—Hansen's Disease

Indian synonym: Korh, Kusth.

Leprosy is a chronic, infectious disease caused by *Mycobacterium leprae*. Its incubation period varies from 6 months to 20 years. It principally affects the skin and peripheral nerves. It is one of the oldest diseases of humanity. Leprosy has also been described in *Charaka Samhita* written in 800 BC. In practice, the name Hansen's disease is preferred to leprosy to avoid prejudice and bias amongst laymen.

Incidence: The incidence of leprosy is high in Central Africa, India, Suriname, Guinea, Burma and parts of Papua, New Guinea. This disease is rarely encountered in cold countries, polar regions and in deserts. According to the Union Health Ministry, despite India being declared "Leprosy Eliminated" in 2005, the country still accounts for about 52% of the world's new leprosy patients. It is noted that earlier gains made in the leprosy programme in India were reversed during the COVID-19 pandemic as case detection dropped significantly and the decline in detection has led to an increase in patients with grade 2 disabilities. Broadly speaking, the incidence of leprosy is high in the south-eastern parts and low in the north-western parts of our country. Tamil Nadu alone has about one-third of the total leprosy cases in India.

Etiology: Leprosy is caused by *Mycobacterium leprae* or Hansen's bacillus after the name of the discoverer, Gerhard Henrik Armauer Hansen. They are pleomorphic, straight or curved, acid-fast, rod-like bacteria occurring in clumps like bunches of cigars inside the phagocytes termed lepra cells. The size varies from 1.5 to 5 μ by 0.2 to 0.5 μ. Lepra bacilli resemble tubercle and smegma bacilli which are both acid-fast. Attempts to grow lepra bacilli in the Armadillo have been successful in Venezuela and other places. Man is the only known source of infection, though cockroaches, etc. have been blamed for spreading the disease. Prolonged and close contact is ideal for its transmission. Transmission by short and intimate contacts has also been reported. Exposure to lepromatous cases results in 4–11 times more effective transmission as compared with exposure to non-lepromatous cases.

The skin is believed to be the common portal of entry. Weddell and Palmaer believe that *Mycobacterium leprae* enter through the upper respiratory and intestinal tract and disseminate through the blood stream. Indirect transmission may occur through wearing an infective patient's clothes and from articles of daily use. Leprosy is not inherited. There is no age bar to the incidence of leprosy. Leprosy affects more males than females. There is no difference in the incidence of leprosy between the ABO blood groups. Neither diet nor climate play an important role in the epidemiology of leprosy. Over-population, over-crowding and inadequate housing lead to intimate and more frequent contacts and favour the spread of leprosy. The epidemiology of leprosy depends upon the infectivity of the patient, susceptibility of the infected and proximity of the two.

Classification: Indian classification (1955) is based on clinical criteria, bacteriological examination and histopathological findings. It is very useful in clinical practice. Jopling's classification is based on the immunological status of the patient. Tuberculoid (TT) and lepromatous (LL) types are considered the two stable determined polar ends of the spectrum; borderline tuberculoid (BT), borderline lepromatous (BL) and borderline-borderline (BB) are considered immunologically unstable and may swing into either polar variety. Indeterminate is undetermined stage in evolution. **Table 17.1** help to understand the relationship between the clinical patterns and immunological status.

Evolution of Leprosy Lesions

A significant number of people, especially children living with leprosy patients harbour *Mycobacterium leprae* in the skin, without any clinical manifestations. This is the 'silent phase' of infection. In people with low resistance, the silent phase leads to the indeterminate phase and a primary lesion is formed. Spontaneous regression occurs in cases having high resistance. Depending upon the immunological response, the primary lesion may progress to non-lepromatous, borderline or lepromatous leprosy. In the tuberculoid forms, histiocytes are turned into epithelioid cells, while in the lepromatous form they are gradually turned into foamy lepra cells, viz: 'Virchow's cells'. Borderline lesions present mixed characters. According to Muir, the tuberculoid form may pass into the lepromatous form. Occasionally, the primary lesion may be absent and the silent phase may directly lead to tuberculoid or lepromatous leprosy.

Immunity: Humoral immune response appears to be unaffected; there is depressed cell mediated immunity. Degree of depression varies. In lepromatous leprosy, immunoglobulin levels are raised. ANA, Rheumatoid factor and even LE cells may be seen **(Fig. 17.1)**.

Classification and Clinical Features

Classification of leprosy is shown in **Table 17.1** and their clinical features are discussed as follows.

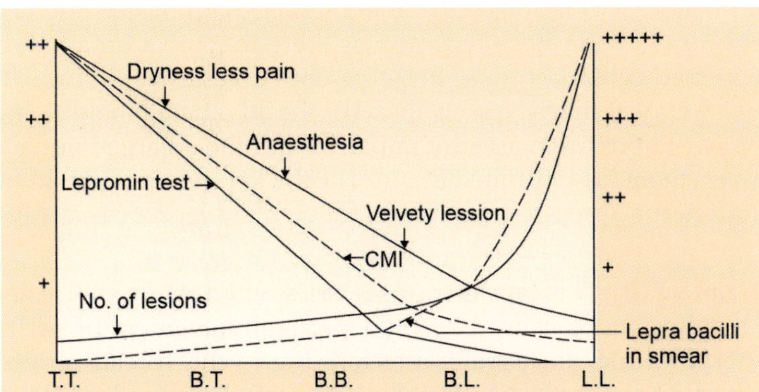

Fig. 17.1: Immunity and clinical features in different types of leprosy

Table 17.1: Classification of leprosy

Tuberculoid	Borderline	Lepromatous
Stable and high resistance	Immunologically unstable	Stable but low resistance and depressed (CMI)
Tuberculoid (TT)	Borderline lepromamatous (BL), Borderline tuberculoid (BT), Borderline borderline (BB), Neuritic, Maculo-anaesthetic (MA), Indeterminate (I)	Lepromatous (LL)

Indeterminate leprosy (I): Lesions of leprosy usually evolve from an indeterminate form comprising pale or pinkish erythematous macules. The number, size and location may vary considerably. Indeterminate lesions frequently show impairment of sensation. The edges may or may not be well defined. Bacilli are usually absent or scanty on routine examination. The lepromin test may be either negative or positive. The indeterminate form may pass into other forms of leprosy, may continue unchanged or may even regress.

Maculo-anaesthetic Leprosy (MA): This is the most benign form of leprosy. The lesions are few, asymmetrical, flat, hypopigmented, well-defined and anaesthetic. The integument is dry and rough; hair is lost in the patches. The lesions are not raised above the surface of the skin. Routine smears from the lesions are almost always negative. A small number of bacilli may be found by concentration method. The histological picture is non-specific and does not present the typical tuberculoid pattern. The lepromin test is usually moderately positive.

Tuberculoid leprosy (T): The WHO Expert Committee's report (1953), defined tuberculoid leprosy as a benign form, infrequently positive on bacteriological examination, presenting erythematous skin lesions which are either marginally or entirely raised and are almost always positive to lepromin. The tuberculoid form (T) may be subdivided into major (TM) and minor (Tm) varieties. The differences are of degree only; there is no fundamental difference between these two varieties. Tuberculoid minor (Tm) lesions are slightly elevated, anaesthetic and finely pebbled. In the tuberculoid minor variety, anaesthesia and enlargement of the regional cutaneous nerves are less marked than in the tuberculoid major lesions. This form has been termed as 'minor lepride' by Cochrane.

Tuberculoid major (TM) lesions are markedly raised, infiltrated and erythematous. The entire lesion may be uniformly raised or there may be a broad and thick outer zone with depressed central portion. In a case with excessive activity, scaling is seen. Pioneer tubercles may at times be seen ahead of the advancing margin. In tuberculoid major leprosy, sensations are markedly impaired and the enlarged nerve can at times be traced to an erythemato-infiltrated lesion. The thickening may go into caseation and liquefaction and nerve abscesses may form. Tuberculoid leprosy is always positive to lepromin.

Polyneuritic leprosy (P): This type comprises cases without any skin lesions, but with polyneuritic manifestations caused by the leprous involvement of peripheral nerve trunks. The nerve trunks are usually affected due to the spread of infection along cutaneous nerves. The commonly affected nerves are ulnar, median, lateral popliteal, posterior tibial, fifth and seventh cranial nerves. In contrast to other forms of neuritis, in polyneuritic leprosy, sensory changes are more marked than the motor changes. Deep reflexes like knee jerks are never lost in leprosy. In cases of polyneuritic leprosy, anaesthesia starts peripherally and extends up the affected limb along the distribution of the peripheral nerve. In leprosy, sensations of temperature and pain are usually lost earlier than the sensation of touch and pressure. Heaviness, tingling and numbness might be present and acute inflammation of the affected nerve may lead to severe neuralgic pain. In cases of leprosy, motor involvement may lead to paresis, hypotonia and atrophy, particularly of the muscles of the hand and feet. The paralysis of muscles leads to deformities like claw-hand, claw toes, wrist-drop, etc. Trophic changes occurring in case of leprosy are due to vasomotor changes resulting from nerve involvement. These include formation of anhidrotic, dry and glossy skin, blisters, trophic ulcers and decalcification as well as absorption of small bones of the hands and feet.

Borderline leprosy (B): It is an unstable form belonging to the intermediate group and may pass into the lepromatous type. It is characterized by erythematous, raised lesions, sloping towards the periphery and presenting an 'inverted saucer appearance'. Anaesthesia may be present. Skin lesions usually have asymmetrical distribution. They are bacteriologically positive but globi are either few or absent. The lepromin test is generally negative.

Lepromatous leprosy (L): In this type, the patient has low resistance and *Mycobacterium leprae* multiply in astronomical numbers. The chief clinical signs are in the skin and mucous membranes. From the lesions in the skin and mucosa, through blood and lymphatics, *Mycobacterium leprae* enter reticulo-endothelial cells of the lymph nodes, spleen, liver, bone marrow, testes and nerves. Rarely, tendons, cornea, choroid, bone, adrenal glands and tooth pulp may also take up lepra bacilli. Although lepromata may be found in all these sites, local signs and symptoms are lacking except when the testes are affected. Involvement of the testes might lead to impotency, sterility and enlargement of breasts in males. In lepromatous leprosy, the loss of the sweat function may be marked on the extremities, while the trunk and face may show compensatory hyperhidrosis. Depending upon the spread or progression of the disease and its severity, lepromatous leprosy has been subdivided into L1, L2 and L3 forms.

Lepromatous macules (L1) have a smooth shiny surface and a velvety feel, while the margins are indistinct and merge imperceptibly with the surrounding skin. They may appear faintly hypopigmented or coppery brown or infiltrated. Except in the very early prelepromatous phase, bacilli can always be easily detected by routine methods. The lepromin reaction is negative. Usually there is no sensory loss.

Lepromatous infiltration (L2) is a step ahead of its macular form. As a matter of fact. all lepromatous lesions are infiltrated, but infiltration is negligible in the macular form. Infiltrated skin is erythematous, thickened and shiny. In late cases, the eyebrows are lost. Infiltrated plaques are soft, velvety and slope towards the periphery. Sensory impairment is negligible, but *Mycobacterium leprae* can be easily found with the routine methods. Almost the whole of the integument may be involved. On healing, dry xerodermic skin may be left behind.

Lepromatous nodules (L3) denote advanced leprosy **(Table 17.2)**. Nodules do not appear *per se*, but are due to the marked localized aggregation of the infiltrate. Usually starting on the ears, they may crop up on the face, trunk and extremities. They may be

Table 17.2: Differentiating features of different varieties of leprosy

Differentiating	*Lepromatous*	*Tuberculoid*	*Borderline*	*Polyneuritic*	*Maculo-anaesthetic*	*Indeterminate*
Lesions	Small multiple, bilaterally symmetrical, glossy, velvety, inverted saucer-shaped patches or nodules fading at periphery; may or may not be anaesthetic	One or more big, asymmetrically placed, dry, erythematous, anaesthetic macules with well-defined border or the margin only is raised	Lesions as in both major varieties are seen	No skin lesion in primary type. An anaesthesia in the distribution of nerve	Few asymmetrically placed, hypopigmented, well-defined anaesthetic macules with hair loss on them. No or slight erythema or infiltration	Pale or pink, poorly defined macules, not necessarily anaesthetic. Not raised above surface
Nerves	Not usually, but in later stages may be grossly thickened and tender	Regional nerves and also others are thickened and tender	May or may not be affected	Thickened tender nerves and nerve abcesses may be seen	Regional nerves are thickened	None
Slit smear	Teeming with AFB infective	AFB may be found only at times from margin. Usually not infective	Depends on the nature of the lesion whtere from it is taken. Infective for all practical purposes	Ordinarily negative but may be seen in smears from the nerve itself	Almost always negative by routine method. Concentration method may show some AFB	±
Lepromin test (Mitsuda's)	Always negative	Strongly +ve	Usually -ve but may also be +ve, specially during activity	Usually +ve	Moderately positive	Positive, may also be negative

(Contd.)

Table 17.2: Differentiating features of different varieties of leprosy *(Contd).*

Differentiating	*Lepromatous*	*Tuberculoid*	*Borderline*	*Polyneuritic*	*Maculo-anaesthetic*	*Indeterminate*
Special features	Leonine face; loss of eyebrows; affection of mucous membrane; hoarseness of voice; nasal bleeding. Gynaecomastia and testicular atrophy and ocular involvement	Trophic changes in the form of wasting of small muscles, perforating ulcers, contractures, absoption of bones, etc. Nerve abscesses	According to the turn it takes whether tuberculoid or lepromatous	Sensory changes more marked than motor. Deep reflexes, e.g. knee jerk, etc. are never lost	Nil	Nil
Histology	Characteristic features is foam cells; AFB can be demonstrated. A thin sub-spidermal zone is spared	Non-caseating granuloma with a tubercle consisting of epithelioid and giant cells of Langerhans type. Sub-epidermal zone affected, Globi are either absent or few	Changes of both type may be seen. Sub-epidermal zone is not affected. Globi are either absent or few	Infiltration around the affected nerve	Non-specific. Slight infiltration around nerve endings and appendages	Only slight infiltration in upper dermis.
Course and prognosis	The most malignant form; slow and steady course with reactions	Due to good resistance, prognosis is very good. Reactions less often.	May pass to any of the major forms but usually lepromatous	May go both ways but mostly to tuberculoid form	Most benign of all; usually takes the form of tuberculoid	May either proceed to any major form or regress by itself

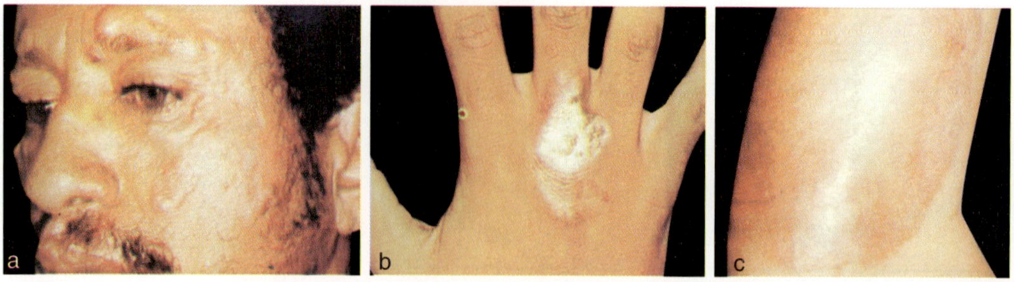

Fig. 17.2: (a) Lepromatous leprosy; (b) Tuberculoid leprosy; (c) Nerve abscess—Ulnar nerve

small or large, free or fixed, sessile or pedunculated. Nodules might get either absorbed or ulcerated (lepromatous ulcers) **(Fig. 17.2)**. In the lepromatous type, ocular, nasal, oral, pharyngeo-laryngeal and tracheo-bronchial mucous membranes are frequently affected. The affected mucosa may show infiltration, nodulation and ulceration. Lucio's phenomenon consists of bullous and ulcerative lesions due to necrosis, causing considerable misery to the patient.

Reactions in Leprosy

Broadly speaking, reactions comprise acute, subacute or recurring exacerbations in the course of this chronic disease. Exacerbations may occur in any form of leprosy. According to Dharmendra, although the exact cause of reactions is not known, reactions in non-lepromatous cases are probably allergic and in lepromatous cases toxic in origin. It might be due to increased concentration of DDS in tissues and skin. Smallpox vaccination, typhoid, malaria, influenza, malnutrition, pregnancy, delivery, sulphonamides and iodides may precipitate reactions in cases of leprosy.

Reaction in non-lepromatous leprosy: Existing lesions may show aggravation and fresh lesions might crop up. Regional nerves may become tender and painful.

Reactions in lepromatous leprosy: These reactions are usually associated with fever, malaise, body-aches, oedema of hands and feet, epistaxis and in acute cases, the patient is severely ill. Existing lesions show exacerbation. Nodules may show vesiculation, suppuration and ulceration. Multiple symmetrical, reddish, disseminated nodules may appear on the body. These are called rose spot nodules or erythema nodosum leprosum (ENL). ENL lesions may show recurrence and suppuration. ENL may be acute, sub-acute, or chronic. In some cases of reactions, subcutaneous tender lumps are formed. Lucio's phenomenon or lazarine leprosy is a peculiar but extreme reaction in leprosy. Nodules break down to produce deep ulcers, scars, bullae and miserable appearance. Other manifestations associated with reactions in leprosy are acute neuritis, arthritis, bursitis, orchitis, iritis, iridocyclitis, gynaecomastia, lymphadenitis and enlargement of the liver and spleen.

Deformities in Leprosy

Early diagnosis and proper treatment can help considerably in preventing various organ deformities classified in **Table 17.3**.

Face: Facies leonina is due to multiple nodules appearing on the face. It is characteristic of lepromatous leprosy, while the mask face is due to facial nerve paralysis and is typical

Table 17.3: Topographical classification of deformities occurring in leprosy	
Face	Mask face, facies leonina, sagging face, lagophthalmos, loss of eyebrows, perforated nose, depressed nose, ear deformities, e.g. nodules on ear, and elongated lobule. Perforation of the palate.
Hands	Claw-hand, wrist-drop, neuropathic ulcers, absorption of digits, thumb web contracture, hollowing of interosseous spaces and swollen hands.
Feet	Neuropathic ulcers, foot-drop, inversion of foot, clawing of toes, absorption of toes, collapsed foot and swollen foot.
Other deformities	Gynaecomastia.

of tuberculoid leprosy. Sagging face is due to the rapid disappearance of lepromatous infiltrate under the influence of sulphones. Lagophthalmos is caused by the selective paralysis of the zygomatic branch of the facial nerve. Loss of eyebrows is due to the lepromatous infiltration of the hair follicles.

Nasal deformities are due to the invasion and destruction of nasal tissues by *Mycobacterium leprae*. The depressed nose is due to destruction of the nasal septum while perforation is due to the circumscribed gangrenous involvement of the nasal tissue. In advanced cases, the nasal mucosa is replaced by scar tissue which pulls the nose down on the face.

Perforation of the palate, either hard or soft or both, may occur in leprosy. It is due to circumscribed gangrenous destruction caused by *Mycobacterium leprae*. The patient may complain of regurgitation of food and may have the typical speech due to incompetent palate.

Hands: The claw-hand is a characteristic hand deformity. In it, the *metacarpo phalangeal* joints are hyperextended and the interphalangeal joints are flexed. In the ulnar claw hand, the little and ring fingers are affected. Clawing of all fingers is seen in high ulnar and low median nerve paralysis occurring together **(Fig. 17.3)**.

Thumb-web contracture is the most common complication of paralysis of the thumb. The disuse or overuse of the finger tips and sepsis are important factors underlying the absorption of the digits seen in cases of leprosy. Wrist-drop is due to radial nerve paralysis and occurs infrequently.

Neuropathic or trophic ulcers and hollowing of interosseus spaces are commonly encountered in India.

Feet: Neuropathic ulcers are very commonly seen in patients coming from rural areas. Plantar ulcers, trophic ulcers and perforating ulcers, are the various synonyms used for this condition. Factors responsible for these ulcers are analgesia, paralysis of intrinsic muscles, strain due to walking and trauma due to stones,

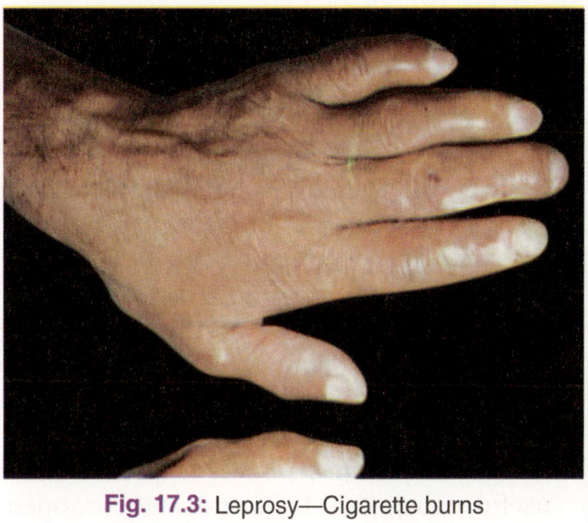

Fig. 17.3: Leprosy—Cigarette burns

nails and pointed objects. Neuropathic ulcers may be single or multiple, localized or extensive. They may penetrate even through the whole thickness of the foot (Fig. 17.4).

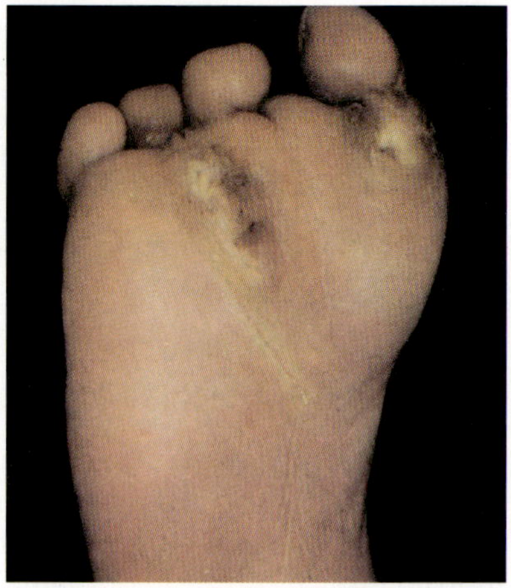

Fig. 17.4: Leprosy—Trophic ulcer

Foot-drop: Paralysis of the common peroneal nerve at the neck of the fibula may lead to foot-drop. Patients cannot lift up the foot and have a high-stepping gait.

Claw-toes result from posterior tibial neuritis. It is due to the paralysis of the intrinsic muscles supplied by the posterior tibial nerve. Claw-toes may be stiff or mobile. Swollen foot, collapsed foot and absorption of toes are the other deformities.

Breast: Gynaecomastia or swelling of the male breast is a very embarrassing deformity caused by leprous destruction of the testes resulting in proliferation of stroma and ducts of the mammary glands. It is not generally due to leprous infiltration of the male breast, though mild infiltration of nipples is seen.

Investigations

It is best to point out at the onset that the diagnosis of leprosy is mainly on clinical grounds. Most cases escape the notice of general practitioners and physicians because they forget to consider this disease in the differential diagnosis. The following tests are useful in diagnosis of leprosy:

1. *Sensations:* In every suspicious case of leprosy, the sensations must be tested on the patches as well as on the extremities. Most helpful in diagnosis are the sensations of pain and temperature (hot and cold). The latter is tested with two test tubes—one contains hot water and the other cold.
2. *Bacterial demonstration of lepra bacilli.* This is not essential for diagnosis, but its value lies in establishing whether or not a case is infectious and its progress requires to be watched. The skin, nasal mucosa and even buccal granulomas are selected for such examination. The slit method is usually adopted for making a smear of tissue cells from the affected skin, ear lobules or nose. The slide is stained with Ziehl–Neelsen method, the precaution being taken that the discoloration with acid is carried out only for a short while till the film turns slightly pink. The slide should be declared positive only when numerous lepra bacilli are seen. For a nasal smear, the mucosa on the anterior part of the septum should be scraped with a scalpel or probed hard with a swab stick, bleeding being avoided.
3. *Serology:* VDRL is positive in advanced cases of lepromatous leprosy; otherwise, only doubtful or weakly positive reactions are obtained. Concurrent infection with syphilis or yaws should be considered in cases that show a strongly positive blood serology. In lepromatous leprosy LE cells, anti-nuclear factor, rheumatoid factor and cryoglobulins may be present.
4. *Histological examination:* It is helpful in classifying the disease but only sometimes useful in diagnosis. Epidermis and the appendages show atrophy, more in advanced

cases. In the lepromatous variety, infiltration in the corium is diffuse. and it consists of mainly histiocytes with vacuolation (foam cells of Virchow). Between these lepra cells small round cells and fibroblasts may be seen. The latter increase as the lesions resolve. Lepra bacilli are present in abundance.

In the tuberculoid form, the infiltration is focal and tubercles consisting of epithelioid cells, lymphocytes and giant cells are seen. In practice these two typical pictures are less commonly seen compared with simple inflammatory infiltrate seen in a large proportion of cases. Infiltrate consists of small round cells, an occasional epithelioid cell and fibrocytes. This infiltrate is localized around blood vessels and other skin appendages. At this stage, diagnosis of leprosy is difficult on histopathological examination alone. In the intermediate variety, few vacuolated cells, many lepra bacilli and a non-specific inflammatory infiltrate are found.

5. *Lepromin test:* An immunological test for leprosy was first demonstrated by Mitsuda. Two types of antigens are used for this—Dharmendra's and Mitsuda's (modified by Wade). Intradermal injection of Mitsuda's antigen is followed by an early (after 48 hours) and a late (after 7 days) response. The early reaction is represented by erythema and infiltration while late, by induration and nodulation. Positivity of the lepromin test is marked by the appearance of a nodule after seven days which is persistent and progressive. It enlarges and ulcerates after 3–4 weeks. Its value is mainly prognostic. It also helps in the categorization of cases—tuberculoid (strongly), maculo-anaesthetic and polyneuritic types, i.e. in high resistance varieties, while always negative in the lepromatous type. It may also be positive in healthy individuals and contacts. When the patient has recovered from lepromatous leprosy, the hitherto negative test becomes positive. Hence, its usefulness as a therapeutic index.
6. *Blood picture:* ESR is raised considerably in severe forms of the disease. Its value is only prognostic. In reactional and lepromatous leprosy, the electrophoretic pattern of serum proteins is affected; it is accompanied by anaemia.

Diagnosis

It is not difficult if leprosy is borne in mind while practicing in tropical countries and endemic areas.

The characteristic features are:

- Hypo-pigmented and hypo-anaesthetic macules.
- Thickened nerves and sensory changes in the distribution of such nerves.
- Trophic changes in the integument. Trophic ulcers.
- Indurated, erythematous, velvety plaques or nodules or ulcers.
- Deformities of the hands, the feet and perforation of the nasal septum, etc.
- History of nasal bleeding.
- History reveals contact.
- Demonstration of lepra bacilli.
- Biopsy.

Maculo-anaesthetic lesions must be differentiated from vitiligo, pityriasis versicolor, naevus achromicus, syphilitic leucomelanoderma, etc.

Leprotic neuritis should be distinguished from other causes of neuritis, particularly from progressive hypertrophic polyneuritis. The latter is a heredo-familial, progressive and bilaterally symmetrical neuritis accompanied by thickened nerves. Peripheral neuritis. especially the diabetic variety, must also be borne in mind in the differential diagnosis.

Trophic ulcers of leprosy must be distinguished from those produced by tabes dorsalis, diabetes and syringomyelia.

The differential diagnosis of lesions in lepromatous leprosy is made from chronic urticaria, psoriasis, syphilis and other infective granulomata.

Prognosis and Course

Leprosy is a chronic disease with slow ups and downs; only occasionally is a lepra reaction seen. The lepromatous form is malignant and contagious; there is no tendency to self-arrest or regression. When the infection clears up, it leaves atrophic, anaesthetic or shiny, wrinkled scars, deformities and trophic ulcers. Sometimes, the neural symptoms increase with the subsidence of the disease due to subsequent fibrosis (paradoxical reaction). Neural dissection is being tried, with some success, to prevent neural strangulation. The prognosis in leprosy has improved considerably since sulphones, rifampicin and lamprene have come into use. Today, a case can be cured except for the sequelae of the disease. The outlook is better in the neural than in the lepromatous variety, because of the natural resistance of the body in the former. Intercurrent infection, poor health, advanced age, the susceptibility of childhood, pregnancy, recurrent lepra reactions and sensitivity to drugs, all have an unfavourable influence on the outlook of the disease. The resultant deformities are a definite handicap; modern surgical repair may prove a boon to patients left with these. The lepromin test is of prognostic value; a positive lepromin test suggests the high resistance of the individual and so better the chances of recovery.

Before the treatment of leprosy is started, the physician in charge must establish the following:

1. The clinical variety—neural, tuberculoid lepromatous, indeterminate, lepra reaction, etc.
2. The infectiousness of the case—bacteriological demonstration of the bacilli in the nasal smear, skin nodules and ulcers, etc.; positiveness implies that the case is infectious. Further cases must be divided into multibacillary or paucibacillary types.
3. The severity and activity of the disease judged by the number of lesions and whether or not new ones are cropping up.

Treatment

Leprosy patients should be treated with patience, perseverance and understanding. Proper attention should be paid to diet and general health. Attempt should be made to isolate infectious cases. They should be told to keep their beds, clothing, towels and toilet things separate and to avoid close contact with others specially with infants and children.

From the therapy point of view leprosy is divided into two types—paucibacillary and multibacillary. Paucibacillary refers to patients with a bacterial index (Bl) of less than 2 on the Ridley scale at all sites and multibacillary to patients with BI of 2+ or more at any site. Thus, paucibacillary would usually include all indeterminate, tuberculoid and most borderline-tuberculoid cases, and multibacillary all the others.

Aims of therapy are interruption of transmission of infection, to eliminate all viable M. leprae from the body in as short period of time as possible and to prevent deformities and rehabilitation. Following drugs are usually employed:

Dapsone (DDS): At present DDS is the drug of choice for leprosy. It is the cheapest and the best available drug. Animal experiments have shown that—DDS is also completely absorbed in the gastrointestinal tract. Studies have shown that the concentration of DDS in the affected skin is about 10 times more than in the normal skin. Sulphones possess cumulative action and are retained in the liver, skin, muscles and kidneys. Dose is 50–100 mg DDS orally daily for 3–10 years, 6 days a week. It does not affect the intrauterine foetus; hence may be continued during pregnancy (Jopling).

The possibility of *Mycobacterium leprae* developing resistance to DDS is uncommon. DDS may lead to anaemia, leucopenia, drug fever, pigmentation, hepatitis, dermatitis and psychosis.

Clofazimine (CLF): It is an imino-phenazine derivative which has been extensively used with success in lepromatous leprosy and lepra reactions. It is a drug of choice in sulfone resistant and intolerance cases. Dosage is 100–300 mg daily or biweekly. Skin pigmentation and xeroderma are definite draw backs in patients taking clofazimine. Incidence of neuritis and ENL is much less in patients taking clofazimine.

Rifampicin (RFM): It is a semi-synthetic, broad—spectrum, bactericidal but expensive. It is absorbed rapidly if taken on empty stomach. Biological half-life is approx. 3 hours. Dose is 300–600 mg administered in capsule form 1/2 hour before breakfast. It produces reddish-orange urine, faeces, saliva, sputum, sweat and tears. Adverse effects are weakness, leg pains, gastrointestinal upset, stomatitis, purpura and hepatitis. Intermittent administration produces 'Flu' like syndrome, anaphylactic shock, anaemia and renal failure. The drugs available for leprosy can be divided into two groups–primary and secondary. The primary drugs includes dapsone, rifampicin, clofazimine and ethionamide/prothionamide. Secondary drugs consist of thiacetazone, thiambutosone. long acting sulfonamides and certain fluoroquinolones.

Ethionamide (ETH) and prothionamide (PTH): They are bactericidal drugs killing most of the bacteria in 4–5 days. PTH is better tolerated than ETH. Dose of 250–500 mg is sufficient.

A combination of DDS, INH and thiacetazone is found to be only slightly less effective than rifampicin and DDS after 2 years of therapy. The significance of INH in the treatment of leprosy is often underrated. As a component of combination, it also contributes to prevent resistance.

Fluoroquinolones: Pefloxacin 400 mg BD and Ofloxacin 200 mg BD are commercially available in the management of leprosy and several gram-positive infections. They are bactericidal to the extent that in about 22 days, 99% of the bacilli can be eliminated. Side-effects like depression of the haemopoietic system are rather few. They are particularly useful in patients with resistance to rifampicin, which is steadily increasing. Thus they can be used as the first line of therapy.

There is lot of controversy about drug management of leprosy regarding the combination, and duration of treatment. Resistant strains have developed because of use of monotherapy, irregular multidrug therapy and use in suboptimal dose.

Multidrug therapy is recommended both for paucibacillary and multibacillary cases of leprosy to prevent drug resistance. WHO study group recommendation (1982) is as follows:

PB leprosy—Rifampicin 600 mg once monthly for 6 months, supervised, plus dapsone 100 mg (1–2 mg/kg body weight) daily, self-administered, for 6 months.

MB leprosy—Rifampicin 600 mg once monthly, supervised, plus dapsone 100 mg daily, self-administered, plus clofazimine 300 mg once-monthly, supervised, and 50 mg daily self-administered. The duration of treatment should be at least two years and be continued, wherever possible, upto smear negativity. Where clofazimine is totally unacceptable owing to the coloration of skin lesions that it causes, its replacement by 250–375 mg self-administered daily doses ethionamide/prothionamide should be considered.

The two standard regimens have been endorsed by the WHO Expert Committee on Leprosy (1988), except that substitution of ethionamide/protionamide for clofazimine was not recommended because of potential serious toxic side-effects.

Although in vogue, the WHO regimen for pauci- and multibacillary therapy involving intermittent use of Rifampicin has time and again shown the development of drug-resistance. This may be a serious development and hamper the National Leprosy Eradication Programme. Hence we have discarded it. Currently we are using following regimen with success:

1. Multibacillary leprosy
   - Pefloxacin 400 mg twice daily for 3–6 months
   - Followed by clofazimine 100 mg and dapsone 100 mg daily for one year
   - Followed by only dapsone 100 mg for 3–5 years till bacterio-negativity

2. Paucibacillary leprosy
   - Pefloxacin 400 mg twice a day for 1–2 months
   - Followed by Dapsone 100 mg daily for one to 2 years.

Treatment of lepra reactions: It consists in removing the precipitating cause. During the reaction, sulphones may be withdrawn or dosage reduced. Corticosteroids are singularly effective in bringing down the reactions, but relapses are common. In refractory cases, corticosteroids should be used judiciously, either orally or parenterally in daily doses of 15–30 mg prednisolone or its equivalent. As the improvement sets in, the initial high dose should gradually be reduced.

Pefloxacin, complete bed rest and salicylates with or without steroids control majority of lepra reactions in a short time. In other cases, a course of clofazimine, Thalidomide or chloroquine or antimony may be dried. In steroid dependent cases, thalidomide is the drug of choice.

Physiotherapy and plastic surgery: Physiotherapy includes oil massage, wax baths, exercises, appliances and splints. Exercises consist of passive, free-active, and assisted active movements. Oil massage is useful in increasing the circulation and keeping the joints free and straightening the claw-hand. Wax baths also stimulate the circulation, increase the tone of the muscles and soften the skin. Splints are useful in cases of deformities for maintaining the progress made by operations, exercises and massage. By devising a number of tendon transfer operations, Paul Brand and Fritschi have helped these patients considerably. Reconstructive surgery and physiotherapy today play a vital role in the management of deformities and disabilities occurring in leprosy patients. Surgical decompression and hydrocortisone infiltration of nerves are useful in neuritis.

Follow-up

This is very important for complete cure and control of the disease. Unfortunately, this aspect of treatment gets scarce attention from patients themselves and to some extent from physicians, too. Frankly speaking, these patients need to be watched for their whole lives. But for practical purposes a tuberculoid leprosy case should be followed (in terms of bacteriological and clinical signs) for at least 7–10 years, or two years after an apparent cure of the disease, whichever is the longer. This period goes up to 10–20 years in cases of lepromatous leprosy. Cases have been seen by the authors, who developed reaction after several years of completion of sulphone therapy.

Besides this, the relatives and contacts in the family should be checked up periodically. Some workers suggest giving sulphones as a prophylactic measure. Children should be vaccinated with BCG.

Control of the Disease

Being a contagious and communicable disease, control and eradication is indispensable for the well-being of society. As 1,20,000 to 1,30,000 new cases of leprosy are reported every year in India, it warrants an aggressive approach in overall control of the disease burden.

The control of leprosy would require the following measures:

1. Survey of a community, village, district or state.
2. Education of the masses regarding the etiology, prognosis and treatment and improvement of socio-economic status.
3. Detection of patients and their treatment as early as possible.
4. Preventive measure like BCG vaccination and DDS prophylaxis. Operational efficiency and utilization of para-medical staff.

The chemo-prophylaxis value of DDS has been accepted and the contacts of open cases should receive sulphones in the following dosage:

Above the age of 12 years	75 mg biweekly
6–12 years	50 mg biweekly
2–5 years	25 mg biweekly

This is administered for 2 years after the contact with the source is discontinued or the case becomes non-infectious.

Immunotherapy, once it becomes available, shall be the ultimate answer.

Rehabilitation

It is very essential for leprosy patients because of the bias and prejudice amongst the public and deformities suffered by the patients. It consists in the following measures:

i. Early detection and treatment.

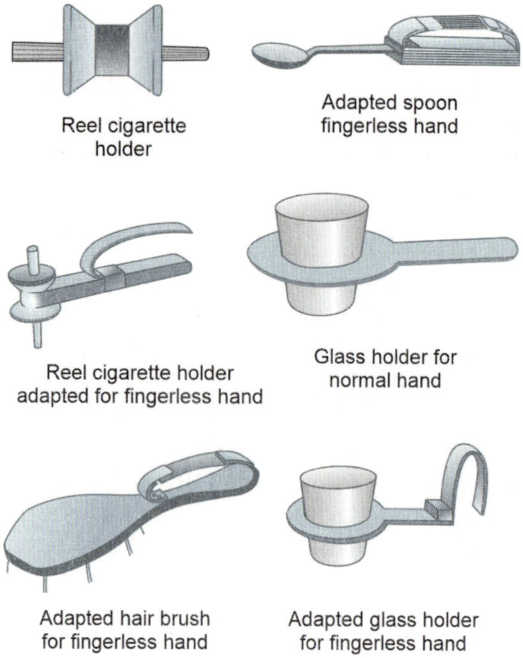

Fig. 17.5: Appliances for leprosy patients

ii. Prevention and treatment of deformities.

iii. Training in suitable crafts and vocations in special leprosy colonies, villages or leprasoriums.

iv. Use of special devices and equipment for patients with limb deformities **(Fig. 17.5)**.

Chapter

18

Syphilis

Syphilis is specific, highly contagious disease, caused by the spirochaete, *Treponema pallidum*, found all over the world; confined only to the human beings of all ages and both sexes (males more than females); with a high morbidity but low direct mortality rate; acquired usually by sexual intercourse, and sometimes accidentally, and also capable of involving almost all structures in the body; distinguished by florid manifestations and years of complete latency; capable of simulating many diseases; transmissible to offsprings; curable by penicillin.

Etiology

Syphilis is caused by a spiral organism, *Treponema pallidum*, discovered by Fritz Schaudinn and E Hoffmann on March 3, 1905. The organism is corkscrew shaped, 0.25 micron in diameter, the length varying from 6 to 14 microns, with an average of 7 microns (the thickness of a red blood corpuscle) having usually about 6–14 spirals. It can be seen only under the dark-field microscope as a shining, silver corkscrew, against a dark background, with characteristic movements of propulsion, rotation on its own axis and angulation; the special characteristic is its ability to keep the coils in shape.

Mode of Infection

There are four modes of infection, namely:

1. Direct.
2. Indirect.
3. Accidental.
4. Congenital

The most common way in which infection sets in is through direct contact (90–95%), and this is usually by sexual intercourse. Kissing and fondling the genitalia can produce extra-genital chancres on the lips, fingers and nipples.

The discharge from the early lesions of syphilis (primary and secondary stages) is found teeming with spirochaetes; hence the lesions are infectious. So, they must be handled with care. After about five years, the late lesions (tertiary stage) are practically non-infectious except in pregnant women.

Course of Untreated Syphilis

The spirochaetes usually enter the body through minute abrasions in the body, either on the skin or mucous membrane; they are also capable of penetrating the unbroken skin or mucous membrane. They invade the perivascular lymphatics and reach the regional lymph glands within a few hours after infection. The spirochaetes then enter the circulation, multiply and lodge themselves in different tissues.

While the spirochaetes invade the body, local reaction occurs at the site from which the spirochaetes made their entrance. This is called the primary lesion or chancre. The disease passes through the following stages: Early syphilis consisting of the primary, the secondary and the early asymptomatic infection which is known as latent syphilis; Late syphilis which denotes all the other manifestations of syphilis occurring after more than four years of infection.

Pathology: The typical histopathology consists of perivascular infiltration with plasma cells, lymphocytes, and histiocytes; the other features vary with the stage and lesion.

General diagnosis: After eliciting a history of exposure and the subsequent development of primary lesion occurring after the characteristic incubation period, a thorough clinical examination should be made. In experienced hands, these give a clue or a strong suspicion of syphilitic infection which should be confirmed by laboratory tests.

1. The dark-ground illumination test for *Treponema pallidum* in the serum from the sores.
2. VDRL test on the blood serum, or cerebrospinal fluid.

Serological tests for syphilis (STS) become positive about 8–10 weeks after exposure. So, they may be negative in primary syphilis, but are usually positive in secondary (95–100%) and tertiary syphilis (80%). Sometimes these tests become positive in leprosy, malaria, yaws, etc. Therefore, one must be careful in interpreting them. The problem of biological false-positive reactions obtained with VDRL has been considerably solved by the introduction of specific treponemal antigen. The various tests in vogue are the *Treponema pallidum* immobilization test (TPI); the *Treponema pallidum* agglutination test (TPA); the *Treponema pallidum* immune adherence test (TPIA), the fluorescent antibody test (FTA) and the *Treponema pallidum* complement fixation test (TPCF).

PRIMARY SYPHILIS

Synonyms: Chancre, Hunterian chancre, primary chancre or sore, hard chancre.

Incubation period: It is the period between the inoculation of the spirochaetes at the time of exposure and the manifestation of the sore. The usual period being 2–3 weeks; it can range from 10 to 90 days.

Clinical features: Chancre is usually the first recognisable sign of syphilis. It starts at the point of traumatic erosion. The chancre develops on an eroded point, balanitis, or on lesions of herpes and scabies. It is usually single, ham-coloured, relatively painless with an indurated base and pink areola, discharging serous fluid; with a painless, characteristic, bilateral enlargement of the regional lymph glands which are shotty, discrete and painless. It usually occurs on the genitalia (about 95%) and rarely extra-genital (about 5%). The common sites in the male are the coronal sulcus, prepuce, glans, frenulum, meatus, etc. and in the female, the cervix, labia majora and minora, fourchette, urethra, clitoris, etc. The extragenital chancres are seen usually on the lips, tongue, tonsils, anal region, fingers, breasts, eyelids, and may occur on other parts of the body also.

Varieties: Chancres may be of different types—the Hunterian chancre, the erosive chancre, the ulcerative, the phagedenic, the phimotic meatal and the mixed type depending on the situation, shape, induration and whether or not secondary infection is present.

Diagnosis: As already mentioned above, the diagnosis depends on the history of exposure, the characteristic incubation period, and clinical findings. It is confirmed by a positive dark-ground illumination test for *Treponema pallidum* and the performance of a VDRL test, which may be negative or positive depending on the time when it was performed.

Differential diagnosis: The chancre should be differentiated from chancroid (soft chancre), granuloma venereum, herpes progenitalis, contact dermatitis, scabies, the primary lesion of lymphogranuloma venereum, pyogenic ulcer and epithelioma. For details, refer to **Table 18.1**.

SECONDARY SYPHILIS

The manifestations of secondary syphilis occur, usually, within six months after the primary stage. The primary sore may or may not be present. But the VDRL test is always positive. This stage is characterized by a rash, adenitis and constitutional symptoms which are manifested usually, as general malaise, fever, headaches, vague pains and arthralgia which is worse at night. The manifestations of secondary syphilis affect, most commonly, the skin and the mucous membranes; the other structures are involved less frequently.

The common characteristic features of skin lesions in secondary syphilis are:

1. A rash which is generalized and bilaterally symmetrical in distribution.
2. Reddish or coppery in colour (difficult to make out in dark-skinned people).
3. Pleomorphic appearance, i.e. different varieties of skin lesions occurring at the same time.
4. Induration and infiltration.
5. Itching is characteristically absent.
6. Accompanying adenopathy.
7. The presence of *Treponema pallidum* in the dark-ground preparation.
8. On healing, they leave faint stains. There is atrophy and scarring only in advanced cases.

Macular Syphilide

It is a generalized, faint rash occurring on the trunk, extremities, palms of the hands and soles of the feet. It fades on pressure. The macules vary in size from about 0.5–1 cm. This rash, when viewed from an oblique angle, is very apparent.

Differential Diagnosis

- *Measles:* It starts with fever, coryza, conjunctivitis, Koplik's spots, and the rash is typical.
- *Drug rash:* The history reveals the patient having taken some drug prior to the development of the rash which is generalized and itchy. The rash subsides when the drug is withdrawn.
- *Leprosy:* The lesions are associated with thickened nerves and anaesthesia.
- *Pityriasis rosea:* A herald patch, a typical rash along the ribs, the macules show cigarette-paper-like scaling pointing towards the centre. The VDRL test is negative.
- *Pityriasis versicolor:* Hypopigmented macules with furfuraceous scaling.

Table 18.1: Distinguishing features of common genital lesions

	Primary sore of syphilis	*Ulcers-chancroid*	*Herpes genitalis*	*Contact dermatitis*	*Epithelioma*	*Granuloma*	*Lympho-granuloma*
1. History	IP 4–10 weeks; only one attack	IP 3–5 days Only one of two attacks	IP. 1–3 days Recurrent	12–72 hours May be recurrent	History of months and years. single attack	Ip, 2–60 days, single	IP one week. Single
2. Number of lesions	Single	Multiple	Multiple	Usually multiple	Single	Single	Single
3. Site–male	Glands, prepuce, body of penis and scrotum	Fraenum, corona, glans, prepuce Rare-labia	Glans, pre-prepuce, body of penis	Glans, prepuce and shaft of penis	Glans	Prepuce and glans penis	Genital and anorectal region
Female	Labia, clitoris and fourchette		Labia, vulva, mons pubis	Labia and vulva	Labia		
4. Characters	Indurated and painless ulcer	Shallow ulcers with ragged margins, painful. No induration	Superficial vesicles and erosions. Painful	Erythema, vesicles, oozing and itching	Indurated, fungating, slowly enlarging mass	Raw, beefy granuloma	Primary lesion may not be noticed
5. Associated features	Painless shotty glands, mucous patches and skin rash	Bubo	Nil	History of use of contraceptives, douches, pads, etc.	Regional lymph gland may be affected	Regional glands not involved	Unilateral inguinal adenitis; bubo; elephantiasis, esthiomene; strictures
6. Diagnostic tests	Dark-ground examination. Later serological tests	Smear, culture, Ito reenstierna test	Smear -ve virus rarely grown	Patch test	Smear	Biopsy	Elementary bodies in smear; Frei's test, increased globulin in blood; complement fixation +ve
7. Causative organism	*Spirochaeta pallida*	*Bacillus ducreyi*	Virus	Chemicals	Nil	Donovan bodies	Virus

Maculopapular Syphilides

These are a transition between macular and papular lesions, the papules being situated at the centre of the macule.

Papular Syphilides

They affect the trunk, extremities, palms of the hands and soles of the feet. On the face, they have a special predilection to be present along the hair margin; they go by the name of corona veneris. This is to be distinguished from corona seborrhoeica and corona psoriatica. On the palms and the soles, they may assume a pigmentary appearance, or present themselves as maculopapules or squamous patches with infiltrated edges. The other varieties derive their names from their configurations. Scaly lesions (Psoriasiform syphilides) resemble psoriasis, except that there is induration, the scales are less silvery, the surface not so smooth; other stigmata of syphilis are present, and the VDRL is positive. Annular syphilides are arranged in circles, as the name indicates. The lesions have a special predilection for the face, neck and genitalia. The differential diagnosis is made from other annular eruptions like leprosy, ringworm, psoriasis, lichen annularis, seborrhoeic dermatitis, etc. Corymbose syphilides consist of a large central papule surrounded by small satellite lesions.

Condylomata lata are usually large, hypertrophic, papular syphilides with a moist, greyish plaque, situated in moist areas like the genitalia, crural and anal regions and the axillae. These must be differentiated from condylomata acuminatum and external piles. Framboesiform syphilides are seen over the trunk and extremities, either as generalized or grouped follicular miliary papules. The ulcerative type of lesions are not common, and are known as ecthymatous and rupioid syphilides, the ecthymatous being flat and crusted and the rupioid having a punched-out ulcer with lamellated crust described as "oyster-shell" shaped. Pustular syphilides are not a common variety.

Syphilitic leucomelanoderma is a combination of hyperpigmentation and depigmentation. It is a rare condition occurring on the sides of the neck, on the upper part of the chest and on the palms of the hands and the soles of the feet.

Mucous patches are oral lesions found on the lips, cheeks, tongue, palate, tonsils and fauces. These are oval or circular, slightly raised patches, covered by a greyish sodden membrane. Superficial ulcers in the form of snail-track ulcers are occasionally seen.

Differential Diagnosis of Mucous Patches

Aphthous stomatitis	Small, round, painful, yellow erosions distributed all over the buccal mucosa.
Lichen planus	Violaceous, flat-topped, polyhedral, itchy papules on the skin, particular on the wrist and legs. In the mouth, dull white spots and streaks on the inside of the cheeks or tongue.
Erythema multiforme	Oedematous, multicoloured macules bilaterally and symmetrically distributed on the hands, forearms, and less so, on the feet. In the mouth, the lesions are uncommon. If they occur, they produce extensive, superficial erosions.
Pemphigus	Bullae and erosions in the mouth and on the skin.
Leukoplakia	A single hypertrophic patch or plaque. No cutaneous lesions. The VDRL and dark-ground examination are negative.

Affections of the Bones and Joints

Bones, joints and the surrounding structures may be affected. A common feature is localized periosteitis, affecting usually the anterior surface of the tibia which exhibits itself as a painful and tender swelling. Other features are vague bone pains with nocturnal exacerbations and bilateral arthralgia. Other rare manifestations are tenosynovitis and bursitis.

Affections of Hair and Nails

Alopecia: The loss of hair during secondary syphilis is patchy, giving rise to a moth-eaten appearance, particularly over the back and sides of the scalp. This has to be distinguished from alopecia areata in which patches, completely denuded of hair, are present. Another condition to be excluded is tinea capitis, in which well-defined, circular patches of alopecia, with dull, greyish scales and dull, broken hair are seen.

Onychia and paronychia: Syphilitic nail changes are not so common. They occur as onychia in association with paronychia and dactylitis. This combination distinguishes the condition from such causes as ringworm, psoriasis, etc.

Affection of the Central Nervous System

Neuritis of the eighth nerve with tinnitus may occur. Basal meningitis with the concomitant symptom of headache, and sometimes, with the involvement of the nerves, particularly the seventh, are observed. The cerebrospinal fluid, if examined at this stage, shows definite changes.

Ocular Affections

Iritis occurs during the secondary stage of syphilis; it is more common in inadequately treated cases. The usual signs and symptoms are circumcorneal congestion, photophobia, pain and dimness of vision; later the condition gives rise to irregularity of the pupil. Neuroretinitis also occurs, but is usually diagnosed only on routine fundus examination, as the patient does not complain, and the condition disappears under routine treatment.

Relapse in Syphilis

A relapse usually occurs within two years, particularly in irregularly or inadequately treated cases of syphilis. The relapse may take any of the following forms:

1. *Serological relapse:* The blood VDRL test becoming positive in higher titres than before.
2. *Mucocutaneous relapse:* Recurrence of the chancre in its original place called the chancre redux, or recurrence of muco-cutaneous lesions, both showing *Treponema pallidum* in the serum.
3. *Osseous relapse:* Occurrence of osteitis and periosteitis.
4. *Neuro-relapse:* In the form of asymptomatic neurosyphilis of neuro-recurrence.
5. *Ocular relapse:* Occurring as iritis, iridocyclitis or neuro-retinitis.
6. *Visceral relapse:* As hepatitis.
7. An apparently healthy mother with negative serology giving birth to a syphilitic child; or infection in the sex partner, without any clinical or serological relapse in the patient.

LATENT SYPHILIS

Latent syphilis may be described as the asymptomatic stage of syphilis in a patient with a definite history revealing the contraction of the disease, but exhibiting only a reactive serology, after all causes of biological false-positive reactions and other manifestations of syphilis have been excluded by a thorough clinical, radiological and cerebrospinal fluid examination. These would help to exclude any external manifestation, affection of the heart and the vessels and any changes in the cerebrospinal fluid respectively.

Latent syphilis may be either early or late; and it may either progress and develop signs and symptoms of late syphilis, or persist as latent syphilis, or have a spontaneous cure, as reported by Bruusgaard.

LATE SYPHILIS

The late or tertiary stage of syphilis is manifested by the appearance of lesions of benign late syphilis of the skin, mucous membranes, bones, joints, tendons and viscera and/ or of the cardiovascular and nervous system.

As time passes, the number of spirochaetes is reduced greatly due to the tissue reaction and the natural defences of the human body coming into action, and state of allergy may be established between the tissues and the spirochaetes giving rise to the various types of lesions. These lesions generally occur four or more years after the infection has been contracted, depending on the structure affected.

Classification: The lesions may be classified as follows:

1. Benign late syphilis.
2. Visceral syphilis.
3. Cardiovascular syphilis.
4. Neuro-syphilis.

BENIGN LATE SYPHILIS

This may affect the skin, mucous membranes, bones, joints, muscles, tendons and bursae, etc. The tertiary skin lesions are characterized by their asymmetry, by the occurrence of a single or few lesions which are indolent, indurated and arranged in an archiform manner; with or without ulceration; with a tendency to central healing and peripheral spread and hyperpigmentation. On healing, the lesions leave thin, papery, atrophic scars.

Cutaneous lesions: They may manifest themselves in any of the following forms: nodulocutaneous, noduloulcerative, gummata, juxta-articular nodes.

The nodulo-cutaneous type is characterized by non-ulcerated, gummatous infiltrations of the skin which do not break down. The noduloulcerative type consists of nodular lesions mixed with ulcerated ones which are relatively deep. A gumma is either cutaneous or subcutaneous swelling, which may subside under treatment or develop a central softening discharging thin pus, and later, leaving an ulcer with its characteristic punched-out margin and a "wash-leather" slough covering its base. Juxta-articular nodes are usually multiple, fibrous, painless, slow-growing subcutaneous nodules of varying sizes, found commonly over the knees, elbows, and hips. They may also be found over the other joints.

Differential diagnosis of Gumma

Varicose ulcer: Usually single, and associated with varicose veins, occurring on the lower third of the leg; the edges are surrounded by eczematous changes; the STS are negative.

Lupus vulgaris: Apple-jelly nodules are present; the edges are irregular; the course is extremely chronic, and lasts over years; the serology is negative; there is evidence of tuberculosis elsewhere; typical histopathology etc. Lupus vulgaris destroys cartilages, while syphilis destroys bones.

Ringworm: More superficial, with vesicular margin; itching is marked, and fungus can be demonstrated from the scraping.

Dermatitis: Greasy scales over face and scalp and on the presternal and inter- *seborrhoeica* scapular regions with a negative blood serology.

Psoriasis: Seen more on the extensor aspects of the limbs and scalp; silvery scales, which when removed exhibit typical capillary haemorrhage; and negative blood serology.

Leprosy: Affects the face, eyebrows and ears; thickening of the ulnar nerves; atrophy of the interossei muscles; areas of depigmentation and anaesthesia; the nasal smear and slit biopsy may show lepra bacilli. Histopathology is characteristic.

Epithelioma: Usually found in elderly people; hard and indurated, easily bleeding ulceration with everted edges. Biopsy confirms malignancy.

Palmar syphilides: Occurring on the palms and soles, they are scaly, nodular or gummatous. They are usually unilateral and exhibit some degree of infiltration. Palmar syphilides (both secondary and tertiary) are frequent in practice and are usually characteristic. The early lesions are usually bilateral, and the late ones, unilateral.

Differential Diagnosis of Palmar Syphilides

Ringworm: Hyperkeratotic or vesicular types are seen. Tinea of the nails, feet and glabrous skin may be present as well. The margins of tinea palmaris patches are usually inflammatory, and fungus can be demonstrated.

Psoriasis: Bilaterally symmetrical; psoriatic patches elsewhere; typical changes in the nails. Pustules may also occur.

Arsenical keratosis: Dew-drop pigmentation of the trunk. The palmar lesions are bilateral, and keratotic nodules may be seen; History of arsenic administration.

Eczema: Itching and vesiculation are present. On the palms, eczema is rare. History of contact with chemicals and subsequent irritation.

Chronic lesions on the palms usually indicate syphilis. A search for other stigmata should be made, and a VDRL test ordered.

Mucous Membrane Lesions

The common lesions are the gummata found in the mouth, pharynx and nose. They occur mainly over the palate, fauces, posterior pharyngeal wall, nose, tongue, lips and the inside of the cheeks. Ultimately, the gummata may lead to ulceration and perforation. The perforation of the palate may result in regurgitation of fluids, and may also produce a nasal twang in the voice. One other late manifestation of syphilis is leukoplakia of the angles of the mouth and tongue.

Lesions of Bones, Joints, Muscles, Tendons, Bursae, etc.

Bones: The common lesions are periosteitis, osteitis and osteomyelitis affecting the long bones, the skull and the shoulder girdle. Clinically, a perforated palate, saddle nose (depressed bridge of nose) and bossy thickening of the cranial and leg bones are some of the typical features.

Joints: Arthritis and synovitis may occur in late syphilis. But the most common lesion is the Charcot's joint of tabes dorsalis. This is a neuropathic condition usually affecting the larger joints such as those of the knees, hips, ankles, shoulders and elbows. It is a painless, hypertrophic, osteoarthritic affection, with triple displacement of the affected joint. An X-ray will show destruction of the bones with areas of rarefaction and hypertrophy, along with loose bodies in the joint described as "bag of bones"

Muscles, tendons and bursae: Affection of these is not common, except of the patella bursa, which is sometimes observed.

Visceral Syphilis

Lesions are seen more frequently in the liver and testes than in the other viscera.

Liver: The common type is gummata of the liver, and the less common type is interstitial fibrosis. The gummata are of varying sizes secondary fibrosis and scarring give rise to the characteristic "Hepar lobatum." This is to be differentiated from secondary carcinoma, hepatic abscess, cirrhosis of the liver and hydatid cyst of the liver.

Testes: Late syphilis manifests itself as gumma of the testes, and diffuse interstitial fibrosis. The diffuse. interstitial fibrosis is characterized by an increase in the size and weight of the testes, accompanied by the complete loss of testicular sensation. Gumma of the testes is less common; it may be associated with diffuse interstitial fibrosis. It produces a localized swelling which becomes adherent to the scrotum, and breaks down, resulting in gummatous ulceration.

Cardiovascular Syphilis

It usually occurs 10–30 years after the initial infection. It is more common in males than in females. Physical exertion seems to make people more prone to develop cardiovascular lesions. The blood serology is positive in about 80% of cases.

The most common affection is that of the aorta, in the form of aortitis, aortic regurgitation and aneurysmal formation. The heart muscle may also be affected. The veins are rarely affected. The prognosis of cardiovascular syphilis is, as a general rule, bad.

NEUROSYPHILIS

The central nervous system is invaded by the *Treponema pallidum* during the generalization stage of infection; this forms one of the most important causes of the organic disease of the nervous system. Males are affected more than females. Irregular and inadequate treatment may increase the incidence of neurosyphilis. The most common period for the onset of the signs and symptoms is from 10 to 15 years after infection has been contracted.

Patients having symptoms like ataxia, headaches, lightening pains, paraesthesias, visual disturbances, bladder symptoms and speech defects, have to be carefully examined. A thorough clinical examination should be carried out, along with the VDRL test, cerebrospinal fluid examination and Lange's colloidal gold curve.

The common neurological affections are tabes dorsalis, general paralysis of the insane, optic atrophy and meningovascular syphilis.

CONGENITAL SYPHILIS

Syphilis acquired by the foetus in uterus from the mother is called congenital or prenatal syphilis.

The foetus is infected via the transplacental route by *Treponema pallidum*, usually after the fourth month. The chances of infection are greatest in early syphilis, diminishing with time.

The clinical features of syphilis tend to become less severe during pregnancy. Repeated miscarriages, stillbirths, premature deliveries and neonatal deaths are good indications of syphilitic infection **(Table 18.2)**.

The only means of diagnosing syphilis in a pregnant woman, in the absence of clinical signs, is by a routine blood serological examination during the early and late stages

Table 18.2: Clinical features of congenital syphilis

Early (within 2 years)	*Late (after 2 years)*
Wasting, irritability, fever, "old man" facies Macular, papular and bullous lesions of the skin	Saddle nose, Sabre tibia Periosteitis and osteitis (8–10 years) Clutton's joints.
Snuffles, Rhagades Laryngitis (cracked aphonic cry)	Teeth Hutchinson's incisors Moon's molars
Onychia Adenopathy	Eye Iritis
Periosteitis, osteochondritis (Parrot's pseudoparalysis) and osteitis	Interstitial keratitis Choroiditis Optic atrophy
Dactylitis Cranio-tabes Parrot's nodes	Ear Suppurative otitis media Eighth nerve deafness Vertigo and tinnitus
Nervous system	**Nervous system**
Basal meningitis hydrocephalus	Meningitis Hydrocephalus Epilepsy
Visceral	Mental deficiency Vascular lesions Parenchymatous lesions
Enlargement of liver and spleen "White pneumonia"	Juvenile paresis Juvenile tabes

of pregnancy. An early diagnosis followed by adequate treatment is the only effective way of preventing congenital syphilis.

Signs: They may be classified as early, occurring before the age of two and late, occurring at a time later. As a general rule, the early manifestations resemble the lesions of secondary syphilis, and the late ones, those of the tertiary stage.

The cutaneous lesions of congenital syphilis are very characteristic. Within the first seven days of birth, a bullous eruption (syphilitic pemphigus) may develop. It consists of bullae distributed bilaterally and symmetrically on the front of the wrists, palms, ankles and soles; later, bullae develop on other parts of the body. Other features of congenital syphilis are usually present. The differential diagnosis is made from impetigo contagiosa in which the eruption develops at a later age, the history reveals contact with an infective case and the lesions are asymmetrical and the child is quite healthy to begin with.

Later, a maculopapular rash may develop all over or on the buttocks, where it may resemble napkin rash. Even condylomata lata may be found. The palms of the hands and the soles of the feet are usually shiny, and may also show a maculopapular eruption.

In the late type of congenital syphilis, nodulocutaneous and gummatous lesions are found.

Diagnosis: In the early stages, diagnosis is established by a careful examination followed by the demonstration of *Treponema pallidum* in the lesions, and by serological test of the parents and child.

Immediately after birth, the diagnosis is assisted by an examination of the placenta, which shows characteristic features, viz., it is pale, greasy and bulky (weighing more than one-fourth of the foetal body weight). *Treponema pallidum* can be demonstrated in a smear from the umbilical vein.

An X-ray examination of the long bones reveals characteristic features.

Late cases are diagnosed with the assistance of a carefully elicited history, clinical manifestations, serological findings and examination of the parents. The X-ray examination of the long bones and the unerupted incisors gives conclusive evidence.

Prognosis of Syphilis

The outlook in syphilis, as in other venereal diseases, has changed for the better since penicillin and several broad-spectrum antibiotics have come into use. Now syphilis can, almost always, be completely cured in the early stages; in late syphilis, the progress of the disease can be controlled, but the damage done cannot be repaired or undone. For this reason, treatment of early syphilis is essential. Besides, detection and treatment of early cases reduces infectivity; the disease in its early stages is highly infectious. The same applies to congenital syphilis, which is a preventable disease.

It is possible to prevent syphilis by: Tracing contacts, treating cases early and educating people in taking prophylactic measures. In USA, UK and Scandinavian countries, the incidence of venereal disease has been considerably reduced and their spread controlled.

Treatment of Syphilis

Prophylactic: Prevention is better than cure, more so, with a communicable and seriously incapacitating disease like syphilis. The prophylaxis consists in treating early syphilis cases to reduce infectivity and in tracing the contacts. Every case of syphilis has as its source, a previous case. Careful investigation will bring to light not only the source, but also all other individuals infected by that source, along with the case under study. Since the incubation period is about four weeks, all sexual contacts made by the patient in the last 4–8 weeks must be identified, examined and investigated.

As already mentioned, the presence of unregistered prostitutes in Asiatic countries, and the general reticence of the people, who will not speak up, are two great obstacles in the way of successful contact tracing. Even so, good results can be obtained if there is teamwork between venereologists, nurses, social workers and health agencies. Perseverance, tact and discretion should be the watchwords of those engaged in the search; then only, can there be any hope of success. The other preventive measures taken against syphilis are the use of the condom during sexual intercourse and washing of the genitalia after the intercourse with potassium permanganate or mercuric bichloride lotion.

Curative: The treatment of syphilis should be early, continuous and adequate **(Table 18.3)**. This will render the early lesions non-contagious and control the progress of the disease thus preventing late manifestations. Irregular and inadequate therapy leads, later on, to complication; this must be borne in mind. There is no place for routine therapy. Every case should be individualized according to the stage of the disease and the type of lesions present.

The drug of choice is penicillin.

No major or serious toxic manifestations have been observed. The most common reaction observed is the Jarish–Herxheimer reaction manifested in fever rising to 102–104°F, which may be associated with the exacerbation of the symptoms and signs.

Table 18.3: Drug therapy of syphilis

Stages	*Benzathine penicillin*	*Procaine penicillin*	*Other drugs*
Early	2.4 mega units IM single dose	4.8 mega units (0.6 mega unit daily IM for 8 days)	Tetracycline 2 g per day in divided doses for 15 days (except in pregnancy). Erythromycin 2 g per day in divided doses for 15 days. Most antibiotics except, amino-glycoside group are treponemocidal but are not thoroughly evaluated.
Late	7.2 mega units IM (1.2 mega units alternate days for 6 injections)	9.6 mega units (0.6 mega units daily IM for 16 days).	Normally double duration of treatment is required in late syphilis.
Congenital	50,000 units IM single dose (if CSF normal)	Aqueous penicillin G. 50,000 units per kg body weight in 2 divided doses for 10 days	

It has been observed that the severity or otherwise of the reaction does not depend upon the dosage.

In cases where serious consequences can develop, e.g. in late syphilis of the larynx, cardiovascular and neurosyphilis, a preliminary preparation of the patient with iodides and bismuth is recommended. In some cases, a course of bismuth IM (1–2 cc 10% suspension) and arsenic (mepharside 0.03–0.06 g), IV weekly for 8–10 weeks may have to be given after the course of penicillin has been completed. Since these are toxic metals, views differ regarding their use. According to some authorities, penicillin alone is enough; according to others in secondary and tertiary syphilis, a course of penicillin must be followed by bismuth (one or two courses) and possibly arsenic as well. Fever therapy with drugs or artificially produced malaria is indicated in resistant cases of neurosyphilis. Local treatment of chancre and other open lesions consists in dressing the lesions with mild antiseptics. The use of penicillin ointment is to be discouraged.

In all cases of relapses, the courses recommended may be repeated.

Follow-up: All cases of syphilis should be watched regularly for at least two to three years. During this period the blood serological examination should be performed once in 3 months for the first year, and once in 6 months for two years. A cerebrospinal fluid examination should be performed in 6 months, and then again in 2 years after finishing the therapy.

For more information on syphilis, special works on venereal diseases should be consulted.

Chapter

19 Chancroid, Granuloma Inguinale, Lymphogranuloma Venereum, Gonorrhoea and AIDS

CHANCROID

Synonym: Soft chancre, soft sore.

It is an uncommon venereal disease compared with syphilis or gonorrhoea. Nevertheless, one comes across it quite frequently, chancroid being the third most common venereal disease. The incidence of this disease is greater in tropical countries than in countries that have temperate or cold climates. The people most commonly affected are usually those whose economic status is low and those negligent of personal hygiene. The disease is very common among males. Very few female cases are seen, although such cases have been known to act as asymptomatic carriers of infection.

Etiology: The causative organism is *Haemophilus ducreyi* or Ducrey's bacillus which is gram-negative *Streptobacillus*, 1.5 μ by 0.5 μ, found in small groups or chains, usually outside the cells. Infection is transmitted by sexual contact in the great majority of cases, although accidental infection by infected material is possible.

Clinical features: In the male, the lesions usually appear near the frenum (junction of the prepucial skin with the glans), on the corona, the under-surface of the prepuce, glans penis and on the external urinary meatus. In the female, the infection rarely shows lesions; but when present, ulcers are seen on the labia, or in the fold between the inner surface of the thigh and the groin. Occasionally, the urinary meatus may be affected. The incubation period is 3–5 days, may be as short as 24 hours.

Chancroid starts as a small papule, which increases in size and becomes a pustule. This pustule breaks down to form a shallow ulcer with ragged, irregular margins; its floor is raw, of pale red colour, and has a typical sieve-like appearance. The ulcer is always free of induration and bleeds freely on friction with clothes or physical manipulation.

Many more such lesions develop on the surrounding areas as described above, by the process of autoinoculation. These multiple lesions present a rosette appearance. They may fuse with each other forming large ragged areas. An extragenital spread is uncommon. The constitutional symptoms consist of acute pain and tenderness in the affected areas; occasional headaches, and slight pyrexia, especially when superadded infection with pyogenic organisms takes place; this also results in spreading the local lesions.

Complications:

1. *Inflammatory phimosis:* Due to oedema of the prepuce causing difficulty in retraction. Haemorrhage from the frenal artery may also occur.

2. *Bubo formation:* It is the usual sequela of the disease. The bubo starts firstly as a painful enlargement of the inguinal glands usually. The swelling is smooth, globular and tender to touch. After a few days softening and fluctuation occur, and finally ulceration takes place with the rupture of the overlying skin by a single opening (cf. LGV bubo which has multiple openings). The ulcer formed has, once again, ragged margins and a dirty, sloughy base; it continues to discharge serosanguinous and purulent material.
3. *Balanitis* and balano-posthitis which is particularly common amongst non-circumcised persons.
4. *Phagedena:* This is the most dreaded complication. It results from secondary infection with microorganisms like Vincent's spirilla and fusiform bacillus. The lesion becomes very ugly and foul smelling and the margins almost black, and spreads rapidly.

Diagnosis: The diagnosis is arrived at by:
1. The typical clinical features.
2. A history of exposure, and the appearance of sores within the incubation period.
3. A smear examination of material taken from the deeper parts of the margin of the ulcer and by staining this with Gram's stain.
4. A culture examination by a swab rubbed on a suitable medium in which defibrinated rabbit blood is added.
5. The ITO-Reenstierna test: This is done by an intradermal injection of 0. 1–0.2 cc of vaccine prepared from the pus to an infected case. A positive reaction is indicated if after 48 hours the site that has been injected with vaccine shows a papule of 5 mm diameter with erythema all around.
6. The dark-ground illumination test for spirochaetes of syphilis, and also a serological test for syphilis should form a routine diagnostic procedure to rule out any concomitant infection.

Differential diagnosis: It is to be made from all diseases causing an inflammatory genital lesion (a sore), viz., primary sore of syphilis, herpes progenitalis, dermatitis resulting from irritants or medicines, epithelioma, granuloma venereum and lymphogranuloma venereum (for distinguishing features, refer to **Table 18.1**). In scabies, secondary pyoderma may produce boils and pyogenic ulcers, but features like nocturnal pruritus and burrows are obvious. Chancroid bubo is differentiated from lymphogranuloma venereum bubo in **Table 19.1**.

Treatment: The treatment resolves itself into:
a. Local applications.
b. Systemic medication.
c. Treatment of complications.

Local Application

(1) The affected parts should be washed with a warm antiseptic, e.g. potassium permanganate (1:8,000 aqueous solution), (2) Bacitracin and soframycin topical creams can also be applied with advantage, but penicillin has no action. Preferably however, antibiotics should be avoided because they interfere with dark field examination later on.

Table 19.1: Difference between lymphogranuloma venereum bubo and chancroid bubo

Lymphogranuloma venereum bubo	*Chancroid bubo*
1. The primary lesion is absent or healed.	1. The primary lesion is always present.
2. Slow evolution.	2. Quick evolution.
3. Involvement of several glands.	3. Involvement of a single gland only.
4. Iliac adenopathy is invariably present.	4. Iliac adenopathy is absent.
5. Multiple areas of fluctuation.	5. Single fluctuant swelling.
6. The skin is thickened and rugose. The bubo retains its shape after rupture.	6. The skin is thin and collapses when the abscess bursts.
7. The pus is sterile. The elementary bodies may be demonstrated by special staining.	7. Ducrey bacilli may be demonstrated in the pus, or scraping from the wall of abscess.
8. Frei test is positive.	8. Ito-Reenstierna test is positive.
9. Complement fixation test is positive.	9. Complement fixation test is negative.
10. Hyperglobulinemia is a constant feature.	10. No change in the serum proteins.

Systemic Medication

Sulphonamides, e.g. trimethoprim and sulphamethoxazole or Septran (P) should be administered internally in their usual dosage for about a week.

Most cases improve on this therapy, but those that resist it should be given streptomycin 0.5 g twice daily for about a week, and then 1 g bi-weekly for 2–3 weeks. These medicines have no effect on syphilitic infection; hence, they can be safely used even if the dark-ground examination for spirochaetes, and an STS of the blood are delayed by some days. Penicillin has no effect on the chancroid, but broad-spectrum antibiotic like tetracycline, minocycline, erythromycin 2 g daily for 7–10 days are useful in resistant cases.

Patient should be followed for at least 6 months to detect concomitant syphilitic infection.

Treatment of Complications

1. *Inflammatory phimosis*: This requires use of repeated compresses of Condy's lotion, and the wearing of suspensory bandage to obviate a gravitational effect on the dependent part. If the condition persists, a dorsal slit with a sharp pair of scissors or a knife is made (a cut on the upper part of the prepuce). A dorsal slit is preferable, because there are no main vessels in this region, and the danger of haemorrhage is obviated. When a dorsal slit is made, slight bleeding and oozing occurs and congestion is removed, and the prepuce can be retracted, exposing any ulcer underneath, which can be treated with Condy's soaks. An ideal treatment is circumcision.
2. *Bubo*: When the glands are enlarged, local heat should be applied. Once fluctuation has taken place, then instead of waiting for the abscess to burst, it is better to aspirate the pus.
3. *Balanitis and balanoposthitis*: It clears up with cold compresses, cleaning the affected part with Condy's fluid, and the systemic use of sulphadiazine or any of the broad-spectrum antibiotics.

4. *Phagedaena*: Broad-spectrum antibiotics must be employed in fairly large doses to control the spreading infection. Amputation may have to be resorted to in very bad and advanced cases.

GRANULOMA INGUINALE

Several confusing synonyms exist; but it is always preferable to know one name and be sure of it. It is a chronic, mildly contagious disease, caused by *Klebsiella granulomatis* or *Calymmatobacterium granulomatis* (distinct from Leishman–Donovan bodies, which cause leishmaniasis). They are gram-negative, encapsulated bodies present mostly inside the mononuclear cells. The disease is transmitted either through sexual contact with an infected individual or by infected vectors. It is mostly venereal in origin.

Incubation period: It varies from 8 to 60 days.

Clinical features: The lesions occur mainly on the genitalia. In the male, the prepuce and glans penis, and in the female, the labia are the sites of choice. The disease begins in the form of a papule which soon becomes a nodule; this progresses slowly to take the form of an ulcer or a papillomatous and vegetative nodule. Lesions in granuloma inguinale are characteristically raw, red and beefy in appearance. Elephantiasis of the labia, penis or scrotum may also occur. The mucous membranes and viscera are usually spared. The regional lymph glands are not involved but pseudobubo may be seen. The course of the disease is slow and prolonged in the absence of modern treatment; the prognosis, though, has improved remarkably since antibiotics have come into use.

Diagnosis: It is confirmed by the demonstration of Donovan bodies in the lesions. Cultures and animal inoculations are, generally speaking, not helpful; serological tests for syphilis, however, should always be carried out to exclude syphilis, the most important of the venereal diseases. Sometimes, it may resemble epithelioma, hence careful examination is necessary.

Treatment: It is specific and consists in:

1. A course of streptomycin 1.0 g twice a day, intramuscularly for 10 days. When administering streptomycin, what must be remembered are the toxic symptoms produced, like giddiness, tinnitus, deafness and dermatitis.
2. Locally, antibiotic creams like bacitracin are helpful.
3. Gloves should be worn while dressing the affected part. Penicillin and sulphonamides have no action.

Very good results have been reported with the systemic use of chloramphenicol and tetracycline. Since these are also successful against lympho-granuloma venereum, chancroid, gonorrhoea and even syphilis, all venereal diseases, they have become particularly important in treatment.

LYMPHOGRANULOMA VENEREUM

It is a contagious, venereal granuloma differing from granuloma inguinale in one important aspect; it rapidly involves the lymphatic system. It is caused by *Chlamydia* which is similar to *Chlamydia trachomatis* organism, of 0.25×0.5 µ size.

Mode of infection: Infection is transmitted by sexual intercourse. Medical practitioners, nurses and laboratory workers can accidentally pick up the disease by handling infected material.

Usually young adults are affected; but no age is exempt. Localization of the disease differs in the two sexes; in the female, the genital and/or the anorectal regions are pre dominantly involved; in the male, the inguinal region. This is because of the difference in lymphatic drainage in the two sexes. Females are often asymptomatic carriers of the disease.

Incubation period: It is ordinarily about a week.

Clinical features: The primary lesion is frequently not noticed by the patient. The most common type of primary lesion is the superficial, painless vesicle which lasts a short while, and heals without scarring. In a small percentage of cases, the initial vesicular lesion progresses into an ulcer or a bacterial urethritis. In the male, the primary lesions usually occur on the corona and prepuce; in the female, the lesions are seen usually on the fourchette, the posterior half of the labia majora and the posterior wall of the vagina. Often the primary lesions may be unnoticed.

One to three weeks after the primary lesion (on an average about two weeks after exposure), subacute inguinal adenitis develops. The adenitis is usually unilateral. To begin with, the glands are painful, tender, swollen and elastic. Soon they become matted and begin to soften, producing suppuration (bubo). Less commonly, the adenitis becomes chronic and indolent. The pelvic and iliac lymphatics may also be involved, but they rarely suppurate. The adenitis is accompanied by constitutional disturbance. The patient feels weak and feverish, suffers from headache and loss of appetite.

The adenitis is followed later by chronic genital and anorectal manifestations produced by hyperplastic or ulcerative changes or such as result from interference with the lymphatic system. Elephantiasis of the genitalia (esthiomene), rectal and vaginal strictures and chronic ulceration are the common late effects.

Manifestations of lymphogranuloma venereum are rarely seen extragenitally. One sometimes comes across an erythema multiforme-like rash. The eyes, lungs and the meningeal membrane of the brain are rarely involved.

Prognosis: Lymphogranuloma venereum is a slowly progressive disease, resulting in considerable mutilation of the genitalia, anus and rectum, and hence, causes a great deal of misery. Delay in treatment results in disfiguring and troublesome sequelae left by the healed lesions. So, a quick diagnosis and immediate treatment are essential. The outlook is good if treatment is given in time and correctly.

Diagnosis: It is confirmed by:

1. The demonstration of elementary bodies in the smears of bubo pus by Giemsa's stain.
2. The Frei's intradermal test.
3. The complement fixation test is usually positive.
4. The blood shows an increased level of serum globulin. An STS should be done to exclude any concomitant infection with syphilis.

Treatment: It has changed considerably in the last two decades.

1. With the advent of broad-spectrum antibiotics like chloramphenicol and tetracycline the gloomy outlook of the past has been superseded by the bright one of the present.

Sulphonamides are not only effective but cheap in mass treatment. The rule is to give sufficiently large doses for 7–10 days in acute and subacute cases; in chronic and complicated cases, sulphonamides may have to be administered intermittently, over long periods (10–90 days).

2. Surgical help is valuable when there are complications like anal stricture and ano-rectal syndrome. Corticosteroids have also been used with advantage in such cases.
3. The general health of the patient should be maintained.
4. It is very important to find out the source of infection.

GONORRHOEA

Gonorrhoea is a sexually transmitted disease caused by *Neisseria gonorrhoeae*, affects both males and females. It can produce acute signs and symptoms, and may sometime disseminate to other parts of body. The incidence of the disease seems to be on the decline due to increased awareness about personal hygiene, use of condom due to fear of AIDS and frequent use of antibiotics for throat and other infections which may suppress gonococci.

Causative organism: *Neisseria gonorrhoeae* is a gram-negative, kidney-shaped diplococci which is morphologically similar to *Neisseria meningitidis*.

Incubation period: The infection usually results from sexual intercourse with an infected person and non-venereal transmission is quite rare. The incubation period is usually 3–5 days, but it may range from 1 day to less than 2 weeks. The paucity of symptoms in females can sometimes give an erroneous impression of a longer incubation period.

Clinical features: The symptoms are very common in males, while they may be less defined in females. The patient complains of burning sensation in the urethra, copious purulent discharge per urethra and discomfort in passing urine. They may have constitutional symptoms and frequency of urine. The examination of males reveals profuse, yellowish purulent discharge, angry-looking urethral orifice and tenderness along the urethra. Sometimes phimosis can occur due to profuse discharge under the prepuce. The involvement of local glands in relation to male genital tract can cause extension of symptoms. Acute prostatitis, although uncommon, may cause general malaise, perineal aching, and suprapubic discomfort. Rarely, prostatic abscess causes terminal dysuria, rectal tenesmus. Partly treated gonorrhoea can lead to chronic prostatitis. Homosexual males can show proctitis in the passive partner, resulting in burning pain in anorectum, tenesmus and blood and mucopus in stools.

Gonococcal infection of the female genital tract is often asymptomatic. Urethritis is accompanied by dysuria, but the urethral discharge is often scanty or absent. Cervitis can cause vague low backache and abdominal discomfort. Profuse, purulent cervical secretion can manifest as vaginal discharge.

Haematogenous spread of gonorrhoea to sites remote from the focus of infection is the cause of metastatic general complications. They include arthritis, anterior uveitis, meningitis, endocarditis, myocarditis, pericarditis, hepatitis and perihepatitis.

Oropharyngeal gonorrhoea: Among patients suffering from gonorrhoea the frequency of pharyngeal gonorrhoea appears to be about 5% in heterosexual males, 10% in females and 20% homosexual males. Oral sex is a common culprit.

Anorectal gonorrhoea: It nearly always results from anal coitus in passive homosexuals. Perianal abscess, ischiorectal abscess or anal fissure are rarely found in association with this condition.

Gonorrhoea in children: In girls before the age of puberty, the vaginal mucosa is more susceptible to gonococcal infection than that of the adult. Thus, gonococcal infection usually presents as an acute vulvovaginitis. It is also a feature of child abuse, which in boys may present as anorectal gonorrhoea.

Complications: The spread of gonococci to local glands and other parts of genitourethra can complicate a non-treated infection. In addition, the systemic spread of the. organism by haematogenous route can cause serious metastatic complication . Chronic gonorrhoea is a disputable entity, but has been often recorded. **Table 19.2** depicts the magnitude of the disease produced by this gonococci and its complications.

General complications: Arthritis, dermatitis, anterior uveitis, myocarditis, endocarditis, pericarditis, meningitis, hepatitis, perihepatitis.

Diagnosis

1. *Clinical presentation:* The disease has an acute onset, with copious purulent discharge coming out of urethra. In males, tenderness can be demonstrated throughout the penile urethra.
2. *Two glass test:* A common outpatient procedure prevalent for decades is a two glass test, where the patient is asked to void first half urine in one glass and the remaining in the second glass. It is used to know the extent of infection. If urine in the first glass shows haziness, it means involvement of anterior urethra. If both glasses show haziness, the posterior urethra is also affected.
3. *Gram's smear of discharge:* The material from the site of infection is taken by a sterile platinum loop, spread on a glass slide and gently heated before staining with Gram's stain. Gram-negative intracellular diplococci can be demonstrated inside the polymorphonuclear leucocytes.

Table 19.2: Gonorrhoea in men and women

Site of infection	*Local complications*
Affliction in men:	
Anterior urethra	Tysonitis, littritis, peri- and paraurethral abscess, cowperitis, stricture of urethra
Posterior urethra	Prostatitis (acute/chronic), vesiculitis, epididymitis, trigonitis
Affliction in women:	Skenitis, periurethral abscess
Urethra, cervix uteri	Salpingo-oophoritis, parametritis, pelvic abscess and peritonitis
Bartholin's glands	Bartholin's abscess
Affliction both in men and women:	
Anorectum, conjunctivae, oropharynx	
Affliction in children:	
Vulva and vagina, anorectum	
Conjunctivae	Suppurative panophthalmitis, blindness

4. *Culture of gonococci:* The bacteria can be cultured and characterized in specialized media like modified Thayer–Martin medium. After inoculation, the plates/slopes are incubated in an atmosphere of 10% carbon dioxide. Oxidase test can confirm a gonococcal colony by turning it pink which rapidly turns purple. However, it can ferment only glucose **(Table 19.3)**.

Differential diagnosis: Gonococcal urethritis has to be differentiated from other non-gonococcal urethritis and genital infections. The discharge in these conditions is scanty and nonpurulent. Causes of non-gonococcal urethritis are summarized in **Table 19.4**.

Treatment and follow-up: The patient should be advised to take plenty of oral fluids including water. He should avoid heavy exercise and take rest. The sheet anchor drug is procine benzyl penicillin. A single shot of 48 lac units of this drug through intramuscular route is enough for uncomplicated gonorrhoeae caused by gonococci sensitive to penicillin. However, if gonorrhoea is caused by penicillinase-producing *N. gonorrhoeae* (PPNG), cephalosporins (cefoxitin, cefotaxime and ceftriaxone) in combination with probenecid are the drugs of choice. Alternative drugs are tetracycline 3–4 g per day or erythromycin 2–3 g per day in four divided doses for a period of 5–7 days is usually effective. Other drugs include minocycline (200 mg per day) or doxycycline (200 mg per day) for 5 days.

Follow-up of the treated patient is very important to prevent chronic gonorrhoea and its complications. The patient is followed on 4th, 7th, 10th, 14th, and 28th days of treatment. A prostatic massage is done only on 28th day of treatment to rule out affection of prostate gland. As syphilis can be masked by the preceding antibiotics, VDRL test is also done on 28th day and 3rd month of treatment.

Table 19.3: Fermentation reactions of *Neisseria*

	Glucose	*Maltose*	*Sucrose*	*Lactose*
N. gonorrhoeae	+	–	–	–
N. meningitidis	+	+	–	–
N. catarrhalis	–	–	–	–
N. pharyngis sicca	+	+	+	–
N. lactamica	+	+	–	+

Table 19.4: Causes of non-gonococcal urethritis (NGU)

Chlamydia trachomatis	30–40%
Ureaplasma urealyticum	2–5%
Trichomonas vaginalis	2–5%
Secondary to bacterial UTI	1–2%
Herpes simplex	1–2%
Miscellaneous and non-specific (traumatic, chemical, neoplastic stricture, foreign body, mycotic)	50%

AIDS

The acquired immunodeficiency syndrome (AIDS) was discovered in the United States in the early months of the year 1981.

Key statistics related to AIDS (as of September 2020):

1. Global HIV/AIDS Prevalence: According to UNAIDS, an estimated 38 million people were living with HIV globally in 2020.
2. New HIV Infections: In 2020, there were approximately 1.5 million new HIV infections worldwide.
3. AIDS-related Deaths: The number of AIDS-related deaths was estimated at 690,000 in 2020.
4. Regional Distribution: Sub-Saharan Africa remains the most heavily affected region, with about two-thirds of all people living with HIV residing there.
5. Treatment Coverage: Approximately 27.4 million people worldwide were accessing antiretroviral therapy (ART) for HIV by the end of 2020, representing about 73% of people living with HIV globally.

AIDS, as the name implies is a peculiar acquired type of immunodeficiency, with consequential development of unusual and severe infections, and bizarre neoplasms, which occur in healthy individuals without a known cause of immunodeficiency.

The population groups at risk: Fortunately, AIDS has almost exclusively been a disease of certain 'at risk' groups of population viz:

a. Homosexuals
b. Parenteral drug abusers
c. Haitians
d. Haemophilics
e. Those receiving repeated blood product transfusions.
f. Heterosexual partners of AIDS victims
g. Offsprings of AIDS victims
h. Other contacts of AIDS vicitims, like the laboratory technicians and doctors.

The causative agent: The etiology of AIDS is now well established. It is caused by a retrovirus, the human T-cell-leukaemia (lymphotropic) virus (HTLV) number III, designated subsequently as HIV-1. It selectively attacks the helper/inducer (OKT4-Leu3a+) lymphocytes of human blood system.

Incubation period: The incubation period of AIDS appears to be quite variable. In general, it is thought to vary from 15 to 28 months. In infants, it is found to be shorter (8 months). Acute HIV infection is now getting more and more recognizable. The illness is of variable severity with fever, malaise, headache, sore throat, tenderness and slight enlargement of lymph nodes, arthralgia, abdominal pain, asymptomatic maculopapular eruption and diarrhoea.

Clinical features: As earlier mentioned, AIDS denotes an acquired immunodeficiency state of the body. The clinical reflection of this syndrome, thus, will only be secondary infections and unusual malignancies.

The CDC classification of HIV disease is as follows:

Group I	Acute infection
Group II	Asymptomatic infection
Group III	Persistent generalized lymphadenopathy.

Group IV A: Constitutional upset-fever, fatigue, losing weight.
B: Neurological disturbances.
C: Secondary infectious disease-protozoal, viral, fungal, bacterial.
D: Malignancy features like Kaposi's sarcoma.
E: Other conditions.

Diagnosis: It can be done either by isolation of HIV-1 or by demonstration of antibodies to HIV-1 (Western electroblot test or ELISA test). Other laboratory parameter, will reveal extreme reduction of T4 (helper) lymphocytes in blood.

Treatment: It is still very unsatisfactory. Although no vaccine has been effective in providing immunity against AIDS, several drugs have shown to be useful against the virus. Of them the main drug is zidovudine, given in the dose of 200 mg 6 times a day for 3 months, tapered onto a lower dose for a variable period of time. However, prevention still remains the sheet anchor of the disease.

Chapter

20

Erythemato-squamous and Lichenoid Eruptions

PSORIASIS

It is a common, chronic and non-infectious skin disease characterized by well-defined slightly raised, dry erythematous macules with silvery scales and typical extensor distribution.

Etiology: It is world-wide in distribution. Contrary to earlier belief, it is fairly common in the tropics; though undoubtedly, it is more prevalent in the temperate climate. Psoriasis is a chronic disease; its course is punctuated by intermissions and remissions. Attacks are more common in winter than summer; the eruption has a natural tendency to clear up with the warm weather. In the tropics, a fair number of attacks develop in the monsoon (rainy season).

The exact etiology is still unknown. According to most workers, it is a heredo-familial disease brought on by stress, viz., anxiety, mental trauma, fever, physical injury, digestive upsets, etc. on a genetic constitution. Transmission is by a single, irregularly dominant gene. Recent histochemical studies and also studies of vasculature, neural population and family tree have provided double proof of genetic transmission. Streptococcal infection, presence of diabetes, and purines in the diet are the other precipitating factors. Pressure and trauma seem to determine the localization of psoriasis.

Pathology: Psoriasis appears to be largely a disorder of keratinization. The basic defect is rapid replacement of epidermis in psoriatic lesion (3–4 days instead of 28 days in normal skin). In addition, there are marked vascular changes in upper dermis in the form of tortuosity and dilatation. Recently, the presence of abnormal neural cells has been demonstrated in psoriatic plaques.

Histochemical studies have revealed an increase in both oxidative and anaerobic metabolism with increased pentose, glycogen, purines, sulphydral groups and soluble proteins and a decrease in activity of dipeptidases.

It has been discovered that apparently normal skin of both the psoriatics and their relations show these changes in miniature—'Latent psoriasis'.

Histology is characteristic and consists of (i) parakeratosis, (ii) thinning of suprapapillary portion of the stratum malpighii, (iii) elongation of ridges, (iv) oedema and clubbing of papillae, (v) microabscesses of Munro, (vi) dilated and tortuous capillaries in upper dermis, (vii) oedema and round-cell infiltration in the papillae and upper dermis.

Clinical features: Typical distribution is extensor. The areas commonly affected are the scalp, back of elbows, front of knees and legs and the lower part of the back of the

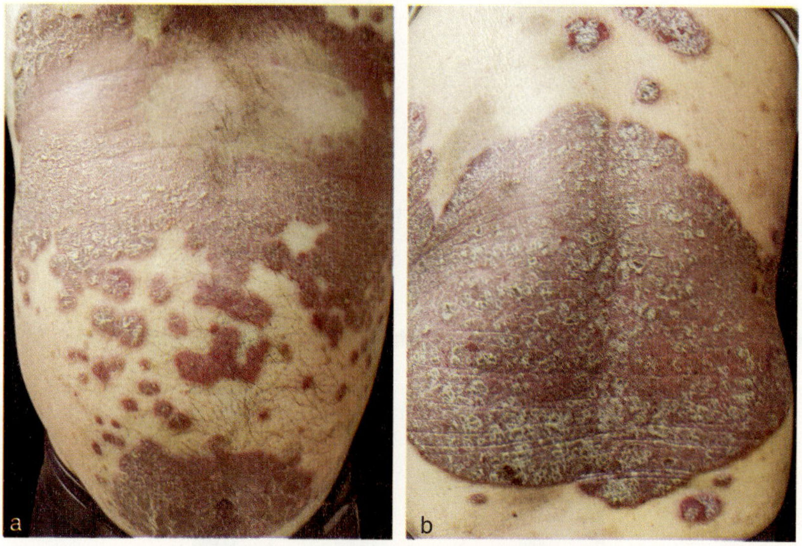

Fig 20.1: Psoriasis vulgaris: (a) Front; (b) Back

trunk. The nails, the palms and the soles may also be affected in the average case; but the mucous membranes may be rarely involved.

Clinically, psoriasis exhibits itself as dry, well-defined macules, papules and plaques of erythema with layer of silvery scales. The typical lesions are coin-shaped; by confluence, big plaques of the size of the palm of a hand (or even bigger) or figurate areas may be formed **(Fig. 20.1)**. When a psoriatic lesion is scratched with the point of a dissecting forceps, a candle-grease-like scale can be repeatedly produced even from the non-scaling lesions. This is called the **candle-grease sign (Signe de la tâche de bougie)**. The complete removal of a scale produces pinpoint bleeding **(Auspitz sign)**. The lesions are slightly raised above the surface of the skin, but there is no induration. Psoriasis is normally characterized by the absence of itching, but in tropical countries, patients complain of slight or moderate pruritus which, if accompanied by secondary psychogenic stress and lichenification, is more marked. Psoriatic lesions may develop along the scratch lines in the active phase; this is called Koebner's phenomenon (other common diseases in which Koebner's phenomenon occurs are warts and lichen planus). The central clearing of the circular lesions produces ringed lesions—annular psoriasis.

The scalp is involved in almost all cases. It shows thick, scaly papules discretely distributed all over, with intervening areas of normal skin. The lesions are dry, and there is no matting of hair, the latter comes out straight through the scales. Psoriasis of the scalp never causes loss of hair and baldness **(Fig. 20.2)**.

Nails show three types of lesions: (a) pitting, (b) separation of the distal portion of the nail from the nail-bed and walls, and (c) thickening of the nail, accompanied by the collection of hyperkeratotic debris under the nail. The face is relatively spared, but lesions may occur along the scalp border (Corona psoriatica). The palms of the hands are involved more commonly than the soles of the feet. Lesions consist of well-defined patches of hyperkeratosis and fissures, on erythematous bases. Lesions are bilaterally symmetrical. Occasionally psoriasis starts on the palms and soles; it may be confined to these areas (Psoriasis inversus).

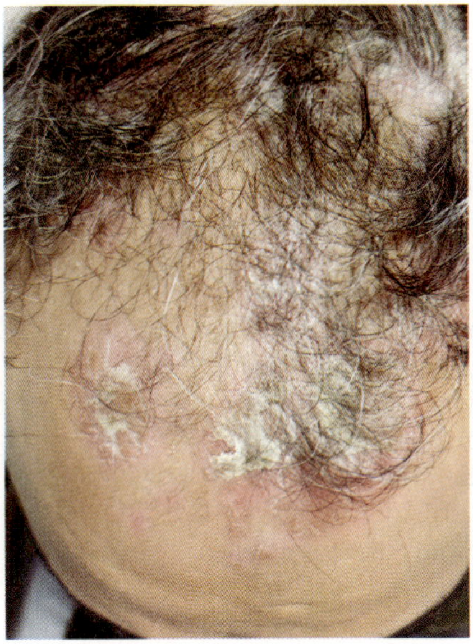

Fig. 20.2: Scalp psoriasis

Pustular Psoriasis

Sometimes, though rarely, psoriatic patients develop generalized pustule formation which may be complicated by arthritis, exfoliation and constitutional symptoms. Lesions may be de novo or on old patches. Pustules may coalesce to form lakes of pus. Condition is precipitated by steroids, iodides, salicylates, etc. Localized psoriasis is confined to palms and soles as pinhead pustules on red exfoliating macules. Differentiation is from tinea, acrodermatitis perstans and bacterid **(Fig. 20.3)**.

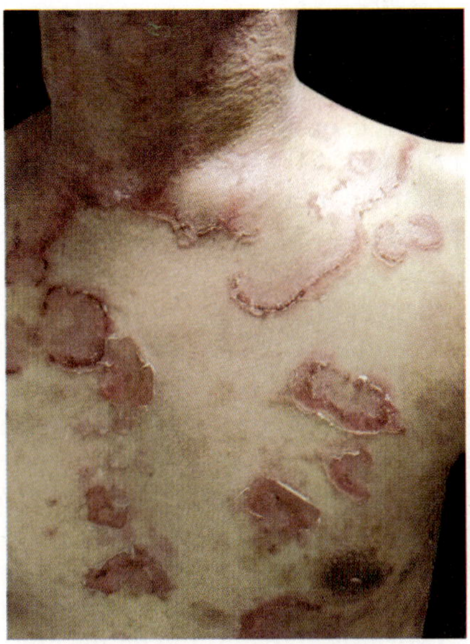

Fig. 20.3: Pustular psoriasis

Flexural Psoriasis

As stated above, the typical distribution of psoriasis is extensor. Occasionally, flexural psoriasis may occur when flexures like the groins, axillae and infra-mammary regions are involved. The lesions lose their dryness in these areas; hence scaling is reduced. Some degree of itching is present in this variety **(Fig. 20.4)**.

Psoriasis Arthropathica

In a small percentage of psoriatic patients, there is involvement of the joints resembling rheumatoid arthritis. This combination is termed psoriasis arthropathica. The joints of the fingers, feet, ankles, knees and sacroiliac are selectively affected; these joints are swollen and painful. The psoriatic eruption and the involvement of the joints may increase or decrease simultaneously. Nail changes are usually present. Radiological changes are characteristic and consist of osteoporosis followed by increased density, diminished joint space, erosion of joint surfaces followed by eventual destruction of the ends of bones. Ultimately, the joints become deformed.

Guttate Psoriasis

Though the normal course of psoriasis is chronic, there occurs occasionally an acute attack in the form of guttate psoriasis. In this variety, small discrete papules develop rapidly all over the body, particularly the trunk **(Fig. 20.5)**, the arms and the thighs. Acute guttate psoriasis is usually precipitated either by an acute illness like tonsillitis or a sharp mental stress or physical injury. It is more common in children than adults.

When a rapid spreading and joining together of individual lesions takes place in psoriasis, it becomes generalized and may produce an erythroderma-like picture viz., generalized erythema and scaling of the whole of the integument **(Fig. 20.6)**. Some typical individual lesions can always be detected in this variety; the history also helps to differentiate it from the other causes of erythroderma (refer to "exfoliative dermatitis" in this chapter).

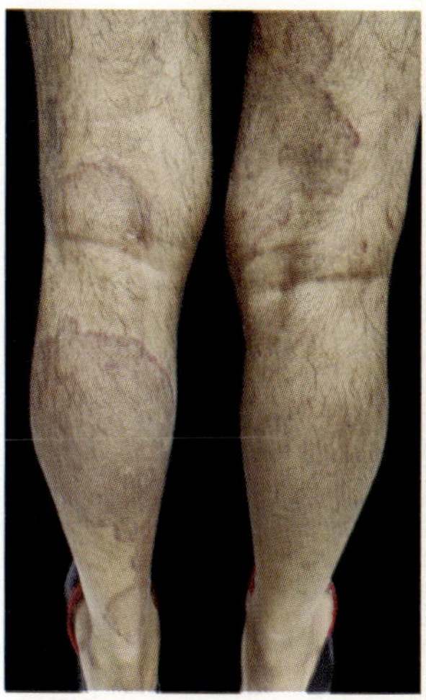

Fig. 20.4: Flexural psoriasis

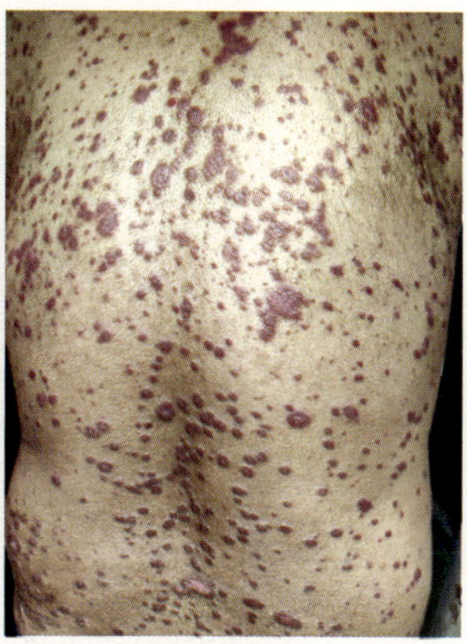

Fig. 20.5: Guttate psoriasis

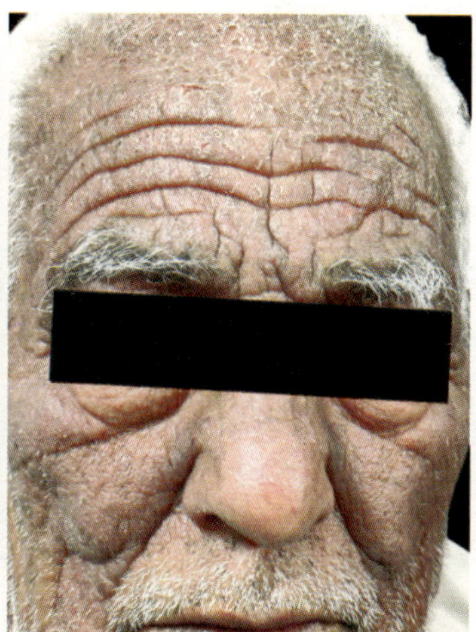

Fig. 20.6: Erythrodermic psoriasis

Diagnosis. It is based upon:

1. The family history of psoriasis.
2. The typical distribution of the lesions on the scalp, elbows, knees, the front of the legs, back and nails.
3. Well-defined, non-indurated, dry, erythematous areas with silvery, layer-upon layer sealing.
4. The candle-grease sign, Koebner' s phenomenon, and pinpoint bleeding upon removal of the scale (Auspitz sign).
5. Little or no itching.
6. History of previous attacks, and seasonal variations of the disease.
7. Typical histopathology.

Differential diagnosis: In the majority of cases, the diagnosis of psoriasis is usually easy if the above-mentioned features are borne in mind. Atypical cases may create diagnostic problems. The following conditions must be particularly considered in differential diagnosis:

Syphilitic psoriasis: The history reveals an illicit exposure and the development of chancre; the rash is less scaly, and shows some degree of induration, mucous patches and lymphadenopathy. The VDRL is positive.

Seborrhoeic dermatitis: The scalp patches are diffuse, ill-defined and moist; the hair is matted and tangled in the crust; the crusts are greasy. Body lesions affect the flexures, the sternal and interscapular regions. Sebopsoriasis is a condition in which features both of psoriasis and seborrhoeic dermatitis art seen as indistinguishable.

Pityriasis rosea: A short history, centripetal distribution, a herald patch and typical oval lesions with cigarette-paper-like, centrifugal scaling.

The flexural lesions must be distinguished from those in tinea cruris, intertrigo, seborrhoeic dermatitis; the nail lesions, from the lesions in tinea unguium, eczema, paronychia and syphilis; the palmar lesions. from the other causes of hyperkeratosis; the guttate variety, from lichen planus, and the erythroderma type from the other causes of erythroderma.

Prognosis: A permanent cure is not yet known, though individual attacks can, almost always, be controlled satisfactorily. Disease is non-infectious. General health and longevity are unaffected though the majority of patients suffer from the disease on and off throughout their lives. The course is chronic with varying periods of intermission (from weeks to years). The outlook is never either sure or bright, but one should avoid an attitude of defeatism. The whole position must be explained to the patient, and then he should be encouraged to persist with the treatment till all the lesions have disappeared; this brings down the relapse rate. The disease does not leave scars. There is only faint staining which disappears slowly. The nails gradually assume their normal appearance in months after the attack has aborted.

Flexural, erythrodermic and pustular psoriasis take longer to heal than the typical variety. The palmar and nail lesions are rather resistant to treatment.

Complications in psoriasis are infrequent. The conditions which can complicate psoriasis are joint involvement (psoriasis arthropathica) which can cause disability, even crippling; exfoliative dermatitis; eczematization caused by scratching an infection or the use of irritants; lichenification brought on by scratching in neurotic individuals.

Treatment: It is unsatisfactory in the sense that cure is out of question as the cause is unknown; hence the treatment is only palliative. The treatment should lay stress on:

1. Impressing upon the patient that the treatment should be continued till the last lesion has disappeared. In this respect, the scalp should not be forgotten. The relapse rate is low, if the attack is completely controlled.
2. The general health of the patient should be maintained, and the exciting causes studied and eliminated, as far as possible. The patient's life should be regulated so that no undue stress affects either body or mind.
3. A moderate, warm climate, frequent sunbaths before the onset of the winter, and visits to sulphur springs, all of which are useful in bringing down the relapse rate. Natural sulphur baths should be taken during the holidays, especially in the winter.

As regards the treatment of individual attacks, methods vary from clinic to clinic and dermatologist to dermatologist. The accepted line of therapy, however, is as follows:

a. ***Diet:*** The cutting down of fats, animal proteins and the quantity of food consumed.

b. ***Systemic treatment***

1. *Withania somnifera* (*Ashwagandha*). In the author's experience, it gives good results. It is an anti-stress herb; it helps to improve physical and mental health.
2. Corticosteroids and ACTH. The only indications are acute guttate, erythrodermic and arthropathic psoriasis. Its use should be avoided in psoriasis vulgaris because of the risk of a relapse, which may follow its withdrawal and serious side-effects.
3. Stimulants in depressive individuals. Dexidrine, Ritalin (P) and Orabolin (P) are the preparations usually recommended.

   Non-specific stimulants like auto-haemotherapy (3–10 cc in gradually increasing doses), milk injections (3–6 cc), crude liver extract, etc. These stimulants are better avoided in very ill patients and erythroderma and arthropathic psoriasis; discoid psoriasis (where the disease is not actively increasing) is the only condition for which these can be safely employed.

   Non-specific agents like calcium gluconate, calcium sandosten (P), vitamin B, etc. are helpful in controlling the progress of the disease. The last one is prescribed along with vitamin A (100,000 IU) biweekly.
4. Use of folic acid antagonists like methotrexate 2.5–5.0 mg thrice 12 hourly doses, once a week in selected recalcitrant cases. These drugs should be avoided in hypertensive people, diabetics or those with liver or kidney disease or in pregnant women. They are toxic drugs; hence should be used with care. Retinoid (Etretinate) may be used in severe cases; cyclosporin A is worth a trial in obstinate cases.

   Indomethacin and Spa treatment are useful in psoriatic arthritis. Psoralens in conjunction with UVA (PUVA) or sunlight is recommended by some as photochemotherapy. Newer biological drugs have shown promising results in selective and properly tested individuals.
5. Vitamin D2–calciferol, sterogyl 15 (P) is sometimes recommended in resistant cases, with beneficial results. Dosage is 600,000 IU weekly. Calcipotriol cream analogue of vitamin D is useful but expensive topical therapy.

c. ***Local treatment:*** No active stimulant or irritant treatment should be employed while the disease is in the acute stage and new lesions are developing. The same principle applies to systemic treatment.

1. Salicylic acid 1%, in vaseline or eucerine, to the lesions, in acute guttate and erythrodermic psoriasis.
2. Salicylic acid 2%, hydrarg ammoniate 5 and 1% pix liquida in a vaseline base, to the chronic discoid lesions; sulphur 1–2% may be used in the place of hydrarg ammoniata. If this simple ointment fails to control the lesions, the next prescription may be recommended.
3. Anthralin derivatives. Chrysorabin 2–8%, cignolin (P) or derobin (P) 0.5–2%, on the patches only, sparing the adjoining healthy skin. These should never be used on the scalp, face and near the genital region because of their irritant properties. Another disadvantage is stains on clothes. Derobin for 4–6 hours is very beneficial.
4. Corticosteroid ointments. They are very beneficial in localized psoriasis, particularly when covered with polythene film (occlusive bandage or saran wrap). Clobetasol is used for the purpose. It is left on for 12–18 hours at a time. Complications of occlusive therapy are pyoderma, prickly heat and danger of fire. When used over large areas, there is hazard of corticosteroid intoxication. Intralesional injections of prednisolone have also been used to clear up small areas of resistant psoriasis. It should be used only for short periods as it causes atrophy of skin, telangiectasia and striae.
5. Sunbath for 15–30 minutes in the morning, UVR exposures in near erythema doses, daily after application of coal tar. Salt water bath, Spa treatment (Dead sea). A ghee (purified butter) massage gives beneficial results.
6. Radiant heat in the arthropathic variety.
7. Psoriasis day care centers (Tar bath → UVR → Anthralin paste) without need for admission. Patience should be the watch-word; slow and steady response is usually more lasting. If PUVA is used, dosage should be properly calibrated, damage to skin and toxicity due to psoralens avoided. Oral psoralens and sunbath are also helpful.

Acute Cases

1. Correction of cause.
2. Calcium gluconate, or vitamin B_{12} or liver extract injections or corticosteroids or *Withania somnifera* (*Ashwagandha*)
3. Rest.
4. 1% acid salicylic ointment.

Only after the spread of this disease has been controlled, is the active stimulant therapeutic regimen adopted.

Chronic Discoid Cases

1. Liquor picis carb or crude tar alternately with butter or oil massage is painted on all the patches; this is followed by early morning sunbath or UVR. *Ammi majus* crushed seeds 1 g or trimethyl psoralen (TMP) taken two hours earlier enhances the healing process. Good results have been reported (Fitzpatrick, et al.), with PUVA-psoralens and UVA (Blacklight)
2. Cold or hot bath according to the climate. A shower is preferable since it avoids soiling and staining the bath tub.

3. Drying, rubbing with a towel and mild oiling.
4. Applying the ointment—Tar or anthralin or clobetasol propionate at night.

In the case of women who do not go to work and want to avoid using messy unguents at night, the ointment could be applied during the day, and removed with a bath in the evening. Clean clothes should be worn after the bath. Minor adjustments must be made to adapt the regimen to the needs of the individual patient.

The erythrodermic type of psoriasis should be treated like other erythrodermas. The arthropathic variety responds best to gold injections. Steroids should be used as a last resort.

PARAPSORIASIS

A blanket term often used as a scapegoat for the ignorance of diagnosis, parapsoriasis is a group of rather infrequent, idiopathic and asymptomatic erythrodermic or scaly maculopapular dermatoses.

In the authors' experience it is a non-specific reaction pattern of the skin which may represent an intermediary stage of definite entities like psoriasis, non-specific dermatitis, lichenoid eruption and mycosis fungoides, etc.

Varieties

a. Guttate types

i. Pityriasis lichenoides chronica usually spares face and scalp. It consists of asymptomatic erythematous round or oval, flat topped papules and runs a chronic course **(Fig. 20.7)**.
ii. Pityriasis lichenoides et varioliformis acuta is considered a separate entity by some. Lesions are scattered macules and papules which may become vesiculopustules or are covered by haemorrhagic crusts which leave superficial scars. There may be

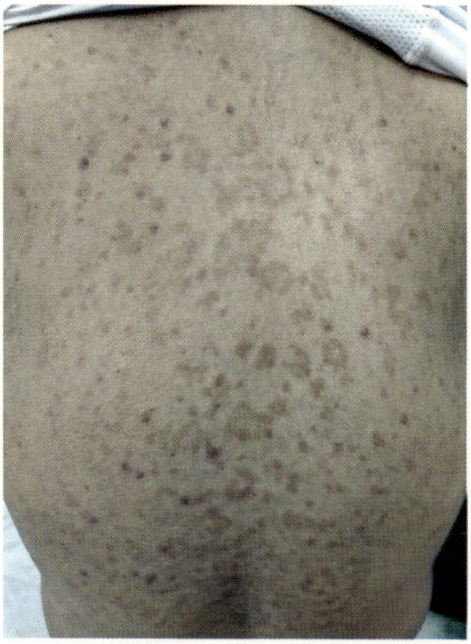

Fig. 20.7: Parapsoriasis: Pityriasis lichenoides chronica

mild constitutional symptoms and generalized lymphadenopathy. Crops may keep on coming for several weeks or years.

b. Erythrodermic types

i. Parakeratosis variegata occurs in middle age as a generalized eruption having clinical appearance between lichen planus and psoriasis in a retiform pattern. Limbs may be the chief site of affection. It is resistant to therapy and may go into mycosis fungoides.

ii. Parapsoriasis en plaque is characterized by a symptomatic, erythemato-squamous, non-infiltrated lesions having a tendency to angulation and finger-like projections, especially on flanks and often showing a yellowish tinge. It may lead to mycosis fungoides.

Histopathology is non-specific.

It should be distinguished from seborrhoeic and discoid dermatitis, both of which are itchy conditions. Other causes of psoriasiform rash, i.e. drugs, syphilis etc. should be kept in mind. In every chronic case of parapsoriasis, reticuloses must be ruled out by histopathological and haematological investigations.

Treatment is unsatisfactory. Calciferol may bring about involution at times. UVR and Thorium X have their advocates. Steroids may be of help in acute cases. Methotrexate has been tried without much avail; tetracyclines are useful in acute guttate cases.

EXFOLIATIVE DERMATITIS

Synonym: Erythroderma.

The above terms imply dermatosis with generalized and universal inflammatory erythema of the skin accompanied by continuous scaling. The skin is thickened and feels hot. The patient becomes extremely sensitive to cold because heat is being continuously lost through the inflamed skin. The hair and nails may fall. Pruritus is constant; hence the patient's movements are restricted. He is extremely uncomfortable and irritable, develops insomnia, grows weak and later becomes emaciated. Emaciation is brought on by irritability, the loss of heat and the loss of proteins through the continuous shedding of scales. Secondary pyoderma, diarrhoea and pneumonia are the usual complications.

Causes and Classification Based upon Etiology

A. Primary:

Newborn and infants

a. Dermatitis exfoliativa neonatorum (Ritter).
b. Erythroderma desquamativum (Leiner).
c. Congenital ichthyosiform erythroderma.

Adults

a. Exfoliative dermatitis (Wilson)
b. Exfoliative dermatitis (Hebra).
c. Epidemic exfoliative dermatitis (Savill).
d. Recurrent scarlatiniform erythroderma.

B. Secondary:

1. Drugs—arsenic, gold, sulphonamides, butazolidine, brufen (P), tegretal (P), anti-tubercular drugs.
2. Reticuloses—mycosis fungoides, leukaemia and Hodgkin's disease.
3. Psoriasis
4. Pemphigus
5. Eczema
6. Pityriasis rubra pilaris

(3–6: Conditions which may progress into erythroderma.)

In practice, secondary erythrodermas are much more common than primary ones and, since the causes can be tackled, the prognosis is, generally speaking, better.

Dermatitis Exfoliativa Neonatorum (Ritter)

It is a rare exfoliative dermatitis of the newborn. It begins within the first few days of life as a red scaly patch, and soon becomes generalized, spreading rapidly over the entire body to produce erythema and exfoliation; occasionally, vesicles, pustules and bullae may develop. The cutaneous lesions are accompanied by mild-to-severe constitutional symptoms. The course extends over a few weeks. The outlook is fair in mild cases, but bad in severe ones. Since antibiotics have come into use; however, the prognosis has improved. The etiology is unknown but the general feeling is, that infection with *Staphylococcus aureus* or drugs used by mother (antenatal or at the time of delivery) may be responsible for the condition.

Erythroderma Desquamativum (Leiner)

It is a rare condition resembling dermatitis exfoliativa neonatorum but with the following differences: (1) It starts later, i.e. between 3 and 8 weeks after birth; (2) There is erythema and scaling as in seborrhoeic dermatitis but no vesiculation. (3) The course is protracted. The etiology is unknown. Gastroenteritis accompanies the disease or precedes it.

Congenital Ichthyosiform Erythroderma

It is a rare heredo-familial, epidermal nevoid condition resembling ichthyosis noticed at birth or sometime after. The characteristic features are: (1) Involvement of the whole integument, especially over the flexures (cubital and popliteal fossae, axillae and the neck), the face, the scalp and the palms of the hands. Redness and dryness of the integument without seasonal variation. It may be complicated by bullous formation. The condition may or may not improve with puberty. It is considered by some as a severe inflammatory form of ichthyosis vulgaris. Use of drugs during pregnancy may be an exciting or aggravating factor.

Primary Exfoliative Dermatitis (Wilson)

Its etiology is unknown; hence it is called primary or idiopathic. It is a rare disease of middle and old age; males are affected more commonly than females. The onset is subacute in the form of a red, scaly plaque on the trunk which spreads to become generalized in a couple of weeks' time. The whole integument is dry, red, inflamed and thickened, accompanied by exfoliation in the form of large scales. The palms of the hands, the soles of the feet, and the scalp are equally involved; nails and hair may be shed. There is pruritus. The erythrodermic skin feels uncomfortable and restricts the movements of the joints. Constitutional complications like pyoderrna, pneumonia and gastrointestinal upsets may develop and prove fatal. The course extends over months and years, marked by ups and downs; eventually, most cases may recover with corticosteroids or Lomodex (IV).

Exfoliative Dermatitis (Hebra)

It differs from Wilson's variety in the following respects: (1) The onset is slow and insidious; it takes months, even longer, for the disease to become generalized. (2) It begins in the flexures. (3) The skin is not too greatly thickened; on the contrary, it may become atrophic. (4) The scaling is finer. (5) The course is chronic, and most cases end fatally. Often, it is difficult to distinguish between the two—Wilson & Hebra's primary exfoliative dermatitis.

Epidemic Exfoliative Dermatitis (Savill)

It is a rare kind of erythroderma occurring in an epidemic form. The cause is, presumably, an infection. One such epidemic occurred in London in 1891; a few others have also been reported.

Recurrent Scarlatiniform Erythroderma

It is an uncommon, scarlet fever-like eruption recurring from time to time, and is presumably, caused by toxins from a septic focus or drugs. The constitutional symptoms are mild, and the rash subsides within about four to eight weeks. The eruption consists of bright-red erythema involving the whole integument, especially the trunk, arms and thighs, when desquamation starts within a day or two of the onset of the eruption, the skin peels off in flakes, and the redness begins to subside.

Secondary Erythrodermas

The two common causes of secondary erythrodermas are drugs and reticuloses; they start as such in comparison with other conditions like psoriasis, eczema, pemphigus and pityriasis rubra pilaris; in the latter group, the erythroderma is only the eventual termination or complication of otherwise different clinical entities. The history helps to separate these two main types of secondary erythrodermas.

The drugs likely to cause erythrodermas are arsenic, gold, sulphonamides, penicillin, butazolidine, Brufen (P), Tegrital (P) and liver extract. To this group may be added indigenous and homeopathic drugs used commonly in Asian countries. According to the authors' experience, indigenous drugs, particularly Ayurvedic kushtas[1] form the single, most common, potent cause of erythroderma in India.

Reticuloses like mycosis fungoides, acute and chronic leukaemias and Hodgkin's disease, may produce an erythrodermic picture in addition to skin tumours, pruritus, and other rashes. The blood picture and histopathological examination of the biopsy will clinch the diagnosis. The point to be emphasized is that, in every case of chronic

[1]An Ayurvedic term used for metallic preparations like arsenic, mercury, gold, silver. Special processes are employed for the 'digestion' of these metals.

erythroderma, a systemic examination, particularly of the spleen, liver and glands should be undertaken, and the primary condition of reticuloses borne in mind.

Psoriasis may eventuate in erythroderma through over-zealous treatment and emotional stresses. Even though the erythroderma becomes generalized, a few discrete, typical psoriatic patches can always be detected.

Eczema may become generalized and universal by extension, dissemination due to auto-sensitization, or may be generalized from the beginning. The diagnosis can always be established by the history, the presence of vesicles and pustules and the detection of moist areas on the removal of scales.

Similarly, pemphigus becomes generalized, particularly pemphigus foliaceous and erythematosus. A few bullae can always be demonstrated, in addition to which, the skin is moist under the scales.

Pityriasis Rubra Pilaris

It is a rare, chronic cutaneous disorder characterized by: (1) Follicular, conical, pinkish papules covered with scales or horny plugs with hair curled on top. These papules are usually found on the back of the fingers and hands. (2) Later, generalized erythema and scaling develop. The eruption rarely becomes universal. The trunk, neck and extremities are commonly involved **(Fig. 20.8)**. The etiology is unknown but all inherited metabolic defect may be the underlying cause. The condition may respond to large doses of vitamin A; this may have to be supplemented with thyroid or corticosteroids.

General diagnosis or of erythroderma: It is based upon: (1) Universal involvement of the skin. (2) Inflammatory redness, scaling and thickening. (3) Constant pruritus.

Prognosis: It depends upon the cause. On the whole, erythrodermas are chronic conditions producing discomfort, irritability, misery, loss of weight, even emaciation. The common complications are: (1) Pyoderma–furunculoses and abscesses. (2) Gastrointestinal upsets, particularly chronic diarrhoea. (3) Pneumonia.

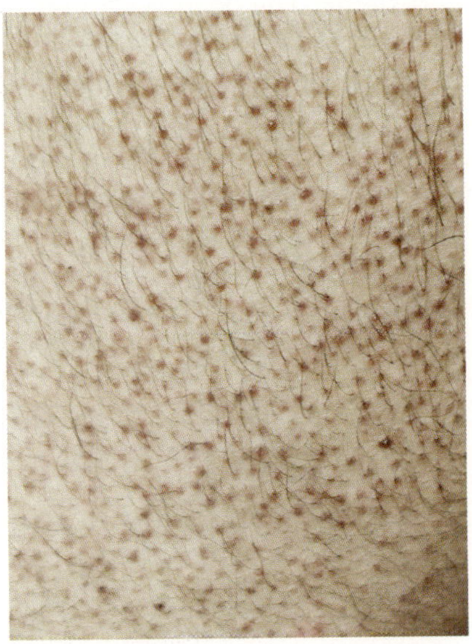

Fig. 20.8: Pityriasis rubra pilaris

Treatment: It consists of:

Specific: It depends upon the cause. In the primary varieties, there is no specific treatment. In the secondary varieties, however, removal of the cause, and specific treatment, do help, viz., the withdrawal and elimination of drugs by BAL, sodium thiosulphate, penicillinase, Lomodex (P), etc.; reticuloses, by X-ray therapy, urethane, radioactive metals, sarcomycin, etc.; pityriasis rubra pilaris, with large doses of vitamin A. Corticosteroids, like prednisone derivatives and ACTH help considerably to cut short the course of most erythrodermas; hence, they save a great deal of misery. Non-specific stimulation with auto-haemotherapy, milk injections and TAB vaccine may be tried in resistant cases. Antibiotics are useful in controlling infantile erythrodermas and complications of exfoliative dermatitis.

General treatment and nursing: The patient is confined to bed in a warm but well-ventilated room. If the patient is afebrile and strong, he can sit on a chair.

The authors prefer to keep the patient up rather than confined to bed. In tropical heat, the room must be air-conditioned, but the patient must be adequately clothed to prevent chills and pulmonary complications. The patient should be kept cheerful and given constant hope. His mind should be well occupied, preferably with reading and games which do not require undue activity.

The diet should include extra proteins and vitamins in the form of meat, chicken, eggs, fish, cheese, salads and fruits to compensate for the loss of these two health-building substances from the skin.

Except in very bad cases, the use of bandages is discouraged. This saves a lot of expense and time; besides, exposed skin heals more quickly than skin that is covered. The patient has a bran bath every morning, followed by cod liver oil or ghee massage. Otherwise, a tar and acid salicylic ointment or a zinc paste is applied all over his body.

The patient is encouraged to apply the medicaments himself; besides giving him independence, this practice exercises the muscles and joints and so prevents contractures, bed sores and gravitational oedema. The head is shaved so that the ointment can be applied with ease.

In weeping cases, a wet application like, for instance, gentian violet lotion 1% is employed. The use of this is indicated only in generalized pemphigus or eczema; but as healing begins to take place, pastes and ointments become more effective. The clothing of the patient should be loose. In case there are ulcers, bullae or weeping from the skin, a mosquito net should be used around the bed to avoid complication with maggots.

A close watch should be kept on the temperature, pulse and respiration. In case these rise, penicillin or other antibiotics should be prescribed along with vitamins and antihistamines.

LICHEN PLANUS

It is a fairly common, irritating disorder of the skin and mucous membranes characterized by purplish or violaceous, polyhedral, flat topped, itchy papules, occurring mostly on the flexor surfaces and in the mouth. The name lichen is derived from the resemblance it has to the purplish lichens that grow on trees in the hills.

It is worldwide in distribution. The incidence is low. It usually affects young and middle-aged people. The disease is non-infectious.

Etiology is unknown. A virus, drug or physical stresses have been blamed. In tropical countries, a lichen-planus-like eruption is often brought about by chloroquine, non-steroidal anti-inflammatory drugs like Brufen. Some of these drugs produce delayed lesions after a latent period of months and insect bites may cause lichen planus tropicalis.

Pathology: It is characteristic and, in a typical lesion, it consists of hyperkeratosis, a patchy increase in the stratum granulosum, acanthosis, shortening of the interpapillary processes, basal cell degeneration, and a well-defined band of round-cell infiltration in the upper corium.

Clinical features: Typically, lichen planus consists of polyhedral, firm, purplish or violaceous papules with shiny, flat tops; very thin, firmly attached scales may be evident on the surface **(Fig. 20.9)**. Faint striation of grey streaks (Wickham's striae) can be seen on the surface of the papules through a magnifying lens. These are best demonstrated after applying oil to the lesion. The papule is about the size of a split pea (sometimes smaller). The papules may become confluent to form plaques. If the papules enlarge with central clearing, rings are formed (lichen planus annularis). Each ring has a clear, pigmented centre with a reddish or purplish lichenoid periphery. Itching is constant, being more so in dark-skinned people living in tropical climates. Itching produces lichen planus papules along the line of scratching—Koebner' s phenomenon—similar to one seen in psoriasis.

The rash is bilateral and symmetrical. It is distributed along the fronts of wrists, the flexor surfaces of the forearms, the abdomen, the legs, the genitalia and the back. In about half the number of cases affected, lesions also occur in the mouth, buccal mucosa, less commonly, on the lips, tongue and genitalia, as dead white spots, streaks and plaques, or like lacy network **(Fig. 20.10)**. The disease is seldom seen on the scalp, the palms of the hands and the soles of the feet. The mucous membrane lesions are usually asymptomatic, but sometimes cause a little burning and irritation.

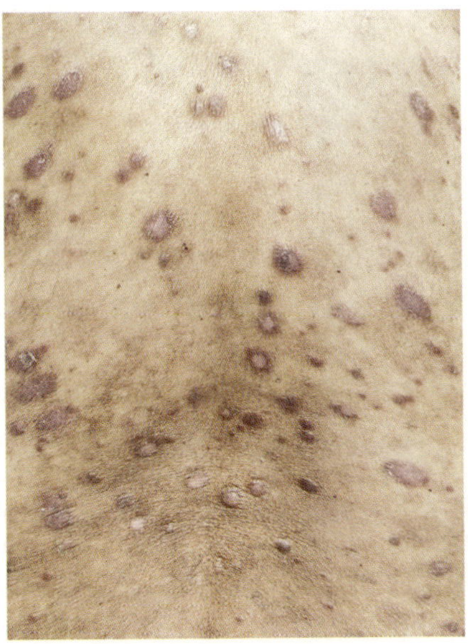

Fig. 20.9: Lichen planus

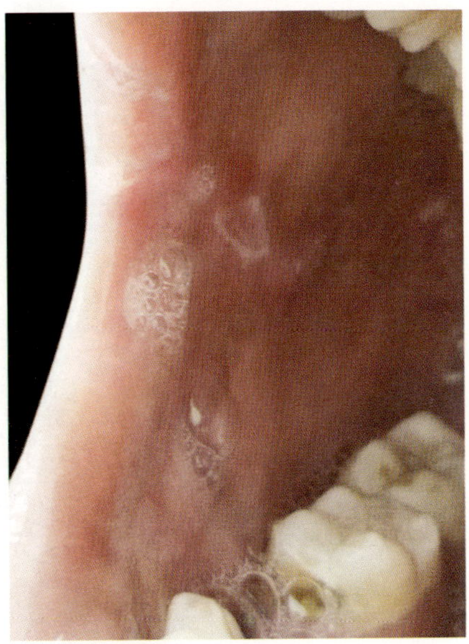

Fig. 20.10: Oral lichen planus

It is usually a chronic disease lasting for several months or years. New lesions appear in crops and then disappear spontaneously, resulting in a pigmented skin which takes long to return to normal. The general health of the patient is not affected. The disease may recur. Nails are affected only in a minority of cases. The first change is seen near the cuticle and gradually it extends forwards with the growth of nail. This results in a nail with rough surface and marked longitudinal striations. If the thinning is severe, the cuticle may grow forward as a pannus. Rarely there may be permanent shedding of the nail.

Variations in Lichen Planus

Annular lichen planus: Here ringed lesions with central clearing and raised firm periphery is typically seen. Lichenoid eruption following an insect bite commonly produces this type of lesion on the exposed parts of the body, particularly the face. The number of lesions vary from 1 to 4 or more.

Acute generalized lichen planus: The onset is sudden, the course short, and the rash is generalized. In the early stages, the eruption may not be typical, but characteristic lesions soon become visible. It may merge into chronic lichen planus.

Lichen planus verrucosus: It occurs as hyperkeratotic, verrucous, violaceous nodules and patches on the legs. It may occur as such, but is usually accompanied by typical lesions on the legs, wrists, forearms, etc. Itching is severe.

Linear or herpes zoster-like lichen planus: The linear form, common in children, is seen on the extremities or the face. The lesions rarely occur along the segmental distribution of nerves; when they do, the condition may be confused with herpes zoster or nevus unius lateralis.

Lichen planopilaris: It is usually seen as acuminate, follicular papules with horny spines, accompanied by flat, lichenoid lesions on the chest, back and upper arms. It may extend to scalp to cause cicatricial alopecia **(Fig. 20.11)**.

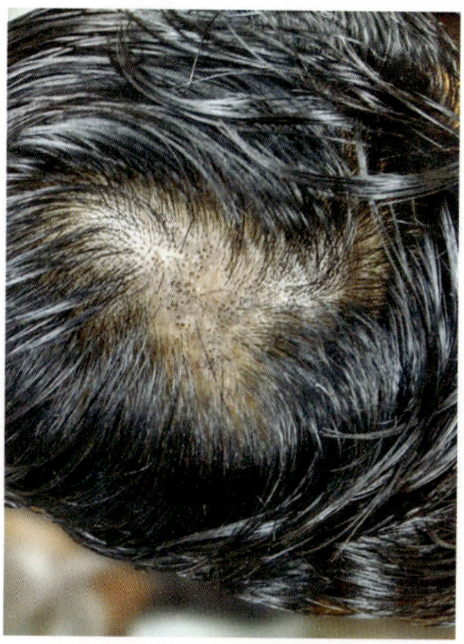

Fig. 20.11: Lichen planopilaris

Bullous form (Lichen pemphigoides) is rare. Bullous lesions on lichenoid bases are the main features. Course is chronic. Healing is with atrophy.

Diagnosis: The diagnosis of lichen planus is based upon:

1. Demonstration of typical lesions—polyhedral, firm violaceous (may be difficult to detect in dark-skinned people), flat-topped papules with Wickham's striae and very thin adherent scales.
2. Distribution on the flexors, genitalia and mouth.
3. Pruritus.
4. A chronic course.
5. A typical histology.

Differential diagnosis: It is made mainly from other lichenoid eruptions, and, less so, from psoriasis, eczema, warts, naevi, pityriasis rubra pilaris. The mucous lesions of lichen planus must be differentiated from the lesions of leukoplakia, the mucous patches of syphilis and aphthous stomatitis. On the scalp it must be distinguished from discoid lupus erythematosus, pseudo-pelade, favus, etc.

Other Lichenoid Eruptions

Lichen scrofulosorum (*see* Chapter 15)

Lichen spinulosus: It is characterized by pin-head sized, follicular, flesh coloured papules with horny spines. The papules are grouped in patches. Children are commonly affected. The sites of affection are the abdomen, buttocks and legs. The condition is asymptomatic, and clears up with a good nourishing diet containing plenty of animal fats, extra vitamins, tonics and the local application of animal fats or cod liver oil.

Lichen syphiliticus: The salient features are follicular papules with induration; slight itching; lymphadenopathy; mucous patches; and a history of exposure. The VDRL is positive.

Lichen simplex chronicus: Lichenification or neurodermatitis is another term used for this kind of lichenoid eruption (*see* Chapter 10).

Lichenoid drug eruptions: These occur commonly in the tropics and in dark-skinned people. An idiosyncrasy to certain drugs, e.g. Brufen (NSAID) arsphenamine, gold, chloroquine, mepacrine, hydroxychloroquine, quinine and certain phenothiazine derivatives, para-amino-salicylic acid, thiazide diuretics and aminophenazole (Daptazole) may result in lichenoid eruption which may simulate lichen planus. Contact with chemicals used in the processing of coloured photographic films may, in sensitized individuals, produce similar eruptions.

Lichen nitidus: It consists of discrete, pink or flesh-coloured, asymptomatic papules, grouped in patches. The typical sites are the genitalia, inner sides of thighs, lower abdomen and at times wrists. No specific treatment is available. It is a benign disease.

Lichen striatus: An uncommon form occurring in children. It usually affects upper limbs and occasionally the legs. Lesions consist of flesh-coloured or darker lichenoid papules arranged in a linear fashion, usually unilateral and along the long axis of a limb. Streak may be only a few centimeters in length or extend along the entire limb suggesting a linear naevus. Histopathology is non-specific. No active treatment is necessary as the eruption has a tendency to disappear spontaneously. Sometimes occlusive corticosteroid dressings are definitely beneficial in aborting the disease.

Lichen urticatus: Syn: Papular urticaria (*see* Chapter 9).

Lichen amyloidoses: (*see* Chapter 25).

Lichen myxoedematosus: A very rare but definite entity, practically independent of thyroid pathology. Lesions consist of discrete, localized papular, annular or discoid, lichenoid plaques. This is associated with infiltration and at times lymphedema. Itching is only minimal. General health is not affected. Basal metabolic rate, erythrocyte sedimentation rate and other tests for metabolic defect are normal except the blood lipids may show slight change. Thyroid extract may benefit an occasional patient.

Lichen sclerosus et atrophicus (*see* Chapter 25).

Prognosis: Lichen planus is a chronic disease lasting for years. The disease occurs usually once in a lifetime; more than one attack may be seen. On involution, there is pigmentation which takes a long time to disappear. There is usually no constitutional disturbance.

Treatment: It is unsatisfactory, since the etiology is not known and a specific remedy is not available. It consists in:

1. Reassurance and, maybe, a relaxing holiday. The use of sedatives is indicated in patients suffering from undue mental tension.
2. Arsenic and mercury are toxic metals to play with in an otherwise benign disease. Antibiotics are ordinarily of no avail. Corticosteroids are useful in acute lichen planus. So is Dapsone in resistant cases.
3. Antihistamines to control pruritus.
4. Soothing ointments preferably 1–5% tar paste. Crude tar is very useful in lichen planus verrucosus. Occlusive clobetasol bandages and intralesional injection of steroids do help in verrucous and hypertrophic form of the disease and also oral lesions.
5. X-ray therapy in small, fractional dose is useful in aborting resistant lesions of localized lichen planus and lichen verrucosus.

PITYRIASIS ROSEA

It is a fairly common, acute generalized disease. Etiology is obscure, though it is believed to be caused by a virus. Both sexes are equally affected; incidence is usually between the ages of 12 and 45.

Pathology: The typical histopathology consists of patchy parakeratosis, epidermal oedema, moderate vascular dilatation and infiltration of upper corium with polymorphs and round cells.

Clinical features: The onset is sudden. There may or may not be any constitutional symptoms like fever, malaise, etc.

The first sign is a herald patch on the shoulder or the arm. It consists of a small erythematous area, about the size of the palm of a hand, with little scaling and itching. About 5–8 days later, a generalized eruption develops on the trunk, upper arms, upper part of the thighs and the neck. Typically, it consists of oval macules of erythema; on the sides and back of the trunk, the macules are distributed along the ribs. Within

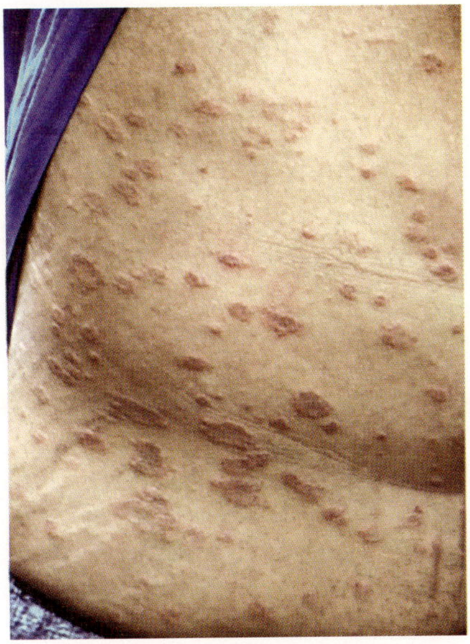

Fig. 20.12: Pityriasis rosea

a few days these macules begin to peel, and become slightly wrinkled. Scaling is typical, cigarette-paper-like, with the free edge of the scale pointing towards the centre **(Fig. 20.12)**.

The course of the disease is about 6–12 weeks. It heals spontaneously, and does not leave scars. Second attacks are rare.

There is slight or moderate itching depending upon climatic conditions.

Differential diagnosis: It is from allergic rash, syphilides, psoriasis and seborrhoeic dermatitis. Single attack, sudden onset with a herald patch, typical rash and histopathology help to establish the diagnosis. Blood serology should be done in a suspicious case.

Treatment: There is no specific treatment. Calamine cream and antihistaminics help to control it. Severe cases may require corticosteroids and antibiotics.

Chapter 21

Drug Eruptions—Dermatitis Medicamentosa

INTRODUCTION

Until a few decades ago, the contemporary physicians had only "pop-gun" pharmacies. However, due to the rapid advance of science in the last few decades, conditions have changed and a multitude of powerful and potent drugs have been added to the pharmacopeia for the treatment of cutaneous as well as systemic disorders. Hand in hand with the progress of science, the hazard of drug rashes has also increased, especially because large number of proprietary preparations are now so easily available to the public. Besides obvious drug eruptions, drugs cause, hidden from eyes, a variety of biochemical, metabolic and immunological changes and also latent eruptions appearing months after discontinuance of use. Several auto-immune reactions are being blamed to drugs.

Definition

Drug eruption or dermatitis medicamentosa implies a cutaneous eruption that has developed from the use of a drug systemically, viz., by mouth, inhalation or parenterally. It must be distinguished from contact dermatitis which is produced by the irritant or sensitizing effect of a drug applied topically.

Common examples of a chemical drug dermatitis are sulphonamide and Furacin (P) contact dermatitis produced by their application to a wound. Further, conditions like drug reactions (e.g. ocular reaction due to chloroquine), teratogenic effects of drugs taken during pregnancy causing developmental defects (thalidomide, methotrexate, steroids, antimalarials; phenothiazine, phenylbutazone, atromid-P, etc.) and skin reactions due to chemicals in food, e.g. margarine disease, Taiwan and Spanish epidemics must be differentiated from true drug eruption. The latter have not only produced acute rashes but also melanosis and scleroderma-like pictures subsequently.

Mode of Action

There are several modes of action:

1. ***Pharmacological action:*** When drugs are used in larger doses than is pharmacologically permissible, they produce toxicity with cutaneous symptoms, e.g. heavy metals like gold, arsenic and mercury, etc.
2. ***Hypersensitivity:*** It refers to the hypersensitivity of an individual to any particular drug used. The patient may be hypersensitive, allergic or idiosyncratic. Familiar examples of hypersensitivity would be urticaria and angioneurotic oedema resulting from penicillin, and serum reactions.

3. ***Biotropism:*** A drug eruption may be the combined effect of the drug and the toxin produced by the pathological process for which the particular drug has been administered, e.g., erythema nodosum brought on by sulphonamides given for streptococcal tonsillitis. It may also be due to the action of a toxin which may have been liberated from the site of the disease under treatment, by the action of the drug; but, the latter hypothesis is difficult to prove in practice.

Perhaps untoward effects of drugs may be best grouped under the headings suggested by Rosenheim (1958):

1. Overdosage
2. Intolerance
3. Side-effects
4. Secondary effects
5. Idiosyncrasy
6. Hypersensitivity—allergic reactions

It is not always easy to decide into which group a particular effect should be placed and several effects may be present in the same patient (Calnan).

Drug Reactions vs Allergy

Drug reactions are very common but not all of them are allergic as is generally thought. Their mechanism is unknown. Even when the circumstantial evidence suggests an immunological nature of reaction, no proof can be advanced to confirm it. However, techniques like Shelley's basophil degranulation test, haemagglutination and gel diffusion tests have their limitations.

Diagnosis

It is based upon the following criteria:

1. The history reveals that the patient has recently taken a drug; and immediately after, the eruption has occurred as a direct result of it. In certain cases, the eruption may be delayed, as when heavy metals are taken.
2. The eruption disappears on the withdrawal of the drug. This constitutes a reliable clinical method of clinching the diagnosis. Exceptions to this rule are: melanodermas and erythrodermas which take a long time to disappear.
3. A previous history of a similar eruption.
4. A drug eruption is usually bilaterally symmetrical, and widespread in distribution, except when it is a fixed drug eruption.

In establishing the diagnosis, patch tests are not applicable. Intradermal tests are useful only in case of few drugs like penicillin, sera, etc.

Laboratory evaluation of drug eruptions is very expensive and not very reliable. The various tests that can be performed are basophil degranulation tests, lymphocyte culture test, macrophage migration inhibition factor, radioallergosorbent test and skin testing.

Quite often the patient drugs himself with so-called harmless drugs like Anacin (P), phenolphthalein containing proprietary medicines such as Brooklax (P), Castophene (P), etc. His memory at times is unreliable, but repeated questioning and observation will often bear fruit. Secondary pigmentary changes, and the erythrodermic type of eruption resulting from heavy metals, do not subside immediately after the drug in question has been withdrawn. This aspect of dermatitis medicamentosa should be borne in mind. Although, the points mentioned above undoubtedly help to establish the diagnosis of eruptions in a large percentage of cases, the behaviour of many a drug eruption is so complex and atypical that it can include almost any type of cutaneous lesion, and may simulate any kind of skin disease. Further the subject is complicated by use of food additives and their cross sensitization with drugs.

A drug rash may be accompanied by constitutional symptoms like fever, aches and pains. There may be involvement of other organs resulting in jaundice, nephritis, blood dyscrasias, etc.

As Sherlock Holmes puts it: "Life often hangs by a thread". Minute observation to elicit evidence pays dividends, and may at times be a question of life and death for the patient. In the history-taking of dermatological cases, detailed questioning about the drugs taken on their own, as a habit, or otherwise administration by any physician, is very important. Undoubtedly, the administration of drugs, particularly the proprietary ones, carries both risk and responsibility; therefore, the physician must be heedful of their cutaneous reactions.

Special Hazards in Tropical Countries

In tropical countries, drug eruptions are very common for several reasons (Peterkin):

a. The use of drugs for tropical ailments, e.g. quinine, mepacrine, sulphones and Hetrazan (P).
b. The strong sun, and the exposure of the skin to it, e.g. sulphonamides produce photosensitivity.
c. The greater excretion of drugs through the skin due to excessive sweating.
d. The practice of quackery and pseudo-scientific medicine. In the authors' experience, the latter constitutes the greatest problem in the developing countries. The use of 'Kushtas' containing heavy metals, by indigenous practitioners, together with the easy accessibility of patent as well as indigenous drugs to the public, constitute a serious threat, because they can cause severe dermatoses. The authors have seen some of the worst dermatoses caused by homeopathic drugs.

Besides the use of potent drugs, there are several other reasons why the incidence of drug eruptions is on the increase (Sheldon). These are:

a. The drugs which are used systemically, are also employed locally, e.g. sulphonamides, penicillin. This has an unduly sensitizing effect upon the skin.
b. The intermittent use of drugs, e.g. sulphonamides and penicillin repeated from time to time, tend to produce sensitization.
c. People have begun to use more and more drugs for minor ailments through knowledge gained by reading advertisement of the patent drugs in newspapers, magazines and by listening in to the commercial radio.

CLASSIFICATION

A complete list of the drugs which can produce eruptions is beyond the scope of this book. However, an attempt is made here to classify cutaneous disorders brought about by drugs (Table 21.1).

Common causes of drug eruptions are sulphonamides, antibiotics, salicylates, barbiturates, ibuprofen (NSAIDs), antidepressants and tranquillizers. Though heavy

Table 21.1: Type of drug reactions along with their incriminating drugs

Type of lesion	*Important incriminating drugs*
Acneiform (Fig. 21.1)	Iodides bromides, hydantoin, steroids, pills, androgens, dianabol (P), INH
Eczematoid	Butazolidine (P), sulphonamides, penicillin extract, chlorthiazide, arsenic, mercury, gold, methyldopa
Erythematous	Salicylates, belladona, barbiturates, penicillin, sulphonamides, sulfones, chlorpromazine, chlorothiazide, anticonvulsants, griseofulvin, phenylbutazone
Erythema multiforme (Fig. 21.2)	Sulphonamides, barbiturates, phenothiazine, butazolidine, salicylates
Exfoliative dermatitis	Arsenic, mercury, gold, penicillin, sulphonamides, chloroquine, hydantoins, phenylbutazone PAS, sulphonylureas, tegritol (P)
Fixed drug eruption	Sulphonamides, phenolphthalein, aspirin, barbiturates, dapsone, tetracyclines, quinine, phenylbutazone, chlordiazepoxide
Granulomatous	Iodides, bromides.
Lichenoid	Quinine, chloroquine, gold, phenothiazine PAS, chlorothiazide, methyldopa, Ibuprofen
LE like	Hydralazine, griseofulvin, procainamide, quinidine, H. hydantoins, D-penicillamine, sulphonamides, tetracyclines and oral contraceptive pills
Photosensitization	Chlorpromazine, promethazine, sulphonamides, sulphonylureas, griseofulvin, chlorothiazide, antihypertensives, tranquillizers, Ledermycin (P)
Pigmentary	Heavy metals, sulphonamides, declomycin, hydantoin, chlorpromazine
Psoriasiform	Sulphonamides, mepacrine, chloroquine
Purpuric	Salicylates, anti-convulsants, barbiturates, sulphonamides, meprobamate
Pustular	Iodides, bromides
Urticarial	Penicillin, aspirin, animal sera, toxoids, vaccines, meprobamate, furoxone, NSAID
Vesiculobullous	Iodides, bromides, penicillin, sulphonamides, butazolidine derivatives, barbiurates, nalidixic acid
Oral lesions (bullous purpuric, hypertrophic and inflammatory)	Broad-spectrum antibiotics, aminopterin butazolidine, sulphonamides, hydantoins

metals are responsible for many severe skin reactions, incidence is low in practice because their use has been replaced by other safer drugs. Dermatologists see many cases of drug eruptions due to. butazolidine, chlorothiazide, newer hypotensives and oral antidiabetic drugs resulting in lichenoid eruption, keratoderma or dyshidrosis sicca-like picture.

Sulphonamides: They are used extensively both in dermatological and general medical practice. The skin lesions produced by sulphonamides are of various types, and vary in severity. The milder manifestations include pruritus, not morbilliform, scarlatiniform and erythema multiforme. Cross sensitization is a very common phenomenon.

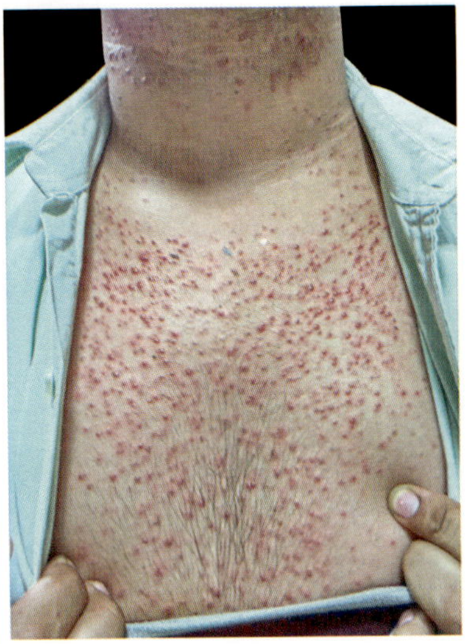

Fig. 21.1: Acneiform eruptions

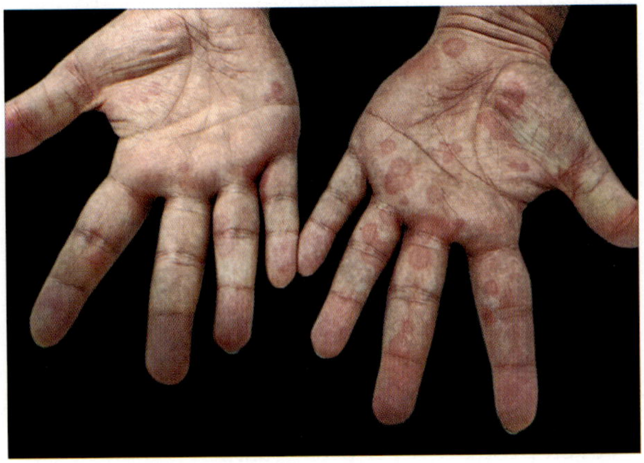

Fig. 21.2: Erythema multiforme

Photosensitization is localized to areas exposed to light. It occurs in a mild form, as an erythematopapular rash or as a bullous eruption.

Antibiotics: They account for a large number of drug rashes owing to their extensive use. Penicillin is the most commonly misused drug in this group. The most dreaded penicillin reaction is anaphylactoid shock. Several deaths have occurred in this manner. This can be prevented by waiting for 3–5 minutes after the patient has been injected with the first drop of penicillin. If there is no reaction during this waiting period, the rest of the drug can be injected.

Urticarial reaction: It occurs any time within ten days of starting the penicillin treatment. The severity of the reaction is variable. Severe reactions are frequently accompanied by joint pains, lymphadenopathy and a feverish feeling.

Erythematovesicular or ide-like reactions (pompholyx), particularly in individuals with fungus affections. On healing there is peeling.

Purpuric and bullous reaction: It mimics acute pemphigus. Exfoliative dermatitis may also develop, but this is rare. Hyperegic reactions like angiitis or necrotizing angiitis (Rajam) may also develop but rarely. They are characterized by maculopapular, vesicular and bullous eruptions, petechial haemorrhages, ulcers and protracted illness which may prove fatal.

In the majority of cases, fortunately, the reaction is mild, and subsides on the withdrawal of the drug; only in a minority of cases, does the serious illness continue and prove fatal. Compulsory intradermal tests with penicillin before its use, have helped us to prevent penicillin reactions. Tetracyclines may cause exanthematous eruption, urticaria, bullous reaction, pigmentation and fixed drug eruption.

The prolonged use of broad-spectrum antibiotics predisposes to moniliasis of the mouth and the skin, vitamin B deficiency syndrome (angular stomatitis, cheilitis, glossitis, swelling and exfoliation of the oral epithelium) and itching of the. scrotum, perianal and vulval regions. Ledermycin (P) has a tendency to cause photosensitivity and photo-onycholysis. Ampicillin may cause erythema multiforme-like eruption. Supplementing of these antibiotics with nystatin and vitamins, particularly vitamin B complex, has helped to prevent untoward reactions and rashes. Griseofulvin rarely produces a drug rash but occasionally stomatitis, erythematous or haemorrhagic rash, LE-like eruption, angioneurotic edema or photosensitivity is seen.

Antimalarials: Quinine usually causes generalized pruritus and a lichenoid eruption. Long continued ingestion of quinine can, occasionally, produce deep brown pigmentation of the buccal mucous membrane, the lower limbs and the glans penis. Mepacrine and chloroquine produce lichenoid and psoriasiform eruptions. Pigmentation of the teeth has also been reported (Peterkin), and so are the white hair following chloroquine therapy. The latter can also precipitate acute attack of porphyria.

Anti-tubercular drugs

1. Streptomycin causes contact eczema. It rarely produces a true drug rash.
2. Para-amino-salicylic acid may cause jaundice and a "non-descript" eruption. It can even produce a purpuric rash.
3. Iso-nicotinic acid hydrazide (INH) may produce polyneuritis or a pellagroid syndrome. The other rashes caused by INH are urticaria; morbilliform, scarlatiniform, purpuric and acne-like lesions.

Analgesics and antipyretics: With salicylates, the common lesions seen are maculopapular, urticarial and fixed-drug eruption. Eczematoid, bullous and haemorrhagic eruptions have been. seen following the use of Irgapyrin (P), Tegritol (P), other non-steroidal anti-inflammatory drugs (NSAIDs) and butazolidine derivatives.

They may produce delayed eruptions especially lichenoid eruptions after a latent period of several months.

Tranquillizers: Because of increasing stress and stains of life, use of tranquillizers has become fairly common in practice. Several preparations are available in the market. Two types of drug rashes come across in practice viz: photosensitivity dermatoses (melanoses of exposed parts, particularly the face and forearms) and lichenoid eruptions. A characteristic eruption consisting of sharply outlined patches of dermatitis on the sides of cheeks has been described due to chlordiazepoxide.

Biologicals: Erythematous rashes following the use of liver extract, Salk vaccine and vitamin B injections have been seen by many workers. Sera are responsible, at times, for severe reactions like urticaria, joint pains and anaphylactoid reactions.

Laxatives: The majority of proprietary laxatives contain phenolphthalein, e.g. brooklax, bicholate, agarol, petrolagar, petrolax and castophene. Considering the number of people who take these laxatives, the proportion of those who develop idiosyncrasies is comparatively low. Phenolphthalein can cause pemphigoid rash, erythema multiforme, and fixed drug eruption.

Fixed-drug eruption: This is a fascinating cutaneous manifestation with characteristic clinical features. The drugs that commonly produce such an eruption are phenolphthalein, tetracyclines, sulphonamides, phenylbutazone, dapsone, quinine, barbiturates, salicylates and chlordiazepoxide. The typical eruption consists of a circumscribed, circular patch or patches of erythema with inflammation of the skin. It may or may not be accompanied by vesicles or blister formation. The eruption may consist of a single patch or several, within 12–72 hours of taking the drug **(Fig. 21.3)**. After the drug is withdrawn, the inflammation subsides leaving behind pigmentation. When the drug is taken again, inflammation in the form of erythema, swelling and vesicle formation appears around the original pigmentation. Either new patches appear in the second or third attack, or the eruption is confined to the original patch, or patches only. When the eruption subsides, deeper pigmentation occurs which takes a long time to fade. Attacks of fixed drug eruptions only subside when the offending drug is permanently withdrawn.

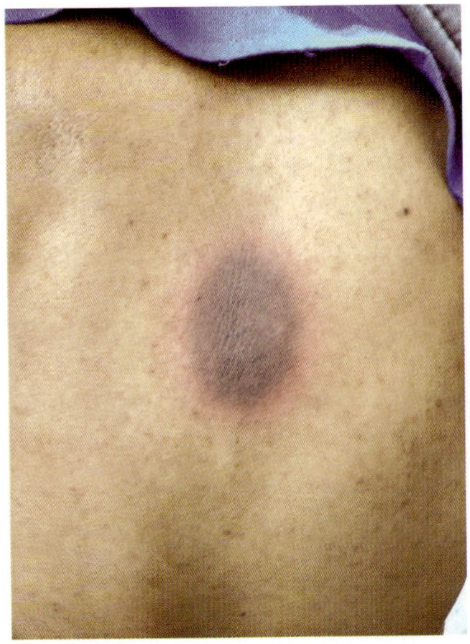

Fig. 21.3: Fixed-drug eruptions

Barbiturates: A few cases of fixed drug eruption and severe intractable urticaria, due to barbiturates have been seen. One also comes across morbilliform, scarlatiniform and erythema multiforme-like lesions which sometimes develop from the use of phenobarbitone.

Chronic pruritus is a frequent complaint amongst opium addicts. Bromides and iodides produce acneiform, bullous and granulomatous lesions mostly on the face, hands and legs.

Arsenicals: With the decline in the use of arsenicals, inorganic and organic, incidence of drug eruptions due to arsenicals has come down considerably. Cutaneous changes take several years to develop. Inorganic arsenicals cause rain drop pigmentation (mottled, follicular, brownish discoloration on trunk and friction sites), punctate keratoses on palms and soles, less so on limbs and trunk, and epitheliomata. Organic arsenicals like arsephena mine cause exfoliative dermatitis which occurs within a couple of weeks of administration. Indian Kushtas and indigenous drugs contain arsenicals and produce cutaneous changes described above.

Anticoagulants: Coumarins cause diffuse alopecia. It is a common but reversible complication. Rarely haemorrhagic bullous eruption is come across.

Phenindione may cause severe hypersensitivity reactions in the form of fever and an itchy erythematous or eczematous eruption which may go into erythroderma. Kidneys and liver may be damaged.

Anticonvulsants: Hydantoin (Dilantin), mesantoin and trimethadione cause erythematous eruption, gingival hyperplasia and hypertrichosis. Erythema multiforme like rash, exfoliative dermatitis and fixed drug eruption have been reported.

Oral antidiabetic drugs: Sulphonylureas can produce maculopapular rash, erythema multiforme, exfoliative dermatitis, photosensitivity and lichenoid rashes. Phenformin (Biguanide) can cause transient erythematous or urticarial rash with itching.

Antihistaminics: They can cause both local contact dermatitis and systemic reaction. Promethazine (Phenergan) is often responsible for photosensitivity and cross-sensitization reactions.

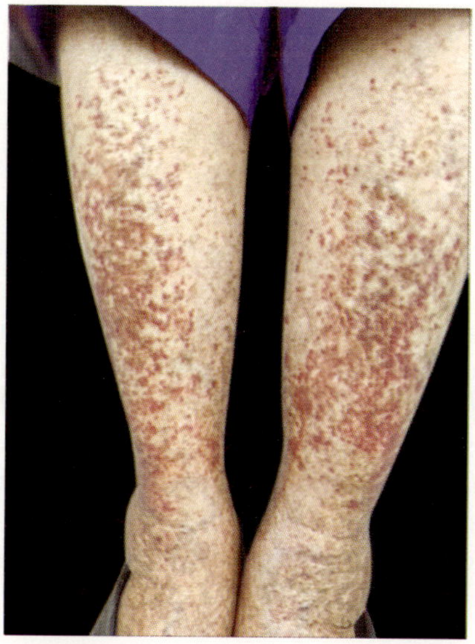

Fig. 21.4: Purpuric eruptions

Allergic reactions to antihistaminics consist of erythematous or urticarial reactions and blood dyscrasias. Benadryl (P) may cause vasculitis.

Anti-thyroid drugs: Thioureas can produce erythematous eruption and urticaria along with fever and blood dyscrasia.

Oral contraceptives: Since their use has become common, many cutaneous side effects have been noted. Exact nature depends upon the individual sensitivity and composition of the oral contraceptive. The common effects are chloasma, acne, photosensitivity, genital moniliasis, alopecia, herpes gestationis and telangiectasia. Some workers have found probable relationship with erythema nodosum, lupus erythematosus, purpura and porphyria **(Fig. 21.4)**.

Drug photosensitivity: Incidence of melanosis, particularly of exposed parts, is fairly common in practice. Common offending groups of drugs are phenothiazine derivatives (tranquillizers, antihypertensive drugs, anthelmintics), diuretics (chlorothiazide), Ledermycin-P, tetracyclines, sulphonamides, psoralens, anti-histaminics (promethazine, chlorpromazine), griseofulvin and sulphonylureas.

Cross-sensitization: With the advances in chemical and pharmaceutical industry, cross-sensitization has become fairly common because of chemical relationship of different groups of drugs, e.g. phenothiazine, anthelmintics, tranquillizers and antihistaminics; sulphonamides and oral anti-diabetic drugs; para-aminophenol group in sulphonamides, benzocaine, para-aminosalicylic acid and para-dyes; Phenergan-P (promethazine), Pyribenzamine-P (tripelennamine) and chloropromazine–different antihistaminics. Hence, care should be exercised in prescribing drugs with similar or closely related formulae. Same applies to food additives.

Course and Prognosis

The course of dermatitis medicamentosa is variable, and is in fact, at times unpredictable. The eruption may last from a few hours to several years. Usually, the drug eruption (except when it is caused by heavy metals) clears up rapidly upon the cessation of the offending drug. Fixed-drug eruptions are very slow in clearing though the acute erythema and colour changes usually fade when the drug is withdrawn, normal pigmentation may not be restored for a long time. Generalized exfoliative dermatitis and extensive bullous eruptions carry a grave prognosis. Lichenoid drug reactions take months to clear up.

Differential Diagnosis

A drug eruption may closely simulate any skin disease. Erythema nodosum, exfoliative dermatitis, acne, SLE, psoriasis and exanthemata are examples of some of the more common dermatoses from which a drug eruption has to be differentiated. It is important for a practitioner to be constantly aware of the capacity drugs have of producing eruptions. Whenever a practitioner treats a cutaneous or systemic disease with drugs, the appearance of any rash should make him ponder: "Is the new eruption one of the side-features of the drug or drugs employed?" If he has the smallest suspicion, that it is so, the suspected drug must be immediately withdrawn.

Treatment

A. Curative

1. The drug must be stopped as soon as the diagnosis has been established, and the patient advised not to use it again unless he has been desensitized. He should also be told to guard against the related group of drugs.
2. The drug must be eliminated from the system as quickly as possible. In the majority of mild cases of drug eruptions, it is just enough to stop the drug, and nature does the rest. But in severe dermatoses, especially the bullous, eczematoid and exfoliative types caused by heavy metals and bromides, the body has to be helped in getting rid of the drug as follows:
   a. In arsenical dermatitis and to a lesser extent in mercurial and gold dermatitis, a course of sodium thiosulphate 10% 10 cc intravenously daily or on alternate days, followed by a course of British-anti-Lewisite (BAL) in short (dimercaptopropanol). The dose is 2.5–6 mg/kg of the body weight, administered one to three times a day for 10 days depending upon the severity of the illness. The usual practice is to give 3 injections of 200 mg, on the first day, two on the second and third days, and then one injection daily upto the 10th day in an average case. Inj. lomodex is also useful as blood lavage.
   b. In penicillin allergic reactions, penicillinase, (Neutrapen-P) 800,000 IU in one or two injections gives excellent results.
3. A general supportive treatment. The health of the patient must be maintained till he recovers, with a good nourishing diet, extra vitamins, etc.
4. Symptomatic treatment.
   a. Antihistaminics are useful in controlling itching and urticarial lesions.
   b. Locally, a bland treatment is the rule. The local applications recommended are exactly on the same principle as those advised for similar cutaneous disease.
   c. Steroids are very valuable in combating inflammatory reactions in all acute drug eruptions. Initially, a high dosage is given, e.g. 30–60 mg of prednisolone per day,

and as the reaction comes under control, the dose is slowly reduced. Usually, a short course extending over two to three weeks suffices. The risk of there being a rebound phenomenon with such a course is negligible. In chronic eczematoid and exfoliative dermatoses, the course should be prolonged till the conditions are completely controlled.

d. The authors have used Peristion-N (P) in the treatment of severe drug eruptions quite successfully.
e. In haemorrhagic eruptions, vitamins C, P and K and calcium gluconate are helpful.

B. Prophylactic

There are six golden rules for the prevention of drug eruptions (modified from Sheldon, *et al.*).

1. Before administering or prescribing any drug, ask yourself: "Is the drug necessary?" Quite often some simple common—sense advice can well replace a bottle of physic or lengthy prescription.
2. Be careful about prescribing for topical use, the drug which are being used systemically, e.g., sulphonamides and penicillin.
3 Ask the patient if he has used the drug before, and with what reactions.
4. Do an intradermal sensitivity test, particularly before using serum and penicillin.
5. Use good substitutes for the sensitizing drugs. The patient should be fully informed about the substitute drugs available.
6. Avoid drugs during pregnancy, particularly in the first 12 weeks. Drugs with teratogenic properties are strictly prohibited.

Chapter

22

Bullous Eruptions

INTRODUCTION

Vesiculobullous eruptions are frequently encountered in heterogenous groups of dermatoses either (i) as primary predominant with essential clinical and histopathological features, or (ii) as a transient secondary event at some stage in the natural evolution of many skin diseases, or (iii) as a feature of some drug reaction.

Basic Mechanism

Disturbances of intercellular coherence in the epidermis or dermoepidermal adherence are the main factors. Such disturbances may basically be caused by different ways which include genetically determined defects, cell lysis by various infective or chemical agents, and immunological reactions often involving very selective sites. In the horny layer, the cells are adherent to each other by desmosomes and intercellular cementing substances. In the Malpighian layer, the intercellular adhesiveness depends mainly on functional integrity of epidermal cell with limited function of intercellular bonds allowing upward epidermal cell migration. Dermoepidermal adhesion is mediated by a well-organized system of fibrillar and laminar structures such as basal lamina, lamina lucida, membranes of basal cells with half-desmosomes and anchoring fibrils attached to collagen network of the dermis.

Clinical Approach

A dermatologist's ability to recognize the group of diseases associated with bullous eruptions is of paramount importance in practice, because the prognosis of these diseases varies, the therapeutic approaches differ. Many of the bullous eruptions are definitely known to be of infective, toxic or allergic origin while the others, like pemphigus and dermatitis herpetiformis have autoimmune etiology. In our experience, an increase in incidence is being recorded. Histopathological studies have, somewhat, improved our understanding of this complex group of diseases, and advances in chemotherapy and corticosteroids have, to a great extent, changed the therapeutic outlook.

A bulla is literally a water bubble. It is synonymous with a big bleb or blister containing serous fluid which may become purulent or haemorrhagic. When confronted with a bullous eruption, answers to the following questions must be sought: Is the eruption localized, regional or generalized? Has it symmetrical or asymmetrical distribution? Is it grouped or discrete, polymorphous or monomorphous? Are the mucous membranes involved? Does the bulla occur as such, or on erythematous base? Are they tense or flaccid, with serous or purulent contents? What are the shapes and sizes of the bulla? Is

Nikolsky's sign positive? Are there any accompanying symptoms like itching or pain? Any accompanying crusting or scaling? What kind of a surface does one see when the roof of a bulla is removed? How is the general health of the individual, and are there any toxic symptoms?

Pemphigus Group of Diseases

The term pemphigus, signifying blister, was formerly applied to every disease of the skin presenting bulla, but at present it is reserved only for a particular group of bullous dermatoses presenting with a distinct histopathology characterized by intraepidermal bulla and acantholysis. The latter consists of Malpighian cells showing characteristic degeneration, intercellular fibrils disappear, the cells become spherical with swollen nuclei and condensed cytoplasm at the periphery (Tzanck cells). These cells soon die and their nuclei become pyknotic and fragmented. It has been suggested that pemphigus may be an auto-immune disorder precipitated or caused by infections, drugs, chemicals, etc. with antibodies bound to the intercellular spaces as demonstrated by direct immunofluorescent technique.

There are four clinical types of pemphigus depending upon site of cleavage formation, amount of fluid and the accompanying epidermal changes:

1. *P. vulgaris*—Cleft is deeply situated between the basal layer and the rest of epidermis and there is sufficient fluid to produce the characteristic bulla.
2. *P. vegetans*—Superficial cleft and proliferative changes producing papillomatous masses.
3. *P. foliaceus*—Subcorneal cleft and little fluid.
4. *P. erythematosus*—abortive phase of pemphigus foliaceus.

In India, the incidence of pemphigus group of diseases is fairly high according to the experience of the authors **(Table 22.1)**.

PEMPHIGUS VULGARIS

It is characterized by the appearance of bulla in crops, mild to severe constitutional symptoms and a bad prognosis. It is worldwide in distribution.

Though the incidence is low, it is the most common cause of chronic bullous eruption. Age and sex are no bars to this ailment. However, individuals in the age group 25–50 years are the usual victims. Though the exact cause is unknown, there is some evidence suggesting autoimmunological basis.

Paraneoplastic pemphigus—pemphigus-like lesions are also reported in patients with internal malignancy. Drugs causing pemphigus vulgaris include D-penicillamine, lithium and captopril.

Etiology: It is an autoimmune disease caused by drugs, chemicals and infections. The causes have to be tackled for effective treatment of the disease.

Pathology: The bullae of pemphigus vulgaris are intra-epidermal and irregular in shape with acute lateral margins. They are formed by the separation of acantholytic epidermal cells (Tzanck cells). Acantholytic cells may be in the bullae cavity. Dermis beneath the bulla shows, number of inflammatory cells including a few lymphocytes and plasma cells.

Clinical features: Bullae are most frequently seen in the mouth and on the face, scalp and trunk though they may occur anywhere on the body.

Table 22.1: Classification of bullous eruptions

Etiological	Infants and children 0–15	Young 15–50	Elderly 50–80
Infective	Impetigo neonatorum, bullous syphiloderma, Reiter's disease, generalized herpes and vaccinia, Kaposi's varicelliform eruption	Epidermophytides, bullous impetigo	
Allergic and toxoallergic	Drug eruptions	Drug eruptions, erythema multiforme, extensive disseminated eczema, Lyell's syndrome, pemphigus	Drug eruptions
Unknown etiology	Infantile or juvenile dermatitis herpetiformis.	Herpes gestationis, dermatitis herpetiformis, subcorneal pustular dermatosis	Pemphigus, pemphigoid, erythema multiforme
Genodermatosis	Epidermolysis bullosa, Darier's disease, incontinentia pigmenti acrodermatitis enteropathica, urticaria pigmentosa, congenital porphyrias.	Familial benign pemphigus Porphyria cutanea tarda	
Local	Contact dermatitis, phytophotodermatitis, trauma–cold, heat, chemical burns. Bites–Insect, stings of jellyfish, (at all ages), nettle rash. Nervous disease: Syringomyelia, Morvan's disease, dermatitis artefacta		[At all ages]

The lesions may be few and sparse, or extensive. The eruption is usually symmetrical. When the mucosa of the mouth and the conjunctivae are severely involved, there is greater severity than when only the skin is affected. The lesions usually appear in crops; however, they may cease to occur for long periods. Some of the bullae are tense and others flaccid. They are usually irregular in shape, and generally develop without primary erythema (Fig. 22.1 and Table 22.2).

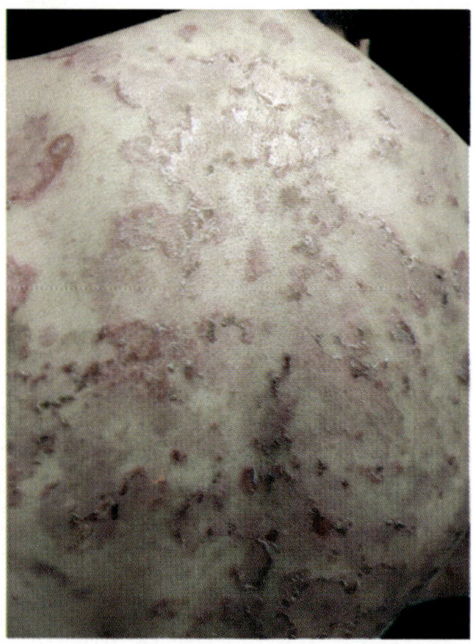

Fig. 22.1: Pemphigus vulgaris

Light pressure on a bulla enlarges it, and the integument will peel off easily under slight or firm sliding pressure. This is called Nikolsky's sign; it signifies splitting of the skin due to acantholysis.

The contents are at first clear and serous, but later may become haemorrhagic or seropurulent. The grouping of the bullae, or ring formation, is not

Table 22.2: Histological classification (after Lever)

I. Intracorneal bullae—Miliarial bulla, e.g. Miliaria crystallina
II. Sub-corneal bullae, e.g. Bullous impetigo, sub-corneal pustular dermatosis
III. Intra-epidermal bullae
  A. Spongiotic bulla, e.g. dermatitis–eczema and pompholyx
  B. Viral bulla, e.g. variola, varicella, herpes simplex and zoster
  C. Acantholytic bullae-Pemphigus (vulgaris, vegetans, foliaceus, erythematosus) and Darier's disease
  D. Miliarial bulla, e.g. *Miliaria rubra*
IV. Subepidermal bulla
  A. Pressure bulla, e.g. bullous pemphigoid, dermatitis herpetiformis, erythema multiforme, epidermolysis bullosa, herpes gestationis, acute pemphigus
  B. Degeneration of basal cell, e.g. lichen planus bullosa
  C. Damage to basal cells and basement membrane, e.g. Burns

uncommon. Usually the bullae rupture, exposing extensive red and raw areas from which considerable loss of serum occurs. Some of them may be covered with crusts. At mucocutaneous junctions and flexures, the denuded areas may develop heaped up crusts and vegetations identical with lesions found in pemphigus vegetans. The disease leaves hyperpigmented scars and stains on healing.

Mucosal lesions: They are encountered practically in all patients. The mouth is most often involved, but denuded areas may be seen on conjunctivae, vagina and nose. Intact bullae are seldom seen. Patients have painful raw areas with detachable shreds of epithelium in the mouth; these may extend to the pharynx and larynx resulting in dysphagia and hoarseness. Lips and gums may be swollen **(Fig. 22.2)**.

The constitutional symptoms are usually slight, the temperature rising when the bullae erupt. However, the absence of pyrexia is a good sign.

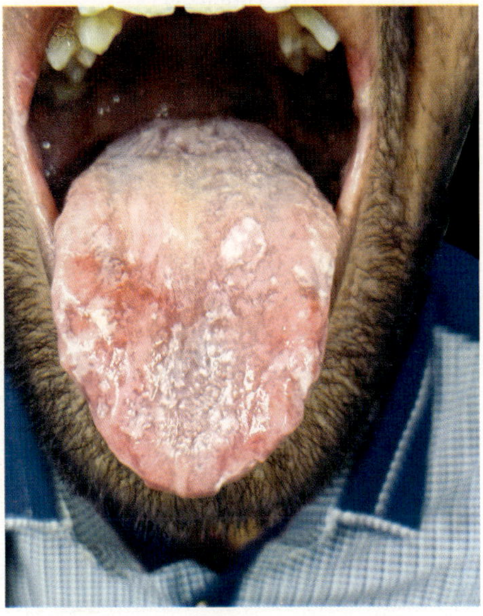

Fig. 22.2: Oral lesions of pemphigus

Hypoproteinemia may result from extensive oozing. Severe hypochromic anaemia and salt depletion are common. With the exception of mild cases, the outcome is usually fatal without treatment. If the throat is affected, there is difficulty in feeding and hence in maintaining the nutrition. There is characteristic offensive odour. There may be leucocytosis and raised blood sedimentation rate.

The disease may be complicated by:
1. Secondary impetigo, ulceration and even gangrene
2. A gastrointestinal upset and debility
3. Lung complications like pneumonia

Any of these complications may be combined with toxaemia and exhaustion which may cause ultimate death.

Diagnosis: Pemphigus may be confused with dermatitis herpetiformis, erythema multiforme and pemphigoid. The following features will serve to distinguish them (**Table 22.3**).

In erythema multiforme bullosum, besides bullae, edematous macules may be seen; lesions are usually bilaterally symmetrical and confined to the extremities; the disease lasts for 3–4 weeks. Bullae develop on erythematous bases.

A drug eruption resulting from the ingestion of phenobarbitone, penicillin, phenolphthalein, iodides and bromides may resemble pemphigus. A history showing that the patient has taken these drugs clinches the diagnosis; moreover, bullous drug rash begins to disappear when the drug is withdrawn.

According to Percival, et al. erythema multiforme bullosum, dermatitis herpetiformis and pemphigus are allied conditions and with time, one condition may easily transform into the other.

The lesion of pemphigus on the buccal mucosa may suggest diphtheria or syphilis. The demonstration of the bacilli in the former, and positive serological tests in the latter, would confirm the diagnosis. In children, pemphigus vulgaris is rare.

Tzanck test: It is carried out by lightly scraping the floor of a bulla after the roof has been removed. The scraped material is spread on a slide, stained with Giemsa's stain, and examined under a microscope for characteristic acantholytic cells. The test is positive in pemphigus vulgaris, foliaceus, vegetans and Senear–Usher syndrome.

Prognosis: It is a chronic disease marked by remissions and exacerbations but may end in death. Corticosteroids, however, can reduce the discomfort caused by the disease, control the clinical lesions. The patient may also can completely recover with treatment. Pyogenic, gastrointestinal and lung complications are serious.

In the case of patients with more mucosal involvement the outlook is more serious than in the case of patients with only cutaneous involvement; furthermore, mouth lesions interfere with nutrition and hence, pose a serious problem.

Treatment: It is rather unsatisfactory because the cause is often unknown and no specific remedy has yet been found.

General treatment: It is along the same lines as the one employed for generalized eczema or exfoliative dermatitis. Good nursing is by far the most essential part of management. The active foci of sepsis should be tackled.

Table 22.3: Differential diagnoses of pemphigus

Differen-tiating	*Differentiating features*	*Dermatitis herpetiformis*	*Pemphigus vulgaris*	*Bullous pemphigoid features*
1.	Age of onset	20–40 years	30–60 years	60–80 years
2.	Itching	Often intense	Usually mild	Common
3.	Arrangement of lesions and their distribution	Mucous membranes are unaffected. Lesions occur in groups. Bilateral and symmetrical distribution on the forearms, scapular region and lower back	Mucous membranes are affected. Asymmetrical distribution. Lesions occur mainly on the face, scalp, trunk and neck	Mucosal involvement rare
4.	Nature of lesions	Polymorphic, erythema present	Large bullae without erythema	Bullae tense, grouped, sometimes haemorrhagic Erythematous plaques
5.	Nikolsky's sign	Negative	Positive	Usually negative
6.	General health	Usually unaffected	Deteriorates gradually	Fair usually
7.	Application of KI (50%) ointment	Applied to healed lesions produces flare up	No effect	Negative
8.	Histopathological features (a) Bullae	Sub-epidermal. Prickle cells normal. Lateral borders of bullae are rounded	Infra-epidermal Acantholysis and degenerative changes in epidermal cells Lateral borders of bullae are acute	Sub-epidermal bulla with acantholysis
	(b) Tzanck cells	Only eosinophils, and a few normal epidermal cells	Typical acantholytic (Tzanck) cell present	Negative
9.	Prognosis	Chronic disease with longevity unaffected	Bad but has improved with corticosteroids	Bad only in people with mucosal involvement
10.	Treatment	Dapsone and sulphapyridine	Corticosteroids cyclophosphamide	Steroids. Occasionally responds to dapsone

The patient must be protected from cold. The diet should be nutritious to maintain his strength. When blisters are present in the mouth, the patient has difficulty in mastication and swallowing. When this is the case, he should be given bland fluids or a semi-solid diet. Causes like focal sepsis, use of chemicals, drugs and food additives should be eradicated. Their proper tackling may cure the case permanently.

Drug Therapy

1. Broad-spectrum antibiotics. Doxycycline, tetracycline, cephalosporidin, cloxacillin, ampicillin are worth trying. The antibiotic should never be given for long periods

because of serious side-effects; furthermore, it should be supplemented with multivitamins.

2. ACTH and/or prednisone derivatives invariably exert a beneficial effect on the bullous lesions and general well -being. Although lifesaving in the majority of cases, they are not curative. Buccal lesions do not respond so well as cutaneous lesions. Cases do show recurrence of stray bullous eruptions even after prolonged periods of remission. Opinions regarding dosage schedule vary; however, it is wiser to start with about 30–80 mg of prednisolone. A prolonged therapy with these drugs is essential and there is always the danger of formidable side-reactions. However, the introduction of triamcinolone and dexamethasone has made the long-term administration of these drugs comparatively free from undesirable side-effects. The dosage of prednisone is gradually reduced in a step-ladder manner till it is finally withdrawn. Usually the drug has to be given in small maintenance doses continuously to prevent relapses. 20–80 units of ACTH may be given in selected cases. Dapsone (P) 100 mg daily is also useful in isolated cases.
3. Cyclophosphamide (Endoxan) or azathioprine (Imuran) in doses of 25–50 mg daily has been used with benefit in selected cases.
4. 250–300 cc of whole blood or plasma transfusion or plasmapheresis. Injection of gold (sodium thiomalate) are beneficial in some cases.
5. Lomodex (P) has been successfully used to reduce toxaemia. It is given as intravenous drip, 500 cc in one or two instalments.
6. Newer biologicals have been shown to give encouraging results.

Pulse therapy for pemphigus includes high dose of prednisolone and cyclophosphamide given in monthly cycles.

Local treatment: Gentian violet 1/2% or silver nitrate lotion is applied on bullae and raw areas. As the lesions start to dry, pastes and creams may be employed. On dry lesions, sterilized vaseline gauze dressing is recommended. The mouth is washed twice a day with Condy 's fluid; lotio gentian violet or boroglycerine is painted afterwards. The eyes must be cleaned with boric acid, and argyrol drops or hydrocortisone eye drops used to prevent keratitis and other eye complications.

Pemphigus Foliaceus

It is a rare chronic type of pemphigus. Adults between 30 and 50 years of age are the usual victims. The exact cause is not known. It may occasionally follow an attack of pemphigus vulgaris.

Clinical features: Characteristic features are flaccid bullae and exfoliating scales. Usually the flaccid bullae develop first on the face; slowly the disease spreads symmetrically till the whole of the integument is covered with bullae. The latter rupture to produce a moist, red, raw and oedematous surface and flake-like plaques of imperfectly keratinized, horny cells. The appearance resembles chronic exfoliative dermatitis except for the presence of flaccid bullae and a moist raw surface. A slight serous exudation often continues to take place giving rise to a peculiar factor. Subsequently, the exfoliative character of the condition predominates. The course of the disease is marked by remissions and exacerbations. The conjunctivae and mucosae may be affected. The scalp may also be involved. It is covered with moist, yellowish scales. The hair may fall. Pyrexia and diarrhoea may develop. However, death may follow an intercurrent infection.

Histopathology: Bulla is high up in the epidermis. Subcorneal cleavage without actual visible bulla formation may occur. Acantholytic cells may be seen loose in the bulla fluid and at its edges. Later there may be acanthosis, hyperkeratosis and parakeratosis. Dermis may show chronic cellular infiltrate in which eosinophils may predominate.

Differential diagnosis: It is made from exfoliative dermatitis, pemphigus vulgaris and generalized eczema. Demonstration of Nikolsky's sign, flaccid bullae and acantholytic cells help in establishing the diagnosis.

Course is chronic (slower than pemphigus vulgaris) and the ultimate prognosis is bad.

Treatment: It is similar to that employed for pemphigus vulgaris. Besides corticosteroids and a tetracycline, endoxan and gold have also been used with benefit.

Causative factors must be properly tackled.

PEMPHIGUS VEGETANS

This is the rarest variety of pemphigus. Individuals of any age group may be affected; however, it usually commences between the ages of 30 and 40. It is more common in females than in males.

Clinical features: The onset is insidious. The initial lesions, in the form of broken bullae, appear on the mucosa of the lips, mouth or nose; later, they develop in the axillae, groins and sometimes on the other parts of the body. When ruptured, the bullae develop into moist, superficial ulcers. The ulcers undergo proliferative changes producing fungoid vegetations with malodorous discharge. The vegetations may also seem to arise *de novo* on the normal skin. Nikolsky's sign is often positive. The constitutional disturbances are minimal, and the disease has a tendency towards long remission. If untreated, the disease becomes widespread and transforms into the vulgaris variety.

Diagnosis: This condition has to be differentiated from a fungating iodide eruption, syphilitic condylomata and pyoderma vegetans. Differentiation from pyoderma vegetans can sometimes be difficult, the main differentiating feature being the demonstration of flaccid bullae.

Treatment: It is along the same lines as that for pemphigus vulgaris. However, the vegetations should be kept disinfected with local antiseptics. Potassium permanganate baths and silver nitrate 5–10% are helpful. Broad-spectrum antibiotics like ampicillin and erythromycin should be given. X-ray therapy has been reported to inhibit formation of vegetations and, as such, is a valuable adjunct to treatment. In pemphigus vegetans, ACTH and corticosteroids produce a universally favourable response.

PEMPHIGUS ERYTHEMATOSUS

Synonym: Senear–Usher syndrome.

It is an unusual form of pemphigus, presenting features of lupus erythematosus and seborrhoeic dermatitis at different stages. The disease runs a benign course; however, it may later show manifestations of pemphigus vulgaris or foliaceus and end fatally. These varieties may sometimes, though rarely, precede rather than follow pemphigus erythematosus.

Clinical features: The early lesions which are erythematous and crusted, appear on the nose, cheeks and ears, resembling lupus erythematosus both in their location and appearance. However, the lesions exhibit the Nikolsky's sign and a moist, raw surface when the crust is removed. The greasy crust may indicate seborrhoeic dermatitis. These lesions may appear along with bullae on the chest and extremities. The eruption is, to some extent, symmetrical in distribution. Its course is chronic, punctuated by remissions and intermissions. However, the general health of the patient is not affected. Some patients complain of intense itching. The Nikolsky's sign is positive.

Histological picture is like that of pemphigus foliaceus. In older lesions, hyperkeratosis, dyskeratosis and degenerative changes in the cells of stratum granulosum are pronounced. Bullae, if present, are subcorneal in contrast to sub-epidermal bullae of DLE.

This variety of pemphigus is rather resistant to therapy. However, corticosteroids, and aureomycin do help. Systemic therapy is withheld so long as the lesions are localized. Topical betamethasone cream is useful as such or with occlusive dressing in localized cases.

BENIGN PEMPHIGUS OF MUCOUS MEMBRANES

Synonym: Ocular pemphigus, cicatricial pemphigoid.

It is a vary rare condition, and is characterized by the occurrence of a bullous eruption, denuded areas and scarring in the eyes and the mouth, pharynx, nose, vulva and anus with or without minimal involvement of the integument. The bullae occur at epidermo-dermal junction with marked inflammatory reaction and subsequent fibrosis.

The condition is associated with conjunctivitis, with the formation of fibrous adhesions between the palpebral and ocular surfaces, or between the upper and lower palpebral and ocular surfaces, eventually leading to blindness. Vesicles appear on the oral mucosa, coalesce and leave extensive raw areas. The vermilion surface of the lips is spared. The formation of adhesions narrows the oral orifice. Lesions may occur in the mouth, nose or throat. The disease runs a chronic course with remissions and exacerbations.

FAMILIAL BENIGN CHRONIC PEMPHIGUS

Synonym: Hailey–Hailey disease.

It is a heredo-familial disease with basic disturbance in the form of genetically determined fragility of the epidermis resulting in acantholysis, when the skin is subjected to shearing stress. It is autosomal-dominant. Family history is positive in one third of the cases.

Clinical features: It is characterized by vesicular or bullous lesions, which tend to spread peripherally and on rupturing leave behind amber-coloured crusts. On healing, they leave pigmentation without scarring. The lesions occur at flexural or friction sites, e.g. the neck, collar bone, axillary folds, groins, perianal and genital areas and the thighs. Patients usually complain of chaffing at the sites of pressure from clothes. The condition is benign, persisting for many years with occasional remissions which may have no bearing on the treatment or the season. However, exacerbations have occasionally been observed in summer.

Pathology: The histopathological features of the disease are characteristic. There are slits in the basal layer of the epidermis, containing rounded prickle cells resembling corps ronds of Darier's disease.

Treatment is unsatisfactory: Calamine ointment and 1% ichthammol, 0.1% pyragallol may be applied locally. Antibiotics are administered in the phase of secondary infection. Clothing should be soft, smooth and loose. Systemic use of corticosteroids and antibiotics may be effective; they are withheld in mild cases. Excision of involved areas and split thickness grafting have been claimed beneficial in many cases.

BULLOUS PEMPHIGOID

It is considered to be a chronic variant of erythema multiforme. In the absence of established etiology, there is some confusion and controversy about this clinical condition, which is thought to be of auto-immunologic origin.

Clinical features: It is a disease of old age (50–80 years), though cases in younger age groups have also been seen. It is characterized by large, tense, dome-shaped bullae, often preceded by irritating erythematous patches or gyrate urticarial plaques **(Fig. 22.3)**.

Usually, the groins, lower abdomen, thighs, flexor aspects of the upper limbs and axillae show the largest number of lesions. The eruption may remain localized on one region of the body, commonly on the lower limbs, for 2–3 months before becoming widespread. Buccal mucosa is only rarely affected; it is hardly the site of the first lesion in contrast to pemphigus vulgaris. Characteristically, the bullae remain intact for several days and their contents may become blood-stained. After rupture, the healing is usually rapid and there is no tendency for the denuded areas to spread peripherally. General health is usually unaffected.

In recent years many systemic drugs have been found to induce or trigger bullous pemphigoid or eruption resembling bullous pemphigoid (BP-like eruption). These are frusemide, ibuprofen and other NSAID drugs, pencillamine, pencillin and its derivatives. Certain topical medication can also precipitate bullous pemphigoid, i.e. topical fluorouracil, psoralen, ultraviolet-A (PUVA) therapy.

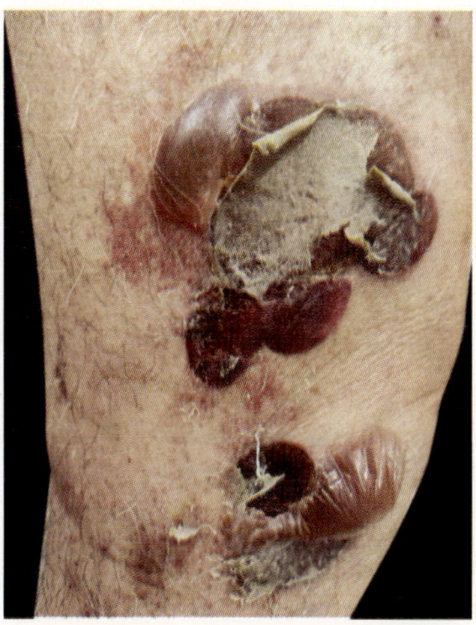

Fig. 22.3: Bullous pemphigoid

Course: It usually runs a benign course but may be fatal in elderly, debilitated people. Some patients may have a single attack persistent for weeks while others have recurrent attacks. Mortality rate is low, especially after the advent of corticosteroids.

Histopathology: Subepidermal pressure bullae without any acantholysis are characteristic. With regeneration of the epidermis at the floor of the bullae, intra-epidermal location may be come across. Usually, the bulla contains a network of fibrin with only a few inflammatory cells. Upper dermis shows oedema with little inflammatory infiltrate.

Treatment: It mainly consists of steroid therapy; initial and maintenance dose is less than in pemphigus vulgaris. Occasionally, pemphigoid responds to sulphone and sulphapyridine. Generally, nutrition of the patient must be maintained. Local treatment consists of application of soothing astringent lotion.

PEMPHIGUS ACUTUS

It is a rare dermatosis. Butchers, pathologists and others engaged in handling dead bodies are the usual victims. Acute pemphigus can also complicate a traumatic wound or vaccination. Various organisms have been blamed for causing the disease including diplococci and the virus of foot and mouth disease. In reality, however, the exact causation is still not established

Clinical features: Onset of the illness is sudden. An infected wound or a minor injury may be the only prodromata. Often, these lesions heal before pemphigus develops. The illness is ushered in by malaise, lassitude and rigor, followed by sudden rise of temperature to about 102–104°F. Bullae of varying sizes appear, initially on the fingers, in the mouth or neck, spreading rapidly particularly to the flexor surfaces of the joints. Occasionally, the bullae are arranged in a linear fashion. Their diameter ranges from one to several centimetres. They may be flaccid or tense and contain serous or haemorrhagic fluid. The bullae may rupture leaving raw surfaces. An extensive surface of the skin may thus become denuded. Severe cases manifest haemorrhagic lesions with purulent exudate on the raw surface, emitting a foetid odour. The conjunctival, oral, pharyngeal and mucosal surface of the rest of the gastrointestinal tract and trachea may be affected. Leucocytosis, with a total count of upto 20,000 or more, and 65–75% polymorphonuclear leucocytes is commonly found. Histologically, bullae are subepidermal and not due to acantholysis. Dermis shows polymorpho-nuclear infiltrate.

Differential diagnosis: It is made from the bullous type of erythema multiforme, impetigo contagiosa and smallpox. Erythema multiforme manifests a milder constitutional disturbance; the eruption is polymorphous, being distributed symmetrically on the extremities. Widely distributed impetigo contagiosa may resemble pemphigus acutus, but it can be differentiated from the latter in that impetigo contagiosa is not associated with constitutional disturbance; the bullae, being smaller than those of pemphigus, dry up to form a characteristic 'honey-coloured crust'. A similar eruption has also been seen in bullous drug eruptions resulting from penicillin, sulphonamide and Irgapyrin (P).

Prognosis: The disease runs a rapid course of a few weeks, and most often, terminates fatally through exhaustion and toxaemia. About 50–70% of patients die within 3–4 weeks. Occasionally patients recover completely, but the disease leaves behind considerable pigmentation. Very rarely, does this acute condition lapse into chronic pemphigus (Andrews).

Treatment: A broad-spectrum antibiotic, like ciprofloxacin should be administered in high doses. Corticosteroids, particularly prednisolone in doses of 40–80 mg is useful. General nursing and symptomatic treatment is of paramount importance. Utmost care should be taken to keep the skin as clean as possible. Locally, mild antiseptics like gentian violet jelly should be used to prevent secondary infection.

LYELL'S SYNDROME

Synonym: Toxic epidermal necrolysis.

It is characterized by acute onset, epidermal separation similar to scalding, flaccid bullae, strongly positive Nikolsky's sign and severe constitutional symptoms. Early lesions are chiefly localized at muco-cutaneous junctions. Attack of fever may accompany the onset.

Laboratory findings are unremarkable. Degenerative toxic changes of nuclear substance of the leucocytes have been noted in the peripheral blood. Usually there is leucocytosis.

Etiology is attributed to some drug intolerance-allergic or hyperergic reaction to phenacetin, barbiturates, penicillin, sulphonamides and primidon. Others attribute it to some toxic factors like staphylococcal infection. It affects all age groups.

Histopathology resembles severe erythema multiforme excepting that necrosis of the epidermis is extensive and diffuse in nature.

Treatment consists in hospitalization, elimination of the cause, high doses of steroids and management of infection with antibiotics.

SUBCORNEAL PUSTULAR DERMATOSIS

It is a chronic, pustular dermatosis, seen mainly in young and middle-aged women. Since it was first described by Sneddon and Wilkinson, several cases have been described all over the world.

Clinical features: Disease occurs chiefly on the abdomen and back in the form of superficial sterile pustules arranged in annular or serpiginous pattern. Mucosal involvement is rare.

Histology: Subcorneal vesicles containing polymorphonuclear cells is the characteristic feature; acantholysis is usually absent. There may be surrounding spongiosis. Upper dermis shows dilated capillaries surrounded by polymorphonuclear cells and a few eosinophils.

Treatment is with sulphones and sulphapyridine. Response to corticosteroids is poor. Prognosis is fair.

CHRONIC BULLOUS DERMATOSIS OF CHILDHOOD

Children of pre-school age are the sufferers from this benign, nonhereditary uncommon disorder, a separate and distinct entity from bullous pemphigoid, erythema multiforme and dermatitis herpetiformis. The etiology of this is unknown.

The disease clinically resembles adult bullous pemphigoid seen usually on lower trunk, inner thighs and pelvic region. Pruritus may be severe or may be absent. Spontaneous remission usually occurs in 2–3 years of onset.

The disease may be responsive to sulphones or sulphapyridine. Some patients need systemic steroid therapy.

FOGO SELVAGEM

Synonym: Brazilian pemphigus.

It is endemic in certain parts of Brazil and may affect several members of the family. It resembles pemphigus foliaceus clinically and histologically. Age of onset is below 30.

Its occurrence in certain areas and its affection of many members of a family led to the belief that it is an infectious disease, but no organism has been isolated.

DERMATITIS HERPETIFORMIS

Synonym: Duhring's disease.

It is a chronic, relapsing, pruriginous dermatosis characterized by the appearance of polymorphic lesions, grouped in clusters. It does not affect the health of the patient.

Etiology: The exact cause is still unknown. Although no age group is immune from this disease, it most frequently affects young adults, being more common in males than females. The patients are extremely susceptible to blister formation when potassium iodide is administered orally.

Pathology: In dermatitis herpetiformis, changes occur primarily in the dermis. They consist of vascular dilatation, oedema and cellular infiltration with a predominance of eosinophils and lymphocytes. The bullae are invariably subepidermal with rounded lateral borders. There is deposit of lgA at the epidermo-dermal junction.

Clinical features: The onset of the disease may be sudden, or may be ushered in by a brief period of malaise, burning sensation in the skin, intense pruritus and occasional neuralgic pains. The eruption is usually polymorphic by nature, and has a characteristic bilaterally symmetrical distribution. The common sites of choice are the scapular regions, sacral region, buttocks, abdomen and forearms. Burning rather than itching is frequent. The eruption usually develops in crops. The general health of the patient remains otherwise unaffected. The eruption usually consists of three components viz., vesicles or small bullae, reddish plaques and pustules.

Vesicles and small bullae: They may be isolated but are often multiple, and arranged in clusters like herpetic vesicles. Bullae may crop up on an erythematous base or on healthy skin. It takes a few days for involution to take place in the lesions. The intensity of itching diminishes after the bullae have ruptured.

Reddish plaques: They are infiltrated, erythematous macules, and may resemble urticarial lesions. They are intensely itchy.

Pustules: Rarely primary in nature, the pustules generally result from secondary infection of vesicles. However, grouped lesions of various types may occur at one time in the same patient. In a full-blown case, vesiculo-bullous lesions predominate.

Involution in the primary lesions produces scales and crusts. Scratching results in excoriations. Found in the late stage are pigmentation and groups of scars. Pigmented scars, *per se* on the lumbo-sacral region are characteristic. The mucosae are involved in rare cases of marked severity. The lesions spare the hands and the feet, usually also the face. The serum from the bullae shows predominance of eosinophils. The blood may also reveal a high eosinophil count. A relationship between DH and coeliac disease has been reported by many authors. Enteropathy is observed in about 70% of the cases and improves steadily on gluten-free diet.

Juvenile dermatitis herpetiformis: It is a special type occurring in children. Starts at about the age of 4 years and clears up by puberty. It is more common in males than females. Lesions are often bullous, non-pruritic and appear on the genitalia. It does not respond to dapsone or sulphapyridine. According to many authorities, it is a type of Juvenile pemphigoid.

Diagnosis: It is based upon:

1. Polymorphous lesions, frequently with grouped vesicles.
2. The symmetrical distribution.
3. The typical distribution on the lumbo-sacral region, scapular region, forearms and abdomen.
4. The fact that the general health of the patient is unaffected.
5. The recurrent nature of the eruption.
6. Intense itching.
7. Typical hyperpigmented scars.
8. Ready response to gluten-free diet, sulphones and sulphapyridine.
9. Typical sub-epidermal bulla histologically.

The disease presents such a characteristic clinical pattern that diagnosis does not present any difficulty. However, differentiation from certain cases of pemphigus and erythema multiforme may prove difficult, and prolonged observation if often required to reach a definite conclusion. The differential diagnosis is made from the following:

Scabies: Multiple cases of pruritus in the family; nocturnal pruritus; itching on the genitals and hands; and presence of burrows.

Erythema multiforme: This is an acute condition of short duration. Pruritus is not as intense as in dermatitis herpetiformis. The lesions are rosy in colour, scattered and not grouped. Constitutional symptoms are more marked. Distribution is more on the periphery of the limbs.

Pemphigus vulgaris: Some authors (Percival, et al.) consider dermatitis herpetiformis (DH) as a variant of pemphigus and erythema multiforme; this view is not accepted universally. The differentiating features between the two conditions have already been dealt with in the previous pages. Some cases of erythema multiforme and dermatitis herpetiformis do end up as pemphigus.

Prognosis: There are good prospects of longevity. But the condition is chronic, marked by a fluctuating course. Some cases clear up rapidly on the removal of the septic focus; others continue for years till the disease wears out or terminates in pemphigus.

Treatment: It consists in:

A. General management and the removal of active septic foci. During the acute phase of the disease, the patient should be advised complete rest.

B. The following drugs help in the treatment:

Dapsone (P) DDS 50–100 mg daily is very effective. It produces dramatic clearance of the lesions and subsidence of itching within a few days. However, vitamin B and iron should also be administered simultaneously.

Sulphonamides: The majority of patients show excellent response to sulphonamides in general and sulphapyridine in particular. It is given in doses of 1–3 g daily.

ACTH and cortisone: Reports on the efficacy of ACTH and cortisone are hopelessly conflicting. Its use should, therefore, be considered after other methods have failed. The same applies to broad-spectrum antibiotics. Tetracyclines have been found effective in the treatment of bullous pemphigoid in a dosage of 2 g daily. Some workers have reported good results with colchicine.

C. Local application. Antipruritic lotion, like 1% phenol in calamine lotion, is helpful.

HERPES GESTATIONIS

Regarded as a variant of dermatitis herpetiformis, this is a rare specific dermatosis occurring in pregnancy or puerperium. The exact etiology of this condition is unknown; but pregnancy is regarded as a precipitating factor, an auto-immune progesterone dermatosis. Oral contraceptives may precipitate an attack.

Clinical features: The onset of the illness usually in the 4th or 5th month of pregnancy may be acute or insidious. The disease is characterized by successive outbreaks of polymorphous cutaneous lesions occurring in clusters. They are roughly symmetrical in distribution, and are associated with intense itching and pigmentation is usually slight. Oral lesions may occur. The eruption may be generalized; however, the face is rarely involved. The disease runs a long course with remissions and exacerbations, often resolving soon after delivery. The disease tends to recur with increasing severity and longer duration in subsequent pregnancies. Occasionally, the disease recurs with each menstrual period. The patients are sensitive to iodides and bromides.

The blood may contain numerous eosinophils. Ultrastructurally, the level of splitting occurs within the lamina lucida.

The skin biopsy shows a sub-epidermal bulla and a dermal inflammatory infiltrate.

Course: The outlook for the mother is usually good. Abortion and stillbirths occur frequently, and foetal mortality is high. Sometimes, though rarely, herpetic lesions may occur in infants born of such patients. After or just before delivery, there is rapid clearance of the lesions.

Treatment: No specific remedy for this disease is as yet known. Progesterone injections 10–20 mg weekly may give the most amount of relief. Pyridoxine in doses of 50–200 mg daily has been tried and given good results. Nicotinic acid may be given along with pyridoxine. Restraint should be exercised in the use of antibiotics and corticosteroids. A therapeutic abortion or caesarian operation is indicated only if the disease is severe and beyond control, and if the patient develops suicidal tendencies. Local treatment consists of 1% phenol in calamine cream.

The main line of treatment is prednisolone in a dosage of 40–60 mg/day. Other drugs that can be used are Daspone and immuno-suppressive agents, but the latter drug should not be used during pregnancy and in mothers breastfeeding their offsprings. Plasmapheresis is indicated in most severe cases.

Chapter

23

Anomalies of Pigmentation

PHYSIOLOGY

Pigmentation of the human skin is dependent upon the local production of melanin by melanocytes (also called melanoblasts) which are dendritic branching cells interspersed between the basal cells of the epidermis. Melanophores are the dermal histiocytes which carry small quantities of the pigment shed by the epidermal melanocytes. In mammalian animals, the pigment melanin occurs in large quantities in both the epidermis and dermis. As we descend the tree of evolution, nucleo-proteins and carotinoids become responsible for pigmentation. Credit goes to the work of Bruno Bloch for elucidating the mode of melanin formation. According to him, melanin is formed from tyrosine through the intermediary stage of di-oxy-phenylalanine (dopa in short). Melanocytes contain enzymes which convert tyrosine into melanin in the following manner:

$$\text{Tyrosine} \xrightarrow{\text{Tyrosinase}} \text{Dopa} \xrightarrow[\text{Copper}]{\text{Dopa oxidase}} \text{Melanin}$$

$$\text{Reduced melanin} \rightleftharpoons \text{Oxidized melanin (Dark)}$$

The ultrastructure of melanocyte and melanin formation has extensively been studied by Fitzpatrick, et al. From the Golgi body of the cell arises a vacuole-like premelanosome which incorporates zinc and becomes melanosome. The latter becomes heavy and loses tyrosinase activity to be transformed into melanin granule.

The quantity of melanin in the skin varies from individual to individual, and race to race, and also, from time to time. People living in temperate and cold climates tend to have fairer (lightly pigmented) skins than those living in sunny and warmer places. Blondes have fairer skins than brunettes.

Melanin formation is physiologically under the control of melanocyte-stimulating hormone (MSH) of the pituitary gland. The sun, UV rays, X-rays, photosensitizing agents, etc. stimulate melanin formation, while ascorbic acid tends to reduce it. Special dopa and tyrosine staining and also tissue culture have helped us to understand the mechanism of pigmentation in pigmentary disorders.

MELANODERMA (Melanosis or Melanoderma—Increased Formation of Melanin)

Causes

A. *Generalized melanosis*, extensive, diffuse or generalized excessive pigmentation generally due to a systemic, internal cause.

1. Endocrine disorders—Addison's disease, thyrotoxicosis, Simmond's cachexia, ACTH administration.

2. Chronic wasting diseases—cachexia, malaria, kala-azar, tuberculosis, reticulosis, carcinomatosis, anaemia.
3. Nutritional—Pellagra (refer to Chapter 25).
4. Toxic melanosis (Synonym: Melano-dermatitis toxica)—idiopathic, heavy metals like arsenic, gold, silver and drugs like phenothiazines, tranquillizers, Ledermycin (P), sulphonamides, quinine, mepacrine etc. (refer to Chapter 21).
5. Metabolic—Porphyria, ochronosis, haemochromatosis (refer to Chapter 25).

B. *Localized melanosis:* Localized hyperpigmentation is localized or distributed in selective regions. It is usually due to an exogenous cause.
1. Post-inflammatory, particularly following a chronic skin disease or irritation--eczema, tinea cruris, fixed drug eruption, lichen planus, scleroderma, Vagabond's disease and healed lesions of pemphigus vulgaris and photo-sensitization dermatoses like Riehl's melanosis, Berloque dermatitis, parship or babchi* dermatitis.
2. Physiological—sun-tan, heat-tan (refer to Chapter 8).
3. Naevi-naevus pigmentosus (pigmented birth mark), Mongolian spot, urticaria pigmentosa (refer to Chapter 27).
4. Freckles, lentigines, senile lentigenes and chloasma.
5. Miscellaneous: Acanthosis nigricans, incontinentia pigmenti.

Melanosis caused by excessive formation of melanin should be distinguished from:
1. Deposition of blood pigments as in bruising, haematoma, purpura; Schamberg's disease, chronic venous congestion, ephelis ab igne.
2. Deposition of extraneous substances, e.g. heavy metals like lead, silver, arsenic, carotinemia. mepacrine, xanthomatosis (refer to Chapter 25) and tattooing (cosmetic or therapeutic or accidental as in coal miners or resulting from explosions).

Blood pigments and heavy metals can be demonstrated in the skin by different histological techniques, by special stains, the dark-field examination, the spectroscopic and chemical methods. Clinically, acute pigmentation due to deposition of blood pigments must be differentiated from melanosis; in most cases it is easy, because in the former, the colour is bright-red changing to dark-red and then to bluish hue, and thereafter slowly fading away, unless of course, the disease process becomes chronic and haemosiderin deposits take place.

The causes of pigmentation in the mouth are:
1. Addison's disease, Peutz–Jegher's syndrome.
2. Arsenic, other heavy metals and myleran.
3. Cachexia, anaemia particularly pernicious anaemia.
4. Melanoglossia—black hairy tongue.
5. Local irritation, bad oral hygiene, tobacco chewing, bidi smoking.

When studying the anomalies of pigmentation, the following clinical points must be specifically considered: The distribution; the course; the duration; the type of pigmentation, for instance the size, shape and colour; the presence of any associated cutaneous or systemic disease.

*It is a Hindi equivalent for *Psoralea corylifolia*. Indigenous practitioners use it to treat vitiligo.

Later, histological techniques may be employed to establish the etiology. Only conditions important from the dermatological point of view are discussed in this book; for other conditions, reference should be made to textbooks dealing with internal medicine.

FRECKLES

Synonym: Ephelides.

Freckles are a very common anomaly. They are either discrete, grouped or confluent pigmented macules caused by excessive, localized formation of melanin; the size of a freckle, however, varies. It can be anywhere between the size of a pin-head and a split pea (sometimes larger). Freckles occur symmetrically on the exposed parts of the body like the face, neck and forearms; if other parts of the body are exposed, as for instance in sunbathing or when sleeveless blouses are worn, they may also be affected **(Fig. 23.1)**. White people, blondes, red-heads and people with delicate, fair skins are prone to freckles. Hence, dark-skinned people like Indians and Africans rarely develop freckles.

The colour of freckles varies from light-brown to dark-brown, fading when the skin is protected from the sun. For this reason, freckles are most noticeable in the Indian winter and the continental summer. They do not occur on the palms of the hands and the soles of the feet, nor do they become malignant. They begin to appear from the age of 7 and 8, and may persist through life.

Differential Diagnosis

It is made from the following:

Lentigines: They occur on all parts of the body, especially the covered parts like the genitalia, trunk and thighs. They are darker than freckles, do not fade on protection or increase on exposure to the sun. Starting in infancy, they persist for years.

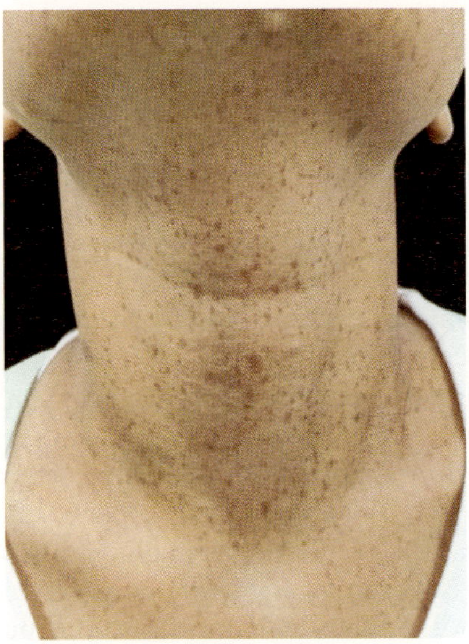

Fig. 23.1: Freckles

Lentigo senilis: They are referred to by the lay people as. 'liver spots'. They occur on the senile skin (at the age of 40–50 or later) as irregular-shaped, pigmented macules slowly increasing in number and size. They are usually found on the exposed parts of the body especially the dorsum of the hands and sometimes, though rarely, the face and the ankles. They are occasionally familial. They never turn malignant.

The other conditions which should be distinguished from freckles are pigmented naevi, xeroderma pigmentosum, etc. **(Table 23.1)**.

Treatment

It is unsatisfactory. It consists mainly in:

1. Protection of the skin from the sun by sunshades or antiactinic creams or lotions, e.g. Paraminol (P), Sol-bar (P), calamine lotion with 5% para-amino benzoic acid, newer physical and chemical sunscreens.
2. Rubbing in an ointment containing 5–10% ammoniated mercury to produce mild exfolfation of freckles, thus lightening the colour. Hydroquinone ointment (2–4%) is also recommended as for chloasma.
3. Hydrogen peroxide application to freckles.
4. Plastic planing has given good results. It is indicated in cases where freckles are a cosmetic blemish and cause psychological embarrassment; otherwise, no treatment is usually indicated. Cauterization-electrical, cryosurgery or chemical should be avoided as it causes scarring which is worse than the original defect.

MELASMA (CHLOASMA)

The Hindustani name is '*Chhaiaan*'. It is a very common pigmentary disorder usually confined to the face. To begin with, it shows as light-brown pigmented patches on the cheeks; it later spreads to the nose, the centre of forehead, the area above the eyebrows, the upper lip and the chin. In early cases; the patches are discrete, bilaterally symmetrical, light mottling **(Fig. 23.2)**.

As the disorder progresses, the patches become confluent, and the whole of the face including even the upper neck may assume a mask-like pigmentation.

Etiology: Common known causes are:

1. Pregnancy, ovarian and uterine disorders. Chloasma due to pregnancy disappears after delivery, but persists in some cases, particularly when it follows an abortion or miscarriage. In a few cases, it has followed the use of oral contraceptive pills, use of Copper T and other contraceptive devices, irregular and scanty periods.
2. Hepatic and gastrointestinal disorders. Chronic diarrhoea, dysentery, colitis and liver disorders frequently account for chloasma.
3. Nutritional. Diet deficient in animal fats, proteins, vegetables and fruits.
4. Cosmetics—powder and creams containing volatile oils, aniline dyes and perfumes may produce chloasma due to their photosensitizing action (phytophoto-dermatitis-Berloque).

Chloasma is more common in women than in men. Middle-aged people are selectively affected, though chloasma can occur at any age between 15 and 50 years. In the majority of people, one or the other of the above-mentioned causes may be found to account for chloasma; in others, no cause can be established. In a few cases, chronic sinusitis and

Table 23.1: Differential diagnosis

Differentiating features	*Freckles*	*Lentigines*	*Senile lentigines 'Liver spots'*	*Pigmented Naevi*	*Xeroderma pigmentosum*
1. Age of onset	7–8 years	0–2 years	40–45 years	At birth or later	0–10 years rarely later
2. Sites	Exposed parts, usually bilateral and symmetrical	Covered parts, bilateral and symmetrical	Dorsum of hands bilateral and symmetrical	Any part. Localized and asymmetrical	Exposed parts especially the face, hands and feet. mostly symmetrical
3. Colour and other clinical features	Discrete, grouped or confluent; light-brown or dark in colour; size pinhead to split pea	Darker than freckles	Irregular shaped, dark in colour	Macules or plaque or papulo-nodule Different colours	Pigmentation, telangiectasia, atrophy, keratosis and epitheliomas
4. Effect of exposures to sun and protection	Increase on exposure; decrease on protection	Nil	Nil	Nil	Aggravation on exposure to sun
5. Malignancy	Never	Very rarely	Nil	Can become malignant	+++
6. Histology	Melanin pigment increased	Thickening of epidermis, rete pegs↑, Dopa +ve cells increased	Hyperkeratosis, rete pegs↑, Dopa +ve cell increased	Naevus cells	Different features according to clinical lesion
7. Any other features	Familial, affects fair coloured people	Indefinite	Familial	Nil	Familial

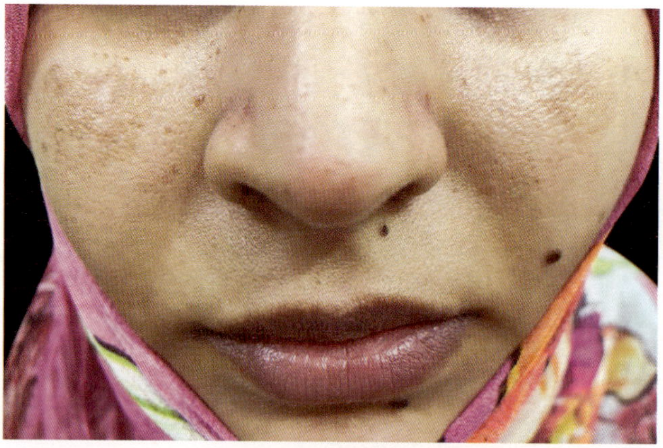

Fig. 23.2: Melasma

persistent seborrhoea may account for the condition. In the authors' view, chloasma is an outward expression of an internal disorder; the latter demands correction while the former draws attention.

Treatment: It is unsatisfactory in cases where the cause is unknown or beyond correction. Some cases disappear spontaneously; others show exacerbations or recessions from time to time. General health of the patient must be improved. Good nourishing diet and regular exercise are helpful. Occasionally serum gonadotrophins may help.

The main treatment is along with same lines as for freckles. Besides, vitamin C and B complex by mouth, short-term and careful use of monobenzyl ether of hydroquinone (MBEH in short) or hydroquinone (2–4%) in lotion or ointment are also beneficial. With the former, care must be exercised for two reasons: Sensitization to MBEH causing-contact dermatitis and complete depigmentation resulting in leucoderma, both at local site and at distant areas. Several workers have used hydroquinone ointment mixed with retinoic acid and fluocinolone ointment in equal parts with some degree of success. Azelaic acid in cream base and beta-carotene application may help some resistant cases.

MELANODERMATITIS TOXICA

A common but distinct pattern of pigmentation is seen frequently in practice. It affects middle-aged persons of both the sexes, but is more common in females. Clinically, a light brown to dark brown or bluish discoloration starts from the temples or forehead and spreads to the periphery of face, central part of nose, pinna of ears, neck-upper part of chest and upper limbs. Mucous membranes are not affected **(Fig. 23.3)**. Lesions are usually non-inflammatory and asymptomatic but in early lesions, erythema and itching may be present. History and routine investigations are not very helpful.

Histopathological changes are not diagnostic but are definite. There is epidermal thinning, flattening of rete pegs, increase of pigment in basal layer and shedding of melanin into dermis where it is seen within and outside the macrophages. There is slight to moderate round cell infiltration.

Cause is usually not known. Patients may have seborrhoeic diathesis; sometimes there is history of intake of photo-sensitizing drugs or food adultration (chemical additives, preservatives, etc.). Melanosis has been reported after the Spanish and Taiwan outbreaks.

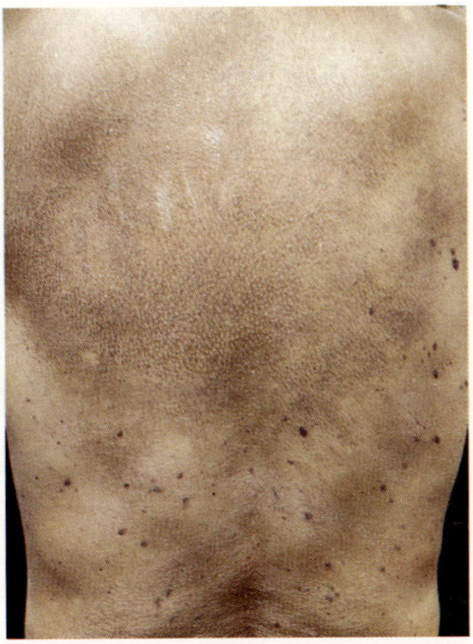

Fig. 23.3: Toxic melanoderma on the back

Treatment is not specific. It mainly consists in eradication of causes, a course of sodium thiosulphate or Lomodex N (P) intravenously, improvement of general health, avoidance of sun, administration of multivitamins and topically a bland lotion or ointment.

Prognosis is fair in symptomatic cases. Idiopathic cases are very resistant to treatment. It takes 12–18 months, or longer for the lesions to disappear.

SEBORRHOEIC MELANOSIS

Pigmentation is typically distributed on seborrhoeic sites, i.e. forehead, beard area, posterior auricular folds, neck, upper part of the chest and upper back. Colour is brownish-black. To begin with pigmentation is follicular, and later streaks or reticular pattern develop. The whole of the face is darker than the rest of the skin including the exposed parts like dorsum of hands. It is accompanied by erythema and itching; the latter can be severe. There is an associated pityriasis capitis, greasy skin and constipation **(Fig. 23.4)**. To correlate seborrhoeic diathesis with melanosis is desirable but may be an over-simplification. It can be difficult to distinguish it from toxic melanosis. Amyloid degeneration, zinc sulphate deficiency and hormonal imbalance have also been blamed.

Treatment consists of controlling the underlying causes.

Prognosis is poor. Condition is usually chronic and resistant to therapy.

PIGMENTATION DUE TO HEAVY METALS

Heavy metals cause generalized pigmentation by increased melanin formation and the deposition of the metals themselves. The common metals causing pigmentation are arsenic, silver, gold and bismuth.

Arsenic: It produces a dew-drop-like, generalized pigmentation. The dew-drop appearance is due to the pigmentation being more marked around the hair follicles than the interfollicular areas. One may come across other features like exfoliative dermatitis,

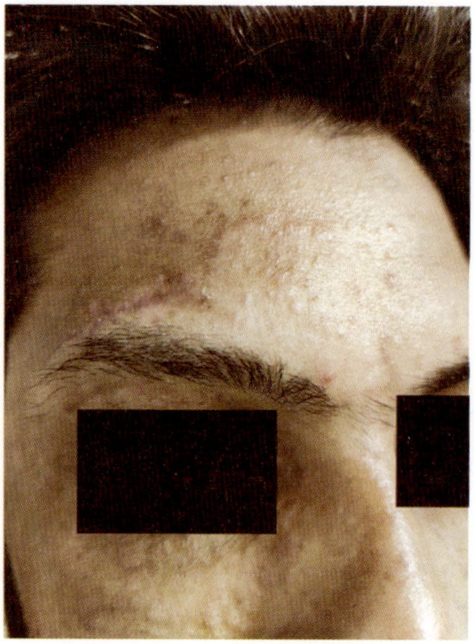

Fig. 23.4: Seborrhoeic melanosis with acne vulgaris lesions

keratoderma of the palms and the soles, even keratoses. The arsenical preparations which produce pigmentation are liquor arsenicalis, arsenic injections and the arsenic 'kushtas' so commonly used by the indigenous practitioners.

Silver (Argyria): Among the common preparations that often give trouble during ingestion are those containing silver nitrate; argyrol and silver arsphenamine. It is surprising that though silver leaves are habitually consumed by Indians and certain other Asiatic people, argyria is uncommon amongst them. Clinically, argyria is seen as bluish or slate-coloured pigmentation starting on the face, hands and finger-nails; it later becomes generalized. The pigmentation is usually permanent.

Gold (Chrysiasis): The offending preparations are the gold salts used intravenously for the treatment of rheumatoid arthritis. Fortunately, they are used very rarely now. As in the case of silver leaves, though gold leaves are habitually ingested by Indians and other Asiatic people, one rarely comes across slate-coloured pigmentation and lichenoid dermatitis.

Bismuth: Used in large doses over long periods, it can produce bismuth lines on the gums, and sometimes, though rarely, diffuse pigmentation.

Mercury: If used locally in cream form, it can cause a local grey or slate-coloured pigmentation.

Artificial jewellery, cocaine injections and tattooing can also cause pigmentation. Pigmentation brought about by heavy metals is usually permanent since the treatment is rather unsatisfactory. The causative agent should be withdrawn, and a course of sodium thiosulphate and/or BAL given. For details, refer to Chapter 21 on 'Drug Eruptions'. The patient should be protected from sunlight.

Localized cases can be helped by surgical excision and plastic surgery.

Main emphasis should be on prevention; discrimination being exercised in the use of heavy metals. Fortunately, with the introduction of safer and more effective therapeutic measures against the diseases treated previously by heavy metals, the incidence of pigmentation due to them has been reduced considerably.

BERLOQUE DERMATITIS

It results from the application of photosensitizing agents like eau de cologne, the juice of Persian limes, bergamot oil and *Ammi majus* followed by an exposure to the sun. The exposed parts of the body like the face, the neck and the forearms are the sites of choice. Initially, there is an erythema followed by well-defined streaks or patches of hyperpigmentation which appear after a latent period of 48 hours or so. The latter takes several weeks or months to disappear naturally. The therapeutic measures so far available are unsatisfactory. The affected part must be protected from sunlight, and the offending agent avoided.

RIEHL'S MELANOSIS

It is seen as streaked, spotted or patchy, brownish-grey pigmentation of the face and the neck. The condition was very common during the World Wars. It occurs usually in middle-aged women. The exact causation is still not established, but the consensus of opinion is that Riehl's melanosis is caused either by the use of synthetic foods lacing in natural fats or by the use of cheap substitute soaps, oils, ointments and cosmetics containing colours or perfumes. These factors predispose the skin to photosensitization, and hence pigmentation.

INCONTINENTIA PIGMENTI (SULZBURGER)

It is a rare autosomal dominant, hereditary disorder seen more frequently in female infants. Within a few weeks of birth, an inflammatory papulo-bullous eruption develops on the trunk and less frequently on the limbs. As the inflammation subsides in a few weeks or months, a bizarre pigmentation with well-defined borders develops which finally fades with the years. This inflammatory and pigmentary disorder may be associated with other congenital defects like those of the teeth and the eyes.

ACANTHOSIS NIGRICANS

It implies papillomatous or verrucous hypertrophy of the skin combined with pigmentation occurring in streaks or patches in the axillae, groins, neck, sub-mammary region and antecubital fossae. It may occur either in a mild or severe form; in the latter, there is accompanying dystrophy of the nails and hair, there being pigmentation of the other parts of the integument as well **(Fig. 23.5)**. There are two varieties of acanthosis nigricans:

1. The juvenile type. It is the benign type. It may be associated with endocrine, metabolic or digestive disorders.
2. The adult type. The prognosis is bad, since it is usually associated with abdominal cancer.

Third variety is known as pseudo-acanthosis nigricans seen in obese individuals. Its course varies according to the weight of the body. The treatment depends upon the primary cause which must be duly addressed. For local defects, salicylic acid ointment, retinoic acid, vitamins and thyroid medication may be tried.

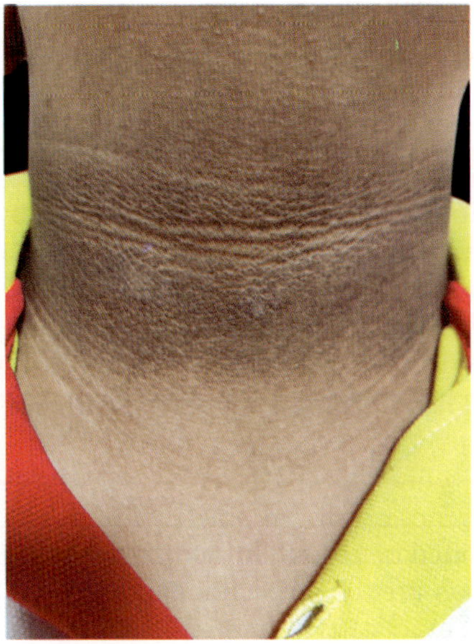

Fig. 23.5: Acanthosis nigricans

CAROTINAEMIA

It implies yellowish discoloration of the integument caused by the excessive consumption of carotin-rich foodstuffs, particularly carrots and oranges. The sites most commonly discoloured are the palms of the hands, the soles of the feet and the naso-labial folds; later, other parts of the body may also be affected. The colour varies from light-yellow to deep-orange. The pigmentation is only temporary, and when the cause is withdrawn from the diet, the colour of the skin returns to normal.

ACHROMIA

Causes

Congenital

1. Albinism—partial or complete (*see* Chapter 27).
2. Naevus depigmentosus (*see* Chapter 27).

Acquired

1. Vitiligo.
2. Occupational—tannery workers and use of chemicals like guanofuracin, amylphenol, quinones (MBEH), etc.
3. Post-inflammatory—leprosy, post-kala-azar dermal leishmaniasis, syphilis, pinta, yaws. Following injury, burns, chronic eczema and morphea.
4. Hypopigmentation in pityriasis alba and pityriasis versicolor.

Whenever one comes across a case of depigmentation, the answer to the following questions must be sought. Is the depigmentation complete or partial? Is it stationary or progressive? At what age did the condition develop—at birth, after or late in life? Is there accompanying loss of sensation, atrophy, scarring, scaling or inflammation? Other features? A blood STS should be done in cases suspected to have endemic syphilis and other spirochaetal infections. Table 23.2 will help in the differential diagnosis of the important depigmentary disorders.

VITILIGO

The Hindustani name is *'phuleri'*. It is an acquired idiopathic depigmentary condition which though worldwide in distribution, is most common in India, Egypt and other tropical countries: It is a source of great social embarrassment to dark-skinned people. It affects all age groups with no predilection to either sex. Many cases start at the age of five, at puberty and at menopause. Its incidence is markedly on the increase.

Clinical features: It is characterized by completely depigmented macules and patches of varying sizes and shapes. Besides loss of colour, there is no other structural change. Early lesion may be pale white and ill-defined. At this stage, Wood' s lamp helps to confirm the diagnosis. Patches enlarge slowly and may affect the whole body, but this involvement is very seldom complete (Fig. 23.6). Any part of the body can be affected but the sites of predilection are the face, dorsa of feet and hands, waist and the legs (Fig. 23.6). Involvement of mucous membranes, especially the lips, is not uncommon; it can precede cutaneous involvement by years. Hair may or may not become depigmented in vitiliginous areas. Patient's skin is susceptible to even minor trauma; it heals with depigmentation (Table 23.2).

At times lesions develop along the distribution of a peripheral nerve, zosteriform vitiligo (Fig. 23.7). It is interesting sometimes to see a bunch of hair turning grey and then followed by loss of pigment in that area of skin. Occasionally, vitiligo develops around pigmented moles—'Halo naevus'.

The onset is slow and the course insidious but enigmatic. It may continue to increase slowly or come to a halt, and then increase again. Cases of spontaneous recovery have

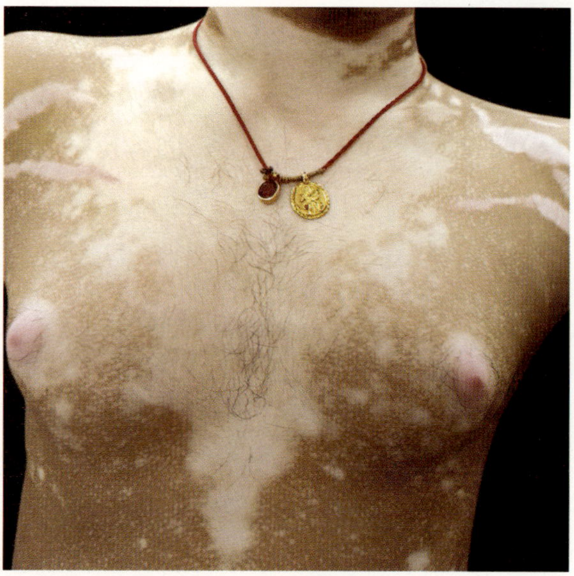

Fig. 23.6: Vitiligo

Table 23.2: Differential diagnosis of common hypo-pigmentary diseases

Distinguishing features	*Albinism*	*Naevus depigmentosus*	*Vitiligo*	*Leprosy*	*Pityriasis versicolor*
1. Age	Congenital, present at birth	Congenital, present at birth	Acquired, any age	Any age	Any age
2. Distribution	Complete or partial	Unilateral	Any area	Any age	Trunk, neck and face
3. Course	Stationary	Does not increase in size or change shape	Progressive	Progressive	Progressive, worse in monsoon and summer
4. Hyperpigmentary border	Nil	Nil	Present	Inflammatory	Nil
5. Heredofamilial	Hereditary	Not hereditary	May be	Nil	Nil
6. Other features	Hair and eyes may be affected	Nil	Nil	Anaesthesia, thickened nerves, nasal bleeding, slit smear and biopsy	Furfuraceous scaling, pin

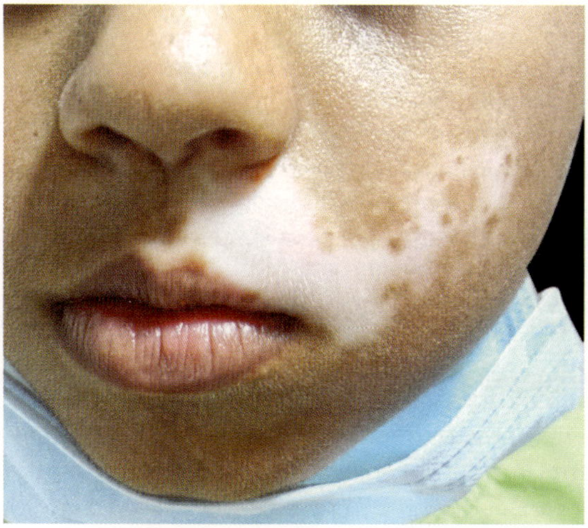

Fig. 23.7: Zosteriform vitiligo

been seen by the authors. According to the authors' experience, the malady usually starts and increases in the summer months in Northern India.

Haemoglobin content of the blood is low and sometimes intestinal parasites and infections can be detected. Patients complain of easy fatiguability.

Classification: Vitiligo has been divided into three stages: Active progressive stage (V1), Quiescent stage (V2) and Repigmenting stage (V3).

Besides classifying the stage of disease, it is useful to decide the variety (acral, vulgaris, zosteriform); severity (localised or extensive) and acuity (insiduous or galloping) or erratic **(Table 23.3)**.

Etiology: It is a feeling of many workers that vitiligo is a multifactorial malady. Genetic predisposition is important, its influence varies from 10 to 35%. Auto-immunity has been blamed but in reality, it is a reaction pattern to drugs, infections and toxin, but not a cause *per se*. Whole of melanocyte system is defective.

Table 23.3: Clinical criteria for classification of vitiligo

Stage of vitiligo	*Clinical features*
Active (V1)	• New lesions developing
	• Lesions increasing in size
	• Border ill-defined
Quiescent/Stable (V_2)	• No new lesions developing
	• Lesions stationary in size
	• Border hyperpigmented and well defined
	• Lesions decreasing in size
Improving (V_3)	• No new lesions developing
	• Border defined and signs of spontaneous repigmentation (follicular and peripheral)
Zosteriformis/segmental	• Unilateral distribution of lesions, preferably along the course of nerves

Important known causative factors are:

a. Nutritional—defects in copper, proteins and vitamins in diet; digestive upsets like amoebiasis, helminthiasis, chronic diarrhoea, dysentery, etc.
b. Endocrines—association with thyrotoxicosis and diabetes
c. Trophoneurosis and autonomic imbalance—emotional stress and strain
d. Infections and toxic products—Enteric fever, ill-health, focal sepsis.
e. Drugs and chemicals like quinones, guanofuracin, amylphenol, chlorthiazide, broadspectrum antibiotics, beta-blockers and chloroquin **(Fig. 23.8)**.

Vitiligo has assumed epidemic proportions in several parts of India especially Gujarat and Rajasthan. Chemicals are known to inhibit melanogenesis, enzymatic actions and several chain biochemical reactions. They can also cause interference with nutrition of the tissues. Hence tie-up of the two—chemicals and nutrition—may provide the answer. Role of food adulterants, industrial chemicals and dyes, contaminating water and foods may be an important causes.

Pathology: A defect in enzyme tyrosinase is held responsible for vitiligo. According to some, melatonin, a substance secreted at nerve ending inhibits tyrosinase, thus interfering in pigment formation; DOPA staining shows that melanocytes are deficient. In active cases, mononuclear hugging at the junction of the lesion and normal skin is a prominent feature (Behl & Pradhan).

Diagnosis: It is usually apparent. In doubtful and early cases, Wood's lamp is of great help in diagnosis. Usually, in macular leprosy, anetoderma, seborrhoeides, pityriasis versicolor and nevoid conditions, its assistance is called for. Vitiligo areas are milky white while others lack this milky white coloration.

Stationary patches are well-defined and have hyperpigmented borders. Sensations are normal, so is texture unless the patches have been irritated with treatment. Absence of scaling, crusting and iching help to eliminate seborrhoeides and pityriasis versicolor. In white anetoderma, lesions are small, well-defined and depressed below the surface of the skin.

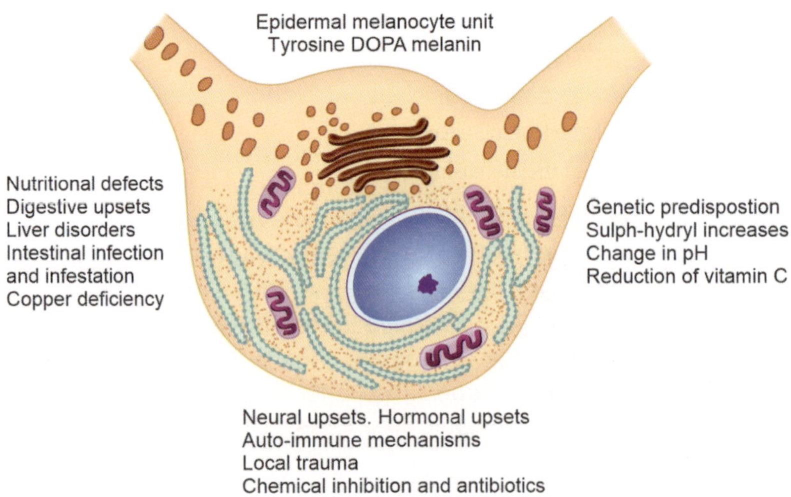

Fig. 23.8: Possible etiological factors in vitiligo

Pinta and syphiltic leuco-melanoderma can be differentiated by other clinical stigmata and positive blood serology.

Leucodermoid is a term coined to describe leucoderma-like lesions at an early stage when the features are not definite and observation is necessary to come to a conclusion.

Prognosis: It has improved considerably in recent years because of better understanding of etiological factors and advances made in therapy. In the extensive trials undertaken by the authors, it was found that the progress of the disease could be controlled in about 90–95% of cases and it could be cured in about 40–90% of selected cases.

Resistant areas

1. Lips, over the joints, acral areas
2. Patches with depigmented hair
3. Patches with thickened integument, scaling and tendency to fibrosis
4. Pale patches with lack of vascularity (do not bleed easily)

Reasons for Poor Response to Treatment

1. Poor nutrition and general health
2. Emotional stress and strain
3. Recurrent/intercurrent infections
4. Prolonged/repeated antibiotic courses
5. Bad disgestion, diarrhoea and dysentery
6. Extensive, galloping variety
7. Leucotrichia/mucosal involvement
8. Endemic areas.
9. Age above 60.

Treatment: At the very outset, the patient and the relatives should be assured about its non-infectious and non-hereditary nature; further that it has no relationship to leprosy whatsoever. This gives immense moral strength to the patient.

Patient should be instructed to avoid physical trauma. As far as possible, broad-spectrum antibiotics should not be prescribed for inter-current illnesses to vitiligo patients.

Therapeutic schedule **(Fig. 23.9)**, which the authors feel very effective, is as follows:

1. Control of etiological factors and improvement of health (mental and physical). The patient's nutritional state is improved as far as possible; this is of particular importance when the vitiligo is active and progressively increasing. Multi-vitamins by mouth and injections of crude liver extract with vitamin B complex are beneficial. In the diet, cheese, butter milk, almonds, figs, germinating grams (which are rich in tyrosinase) and bael fruit (syrup, squash or preserved) are added with benefit. Corticosteroids (both systemic and topical) and ACTH injections are very useful in controlling the progress of disease especially the galloping ones. Geriforte (P), placental extract IM. biweekly and placental extract lotion rubbed in externally thrice daily are useful in active progressive vitiligo. Levamisole 50–150 mg weekly dose has also been found to be useful in some active cases.
2. Copper chloride orally 1–3 mg daily in capsule or mixture or as intravenous injections 200 micrograms twice a week.

This regimen is continued till vitiligo becomes quiescent, i.e. no new lesions develop and margins become hyperpigmented, Usually 2–3 months period is required for attaining this objective in many cases, pigment begins to return during this period. Despite this, few patients continue to get new lesions, while old ones are getting pigmented at the same time. Only, after controlling the activity, are added the following specific measures .

3. *Specific:* Systemic-*Ammi majus* (Meladinine-P), *Psoralea corylifolia* (seeds). Psoralen, Neosoralen, Macsoralen (P): One tablet contains about 10 mg active substance Ammidin and Ammodin and the daily dose is 10–20 mg. It should be followed by exposure to sun two hours later. To achieve this, it is preferable to take the dose early in the morning. Side-effects are a sense of heat in the body, nervousness and sometimes hypertension, giddiness and an allergic eczematoid reaction . If the side-effects are mild, the drug can be continued in small doses. Duration of therapy varies according to patient's needs and can be extended for years. In the authors' experience herbs *Psoralia corylifolia* and *Ammi majus* are more effective and less toxic; of course, they are much cheaper as well.
4. *Local: Ammi majus* or Psoralen (P) ointment, croton oil, babchi (*Psoralea corylifolia*), or bergamot oil locally. All these have photosensitizing action. They produce erythema and, at times, blisters, which are more common in those who have not taken systemic psoralens previously, i.e. whose skin in not acclamatized. When this occurs, further application be stopped and soothing lotion or cream be prescribed. Later, it can be used in a diluted form and less frequently.

   A cream containing 10% para-amino-benzoic acid is applied to the normal skin surrounding the vitiligo, patches, particularly the face, before the paint is used or irradiation given. This helps to avoid disfiguring hyper-pigmentation of the border areas.
5. *UVR.* In stabilized cases, the authors advises patients to use *Ammi majus* paint in the morning and to expose themselves to sunlight 15 minutes later for a few minutes. These patients attend the skin clinic twice a week when placental extract is given intradermally into patches, *Ammi majus* oil is painted on the affected part which is

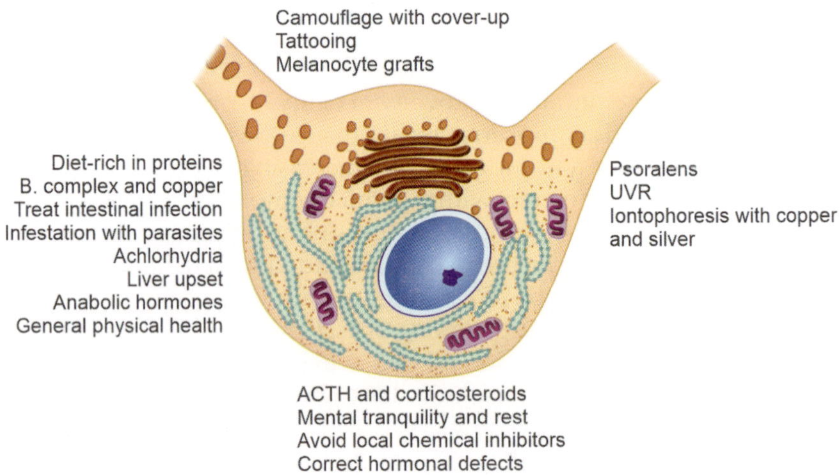

Fig. 23.9: Therapeutic approaches in vitiligo

exposed to UV rays. Cases which were resistant before, respond much better with this regimen.

Principles of Treatment

V1 stage: Correct the cause and give nutritional supportive therapy with B-complex, placental extract, haematinics, rest, etc. Topical aqueous placental extract followed by exposure to sun.

V2 stage: Topical placental extract, psoralens-orally and topically.

V3 stage: If no further improvement with V2 treatment, Autologous Thin Thiersch grafts or Melanocyte culture graft. It takes about 2–4 months to control the progress of the disease. Repigmentation takes from 3 to 12 months. If no further repigmentation, surgery is the answer.

Repigmentation usually starts around the hair follicles and peripherally along the border. The pigmentation appears to be permanent in most cases.

6. Micropigmentation with flesh-coloured dyes may be useful in some cases. To conceal the disfigurement temporarily, the use of a "cover mark", 'cover up', walnut juice, silver nitrate or potassium permanganate is recommended.
7. *Surgery:* In controlled cases defying different measures the authors recommends surgical measures, i.e. melanocyte grafting with Thin Thiersch's autologous grafts under local or general anaesthesia. This technique has been used with success (Behl). For details refer to Chapter 6.

In selected cases, cultured whole thickness grafts or melanocytes suspension gives good results.

OCCUPATIONAL LEUCODERMA (OLIVER)

It is seen on the dorsum of the hands of tannery workers caused by the use of rubber gloves containing agerite alba, monobenzyl ether of hydroquinone (MBEH). The chemical gets dissolved by sweat and acts on the melanocytes in such a way as to interfere with the formation of melanin. In early cases, depigmentation may disappear spontaneously.

LEUKOPATHIA

It was first described as a clinical subtype of vitiligo in Japan and Pacific islands. Hypopigmented macules are seen bilaterally symmetrically on the hands and feet. Condition is hereditary and progressive. We have observed similar picture in our patients.

Hypomelanosis is also seen due to chemicals like hydroquinones, guanofuracin, butyl and amylphenols (disinfectants) and chlorthiazides.

Chapter

24

Collagen Disorders

The group of collagen disorders includes disease involving the dermal collagen, the ground substance with biochemical changes involving the muco-polysaccharides and disturbed auto-immunity. Cutaneous involvement is prominent but multiple systems are involved. Besides, there is a certain overlap in the clinical features.

LUPUS ERYTHEMATOSUS (LE)

There are two distinct forms of LE, viz:

a. Discoid LE (DLE) (localised discoid form, occasionally becoming disseminated).

b. Systemic form (SLE)

However, there are individuals who have susceptibility for both diseases and it is in this group, a conversion from DLE to SLE may be observed.

DISCOID LUPUS ERYTHEMATOSUS

Synonym: Chronic discoid LE (CDLE).

Etiology: A genetic susceptibility to the disease is believed to exist. The precipitating factors include ultraviolet light (UVL), infections, trauma, exposure to cold, stress, pregnancy and drugs (e.g. griseofulvin). Auto-immunity has an important role in causation.

Clinical features: Although any age group may be affected, it is commonly a disease of young adults (peak incidence between 30-40 years). Females are slightly more commonly affected. Characteristic skin lesions develop on the sun-exposed skin of the face and neck. The disease appears slowly as one or more circumscribed erythematous plaques which are moderately infiltrated. The colour varies from bright red to violaceous brown **(Fig. 24.1)**. The surface is smooth in the earliest lesions but soon becomes covered with a thin adherent grey scale; this manifestation of hyperkeratosis is best seen in the follicular orifices, so that horny plug may be visible to the naked eye, and may be seen projecting from the undersurface of the scale (nutmeg appearance) when it is forcibly removed. The lesions enlarge slowly often coalescing, and the picture then consists of an active, fairly well-demarcated edge and a sunken, atrophic centre which may show telangiectasis. Diascopy shows cayenne-pepper appearance. The parts most commonly affected are those which receive the most sunlight, so that the malar prominences and the bridge of the nose frequently show the first changes; when these lesions coalesce, the typical 'butterfly' or 'bat's wing' appearance is produced. Less commonly, lesions of discoid lupus erythematosus may develop on the scalp and if not controlled early

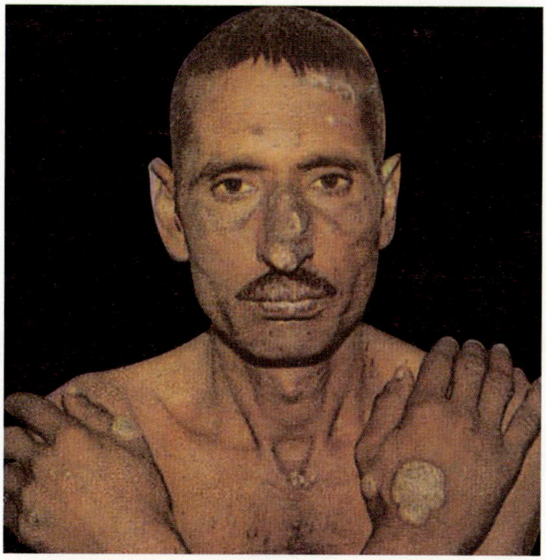

Fig. 24.1: Discoid lupus erythematosus—typical chronic erythematous plaques with adherant scale and follicular plugs-nutmeg appearance

may produce scarring alopecia. Rarely, the disease may be extensive and disseminated, in which case hands and areas normally kept covered with clothes may develop the lesions. Healing of the lesions takes place with atrophy, scarring and depigmentation.

Clinical variants exist and include hypertrophic lesions, 'profundus ' lesions situated in the subcutaneous tissue and associated with panniculitis, 'chilblain lupus' seen in those with poor circulation with resemblance to perniosis (lesions are seen on the nose, ears and fingers) and 'rosacea-like lupus'. Rarely, lesions may develop on the mucous membranes of mouth or eyes and nails may be affected to show crumbling of the nail plates, longitudinal striae and subungual hyperkeratosis.

Histopathology: Any or all of the following changes may be seen: Hyperkeratosis with formation of horny plugs in pilosebaceous orifices, epidermal atrophy, hydropic or liquefaction-degeneration of the basal layer, focal lymphocytic infiltrate around the appendages and dilated blood vessels and hyalinization, oedema, and fibrinoid change in the upper dermis.

Differential diagnosis: In typical cases of CDLE, it is relatively easy to rule out seborrhoeic dermatitis, psoriasis and rosacea. In atypical cases, polymorphic light eruption, lymphocytic infiltrate of Jessner, photo-dermatitis, sarcoidosis and lepromatous leprosy may have to be considered. Late scarring lesions require differentiation from lupus vulgaris, basal and squamous cell carcinoma, and late radiodermatitis. Lichen planus actinicus may resemble CDLE. In the latter, lesions are usually single or a few, well-defined circular macules with pigmented centre and lichenoid border. Lupus vulgaris can be excluded by the absence of tissue paper atrophy, reddish brown colour, apple jelly nodules. Histopathology is usually diagnostic.

Laboratory Findings

i. LE cells and positive ANA test may be expected in about 5% of the cases **(Fig. 24.2)**.

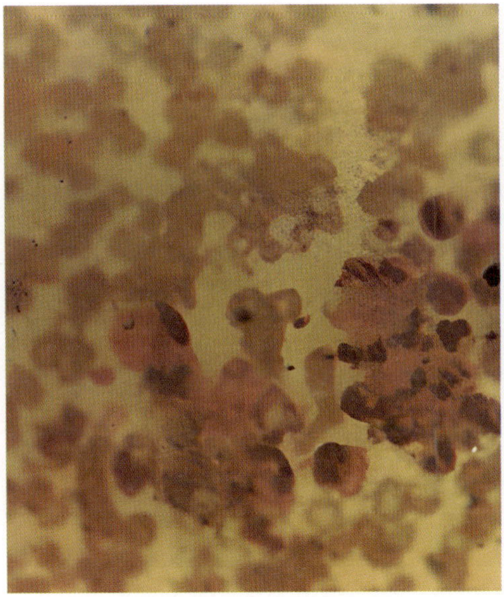

Fig. 24.2: LE cells 10X

ii. Almost all cases will demonstrate a band-like deposition of immuno-globulins (most commonly IgG) along the dermoepidermal junction on direct immunofluorescent examination of the lesional skin. The older the lesion, the thicker the fluorescent band. Non-lesional skin is unaffected.

Prognosis: Spontaneous remission of the disease occurs in some patients. In the rest if untreated, the disease persists. However, therapeutic results are generally satisfactory and the residual damage depends on the severity and the chronicity of the disease. The risk of conversion to SLE is very small, less than 5%, but patients with widespread disease are considered more at risk.

Treatment

1. The patients should be instructed to avoid sunlight as much as possible and to use sun protective preparations. Infections especially of the upper respiratory tract should be promptly controlled. General nutrition should be improved. Indiscriminate use of photosensitising drugs should be strictly avoided.
2. Local application of steroids is the treatment of first choice. They may be applied topically as cream, lotion or impregnated tape, or injected intralesionally. It may take several weeks before further progression of the disease is arrested and complete healing occurs. Topical steroids will limit scarring but will not reverse it.
3. Oral antimalarial, e.g. chloroquine sulphate 200 mg one to three times daily, or hydroxychloroquine 200 mg daily are the second best choice. It may be used in conjuction with topical steroids. Side-effects include retinopathy (dose related), abnormal pigmentation, cutaneous eruptions and neurological changes.
4. The use of systemic steroids is difficult to justify except in disseminated discoid LE. Beta-carotene 50 mg tid and clofazimine (Lamprene) 100 mg daily have been recently tried with some success.

5. Limited disease may be treated with freezing by liquid nitrogen or carbon dioxide snow or phenol application.

SYSTEMIC LUPUS ERYTHEMATOSUS

Etiology: There is unequivocal evidence for the presence of autoantibodies directed against nuclear DNA and other tissue antigens. These autoantibodies form as a result of genetically determined immune imbalance; as a result, B-cells readily synthesize antibodies directed against tissue proteins altered by ultraviolet light, viruses, drugs, e.g. hydralazine, procainamide, quinidine, isoniazid, hydantoins, D-penicillamine, griseofulvin, sulphonamides, tetracycline and oral contraceptives and other unknown factors causing damage by formation of immune complex and cytotoxicity.

Clinical features: SLE is characteristically a disease of young females although other age groups and males are also sometimes affected. The clinical spectrum is wide and variable. The disease may begin insidiously with vague rheumatic pains or other non-specific symptoms, or explosively with rapid onset of symptoms pertaining to multiple systems as well as constitutional symptoms. Because the disease process may affect any system and thereby produce any symptoms, it is quite easy to over-diagnose this entity. To help the clinician in this matter, the American Rheumatism Association (ARA) has developed a set of 14 criteria (Table 24.1); presence of four or more of these criteria in any patient may be taken as indicative of SLE.

Cutaneous involvement occurs in approximately 80% of patients. Photosensitivity is reported by 33% of the patients. The best known is 'butterfly rash'; it is an erythematous blush or maculo-papular eruption occupying the skin of the nose and the cheeks. It is not itchy or painful. Discoid lesions completely indistinguishable from CDLE are commonly seen. Areas of macular erythema, sometimes quite extensive, are common, particularly during severe exacerbations. Hands may show several changes, viz., erythema over the thenar and hypothenar eminences of the palms as well as erythema over the knuckles

Table 24.1: American Rheumatism Association (ARA) criteria for diagnosis of SLE
1. Butterfly rash
2. Lesions resembling CDLE
3. Photosensitivity
4. Alopecia
5. Oral or nasopharyngeal ulceration
6. Raynaud's phenomenon
7. Arthritis (without deformity)
8. LE cells
9. Persistent false positive STS
10. Profuse proteinuria (more than 0.5 g per day)
11. Cellular casts in urine
12. Pleuritis or pericarditis
13. Neurological manifestations, e.g. convulsions
14. Haemolytic anaemia or leucopenia (below 4000/mm^3) or thrombocytopenia

and phalangeal joints, dilated nail fold capillaries, small infarct-like lesions on the fingertips, and lesions resembling chilblains and Osler's nodes. Persistent urticarial lesions have also been documented. Bullae and erosions, especially on lips and buccal mucosa, and leg ulcers may occur. Alopecia is a common feature and is usually diffuse and non-scarring.

The general health is severely impaired especially during exacerbations. Fever is a common feature and may be associated with general malaise and weight loss. Joint manifestations rank as the commonest in SLE. Arthralgia is more common than arthritis. A picture indistinguishable from rheumatoid arthritis (with positive rheumatoid factor) may develop.

Histopathology depends on the type of the cutaneous lesion. More diagnostic features are seen in the chronic lesions and resemble that of CDLE. The acute lesions show more oedema and fibrinoid change in the upper dermis; blood vessels show inflammation and fibrinoid deposits, and 'haematoxylin bodies' in the dermis. The latter are haematoxylin stained, round, homogenous structures, probably the remnants of nuclei from degenerated cells and are thought to correspond with LE bodies.

Laboratory Findings

1. The LE cell phenomenon is positive in about 80% of patients. The LE cell is a polymorphonuclear leucocyte that has ingested a homogenous, basophilic mass-probably nuclear material coated with immunoglobulins.
2. ANA are present in almost all patients.
3. The Farr assay for DNA antibodies specific for SLE as well as quantitative correlate for the disease activity.
4. The level of circulating complement fall during the periods of disease activity.
5. Patients with SLE may also show anaemia, leucopenia, thrombocytopenia, elevated ESR, false positive STS, cryoglobulins and rheumatoid factor.
6. Immunohistology of SLE is characteristic. Unlike CDLE, it shows a band of immunoglobulins and complement components along the dermo-epidermal junction not only in the lesional skin but also in the uninvolved sun-exposed skin.

Differential diagnosis: After syphilis and drug eruptions, SLE is regarded as the greatest mimick. The exact differential diagnosis would depend on the combination of clinical manifestations. However, the ARA criteria, immunohistology and anti-DNA antibody tests should facilitate early and accurate diagnosis in most cases.

Prognosis: The five year survival is above 90% and is improving with better understanding and management of the disease. The clinical course tends to be quite variable. Adverse prognostic factors relate to severity of the disease, onset in childhood and renal involvement. Males are much less commonly affected but carry a worse prognosis than females. Drug induced SLE has the best prognosis.

Treatment

1. General measures are important and include rest, elimination of aggravating factors, e.g. drugs, sun exposure, correction of anaemia and prevention of infections. Symptomatic treatment should be instituted as warranted by the clinical state. For example, aspirin may be used for the rheumatic symptoms, diuretics for cardiac failure or nephrotic syndrome and anticonvulsant drug for epilepsy.

2. The effectiveness of corticosteroids is well established. Moderate to large doses are required in the acute stages of the disease (for example, prednisone 30–60 mg daily) and maintain remission with a much smaller dose. Needless to say that the smallest possible dose should be employed to minimise the risk of side-effects. Levels of serum complement and anti-DNA antibodies are used to adjust the dose of steroids.
3. Chloroquine/hydroxychloroquin may have a steroid sparing effect in some cases and is worth a trial where large doses of steroids are required.
4. Immuno-suppressive and cytotoxic agents like cyclophosphamide (50 mg OD or BD) have been used with success.

SCLERODERMA

The term scleroderma denotes sclerosis- a kind of tethering or hardening of the skin; it is better appreciated by palpation rather than visual inspection. Similar to LE, scleroderma has a limited cutaneous form called morphoea and a systemic form called systemic sclerosis. The distinction between the two is somewhat arbitrary as there are cases of intermediate severity. Although not fully confirmed it is assumed that both morphoea and systemic sclerosis have common etiology and pathogenesis, viz.

1. Disturbed immune regulation. It is suggested that the collagen, in some way, becomes altered and antigenic and thus in predisposed individuals evokes the damaging immune response.
2. Defect in the collagen itself; either there is increased synthesis of collagen or reduced collagenolysis, or there is excessive collagen cross linking.
3. Defect in the vascular system resulting in fibrosis and thickening of the capillaries; the abnormality of vascular tone is related to autonomic dysfunction.

Clinical features: The peak incidence is between the age of 20–50 years. Females are affected three times more often than males.

Morphoea

This may present as solitary plaque, multiple plaques (sometimes referred to as generalized morphoea), linear lesions or small 'guttate' lesions.

Plaque lesions are initially slightly purplish or mauve but after a few weeks the centre of the lesion loses its colour, and develops a thickened waxy ivory appearance with a lilac coloured order; the hair is usually lost in the affected areas and sweating may also be reduced. Hyperpigmentation may develop. Non-pitting oedema may be the initial change in some lesions. There is characteristic feel of the skin; the integument is thickened and cannot be easily pinched or picked up as normal fold between fingers.

Linear lesions are usually seen in children and tend to be unilateral. Characteristic sclerosis is evident but the involvement of the deeper tissues is more likely. 'En coup de sabre' (resembling a scar from a sword cut) is a variant of linear morphoea affecting the scalp and extending onto the face. It is frequently associated with abnormalities of the corresponding mandible, teeth, tongue and skull bones; in extreme cases facial hemiatrophy may develop.

Guttate lesions are multiple small atrophic macules, sometimes pigmented, but otherwise showing sclerosis. They may be indistinguishable from lichen sclerosus et atrophicus.

Generalized morphoea represents more severe disease and raises the fears of systemic involvement. It is essentially plaque morphoea but the plaques may coalesce to form large areas of sclerosis. Viscera are not affected. Trunk and thighs are the areas of common involvement; hands and forearms may be involved. The integument develops a brawny non-pitting oedema, hardening and pigmentation.

Systemic Sclerosis

The initial manifestation is usually non-pitting swelling of the fingers and hands, slowly progressing to tightness and difficulty in clenching fists. Feet may be similarly affected. Further progression of the disease results in a characteristic appearance called 'sclerodactyly' in which the fingers look tapered, the skin is shiny, atrophic and tightly bound and there is periungual telangiectasia. In the subsequent stages, ulcers and stellate scars develop, along with flexion contractures, resorption of bones and calcinosis cutis.

Facial changes are also characteristic and consist of mask-like facies, restricted mouth opening, radial furrows, pinched nose, thin lips and puckered chin. Integument is smooth, thickened and shiny; telangiectasis develops early. Sclerotic changes with pigmentation may develop also over the upper trunk. Sclerotic changes may also affect the mouth. Acral parts are typically affected in contrast to generalized morphoea in which it is predominantly the trunk. Alopecia, anhidrosis and Addisonian pigmentation are the other cutaneous features. In many cases, the initial manifestation is Raynaud' s syndrome.

Systemic involvement becomes evident after a lag period of many months or even years. Oesophageal involvement is the most frequent and causes reduced peristaltic motility with subsequent dysphagia and reflux oesophagitis.

Crest syndrome describes a group of patients who present with calcinosis cutis (C), Raynaud's phenomenon (R), esophageal involvement (E), sclerodactyly (S) and telangiectasis (T). Other important systemic manifestations are heart block and left ventricular hypertrophy, proteinuria, hypertension, progressive uraemia and renal failure, malabsorption syndrome; muscle weakness and arthralgias. Systemic sclerosis spares the central nervous system.

Shulman syndrome is a recently described variant of scleroderma in which the onset of cutaneous sclerosis is acute and rapid and is associated with fascitis, peripheral eosinophlia, hypergammaglobulinemia and other features of systemic sclerosis as described above. Good response to prednisone is also a feature.

Histopathology: The abnormality in the collagen may be so unimpressive as to be easily missed. However, a careful inspection will reveal that the collagen bundles are thickened and closely packed and besides their usual location in the dermis, are also visualized in the subcutaneous zone; the latter represents new collagen. In the early stage a mild lymphocytic infiltrate is present, whilst the late stage is characterized by atrophy of the epidermis and skin appendages, obliterative vascular changes and disappearance of elastic tissue.

Laboratory findings: Antinuclear antibodies (ANA) are found in about 80% of cases of systemic sclerosis. Speckled and nucleolar patterns are specific but homogenous pattern is more common. Rarely LE cells, rheumatoid factor and false positive STS may be found. Other abnormalities include anaemia, elevated ESR and increased gamma globulins. Immuno-histological findings are non-diagnostic.

Differential diagnosis: Patches of sclerosis have to be differentiated from lichen sclerosis et atrophicus and white anetoderma. Generalized scleroderma is to be distinguished from dermatomyositis with sclerodermatous changes, scleroderma and SLE.

Prognosis: Morphoea runs a limited course of few years and leaves minimum cosmetic defect. Generalized morphoea also is no risk to life. However, the prognosis in systemic sclerosis is guarded. Adverse prognostic factors are old patients, male patients, accelerated course, extensive disease and involvement of renal and pulmonary systems. The prognosis of Shulman syndrome is good.

Treatment: There is no satisfactory specific treatment. Topical or intralesional steroids may be beneficial in morphoea. Systemic steroids are effective in Shulman syndrome and may rarely help in the early stages of systemic sclerosis, but are generally of little value. Symptomatic treatment may be employed as indicated. Raynaud's phenomenon is a major problem and requires protection from cold and changes in temperature . Vasodilators, low molecular weight dextran and sympathectomy have been tried. Countless other drugs have been evaluated including cytotoxics and immunosuppressives, but none has proved effective.

Anabolic hormone (Orabolin/Dianabol-P) in conjunction with vasodilator (Duvadilan-P) has been beneficially used. Centellin, a combination of *Centella asiatica* and *Withania somnifera*, has been used effectively in the treatment of scleroderma and keloids.

Oral 1,25-dehydroxy vitamin D3 has been found in high dosage to be beneficial in the treatment of systemic sclerosis and localized scleroderma.

DERMATOMYOSITIS

Dermatomyositis is a rare disease characterized by a distinctive combination of cutaneous and muscular abnormalities along with variable systemic involvement. Its incidence is lower than other collagen diseases.

Etiology: Two age groups are vulnerable; children below the age of 10 years and adults between the age of 40–60 years. Females are affected twice as often as males. The evidence for auto-immunity is least convincing in dermatomyositis. The disease is sometimes seen to follow infections, immunization, drugs or trauma. The association with internal neoplasm is well established and is higher for males and older patients.

Clinical features: Typically, the onset is acute or subacute with fever, malaise, weakness and pain in the muscles, and a characteristic cutaneous eruption. However, some cases may present for the first time in the late stage of the disease with different clinical picture.

Amongst the cutaneous manifestations, heliotrope erythema and oedema of the periorbital skin, often accompanied by a maculo-papular eruption in the butterfly area of the face and extensor surfaces of the extermities is quite diagnostic. Hands show erythematous papules over the dorsal surface of the phalanges and knuckles, and nail fold telangiectasia. Photo-sensitivity, Raynaud's phenomenon and shallow mouth ulcers are inconstant features. In the late stage, appearance resembling poikiloderma or radiodermatitis or scleroderma may be seen. The affected areas show plaques of atrophy, telangiectasia and disturbed pigmentation. Calcification in the skin and muscles is a characteristic finding especially in the childhood cases.

Myositis typically affects the muscles of the proximal limb girdle, i.e. shoulders and hips. The affected muscles are painful, tender and 'doughy' on palpation. The weakness is variable and may present as difficulty in getting out of bed or combing hair. An additional myasthenic component may be present. Other skeletal muscles may be affected causing dysphagia and loss of speech. Myopathy may be accompanied by neuropathy in which case the risk of underlying malignancy is higher. In the late stage the muscles are atrophic, fibrotic and calcified.

The systemic manifestations are less common although any system may be involved. Arthritis, interstitial pneumonitis, arteritic intestinal ulcers, cardiomyopathy, and acute renal failure from precipitates of myoglobulin, are some manifestations worth remembering.

Histopathology: The important changes are seen in the skin, muscles and blood vessels. In the skin, in the early stage, there is oedema and mucin deposition in the dermis, and the picture resembles SLE; in the late stage, the findings include epidermal atrophy with flattening of the rete ridges, liquefaction degeneration of the basal layer, thickened homogenized collagen bundles, and thickened blood vessels. The affected muscles are pale and flabby or firm and fibrotic depending on the stage. The histological features are fragmentation of muscle fibres and loss of cellular detail, basophilia, variable cellular infiltrate and thickened blood vessels.

Laboratory findings: Baseline investigations will reveal elevated ESR and trace of protein and myoglobulin in the urine.

The diagnosis is confirmed by elevation of serum levels of creatine phosphokinase (CPK-MM), which is muscle specific and the levels of which show correlation with disease activity, and aldolase, SGOT and LDH. Urinary excretion of creatine is invariably increased and may be the only abnormality in some cases. Electromyography (EMG) of the affected muscles and a muscle biopsy will further aid in the diagnosis. EMG will show fibrillation and pseudomyotonic discharges.

Differential diagnosis: The cutaneous changes in the acute stage may be confused with SLE, erysipelas and contact dermatitis. The combination of skin and muscle symptoms may be seen in SLE and trichinosis. The myopathy requires differentiation from myasthenia gravis and muscular dystrophy.

Prognosis: This is variable. Dermatomyositis alone carries bad prognosis. Males do worse than females. Calcinosis is a good prognostic sign with regard to long-term survival but is always attended by severe deformities. The disease tends to 'burn out' in a few years.

Treatment: Rest is important in the acute phase. The mainstay of the treatment is oral steroids. Prednisone 40–80 mg should be administered initially and the smallest maintenance dose should be determined according to the severity of the disease and response to treatment Periodic tests for serum enzymes are useful in monitoring the disease activity. Patients should be observed carefully for the possible adverse effects of steroids. In resistant cases, a cytotoxic or antimetabolite may be added. Other symptomatic treatment may be instituted as necessary. In late stages, physiotherapy may help to prevent contractures. In patients over the age of 40 years, a work-up for underlying neoplasm is recommended.

POLYARTERITIS NODOSA

Etiology: The primary abnormality is a necrotizing panarteritis affecting the small and medium-sized arteries. There is evidence for immune complex mechanism; infections and drugs are the most considered sources of antigens. The peak age incidence is in the group of 50–60 years and both sexes are almost equally susceptible.

Clinical features: The overall clinical picture depends on whether the patient has full blown disease with multi-system involvement, or a limited disease with involvement of one or two systems.

In the cutaneous form of the disease, painful, erythematous, subcutaneous nodules appear in crops along the length of the superficial arteries of the lower extremities. These nodules persist for days or weeks and may sometimes ulcerate. Livido reticularis may be an associated finding. In the systemic form, a variety of histologically non-specific lesions may occur, e.g. urticaria, purpura, vesicles and pustules. Common systemic features are pyrexia, hypertension, coronary thrombosis, pericarditis, signs of chronic renal failure, headaches, convulsions, polyneuritis, arthralgia and myalgia.

Histopathology: The specific cutaneous lesions show panarteritis evolving through four stages viz., degeneration, inflammatory cell infiltration, granulation and fibrosis. Similar changes are seen in the blood vessels of other affected organs.

Laboratory findings: Polymorphonuclear leucocytosis, eosinophilia and anaemia may be noted. ESR is usually elevated and provides some measure of disease activity. Urine analysis may reveal protein, RBC or casts. Gammaglobulinemia may be present. The diagnosis is established on histological examination of tissue biopsies from skin, muscle or kidney. LE cells and antinuclear antibodies are usually not found.

Differential diagnosis: This depends on the type and extent of the manifestations. In general SLE, Wegener's granulomatosis. giant cell arteritis and Henoch–Schönlein purpura require differentiation. Granulomatous panarteritis with asthma, pulmonary infiltrates and eosinophilia should suggest Churg–Strauss syndrome.

Prognosis: This depends on the severity and the extent of the disease.

Treatment: Systemic steroids and antibiotics are effective in controlling the disease. The dose has to be determined carefully for each individual patient. Topical steroids may help in the specific cutaneous lesions. Cyclophosphamide (Endoxan-P) is sometimes beneficial.

MISCELLANEOUS DISEASES

Mixed Connective Tissue Disease

This title describes a group of patients who have serum antibodies against ENA (extractable nuclear antigen) and a variety of systemic manifestations common with other collagen diseases. The diagnosis is suggested by an overlap of symptoms and confirmed by the demonstration of ENA antibodies. The importance of diagnosing this entity lies in the finding that the prognosis of MCTD is superior to all other collagen diseases.

Sjögren's Syndrome

This is a triad of xerostomia (dry mouth), xerophthalmia (dry eyes) and collagen disease-rheumatoid arthritis, SLE or systemic sclerosis. It is associated with evidence of autoimmunity in the form of organ specific and non-organ specific auto-antibodies.

Scleredema Adultorum

It is a distinct entity (Bushke). Onset is usually preceded by constitutional upset and infection. Diffuse, symmetrical induration of the integument is noticed on the neck; it spreads to face, shoulders, arms and throat. It takes 4–8 weeks to reach its peak. Induration is non-pitting and wooden-like. Internal organs may be affected.

Occasionally, it is associated with malignancy of the mouth and throat.

Differential diagnosis is from scleroderma. In the latter there is hardening and tethering but not the woody induration. Besides, the distribution is different. Dermatomyositis exhibits typical heliotrope erythema, rash and painful, tender doughy weak musculature.

Sclerema neonatorum affects newborn marasmic children suffering from systemic illness. Exposure to cold brings about hardening of the subcutaneous fat starting from buttocks and spreading to other parts. Integument feels cold and firm; it has whitish and purplish mottling . Prognosis is grave. Treatment consists in improving the general nutrition, keeping the body warm, treating the underlying conditions and use of steroids and antibiotics.

Prognosis: Prognosis of scleredema adultorum is usually good. The condition tends to resolve in 6–24 months.

Treatment: It is unsatisfactory. Iontophoresis, hyaluronidase and pituitary extract may be helpful.

Chapter 25

Miscellaneous Disorders—Metabolic, Nutritional, Vascular, Atrophic and Endocrinal

DIABETES MELLITUS

It is an important metabolic disorder responsible for several cutaneous complications which may attract attention and even be responsible for the diagnosis of diabetes itself.

1. Pruritus of the genitalia (vulva and glans penis) as well as generalized pruritus. Moniliasis and even eczema complicate such pruritus. Diabetic balano-posthitis and vulvitis are a common problem in practice. The former can cause lot of misery in non-circumcised individuals.
2. Furunculoses, carbuncle and other pyodermas.
3. Monilial infection—paronychia, erosio interdigitalis blastomycetica and intertrigo.
4. Xanthoma diabeticorum.
5. Necrobiosis lipoidica diabeticorum.
6. Perforating ulcer and even diabetic gangrene due to atherosclerosis.
7. Polyneuritis, dermopathy, lipodystrophy.

In diabetic patients, use of anti-diabetic drugs may cause certain dermatoses. Insulin causes allergic reactions like pruritus and urticaria; oral antidiabetic drugs may produce drug rashes. Certain lipo-dystrophies and atrophies are seen due to insulin. Psoriasis is supposed to be commoner in diabetics, so is vitiligo.

Treatment consists in controlling the underlying diabetes, regulated diet and exercise, proper personal hygiene and specific measures according to complication. Vascular and neuritic complications demand patience and physiotherapeutic measures.

Diabetic Dermopathy

On the front of legs and less so on other parts of the body are 5–10 mm diameter sized multiple round or oval, reddish maculo-papules with slight scaling and depressed pigmented scars. Diabetic microangiopathy and minor collagen changes are responsible for the condition.

Necrobiosis Lipoidica Diabeticorum

Though it occurs commonly in diabetic individuals with hypercholesteremia, it may also occur in a non-diabetic individual. It is a very rare dystrophy, occurring selectively on the front of legs as well-defined erythematous, infiltrated maculo-papules which become reddish, yellowish, morphea-like plaques. It later atrophies or ulcerates. It is a chronic condition. The histology is characterized by endarteritis obliterans, necrosis and lipoid deposit. The treatment is unsatisfactory. Intralesional triamcinolone or occlusive bandage of corticosteroid ointment may help.

XANTHOMATOSIS

It represents a group of conditions characterized by the formation of yellowish-brown papules and tumours, and often with disturbance of the lipid metabolism. The prognosis and treatment depend upon the individual condition; the diagnosis of the latter is aided by investigations, viz., biopsy, blood cholesterol, triglyceride and lipo-proteins I, II, III, IV and V, urine and blood sugar, liver function tests, etc. Involvement of the cardiovascular system can be judged by the typical abnormalities seen in fundus examination and by electro-cardiographic studies.

Xanthomatosis may be:

a. (i) Primary due to metabolic defect in lipoproteins I, II, III, IV, V (Frederickson) producing xanthoma tuberosum and disseminatum-like pictures. (ii) Proliferation of histiocytes and lipid infiltration as in histioytoma, juvenile xanthogranuloma; Letterer Siwe disease and Hand–Schüller–Christian disease.

b. Secondary to other systemic disorders causing hypercholesteremia, e.g. hepatic disorders, renal diseases, diabetes, myxoedema and pancreatitis.

Xanthelasma or Xanthoma palpebrerum: It consists of round or oval, chrome yellow, infiltrative lesions, the size of which varies from that of lentil seeds to split peas or even bigger. Lesions occur on the upper eyelids, near the inner canthus, less commonly, on the lower eyelids **(Fig. 25.1)**. The blood cholesterol and lipid content may be normal/ raised. Xanthelasma is considered as the yellow signal of cardiovascular disease (athero-sclerosis). Hence, besides cutaneous treatment being given, due attention must be paid to the hidden-from-view but serious coronary disease. Xanthelasma is the most common type of xanthomatosis.

Xanthoma tuberosum: It consists of yellowish to brownish, firm papules, nodules, tumours and infiltrative areas grouped on extensor surfaces, mostly around the elbows, knees and hips. The tendon sheaths, the synovial membranes and the palms of the hands may also be involved. When xanthomatosis develops rapidly, they are called Xanthoma eruptivum. The blood cholesterol and lipid contents are markedly raised. Systemic

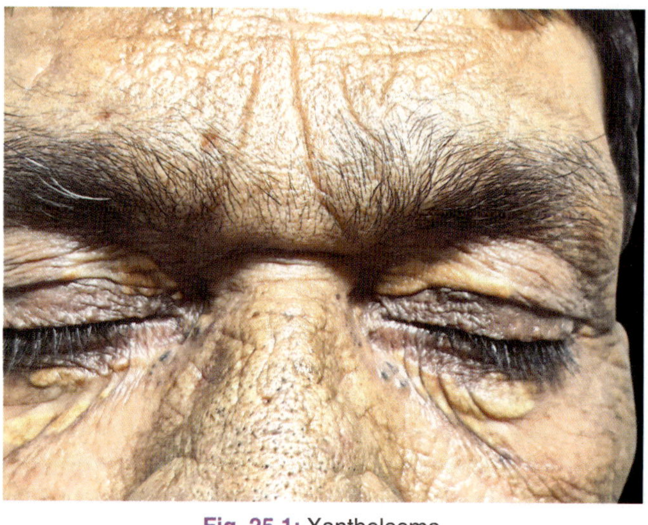

Fig. 25.1: Xanthelasma

lipaemia involves the heart, arteries and liver. When this happens the prognosis is bad; otherwise cutaneous xanthoma tuberosum is an asymptomatic disease. Some of the lesions may involute. The condition may occur at any age, but is seen mostly in adults.

Xanthoma disseminatum: It differs from xanthoma tuberosum in the following ways: (1) The flexures especially the axillae are usually involved. Though diffuse infiltration may occur and lesions on mucous membranes like the pharynx may also be seen. (2) The lesions are fine papules or plaques. (3) The blood cholesterol and lipid metabolism are normal. (4) There is no cardiovascular involvement, hence the prognosis is better.

Juvenile xanthomatosis: It represents xanthoma tuberosum which may be associated with Hand–Schüller–Christian disease.

Xanthoma diabeticorum: It is characterized by: (1) Sudden development and involution. (2) Severe diabetes, raised blood cholesterol and lipid content. (3) Fine or small xanthomatous and inflammatory papules. (4) Lesions on the extensor surfaces and particular involvement of the palms of the hands and the soles of the feet.

Histology of xanthoma lesions is characterized by lipoid deposit in reticuloendothelial cells and even extracellularly. Large histiocytes with foamy cytoplasm and Touton giant cells are typical of xanthoma in a routine paraffin section. Frozen sections stained with scarlet red or Sudan IV demonstrate the presence of lipids. Different xanthomas cannot be differentiated histologically.

Differential diagnosis is made from other yellowish-brown lesions, particularly urtcaria pigmentosa, carotinemia, etc.

Treatment

It consists of:

1. A low calorie, low fat and low cholesterol diet.
2. The administration of choline, methionine and other essential amino acids. Atromid-S (P) orally is benefical in patients with high cholesterol content. Thyroxine, Vit. E, nicotinic acid and oestrogens may be helpful.
3. Treatment of causes like diabetes, liver disease, etc.
4. Local treatment:
   a. Xanthelasma—cauterization with trichloracetic acid. The surrounding skin should be protected. Electro-cautery and curettage are preferred by some workers.
   b. Surgical excision of bigger tumours.
5. Treatment of complications like cardiovascular and hepatic involvement.

GOUT

It is a disorder of purine metabolism with genetic predisposition. Rich diet, excessive alcohol, blood and renal disorders, surgery and emotional strain can cause the disorder. It produces no specific cutaneous disease, only cutaneous tophi and associated ulceration which may present a diagnostic problem. Tophi are seen in the joints and surrounding tissues of feet and ankles, and very rarely in other areas. Tophi are whitish, chalky material composed of sodium urate crystals. Pain of acute gout may also produce confusion. Gout is caused by high uric acid level in the blood and is characterized by intermittent painful monoarthritis; especially of big toe. Treatment consists of low protein diet and drugs like probenecid, colchicine, allopurinol, etc. along with analgesics like indomethacin, ibuprofen and paracetamol.

CALCINOSIS CUTIS

It is very rare disorder characterized by calcification in local lesions like scleroderma and dermatomyositis, in intoxication with vitamin D_2 or hyper-parathyroidism. It may also be idiopathic. The disease may be localized or diffuse. Clinically, bony hard nodules and plaques are felt; these can as well be demonstrated by an X-ray examination and skin biopsy. Lesions are commonly seen over the fingers, knuckles, elbows, knees and other sites of friction and trauma. The treatment is unsatisfactory. It consists of correction of the underlying disease process. Painful nodules can be removed surgically. EDTA (ethylene-diamine-tetra-acetic acid) treatment may be helpful in aborting further calcinosis.

AMYLOIDOSIS CUTIS

It is a rare disorder occurring primarily in the skin, or secondarily, as a result of systemic amyloidosis. In the primary type, one comes across localized or generalized itchy papules, nodules or plaques, yellowish-brown in colour combined with pigmentation. It may also be associated with systemic involvement. Macular amyloidosis is often seen in middle-aged women without any signs of systemic affection (Fig. 25.2). A biopsy and Congo red test (subcutaneous and intravenous) help in diagnosis. The treatment is unsatisfactory. Localized variety of primary cutaneous amyloidosis (lichen amyloidosis) is discussed in Chapter 20 (Fig. 25.3).

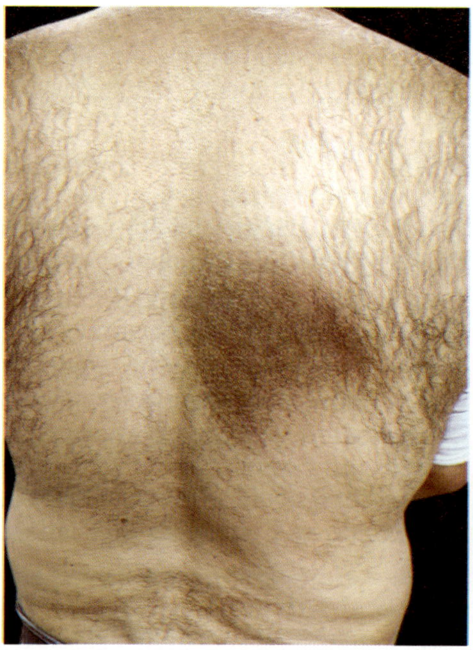

Fig. 25.2: Macular amyloidosis

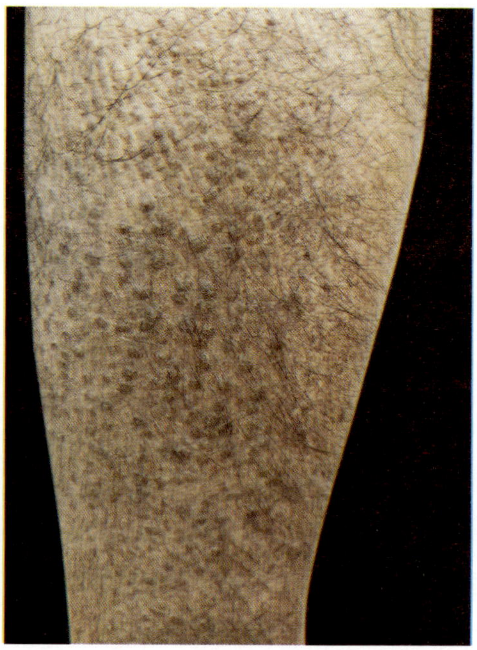

Fig. 25.3: Lichen amyloidosis

MYXOEDEMA

It is characterized by the deposition of mucin in the subcutaneous tissue. Mucin is a protein polysaccharide complex with special staining characteristics. Generalized myxoedema is associated with hypothyroidism. Lichen myxoedematosus is discussed in Chapter 20.

Pre-tibial myxoedema is a specific entity often associated with hyperthyroidism. Clinically, it is seen bilaterally symmetrically over the shin as firm, swollen, non-pitting, round or oval plaque with smooth or papular surface. Treatment of pre-tibial myxoedema consists in tackling associated thyrotoxicosis, and local infiltration with hyaluronidase or triamcinolone.

PORPHYRIA

The term implies disorders of porphyrin metabolism resulting in increased synthesis and also increased levels of porphyrins in blood, urine and stools, may be due to some acquired or genetic enzymatic defect. In the absence of exact knowledge of etiology, classification is unsatifactory.

1. ***Symptomatic porphyria*** includes acute intermittent and acquired porphyria tarda. Besides genetic pre-disposition, liver appears to be involved. It is precipitated by barbiturates especially pentothal, sulphonamides, griseofulvin, alcohol, hydralazine, heavy metals, and chlorinated hydrocarbons (hexachloro-benzene).

   In acute intermittent porphyria is presented with abdominal colicky pain, psychoneurological manifestations (peripheral neuritis, paralysis, psychosis) and porphyrins in the urine (dark coloured urine). Usually there is no photosensitivity and cutaneous features are absent. It is more common in elderly females.

   In acquired porphyria cutanea tarda, patients look weather-beaten; there are vesicles, scars and milia on exposed parts of face, neck and dorsum of hands (**Fig. 25.4**). Photosensitivity and pigmentation appear late in life. Occasionally, Nikolsky's sign may be positive on hands.

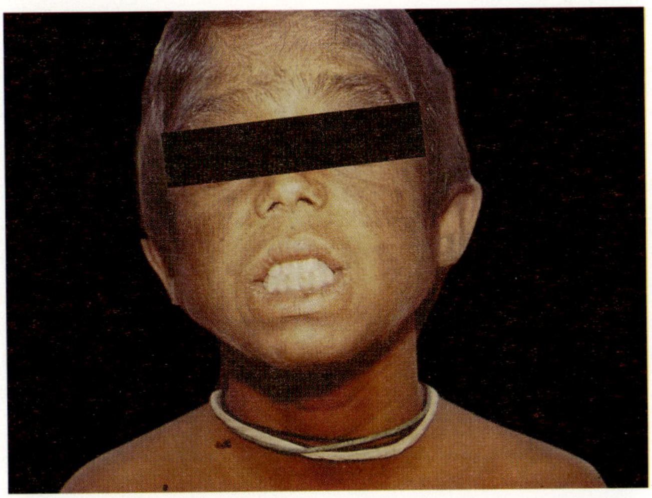

Fig. 25.4: Hypertrichosis seen in porphyria cutanea tarda

2. *Porphyria variegata:* It is heredo-familial, Mendelian dominant. It is frequently seen in South Africa. Characteristic features are photosensitivity, fragile skin and attacks of abdominal colic and psycho-neurotic upsets. In this respect it shows features of acute intermittent porphyria and acquired porphyria cutanea tarda.
3. *Congenital porphyria (Gunther's disease).* It is a rare disease, inherited as Mendelian recessive. Males are predominantly affected . It manifests itself from early childhood. Blisters appear on the exposed parts of the body in the spring and summer; after several years, it may result in severe scarring and mutilation. Deposition of porphyrins on the teeth leads to a pink discoloration. Porphyrins are also deposited in the bones. Sometimes, though rarely, haemolytic anaemia may be associated. Hypertrichosis may also occur. Urine is dark coca-cola shade.
4. *Erythropoietic protoporphyria.* It is a much more common condition than recognized. Clinical features are light sensitive urticaria, burning sensation on exposure to sunlight, oedema and vesicular crusted eruption .

In chronic cases, mild pitting and a few criss-cross scars on the face and somewhat insignificant papules on the back of the hands and fingers appear to be the chief lesions (Magnus).

Cases of photo-sensitivity should be screened for porphyrin metabolic disturbance.

Diagnosis: It is established by the demonstration of porphyrins in the urine by chemical and spectroscopic methods. Under Wood's light, urine fluoroscences red when mixed with acetic acid and amyl alcohol. Quantitative and qualitative estimation of uroporphyrins I and II, coproporphyrins I and III and uroporphyrinogens is a good academic exercise. Blood and stools should also be tested for porphyrins.

Treatment: (1) Protection from sunlight and using an anti-actinic cream. (2) Sodium bicarbonate by mouth- metabolic alkalisation. (3) A course of hydroxychloroquine or desferrioxamine B or carrot juice (Carotene). (4) Chelating agents like dimercaprol and EDTA. Steroids may be life-saving in acute porphyria. EDTA (Ethylene-diamine-tetra-acetic acid) is given in doses of 1 gm by slow intravenous infusion properly diluted with 500 cc of glucose saline. (5) Avoidance of alcohol, barbiturates and other drugs. (6) Splenectomy and phlebotomy may be useful in congenital porphyria.

NUTRITIONAL DISORDERS

Malnutrition

Nutritional disorders are fairly common in the tropical, under-developed countries of Asia. Since most vitamin and other deficiencies affect the skin and mucous membranes before the other parts of the body, a short account of cutaneous lesions thus produced, is given in this book. For details, the reader should refer to reference books on the subject.

Though stress is laid on avitaminosis in the study of nutritional disorders, it should not be forgotten that deficiencies of minerals, proteins and fats are fairly important. For example, it is now realized that the deficiency of fatty acids rather than vitamin A is responsible for follicular keratosis and phrynoderma. Proteins are considered essential for the maintenance of the skin structure; their administration is essential in the treatment of Kwashiorkor's syndrome. Excessive amount of carbohydrates may produce or complicate seborrhoeic conditions. It is presumed by several authorities that copper deficiency may be responsible for the prevalence of vitiligo in some countries and zinc deficiency may produce dermatitis enteropathica-like picture and other dermatoses.

Avitaminosis

It is usually an index of poverty and squalor. The two important factors responsible for avitaminosis are: (1) a poor, unbalanced diet and (2) digestive upsets like chronic diarrhoea, sprue, dysentery and ulcerative colitis. Slimming stunts amongst young ladies may produce malnutrition and proneness to several dermatoses especially chloasma. Rarely inborn, a metabolic defect may be responsible for avitaminosis.

Though deficiencies due to a single vitamin or its component are described, it is very seldom that one comes across anything but multiple vitamin deficiencies in an individual. The use of vitamin is recommended when a deficiency is suspected or feared. Abuse of vitamins is very prevalent in the modern world, particularly among the educated classes; undue commercial propaganda is responsible to a certain extent. This abuse should be discouraged. Indiscriminate medication with vitamins may even result in hypervitaminosis. Hypercalcaemia, calcinosis cutis and even renal calculi are seen in hypervitaminosis. Toxicity with vitamin A may cause deep painful swellings in the limbs, anorexia, dry scaly skin, sparse hair and pruritus.

To sum up, whenever one comes across dry, harsh skin with loss of elasticity, fine wrinkling, abnormal keratinization particularly follicular, haemorrhages, pigmentation of the exposed parts, dry lustreless hair, atrophic nails and involvement of the mucous membranes, one must recognize these as signs of malnutrition-deficiency of vitamins, proteins, fats and minerals in the body. The cause of the deficiency must be looked for in the diet and gastro-intestinal disturbance.

Kwashiorkor's Syndrome

It is specific, severe type of malnutrition particularly of proteins and calories. It is seen occasionally amongst infants and children in India and Africa.

The typical features are:

1. A debilitated, irritable and apathetic child or infant with oedema of the feet.
2. Varnish-like, jet-black, scaly patches on the trunk and limbs. They are cracked at the flexures (crazy-paving appearance).
3. Depigmentation along with areas of hyperpigmentation. Pallor around the mouth and nose.
4. Thinning of hair which tend to become fine and brittle.
5. Nails are thin, ridged and brittle.
6. Photophobia and lacrimation.

It used to be a fatal condition. However, now that its etiology is better understood, outlook has improved. Treatment consists of administration of adequate amounts of milk powder, eggs and extra vitamins. In poor people, soyabean products are useful substitutes.

Pellagra

It is a chronic, nicotinic acid deficiency, characterized by dermatitis, diarrhoea and nervous symptoms. Most cases occur in endemic areas due to use of millet staple diet, which is found to be deficient in nicotinic acid. In the early stages, the symptoms are seasonal. In tropical climates, they start in winter, whereas in temperate climates, they start or tend to become aggravated in summer. The common symptoms and signs are:

Skin: Lesions are selectively present on the exposed parts of the body, and less so, on the sites of friction, viz., the dorsum of hands and forearms up to the level of sleeves, the face, the exposed neckline, V of the chest, the feet and the legs. In the unfortunate unclothed population, almost the whole of the body is involved. The lesions are bilateral and symmetrical; they are well-defined. The subjective symptoms consist of burning and a little itching. The common clinical lesions are erythema, pigmentation and scaling. The integument may show acute or subacute dermatitis, or may appear thin, parchment-like, atrophic and pigmented.

Mucous membranes: Typical features are: A burning sensation and a red tongue with stomatitis. A geographical tongue may be seen in the later stages. Diarrhoea is a very common feature.

Nervous system: Symptoms in the form of neurasthenia, dementia, psychotic features, peripheral neuritis, and signs like subacute, combined degeneration may be seen.

Besides primary nicotinic acid and other vitamin deficiencies in the diet, chronic alcoholism, gastro-intestinal disorders and use of INH (isonicotinic acid hydrazide) may initiate pellagra. Photosensitivity is very charateristic. The diagnosis of pellagra is not difficult in endemic areas. The prognosis is good in well-treated cases.

Treatment: It consists in:

1. Correction of diet and causative factors. The diet should include whole grain cereals, lentils, meat, leafy vegetables, yeast and marmite.
2. Nicotinic acid 50–150 mg TDS by mouth or injections in severe cases.
3. B-complex and multivitamins. Liver extract is also helpful. When there is marked nervous system involvement, vitamin B proves beneficial.
4. Rest and protection from the sun.
5. Locally, zinc or calamine cream for dermatitis **(Table 25.1)**.

Pink's Disease

It is an uncommon disease occurring chiefly in infants and children. It has been attributed to vitamin deficiency and sometimes to mercury poisoning. The characteristic symptoms are:

1. Constitutional—depression, restlessness and irritability; increased sweating; temperature normal or sub-normal; wasting; hypotonia.
2. Cold, swollen, bluish or reddish palms and soles, often described as raw, beefy hands and feet. Recurrent desquamation is a prominent feature.
3. A generalized miliary or erythematous eruption on the trunk.
4. Hair, teeth and nails may be lost.

The outlook is fair with a low mortality. Cases tend to recover in 3–10 weeks, though relapses may occur.

The treatment consists of general management, nourishing food, administering sedatives and extra vitamins. Injection of BAL with corticosteroids may be useful in severe cases.

Table 25.1: Vitamins and the skin

Vitamins	*Requirement daily*	*Sources*	*Physiological action*	*Results of deficiency*	*Remarks*
1. Vitamin A	2000–6000 IU	Milk, butter, ghee, carrots, fish oils, liver, eggs-yolk and green vegetables	Essential for normal epidermal metabolism hence the proper functioning of the epithelial structures	Skin; Dry, harsh skin (phrynoderma with follicular, horny plugs. Follicular keratosis. Eyes: Xerophthalmia. Night blindness, Bitot spots. Defective teeth and nails	Animal fats are lately considered responsible for phrynoderma. Over assimilation of Vitamin A produces toxic symptoms—anaemia, body decalcification, etc. Vitamin A is useful in keratodermas, pityriasis rubra pilaris, etc.
2. Vitamin B	B_1 1–2 mg	Yeast, whole grain, cereals, lentils, meat, liver, rice shavings and leafy vegetables	Essential for carbohydrate metabolism	Beriberi—peripheral neuritis. Cramps, weakness, oedema. Seborrhoeic skin affections. Pellagra (see details below)	
	B_2-nicotinic acid 10–12 mg			Magenta coloured tongue. Angular stomatitis and cheilitis. Seborrhoeic skin affections. Peri-corneal vascularity. No clear-cut symptoms but somewhat related to ariboflavinosis. Macrocytic anaemia	Useful in herpes gestationis
	Riboflavin 1–2 mg				

Contd.

Table 25.1: Vitamins and the skin *(Contd)*.

	Pyridoxine 1–2 mg				
	B_{12} 1 μg				Useful in herpes zoster, psoriasis, etc.
3. Vitamin C	30 mg	Oranges, lemons, tomatoes, green leafy vegetables, sprouted grain, guava, amla	Essential for metabolism of mesoblastic tissues; hence nourishment of capillaries and osteoid tissues.	Scurvy—bleeding and spongy gums, loosening of teeth, purpuric haemorrhages, anaemia, stomatitis	Useful in bleeding diseases and chloasma
4. Vitamin D	500–1500 IU	Milk, butter, ghee, egg-yolk, fish oils	Essential for calcium metabolism and bone formation	Rickets, defective teeth, osteomalacia. No skin lesions	Also produced by the skin from ergosterol by irradiation. Useful in lupus vulgaris. Excessive use produces toxic symptoms—loss of appetite, increased thirst, hypercalcaemia and metastatic calcification.
5. Vitamin E	α, β, tocopherol 1–3 mg	Wheat germ, oatmeal and green vegetables		No skin lesions. Muscular and nervous symptoms have been described	Useful in keratodermas, epidermolysis bullosa
6. Vitamin K		Green vegetables	Essential for prothrombin manufacture by liver	Purpuric haemorrhagves. Bleeding disease	Useful in bleeding disease
7. Vitamin P		Lemon and orange peel	Essential for capillary resistance		Useful in bleeding disease

VASCULAR DISORDERS

Normal vascular supply is essential for proper nutrition of the integument; disturbed circulation produces changes in colour, temperature and tone, congestion, oedema and even necrosis. The arteriolar tone is influenced by the sympathetic supply and the vasomotor centre. Detailed information of peripheral vascular disease is available in textbooks of medicine and surgery, but since the effects of vascular diseases exhibit themselves on the integument, they are discussed here, but briefly.

Gangrene

It implies the death of cutaneous and underlying tissues resulting from interference with nutrition. There are usually two types of gangrene:

1. Dry—in which there is sharply demarcated mummification of the parts. Clinically, the affected part becomes dry, hard, brownish-black, cold and devoid of sensations. Dry gangrene is mainly due to arterial obstruction.
2. Moist—in which the affected part is soft, sodden, purplish cold and devoid of sensations. There is no sharp demarcation. Moist gangrene is due to complete obstruction, and there is secondary bacterial infection.

Gas gangrene is the infection of surgical wounds with gas gangrene organisms.

The common causes of gangrene are interference with the arterial blood supply resulting from arteriosclerosis, diabetes, Buerger's disease, Raynaud's disease, polyarteritis nodosa and ergotism. Physical and chemical trauma may also produce gangrene.

Raynaud's Disease

It is a specific, vaso-spastic disease entity seen more commonly in young adults; it occurs more frequently in females than males. It is limited to the fingers and less so to the toes. Clinically, it is characterized by recurrent arteriolar spasms producing blanching (cold, pale and numbness) followed by asphyxial cyanosis (swollen, blue and painful) of the affected parts brought on by exposure to cold or emotional disturbance. When circulation is restored, there is reactive hyperaemia resulting in redness of the tips of the fingers, warmth and throbbing pain. Typical tricolour appearance of pallor, cyanosis and redness may exist simultaneously in the same individual; this constitutes the classical clinical picture: The paroxysm lasts for two hours or more. Pain is usually present. The condition is bilaterally symmetrical. In severe cases, local necrosis, even gangrene may develop. In chronic cases, the fingers become tapered or even club-shaped; nail dystrophies may also occur.

Occasionally, Raynaud's disease is complicated by the systemic symptoms of haemoglobinuria, amblyopia, etc.

The course is progressive and chronic.

Differential diagnosis: It is made from conditions which can produce Raynaud's phenomena, viz., sclerodactyly, cervical rib, Buerger's disease, arteriosclerosis, syphilitic arteritis, chilblains, acrocyanosis, etc.

Treatment: It consists in protecting the body from cold and the mind from emotional stresses along with improving the general nutrition. Nitrates, acetylcholine, etc. are also beneficial. Orabolin, dianabol, benzoline hydrochloride (Priscol-P) and isoxsuprine hydrochloride (Duvadilan-P) are very helpful. In acute cases, analgesics and antibiotics may be required. Trental (P) is useful stand-by.

Buerger's Disease

It is a rare, chronic inflammatory disease of the arteries and veins resulting in gradual obliteration, selectively affecting the lower limbs of males. The exact cause is unknown; smoking is often held responsible. Cramps, pain and gangrene are the important clinical features. The treatment consists in quiting smoking, Buerger's postural exercise, in keeping the affected parts warm and in using vasodilators. Sympathectomy and surgical amputation are recommended only in extreme cases.

Nodular Vasculitis

Clinical features: It is fairly common in practice, being more common in adult females than males. Lesions are seen on the legs (postero-lateral surfaces, less so anterior), thighs and less so other parts. Lesions start as painful and tender erythema, usually unaccompanied by any constitutional symptoms. It slowly gains in size, frequently it ulcerates to produce a dirty-looking, indolent ulcer. New nodules appear at intervals. They are often better felt than seen. The lesions heal within 2–6 weeks leaving pigmented scars. In ulcerated form, longer time is required for complete healing. ESR may be raised. Rarely, there is systemic involvement.

Etiology: Trauma, septic focus, drugs and stasis are some of the probable causes.

Histology: It shows intense inflammation of the vessels at the junction of dermis and subcutis. There is endothelial proliferation, swelling and inflammation in and around the vessel walls. Features of septitis in the adipose tissue are characteristic.

Differential diagnosis: It is from other nodular lesions viz., panniculitis, erythema nodosum and erythema induratum. In chronic cases, it is desirable to use the term chronic erythema nodosum for these conditions.

Prognosis: It usually does not affect the longevity of life, and the general health of the patients. Acute cases tide over the crisis nicely but chronic cases continue for long periods.

Treatment: In the absence of known cause, treatment is unsatisfactory. Bed rest may be mandatory for few, but rest to the part is essential in all cases. Stasis, if present should be controlled. Steroids and antibiotics in small doses are effective but hazardous in chronic cases. Ulcers should be dressed with mild antiseptics. Cyclophosphamide (Endoxan-P) is useful in some cases.

Schamberg's Disease

Synonym: Progressive pigmented purpuric dermatosis.

The clinical manifestations of capillaritis of unknown origin in upper dermis have been described under various names viz., purpura annularis telangiectoides, purpura pigmentosa chronica, angioma serpiginosum and Schamberg's disease. The last one is the most popular name and the condition is fairly common. Practically speaking they all are the same. Basically they represent different proportions of telengiectasia and pigmentation in the course of long-standing capillaritis, producing different morphological pictures.

Clinical features: More and more cases are being seen with Schamberg's disease in India. It mostly affects legs of adults but may occur at any age. It starts as one or more tiny purpuric spots which enlarge peripherally; with the appearance of more spots, a plaque is formed which in due course, develops dark brown pigmentation having cayenne pepper look. Telangiectasia and a few atrophic areas may also be seen. It may be bilateral but not necessarily symmetrical.

Etiology: Exact cause is not known. Usually there is no other subjective symptom or venous stasis but latter may be a factor in localization of lesions. Standing or sitting in chairs for long hours, use of nylon socks, garters, poor nutrition and focal sepsis are some of the responsible factors. Certain drugs also have been associated with Schamberg's disease and these are acetaminophen, aspirins, carbromals, thiamine and meprobamate.

Histology: There is dilatation and proliferation of capillaries in upper dermis. The endothelium is swollen and inflamed. Extravasated erythrocytes are seen and in older lesions haemosiderin can be demostrated with iron stain. Infiltration with lymphocytes, histiocytes and occasional neutrophil is present specially around capillaries. Epidermis may show atrophy. At times the haemosiderin deposit may invite granulomatous reaction.

Treatment: It is not satisfactory. The measures employed for stasis dermatitis, i.e. crepe bandage, keeping a pillow under the leg at night and calamine or hydrocortisone ointment application may help. Vitamins C, K and P have been prescribed. Septic foci should be treated. Use of nylon socks and garters/suspenders should be discouraged. Foot and leg exercise are useful.

Varicose Veins

It implies a slow or static venous circulation in the lower extremities due to venous varicosities produced by the incompetence of venous valves and increased intravenous pressure. It is mostly gravitational or hypostatic in origin. Middle-aged women are most commonly affected. Varicosity may be confined to the superficial or deep veins; in the majority of cases it affects the long saphenous vein, along with incompetent perforators.

Etiology: Inherent weakness of the venous valves, and standing for long hours, are the important causative factors. Trauma, leg injuries, pregnancy, obesity, pressure on the veins and thrombophlebitis being the other causes.

Clinical features: The common symptoms are swelling of the feet towards the evening; this swelling subsides with rest; the legs become easily fatigued and subject to cramps; there is telangiectases and pigmentation of the skin of the lower parts of the legs and ankles. Lowered vitality and stasis may lead to complications. On physical examination, varicosities are visible; these tend to fill up when the patient stands and disappear when he is in a recumbent position, particularly if the legs are raised. If the valve at the saphenous opening also becomes incompetent, a bruit may be felt on the saphenous vein when the patient coughs. The level to which varicosities have developed, and the extent to which the anastomotic channels have been affected, can be found by tying tourniquets at different levels of the thighs, phlebogram, or injecting fluorescent dye and examination under Wood's lamp.

Complications: They are:

1. Varicose eczema (Fig. 25.5, see Chapter 10).
2. Varicose ulcer. Trauma or infection are the important causes. It is seen typically on the internal malleolus or inner side of the lower third of the leg as oval or irregular, shallow ulcer surrounded by infiltrated and pigmented skin and accompanied by gravitational oedema of the feet. The ulcers usually appear singly and are slow to heal. Pain may or may not be present.
3. Thrombophlebitis.

Treatment: It consists in:

1. Correction of the causes.
2. Prevention of stasis by avoiding standing for long hours, raising the feet while sitting or lying down, wearing elastic stockings or crepe or elastoplast bandages. Leg lifting exercise and yoga are useful.
3. Surgical correction by ligation or stripping of the long saphenous vein and the anastomotic channels. In varicosity of the long saphenous vein, it is ligated flush in level with its junction at the femoral vein. Sclerotherapy is useful in mild and moderate cases.
4. Treatment of complications:
   a. Eczema—infective or chemical along the same lines as the treatment for eczema.
   b. Ulcer—with antiseptic dressing, 20 pc benzyl peroxide and occlusive elastoplast bandaging. Excision and grafting in intractable cases. Hirudoid (p) ointment applied around the ulcer is also helpful. Collagen sheets and Debrisan promote prompt healing of recalcitrant ulcers.
   c. Thrombophlebitis—with antibiotics and anti-coagulants like Tromexan (P).

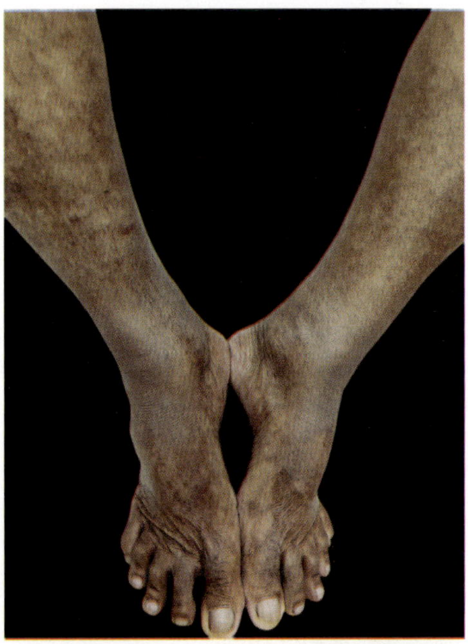

Fig. 25.5: Varicose eczema

Elephantiasis

It implies the gross enlargement or swelling of a part of any limb due to the blocking of the lymphatic system resulting in non-pitting oedema, hypertrophy of the cutaneous and subcutaneous tissues and lymph varices (Fig. 25.6). The common causes of elephantiasis are:

1. ***Elephantiasis nostras***. Recurrent streptococcal infection of the lymphatics, erysipelas and cellulitis. The common sites of affection are the legs and the lips. Castellani attributes it to *Streptococcus metamyceticus*. Initially there is recurring lymphangitis with fever and pain; with passage of time, oedema and elephantiasis develop. *Streptococcus metamyceticus* is a delicate organism which is isolated from the gland juice on neutral 1% creatinin agar.
2. ***Elephantiasis tropica*** is common in the tropics. Cause is filariasis. It is seen mostly on the legs and the genitalia. Streptococcal infection is usually the exciting cause.
3. ***Congenital-Milroy's disease***. It is a rare, heredofamilial disease which usually affects the legs.
4. ***Uncommon causes***. Surgical interference, injuries, cancerous infiltration, lymphogranuloma inguinale, tuberculosis cutis, leprosy, etc.

The outlook in elephantiasis is essentially poor; in an early case, the progress of the disease can be checked if the cause is removed.

Treatment: It consists in:

1. Removing or treating the cause. Hetrazan (P) is recommended for filariasis. A course of penicillin, sulphonamides or broad-spectrum antibiotics, if active streptococcal infection or lymphogranuloma is suspected. Elephantiasis nostras (Castellani) responds best to the special vaccine.
2. Compression by bandage or sling.
3. Diathermy- shortwave or infrared may be helpful.
4. Surgical lymphangioplasty operations.

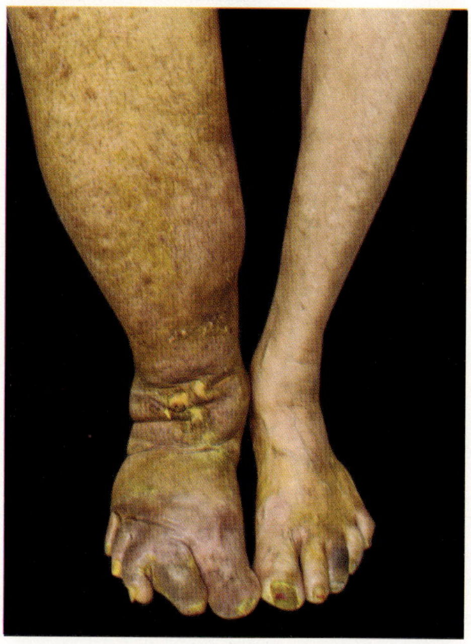

Fig. 25.6: Elephantiasis

Neuritic Atrophy

Atrophy of the integument may occur as such or may be associated with other defects of the skin and/or other organs or systems. When atrophy of the integument is seen in practice, clinician should establish the following points:

Whether the atrophy is localized to the skin, or combined with atrophy or defects of other organs, or associated with hypertrophy or inflammation of the skin; is it diffuse, macular or striate; any associated neuritic disorders.

Once the category or variety of atrophy **(Table 25.2)** is established, clinical diagnosis becomes easy and then an attempt should be made to elicit the cause or causes of the atrophy.

Senile Atrophy

With ageing, cutaneous degeneration sets in affecting the appearance of a person. The integument becomes thin, dry, wrinkled and inelastic; there is diminution or loss of subcutaneous fat, which causes sagging of the skin. On the lateral sides of the eyes, wrinkling may take the appearance of crow's feet. On the back of the neck particularly in farmers and sailors, criss-cross markings produce diamond-shaped areas which may become thickened due to elastic tissue swelling and fragmentation—Cutis rhombodies nuchae. The colour of the skin becomes dull-pale. On the exposed parts appear scattered pigmented macules (Senile lentigines or liver spots). The hair tend to fall off or become thin and lanugo-like. In women, whiskers may grow on the face. Facial contour changes resulting in drooping of the mouth. Sebaceous warts, telangiectasis, particularly de Morgan's spots and senile purpuric haemorrhages may be seen. Malignant neoplasms are common in senile atrophic skin. Senile pruritus may be yet another complication. Wounds, dermatitis and eczema heal with difficulty.

Senile atrophy sets in at about the age of 40–50. It is noticed at an early age on the exposed parts in sailors, farmers and vagabonds. People living in temperate climate

Table 25.2: Classification of atrophies
A. Only atrophy of the skin (without any other associated defect) *Diffuse:* Senile or Premature *Localized:* Macular, striate, acrodermatitis atrophicans, hemiatrophy, white anetoderma
B. Atrophy associated with hypertrophy and/or other defects • Lichen sclerosus et atrophicus • Collagenoses. Poikiloderma • Kraurosis vulvae • Pseudo-xanthoma elasticum • Post-inflammatory as in diseases like lupus erythematosus • Ainhum • Panniculitis • Cutis hyperelastica
C. Atrophy associated with neuritic disorders—Neuritic atrophy
D. Associated with defects of other organs Progeria, Acrogeria, Marfan's syndrome, Werner's syndrome

are less severely affected than those living in the tropics. Premature ageing occurs in hypopituitarism, cachexia, malnutrition, porphyria and xeroderma pigmentosum.

Histology shows flattening of the rete pegs, basophilic degeneration of the collagen, swelling and fragmentation of the elastic tissue.

Treatment: The condition can be prevented or delayed by the methods enumerated in Chapter 7—Aids to a healthy skin. Massaging the skin with vitaminized lanoline or milk cream, use of sex hormones, retinoic acid, proper nutrition and exercises are some of the important therapeutic measures recommended. Dermabrasion, plastic and chemo-surgery may help in reducing wrinkles to a certain extent.

Diffuse Premature Atrophy

Besides premature ageing described above, it is seen in conjunction with atrophy of other organs as in congenital defects, Marfan's syndrome, etc. Diffuse congenital atrophy is usually associated with defects of skeletal system and viscera as in "progeria" (infantile but old). Integument appears wrinkled and atrophic like an old man's but the growth of the body and genitals is like that of an infant. Diffuse atrophy may be confined to extremities as in "acrogeria".

Marfan's syndrome is a congenital and heredo-familial defect consisting of tall body, loose joints, skull and palate deformities, ocular defects and stria atrophica.

Hemiatrophy implies wasting on one side of the body esp. the face. Skin, underlying muscles and bones show atrophy and depression. It may be primary or secondary to morphoea.

Anetoderma

It implies development of small circumscribed areas- macular or linear (striate) atrophy of the skin brought on by degeneration of the elastic tissue due to stretching, pressure, inflammation, malnutrition or interference with the nerve supply. An atrophic integument looks thin, shiny, inelastic, smooth and finally wrinkled. It may be raised in level or depressed. The colour is usually white but may look purplish due to the underlying blood vessels being visible through the atrophic skin. The hair, sweat and sebaceous glands are reduced in the atrophic areas.

a. ***Stria atrophica.*** It is seen on the abdomen, breast, lateral surface of shoulders and thighs as glistening white or purplish lines. The causes are pregnancy, obesity, Cushing's syndrome, malnutrition, collagen disease, use of corticosteroids and adolescence. Incidence is on the increase and it is quite common to see it amongst young, obese kids. Poor nutrition may probably be the cause or lack of exercise or emollient or synthetic clothing.

b. ***Macular atrophy.*** It may be seen as a result of the above mentioned diseases besides syphilis, leprosy, typhoid fever. In a small number of cases, no cause is demonstrable; these cases are termed as Primary or Idiopathic macular atrophy. In the latter, lesions occur on the trunk, shoulders and face. These are of two main varities:

   i. ***Anetoderma of Jadassohnn:*** Lentil to pea-sized macules of loose, shiny, wrinkled skin are visible mainly in females of 20–40 years. Herniation is obvious on palpation and fat may infiltrate these lesions. Lesions remain unchanged throughout life.

   ii. ***Schweninger Buzzi variety:*** Bladder-like new growths appear. By pressure, these growths can be inverted like a hernia into a hole in the corium. On involution, soft depressed scars are left behind.

Primary macular atrophy is slowly progressive. Pin-head or lentil-sized depigmented, flat, or slightly raised macules with fine wrinkling are often seen on the legs and trunk in white anetoderma. Dopa stain shows diminution or absence of melanocytes. There is increase in collagen and decrease in elastic tissue. Another term used is guttate hypomelanosis.

Acrodermatitis Chronica Atrophicans

It is primary, progressive variety of anetoderma affecting the limbs, lower more than upper. It usually affects middle aged, obese women. In the early stages, there are bluish patches or bands of oedematous infiltration on the feet and legs; in the later stages, there are whitish cigarette-paper like atrophic changes. Large areas of the integument may be involved showing marked atrophy. It is rare disorder which may mimic pseudo scleroderma. Microscopy reveals atrophy of the cutis without fibrosis; corium shows lymphocytic infiltration.

Treatment is unsatisfactory. Routine supportive therapy with tonics and vitamins and local massage with vitaminized oil have been recommended but often without success. Some workers have claimed success with large doses of penicillin for 10–14 days. The underlying causes must be studied in each case and an attempt be made to eliminate them.

Neuritic Atrophy

Organic nervous system disorders produce cutaneous lesions, particularly atrophic. Integument exhibits definite sensory changes besides atrophy. The common cutaneous features are glossy, dry, wrinkled skin with diminished hair and sweating (anetoderma neuritica) in nerve injuries, leprosy, etc. Nail, bone and other deformities, accompanied by a glossy skin, may be seen in syringomyelia and Morvan's disease; trophic ulcers in leprosy, tabes dorsalis, syringomyelia, poliomyelitis and diabetes mellitus, etc.

Sometimes, though rarely, there is a peculiar hyperaesthesia or partial anaesthesia/ paraesthesia and spontaneous pain in localized areas of the skin; the latter looks and feels normal. Histology shows no abnormalities. These features are seen in meralgia paraesthetica on the lateral sides of thighs. Leprosy must be eliminated in differential diagnosis. Condition responds to vitamin B-complex injections and massage.

Ainhum

It is a rare disorder, seen usually in black males. A few cases have been described in India. It is characterized by spontaneous falling of the digits particularly the small toes due to primary progressive constriction by fibrous bands. Trauma may be the predisposing cause. A similar condition may develop in leprosy and keratoderma. The treatment is unsatisfactory; it consists in cutting the constricting band in the initial stage and amputation in the advanced stage.

Kraurosis Vulvae

Kraurosis vulvae signifies progressive atrophy coupled with sclerosis of the mucous membrane elements of the vulva.

Clinical features: It is asymptomatic or slightly itchy. The disease process is usually restricted to the true mucous membrane of the vulval region. In the initial stage, there is oedema and redness, accompanied by hyper- or depigmentation. With the progression of atrophy and sclerosis, there is flattening of the features. The clitoris, labia minora and frenum disappear; the labia majora becomes flattened. The mucous membrane appears to be reddish or waxy-white, dry, smooth and shining. The vaginal orifice become stenosed. Similar condition can occur in the male (kraurosis penis/balanitis xerotica obliterans). Kraurosis vulvae may be associated with ulcerative and atrophic lesions of the mouth and tongue.

It may be complicated by secondary lichenification; only then do the adjoining parts of the thighs become involved. Sometimes it is complicated by leukoplakia.

Etiology: Depression of the ovarian function is the most likely cause; hence the condition is usually seen in menopausal women.

Differential diagnosis: It is made from the following:

- ***Senile atrophy:*** It is proportionate to the senile atrophic changes that take place in the integument elsewhere. There is no stenosis.
- ***Lichen simplex:*** Involves more of the cutaneous part of the vulval region than the mucous membrane; no stenosis of the vagina or waxy-white, flattened features;. welldefined area of thickened, pigmented, infiltrated skin with prominent criss-cross marking; marked pruritus; evidence of psychogenic stress particularly sexual.
- ***Leukoplakia:*** Hypertrophic process confined to the mucous membrane; well defined small or large, raised, infiltrated, milky-white patches; danger of malignancy.

The differential diagnosis is also made from lichen sclerosus et atrophicus (*see* below).

Treatment: Since the condition is usually asymptomatic, no treatment is usually indicated. Oestrogens used locally, in the form of an ointment/pessaries, or orally, in the form of tablets, do help in the initial stages. Vitamins particularly vitamin A, tonics and local diathermy are also beneficial. If the complication of leukoplakia sets in, excision of the vulva should be advised.

Lichen Sclerosus et Atrophicus

It is essentially confined to the cutaneous portion of the vulva, anogenital region, trunk and shoulders. It is characterized by irregular, whitish papules and plaques with keratotic plugs or central delling; later white, tissue-paper like, wrinkled patches develop. There is minimal pruritus. The histology is characteristic. It consists of hyperkeratosis, follicular plugging, epidermal atrophy, band of hyalinized collagen below the epidermis, dilated capillaries and a band of round cell infiltration. It is a chronic disease, treatment being unsatisfactory. Hydrocortisone infiltration and 2% testosterone propionate cream are worth trying.

Cutis Hyperelastica

This may be present from an early age and shows in the form of excessive elasticity of the skin which can be stretched like a rubber band (Fig. 25.7). The cause is unknown but it is usually congenital or familial. The Ehlers danlos syndrome may show the following features:

1. Hyper-elasticity of the skin.
2. Hyper-laxity of the joints.
3. Friability of the skin and blood vessels.

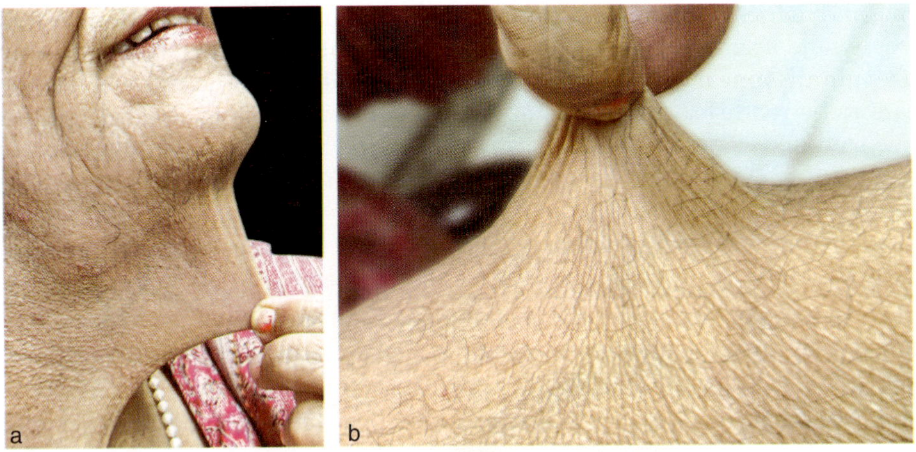

Fig. 25.7: Cutis hyperelastica. (a) Neck; (b) Arm

4. Pseudo-tumour appearance over the knees or site of trauma.

With age, condition may improve slightly or deteriorate. Treatment is unsatisfactory.

Pseudoxanthoma Elasticum

It is a Mendelian recessive, hereditary, degenerative disorder of the elastic tissues; characteristically seen in young females as pale yellowish-coloured, flat, soft and wrinkled papules on the sides of the neck, axillae, abdomen and groins. There may be associated angioid streaks in the retina, psychic disturbances, epilepsy and bleeding tendency. The histopathological features are diagnostic. The condition is asymptomatic, and no specific treatment is known.

Panniculitis

A common form of panniculitis is the nodular, non-suppurative panniculitis (Gilchrist type) which is characterized by nodules and plaques of a dusky colour with underlying hard, sclerotic, easily movable masses, accompanied by relapsing fever and recurrent constitutional symptoms **(Fig. 25.8)**. On resolution, poorly defined, depressed, morphoea-like areas are left behind. Lesions occur mainly on the buttocks and limbs. The etiology is unknown; in every case, a search for a focal sepsis should be made. The treatment is palliative; broad-spectrum antibiotics may be successfully tried in febrile cases.

Poikiloderma

It is characterized by cutaneous atrophy, pigmentation and telangiectasia; it is rarely accompanied by purpuric haemorrhages. The condition is usually chronic and progressive; the appearance of poikiloderma resembles healed, X-ray burns. The important causes of poikiloderma are congenital ectodermal dystrophy, dermatomyositis, reticuloses and arsenical intoxication. It is rarely idiopathic. Poikiloderma of Civatte is a common variety affecting symmetrically the face and neck in middle-aged women. Poikiloderma vasculare atrophicans of Jacobi is associated with poikiloderma-like picture, retiform distribution, keratosis and general pruritus. Telangiectasis may

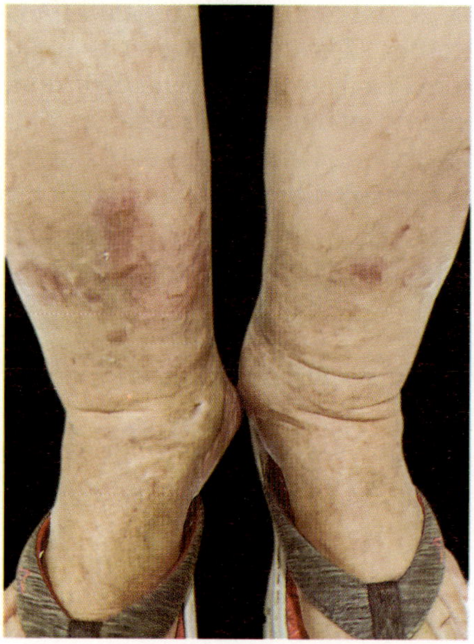

Fig. 25.8: Panniculitis

show capillary haemorrhages. The condition is intractable and the treatment is only symptomatic.

Endocrine Disorders

According to Dunlop, the type and characters of the skin are determined by the endocrine pattern of the individual, besides factors like heredity, nutrition, environment, etc. The mode of action of the endocrines on the skin is shown in Fig. 25.9 and discussed as follows:

Endocrines influence the functions and growth of the skin, sebaceous glands, hair, sweat glands, nails, pigment and dermal tissues. They have been discussed in relevant chapters. Their influence at puberty, menopause and during pregnancy is very pertinent.

Relationship of endocrines to acne vulgaris, chloasma, seborrhoeic dermatitis, itching of pregnancy and pruritus vulvae, etc. is well recognised. Calcinosis in hyperparathyroidism and diabetes in pancreatic affections is discussed in preceding pages. Relationship of endocrines with skin is listed in Table 25.3.

Endocrine Diseases

Acromegaly occurs because of hyper-secretion of growth hormone from anterior pituitary in adult life. Salient features are gigantic hypertrophy of the chin, nose, supraorbital ridges, hands and feet. There is diffuse hypertrophic thickness of the skin, hypertrichosis and hyperpigmentation. The lips and tongue are hypertrophic. There is enlargement of fingertips giving them a drumstick appearance.

Cushing's syndrome is the result of hyperfunction of the basophilic anterior pituitary and adrenocortical tissue. It is seen more commonly in females. The important features are "buffalo type obesity", moon-shaped facies, hypertrichosis, dryness and fragility of the skin, acneiform lesions on face, kyphosis, purplish striae on the abdomen and thighs,

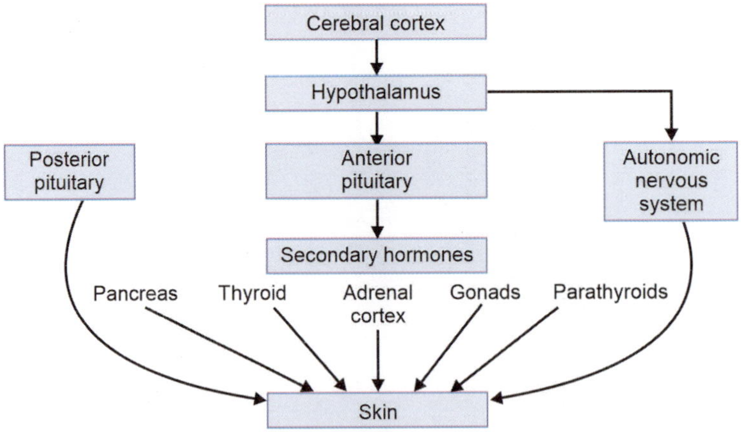

Fig. 25.9: Endocrines and the skin

purpura, echymoses or brownish pigmentation, amenorrhea in females, impotence in males, muscular weakness, hypertension and polycythaemia.

Cretinism is primary thyroid deficiency in foetal life. Skin changes are present either at birth or appear in first few months of life. Integument is cool, dry and pasty white. The lips are pale, thick, coarse and protuberant. The child has a typical face with wide set eyes, flat and broad nose, periorbital puffiness and enlarged tongue. There is poor development of the brain and skeletal system.

Myxoedema is due to lack of secretion of thyroid hormone in middle age. Integument is rough, coarse and dry, which is difficult to pinch especially on the face. It has a dull, puffy expression. Macroglossia and chronic periorbital oedema frequently develop. There is diffuse loss of body hair, the latter become coarse and brittle. Outer one-third of eyebrows are shed.

Hyperthyroidism is due to hypertrophy of thyroid resulting in excessive secretion producing a variety of kin changes. The surface of skin is warm, moist and smooth. The hair is thin, sparse and has downy texture. Palmar erythema and melanoderma are the other features.

Androgen dependent syndrome is caused by the excessive production of adrenal androgens. The skin changes consist of acne, hirsutism, temporal baldness, seborrhoea, enlargement of the clitoris, and decreased size of breasts. Some patients develop hyperpigmentation of the skin, areola, genitalia, palms and buccal mucosa.

Table 25.3: Endocrines and the skin

Endocrine	*Skin*	*Pigmentation*	*Hair*	*Sebaceous and sweat glands*	*Remarks*
I. Pituitary					
a. Physiological	–	–	Growth of pubic and axillary hair	–	Also affected by adrenal cortex
b. Hypopituitarism	In dwarfs, infantile skin. In adults, dry pale, scaly and prematurely senile skin	–	Conspicuous absence of body hair—pubic and axillary. In males, beard and moustache	Atrophic	Starvation produces similar features and also post-partum haemorrhage (Sheehan's syndrome). There is lassitude, anorexia and wasting—body and sexual organs
c. Gigantism and acromegaly	Thickening of skin and sub-cutaneous tissues—thick, coarse, hypertrophic	–	Dark, thick and abundant	Greasy and sweaty. Enlarged pores. Seborrhoea	With burning of disease, features of hypopituitarism set in.
d. Cushing's syndrome	Bloated, plethoric and obese; flame-shaped stria. Buffalo hump. Moon facies, obese trunk and slender limbs				
II. Thyroid					
a. Hyperthyroidism (Grave's disease)	Flushed and moist. Vasodilatation	Dyschromia—hyperpigmentation, depigmentation or both	Excessive growth	Increased seating	May be accompanied by pretibial myxoderma. Loss in weight. Easy excitability
b. Hypothyroidism (myxoedema)	Dry, coarse and may be scaly. Skin cannot be pinched because of infiltration with pseudomucin	–	Tendency for hair to fall especially on the outer thirds of eyebrows. Hair are coarse	Dryness due to dystrophy, and reduced secretions	Also tendency to dystrophy of nails. Puffy oedema of the hands, face and eyelids. Fatigue, obesity and intolerance to cold. Juvenile hypothyroidism is called cretinism

Contd.

Table 25.3: Endocrines and the skin *(Contd)*.

III. Adrenals					
a. Addison's disease	Pale atrophic skin	Hyperpigmentation of skin and mouth	Hair may be diminished	Sweating and grease may be reduced	Loss in weight, low blood pressure, poor appetite and easy fatiguability
b. Hypertrophy (adenoma)	–	–	Excessive growth of pubic and axillary hair	–	Precocious puberty in children
IV. Ovaries					
a. Physiological		Pigmentation of areola, vulva, mouth and face	Growth of scalp hair	Reduction in sebaceous secretion	Increased permeability and so turge-scence of skin
b. Hypogonadism		–	Scalp hair thin and atrophic; may be hypertrichosis, elsewhere same.	–	Rosacea, chloasma, etc.
c. Menopause		–	Same	–	Chloasma, keratoderma climactericum, dermatitis dysmenorrheica, kraurosis vulvae, hirsutism, etc.
V. Androgens					
a. Physiological	–	–	Male sexual hair. Beard, chest and abdomen	Greasy integument and pimples	–
b. Eunuchoidism	Pale and fine	–	Scalp hair dense; rest scanty and fine	Dry, due to atrophic sebaceous glands	No acne or dandruff

Chapter 26

Fevers and Rashes

There is much to be said about a rash: It brings the fever into the limelight.

INTRODUCTION

A rash is a cutaneous eruption produced by the action of an organism or its toxic agents, or other endogenous or extraneous noxious agents. Though a rash is usually generalized and is pathognomonic of exanthemata, the term is often employed to include all cutaneous eruptions.

A rash, on its own, does cause a patient and his attendants anxiety, but when it is accompanied by fever, this anxiety is increased manifold and medical aid is summoned forthwith. These fevers are common and are of a very wide variety.

Before tackling the formidable list of causes of fevers and rashes, we must acquaint ourselves with certain features revealed in the history and examination of patients suffering from these rashes and fevers.

The normal temperature of the human body ranges between 97 and 99°F. A rise in the temperature above 99°F is considered as fever, which may be high, moderate or slight. Special features to be noted are the onset—is the fever insidious or sudden? Is there rigor or chill at the time of the onset? The duration-How long does it last?What is the behaviour of the temperature chart? Are there any constitutional symptoms preceding or accompanying the fever, and if so, are they in any way related to the rash?

The patient must be examined in good light preferably daylight. He must be stripped as completely as circumstances permit for proper examination of the rash. The special points to be noted about the rash are the site of the rash; the manner of spread; the primary lesion, and the secondary lesions resulting from modification; the areas of density. Is the distribution relative or absolute? Any special characters? In what manner does the rash disappear? Any itching or pruritus? Any eruption inside the mouth or other orifices. It is important to enquire whether or not the patient has exposed himself to a similar rash. Have cases with similar rashes occurred in the neighbourhood or family? This question is of particular importance in cases of exanthemata.

The physician should do a complete general examination. This is most essential in a case of fever with rash.

Fevers and rashes are of special importance in tropical countries because of their high incidence and because they are often contagious and eruptive. Diseases take on an epidemic form if due precautions are not taken in time.

The laboratory aids often relied upon are bacteriological; immunological; serological like Widal's, Weil-Felix, etc. and haematological like blood count, blood sedimentation rate.

LIST OF CAUSES OF FEVERS AND RASHES

Fever and rash starting simultaneously or within a week of each other

Acute Illnesses of Short Duration

1. *Exanthemata:* Varicella, scarlet fever, smallpox, monkeypox, typhus, enteric fever, generalized vaccinia, Kaposi's varicelliform eruption.
2. Pyogenic-erysipelas (*see* Chapter 11).
3. Allergic rashes—acute allergy, drug rash, serum sickness, Henoch–Schönlein purpura.
4. Herpes zoster (*see* Chapter 14).
5. Rheumatic fever (*see* Chapter 24)
6. Infectious mononucleosis.
7. Dermatomyositis.

Subacute or Chronic Illnesses of Long Duration

1. Systemic lupus erythematosus (*see* Chapter 24).
2. Tuberculosis of the skin-miliary tuberculosis, papulo-necrotic tuberculides (*see* Chapter 15).
3. Erythema nodosum (*see* Chapter 15).
4. Lepra reaction (*see* Chapter 17).
5. Secondary syphilis (*see* Chapter 18).
6. Polyarteritis nodosa.
7. Panniculitis.

Rashes (or Cutaneous Diseases) Complicated by Fever

1. *Eczema:* Acute dissemination or secondary infection (*see* Chapter 10).
2. *Pemphigus:* Secondary infection (*see* Chapter 22).
3. *Exfoliative dermatitis:* Secondary infection (*see* Chapter 20)
4. Scleroderma with secondary infection (*see* Chapter 24).
5. *Leprosy:* Lepra reaction (*see* Chapter 17).
6. Papulo-necrotic tuberculides (*see* Chapter 15).

Fever (or Systemic Disease) Complicated by Rash

1. Dermatitis medicamentosa complicating any fever.
2. Bacterial endocarditis—petechiae and erythematous rash.
3. Rheumatic fever—erythematous eruptions.
4. Pyaemia—pyaemic abscesses.
5. Secondary carcinomatosis—firm dermal nodules.
6. Reticuloses—Hodgkin' s disease, mycosis fungoides, leukaemia.
7. Gout—chalky tophi.
8. Pulmonary tuberculosis—miliary tuberculosis or ide eruption.

This classification is based on clinical data. There is no sharp demarcation between groups because deviations do occur.

EXANTHEMATA

In scarlet fever, rubella, measles enteric fever and typhus, the rash is erythematous, macular or maculo-papular. In the first three, the eruption appears in the first 4 days of the disease and in the last two the rash appears between the 5th and the 7th day. In chickenpox (varicella) and smallpox, the rash is maculo-papular in the early stage only; it soon becomes vesicular and pustular. In monkeypox, the rashes are in the same stage of development. In the different diseases grouped under exanthemata, the rashes appear within the first seven days of the respective diseases in the following order:

- 1st day: Chickenpox, rubella.
- 2nd day: Scarlet fever.
- 3rd day: Smallpox.
- 4th day : Measles.
- 5th day: Typhus.
- 7th day: Enteric fever.

General discussion of exanthemata. In a book of this nature a detailed discussion of exanthemata will be out of place; the reader should consult textbooks of medicine or infectious fevers to acquaint himself with the details of these diseases. The differentiating features discussed below are for typical unmodified types of eruptive fevers. If the basic features are remembered, the reader can make allowances for deviations. As has been rightly pointed out by Sir James Mackenzie, "When we search for the recondite and obscure, we fail to recognize the simple and obvious".

SMALLPOX

It used to be dreaded in the Asiatic countries. In India, it is now completely eradicated. It occurred both sporadically and epidemically. In a suspected case, the history reveals contact with a smallpox patient, and the absence of vaccination. The incubation period is about 10–14 days. It starts with general malaise, high fever, headache and other constitutional symptoms. The rash starts on the third day of the onset of the symptoms, appearing first on the forehead and gradually spreading downwards. The rash is most prominent on the face, hands and feet, e.g., centrifugal distribution. To begin with it is papular on the third day, transforming into vesicles on the fifth day, and pustules on the eighth day. The vesicles are multilocular and deep-seated. The latter become crusted and later dry up to leave depressed scars (pock marks) **(Fig. 26.1)**. With the appearance of the rash on the third day, the constitutional symptoms begin to subside and the fever comes down, going up again at the pustular stage. In a severe case, death occurs from toxaemia and haemorrhage **(Table 26.1)**.

The course of smallpox can be modified, by a previous vaccination, to a milder type of disease (variola minor). The prophylaxis consists of vaccinating a child within three months of birth, and from time to time, at least every 3–5 years. Due to its eradication, its vaccination is stopped. The curative treatment is rather unsatisfactory. It consists in general management, maintenance of nutrition, control of the pustules with antibiotics, preferably the broad-spectrum ones.

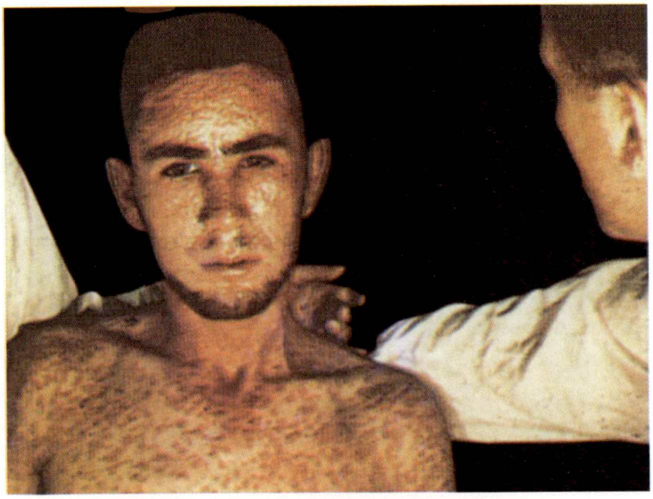

Fig. 26.1: Smallpox—umbilicated vesicles

Table 26.1: Chickenpox and smallpox (the two vesiculo-pustular exanthemata) differentiating features

Differentiating features	*Smallpox*	*Chickenpox*
Incubation period	12–14 days	14–15 days
Prodromal stage	Sudden onset with chill	Slight prodromal symptoms.
Fever	Moderate or high	Mild
Symptoms	Headache, backache, vomiting	Mild
Rash-onset	3rd day of the fever or disease	On the same day as fever
Distribution	Centrifugal-face, forearms and hands, legs and feet are most densely involved. Fewer lesions on the rest of the body	Centripetal-trunk, neck, upper arms and upper thighs are mostly involved
Lesions	Macules-papules-vesicles-pustules-crusts-Pock marks. Individual lesions do not become vesicular till the 3rd day and pustular till the 6th day. Rash is monomorphous at one time; it follows a definite pattern of spread. Vesicles are deep-seated, multilocular and umbilicated	Maculo-papules-vesicles-pustules-scabs. Individual lesions become pustular within 48 hours. Rash appears in crops producing polymorphous appearance, i.e., papules and scabs can be seen in the same area at the same time. Vesicles are superficial and unilocular
Secondary fever	6th day onwards, due to secondary infection	Seldom

CHICKENPOX

It is also called *Varicella*. There is history of contact with a case of chickenpox or herpes zoster. Children are more prone than adults. The mortality rate is low or nil. The characteristic features are the centripetal distribution of the rash involving the trunk, the upper arms, the neck, and upper parts of the thighs; mild constitutional symptoms with a polymorphous eruption (by the time a case is seen). To begin with, the lesions are

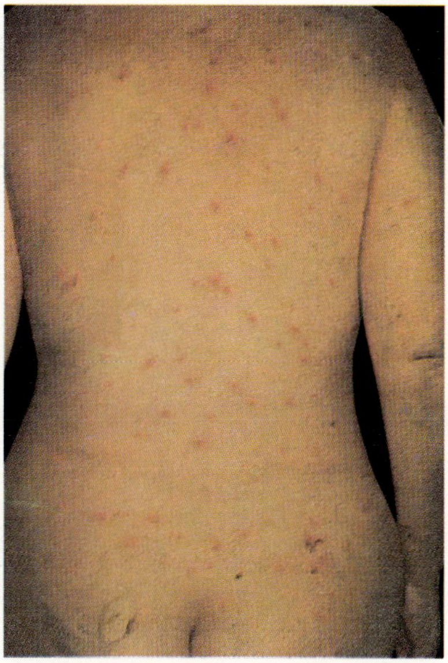

Fig. 26.2: Chickenpox

maculo-papules; these develop into vesicles, pustules and scabs within 48 hours. The eruption appears in several crops; that is how a polymorphous picture is produced (Fig. 26.2). The lesions are superficial compared to those of smallpox; so the disease leaves hardly any or faint scars unless there is secondary infection. Toxaemia and constitutional symptoms are mild (Table 26.1).

The treatment is symptomatic along with oral antiviral drugs—acicolvir, valacyclovir and famciclovir. Preventive vaccination is also routinely given to all children.

MEASLES

Children under two years of age are more frequently attacked. It is a very contagious disease. The incubation period is about 12–14 days. It starts with coryza-like symptoms, i.e., fever, running nose, and conjunctivitis. Koplik's spots on the buccal mucosa are characteristically seen at this stage. A history of contact can easily be elicited. Measles is more common in winter and spring. It starts on the face but spreads to the neck, trunk, arms and legs very quickly, within a span of few hours. The eruption is in the form of discrete and confluent, dark red macules (morbilliform rash) (Table 26.2). The constitutional symptoms are marked when the rash develops, but begin to subside after about 3–4 days, unless the condition is complicated by secondary infection of the upper and lower respiratory tract. There is no specific treatment available except symptomatic management. The points to keep in mind are prevention, and when the disease has already set in, treatment of the secondary infection. Sulphonamides and antibiotics have helped to reduce the mortality rate. Gamma globulin has been introduced with limited success as a prophylactic measure.

GERMAN MEASLES

Synonym: Rubella

Table 26.2: Differentiating features of three erythematous exanthemata (rash appearing in the first 4 days of the disease)

Differentiating features	*Scarlet fever*	*Rubella (German measles)*	*Measles*
Incubation period	3–7 days	17–18 days	10–15 days
Fever and constitutional symptoms	Moderate or high fever with headache and vomiting	Slight or absent	Moderate fever. Child feels miserable
Coryza	Absent	Slight or absent	Definite coryza-like symptoms
Cough	Absent	Rare	Present
Fauces and mouth	Tonsillo-pharyngitis. Typical tongue.	Insignificant Sometimes small, deep pink maculo papules on the soft palate	Gen. injection, and Koplik's spots
Rash: Type	Punctate erythema appearing on the 2nd day of fever	Discrete macules appearing on the 1st day	Fusing maculo-papular blotches appearing on the 4th day. Comes in crops
Colour	Scarlet	Pink	Dull-red
Distribution	Generalized, except face. Face is flushed; circumoral pallor	Generalized, including the circumoral region	Generalized, including circumoral region
Disappearance	Desquamation	Rash appears in crops. No desquamation. Fades in one place before appearing at another	Staining and desquamation
Other points	Pastia's sign	Posterior cervical glands enlarged	Nil
Tests	Dick-positive, becoming negative. Swab for Streptococci +ve, blood-leuco cytosis. Schultz-Charlton +ve	Nil	Leucocytosis, if complicated, by secon dary infection
Cause	Haemolytic streptococci	Virus	Virus

It is a mild variety of an exanthematous eruption, and is caused by a virus. The features are like measles, except that the rash appears on the first day of the illness; further, there is a characteristic lymphatic gland enlargement in the neck, mild general symptoms, a roseolar rash and no Koplik's spots (Tables 26.2 and 26.3). The treatment is the same as for measles. In pregnant females, it can harm the foetus.

Table 26.3: Points of difference between the rashes of typhus and enteric fevers

Differentiating features	*Epidemic typhus fever*	*Enteric fever*
1. Incubation period	12–14 days	12–14 days
2. Prodromal symptoms	Sudden onset. Fever with influenza type of symptoms. Prostration. Stage of invasion lasts up to the 4th or 5th day.	Insidious onset. Step-ladder type of temperature in the 1st week with malaise headache. 2nd week—Continuous temperature. Pea soup stools. Tympanitic abdomen. Temperature settles down by lysis.
3. Rash	(a) Rash is rare before the 4th or 5th day.	Rash, rare before the 7th day.
	(b) Lesions do not appear in successive crops; they persist.	Lesions appear in successive crops.
	(c) Lesions do not invade face.	Lesions may invade face especially in paratyphoid.
	(d) Lesions numerous and of variable size and shape. They tend to aggregate.	Lesions are sparse, discrete. Size and shape are uniform.
	(e) Lesions palpable; disappear on pressure only in the early stage.	Lesions palpable; disappear on pressure throughout their existence.
	(f) Colour dark-pink, rusty-red, slate-grey. Later sub-cuticular mottling and petechial haemorrhages.	Colour rose-pink. May be darker in paratyphoid.
4. Epidemiology	Occurs in louse-infested areas of over-crowding and filth.	Tropical and sub-tropical countries with unhygienic water and milk supply.
5. Nervous symptoms	Stupor, delirium from 5th day onwards. Abrupt defervescence.	Delirium in the 2nd week of the disease.
6. Tests	Weil-Felix agglutination test +ve.	Blood culture +ve in 1st week; Widal's test +ve 8th day onwards
7. Cause	Rickettsia bodies	*Salmonella typhi*
8. Treatment	Chloramphenicol	Chloramphenicol

SCARLET FEVER

It is principally a haemolytic streptococcal tonsillitis associated with glossitis (strawberry, and later raspberry-like tongue), high fever and a scarlatiniform rash (diffuse erythema with bright-red spots scattered on it). The cause of the rash is a toxin. The rash appears on the second day of the fever and is followed typically by desquamation. The clinical diagnosis is confirmed by swab from the throat and a culture of the organisms. Dick's and Schultz Charlton's immunological tests are also helpful. The important complications are otitis media, nephritis, rheumatic fever, and myocarditis. The differential diagnosis of the throat condition is made from diptheritic tonsillitis and streptococcal tonsillitis; of the rash, is made from measles, German measles, drug rashes, syphilis and allergic eruptions **(Tables 26.2 and 26.3)**.

The treatment consists of sulphonamides, penicillin or broad-spectrum antibiotics, complete rest and good nursing. Since the advent of the above mentioned drugs, the use of anti-toxic sera has declined.

INFECTIOUS MONONUCLEOSIS

Synonym: Glandular fever

A rash occurs only in the febrile variety; it is absent in the glandular and anginose types. The main features in the febrile variety of glandular fever are abrupt onset with sore throat; malaise, aches and pains; prolonged fever; enlargement of lymph glands after the third week; a rash which appears during the first week. The rash is characterized by its maculopapular character, appearance in crops and its location on the trunk, and less so on the face. The diagnosis is confirmed by the demonstration of mononuclear leucocytosis, a positive Paul–Bunnel test and raised blood proteins. The treatment is symptomatic.

Chapter 27

Congenital Disorders

To fully understand congenital and developmental disorders, the reader is advised to study Chapter 2 which describes the embryology of the skin and how these anomalies develop. Congenital disorders of the skin are fairly common in practice. When generalized, and even otherwise, they may be associated with systemic disorders, particularly of the nervous system, because of their common ectodermal origin.

Congenital disorders are usually, but not necessarily, present at birth. They may be caused by intrauterine foetal damage by known agents like trauma, toxins, infections or drugs (common examples: syphilis, rubella, thalidomide, etc.). Many developmental defects in embryonic life are of genetic origin and hence, are hereditary.

GENETICS

Genetics is a statistical science based on large pedigrees. The genetic characters depend for their transmission on genes placed on chromosomes. The effects of genes are conditional. What is inherited is a tendency or diathesis to react in a certain way when certain stimuli from the environment impinge upon the organism. Thus there is constant interplay between "nature" and "nurture" to manifest genetic changes.

Terminology in Genetics

Homozygous state: When homologous chromosomes carry similar genes.

Heterozygous state: When homologous chromosomes carry dissimilar genes.

Allele: Genes which occupy homologous loci in homologus chromosomes.

Dominant: When the gene exerts its effect in any state is said to be dominant. It may have variable penetrance and consequently, the expressibility. Common examples are Darier's disease, neurofibromatosis and hereditary keratoderma.

Recessive: The gene expresses itself only in the homologous state. Common examples are complete albinism, ichthyosis (sex-linked), xeroderma pigmentosum.

Intermediate: When heterozygotes manifest traits and homozygous becomes a patient clinically; psoriasis serves as an example.

NAEVI (BIRTH MARKS)

A naevus is defined as a congenital, circumscribed hyperplasia or growth (rarely hypoplasia) of aberrant embryonic nests in the skin. Depending upon the nature of these embryonic nests naevi are classified as follows:

1. **Moles or soft naevi**
   Pigmented flat naevi — Pigmented cellular naevus
   Non-pigmented cellular naevus — Hairy naevus
2. **Epidermal or hard naevi**
   Verrucous naevus — Naevus unius lateris
3. **Vascular naevi (haemangiomas)**
   Spider naevus — Strawberry naevus.
   Port-wine naevus — Cavernous haemangiomas.
4. **Lymphatic naevi (lymphangiomas)**
   Simple lymphangioma — Cavernous lymphangioma
   Cystic lymphangioma
5. **Fibromatous** — Neurofibromatosis
6. **Glandular naevi**
   Adenoma sebaceum — Sebaceous cyst
7. **Mesodermal naevi**
   Blue naevus — Urticaria pigmentosa.
   Mongolian spot

MOLES

They form the most common group of congenital affections. Every individual has one or more. If small in size and few in number they are considered as beauty spots; if too many and large they become cosmetic blemishes warranting treatment. The different types are:

Pigmented Flat Macule

It is caused by hyperplasia of melanocytes in the basal layer of the epidermis; pigment is also found in increased amounts in the prickle cells. Clinically it is seen as a flat, light to dark brown macule; the size varies from that of a lentil seed to the palm of hand (even bigger). Either one or more may occur in a single case, being present at birth or developing later. The macule may increase in size and change shape as the individual grows but usually becomes stationary by the age of about 25. It never turns malignant nor does it ever disappear spontaneously.

Treatment is indicated only if it is present on the face and is large enough to become a cosmetic blemish. The best results are obtained with plastic surgery (excision and skin grafting), laser or dermabrasion.

Cellular Naevus

It is so known because of the presence of special naevus cells, grouped cuboidal or oval or fusiform cells. A naevus cell has homogeneous cytoplasm and a large round vesicular nucleus. A cellular naevus is a circumscribed raised soft papule, macule or plaque. It may be pigmented (contain melanin pigment in melanocytes, prickle cells and also naevus cells) or non-pigmented. If a cellular naevus contains hair it is called a hairy mole which may be pigmented or non-pigmented. When associated with a verrucous surface, it is called a verrucous mole.

Cellular naevus may occur singly or in multiples. The size of an individual lesion is variable, being anywhere between the size of a lentil seed to that of the human palm (even bigger). If a pigmented naevus covers a large part of the body, it is called a giant naevus. The surface of a naevus may be smooth, hairy or verrucous. Any part of the body may be involved. Being hereditary in nature, it may occur in different generations on the same site.

Depending upon the histological position of the naevus cells, a cellular naevus may be junctional (epidermo-dermal), intradermal or compound.

Course: Moles may grow in size or remain stationary. They do not disappear spontaneously. Out of all the naevi, moles (particularly the junctional type) have the greatest tendency to become malignant (melanoma). Though this happens rarely, considering the millions of moles seen, the possibility, all the same, must be borne in mind. Another point needs to be emphasized is that a mole will undergo a malignant change particularly if it is irritated by natural pressure, repeated traumata or bad treatment. Whenever a mole bleeds repeatedly, becomes firmer or darker, or develops a crust, or increases rapidly in size particularly in a person past middle-age, a melanoma should be suspected and an excision biopsy done.

Treatment: It is indicated under two conditions: (1) Constant irritation on pressure sites, viz., hands and beard region. (2) Cosmetic undesirability.

Never cauterize a mole either chemically or electrically. A mole should be removed whole either with a steel knife or a diathermy needle (cutting current) or by plastic surgery. Hair in a hairy mole can be removed by electrolysis.

If malignancy is suspected, an excision biopsy should be undertaken immediately.

EPIDERMAL NAEVI

They imply naevoid hyperplasia of the epidermis particularly the stratum corneum. Naevus cells are absent in a typical epidermal naevus, but occasionally a cellular naevus may be associated with an epidermal naevus to form a verrucous pigmented naevus, i.e. a pigmented naevus with a rough, warty surface (Fig. 27.1).

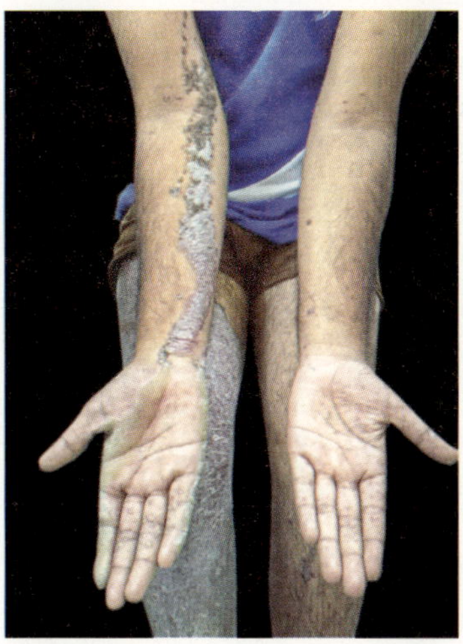

Fig. 27.1: Epidermal nevus (Nevus unius lateris)

Linear naevus (naevus unius lateralis): It is characterized by a linear, usually unilateral, band or streak of naevoid hyperplasia of epidermis which is seen clinically as raised, warty papules, flesh-coloured or slightly darker. It may occur on the neck, the extremities or the trunk; on the latter site, it rarely crosses the middle line.

Linear naevus usually manifests itself within the first year of birth and increases with growth.

Linear naevus should be differentiated from linear lichen planus, linear plane warts and linear psoriasis by the following facts: it is noticed within the first year of birth; its distribution is unilateral; the clinical features are distinctive and so also is the histopathological picture.

Ichthyosis hystrix: It is an exaggerated form of linear naevus.

Course: Though epidermal naevi increase in size with age, they do not become malignant.

Treatment consists in excising the naevus surgically, diathermy (cutting current) or plastic surgery. The authors have had some success with dermabrasion; the cosmetic result has been good, but recurrences can occur, if not removed deep enough. Liquid nitrogen and laser are also useful.

VASCULAR NAEVI

A vascular naevus is a localized congenital hyperplasia of cutaneous vessels and formative vascular tissue. It is usually present at birth or begins within a short time after. It may increase in size with growth, remain stationary, or disappear spontaneously particularly the cavernous variety. Any part of the body may be involved. Vascular naevi may be associated with other congenital affections such as, pigmented moles, adenoma sebaceum and fibromata. Extensive vascular naevi may be associated with haemangioma of the eye or the brain (Sturge–Weber syndrome).

The clinical varieties of vascular naevi are:

Capillary	Spider naevus
	Simple superficial haemangioma
	Port-wine stain (naevus flammeus)
Cavernous	Superficial cavernous-strawberry stain
	Deep cavernous
Mixed	Capillary cavernous haemangioma
	Fibro-angioma
	Lipo-angioma
	Angio-lymphangioma

Differentiation of these sub-types is important because of the varying prognosis and therapeutic measures involved.

Spider naevus: It is found on the cheeks, nose and sometimes other parts of the face as a central bright-red vessel about the size of a pin-point with smaller vessels radiating from it for 3–7 mm. Since this picture resembles the body and legs of the spider, it is called a spider naevus. One or more of these lesions may occur in a single individual. A spider naevus bleeds easily.

Spider naevus may be congenital, but can develop otherwise in cirrhosis of the liver, pregnancy, etc. A spider naevus must be distinguished from dilated capillaries (telangiectasia) which can develop in several skin disorders, particularly rosacea, xeroderma pigmentosum, X-ray burn, hereditary haemorrhagic telangiectasia (Osler's disease which is characterized by recurrent nose bleedings, telangiectasia of the nose and skin), vascular obstruction, de Morgan's spots (senile ectasias-these occur on the trunk in persons past middle-age; the lesions are slightly raised, bright red, lentil-seed-sized papules consisting of masses of dilated capillaries. They do not require any treatment. If cosmetic reasons compel one to do so, the lesion should be removed by electrocoagulation or laser or cryosurgery).

Treatment of spider naevus as well as telangiectasia consists in obliterating the central point with electrolysis or with the epilating current of a diathermy unit. The needle is introduced into the central point of the spider naevus and an epilating current passed through till the central point turns pale. The needle is withdrawn and pressure applied; no bleeding usually occurs. In a certain percentage of cases, other alternate points may be obliterated in the same manner. The results are satisfactory in experienced hands; there is no scarring. 25% saline injection into the spider naevi with a fine needle has also been tried with success.

Simple superficial capillary haemangioma: It is seen as a superficial, circumscribed, pink patch which disappears on pressure or diascopy **(Fig. 27.2)**. It is usually seen on the neck and face. It responds best to thorium X and laser.

Port-wine stain: It is characterized by a red or purple patch which is flush with the skin because only the superficial capillaries are involved. It does not disappear on diascopy or swell up when the child cries. A few naevi may disappear within the first year of birth; otherwise they are usually permanent **(Fig. 27.3)**.

Treatment of a port-wine naevus is very unsatisfactory. The best results are obtained with argon laser, plastic surgery or therapeutic tattooing. If these procedures are not available, the stain can be temporarily masked over with "Cover-up" creams. X-ray therapy is completely contraindicated; CO_2 slush may be helpful in a few cases. Electro-

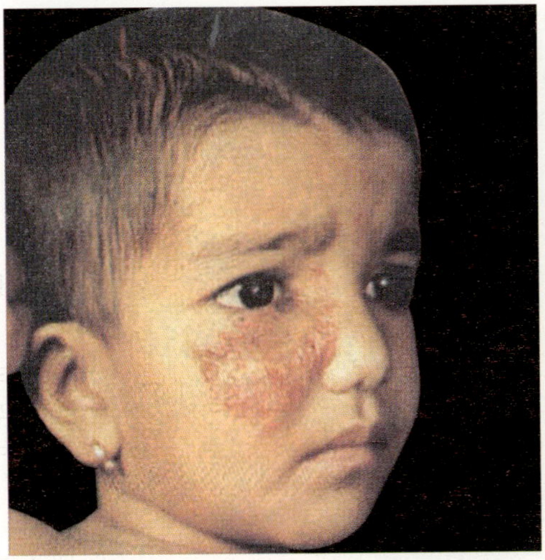

Fig. 27.2: Mixed haemangioma

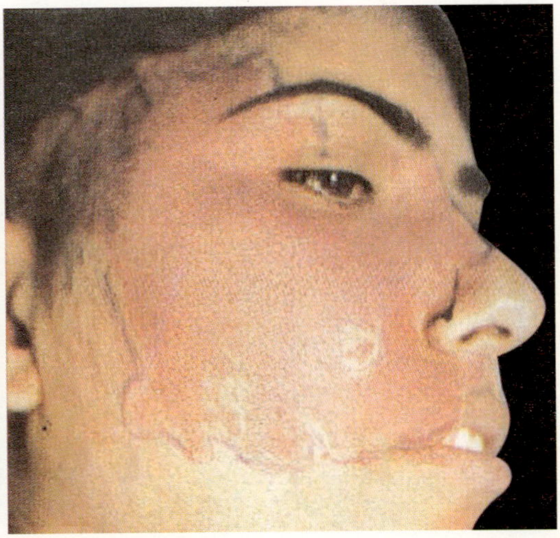

Fig. 27.3: Naevus flammeus involving right side of face

coagulation of deeper tissues with insulated needles has been claimed to give good results.

Strawberry stain: It signifies the dilatation of deeper vessels to form cavernous spaces like those seen in the erectile tissue of the penis. The lesion is well-defined, purple in colour and elevated. The size is about 0.5–2 inches in diameter. It swells up on crying and the cavernous spaces can be emptied by pressure. The naevus bleeds easily when injured; it can become excoriated and secondarily infected. The most common sites are the face, the scalp, the upper extremities and the vulva. They increase in size in the first year or two, but a large majority of them tend to disappear spontaneously by the age of 5, sometimes leaving faint atrophic scars, and at other times, none at all. A cavernous naevus, particularly if it occurs on the vulvar region, rarely becomes malignant.

Treatment in strawberry stain is mostly inactivity and protection from injury and infection. The patient must be periodically observed. Only when the naevus tends to increase rapidly without any evidence of spontaneous regression, should treatment be given preferably after the first year of life. CO_2 snow for 10–20 seconds under pressure gives good results. Small naevi can be surgically excised. Good results have been reported with liquid nitrogen.

Injections of sclerosing solutions, X-ray and radium are also given, particularly in deep, cavernous haemangiomas extending down to the subcutaneous tissue. What should really be borne in mind is that the results of treatment should not be worse than the original affection.

Mixed naevi have mixed features varying with the different combinations; hence treatment also differs with these combinations.

LYMPHANGIOMAS

They are rather rare as compared to haemangiomas. A lymphangioma consists of true hyperplasia of the lymphatic vessels and formative lymphatic tissue; in comparison, lymphangiectasis consists of dilatation of the lymphatic vessels following lymphatic obstruction caused by trauma and infection. A common example is lymphangiectasia following mastectomy and filariasis. Clinically, lymphangiectasia consists of superficial vesicles or soft, deeper nodules, which rupture and discharge lymph intermittently (Fig. 27.4). Obstruction of the deeper lymphatics causes elephantiasis. There are three types of lymphangiomas:

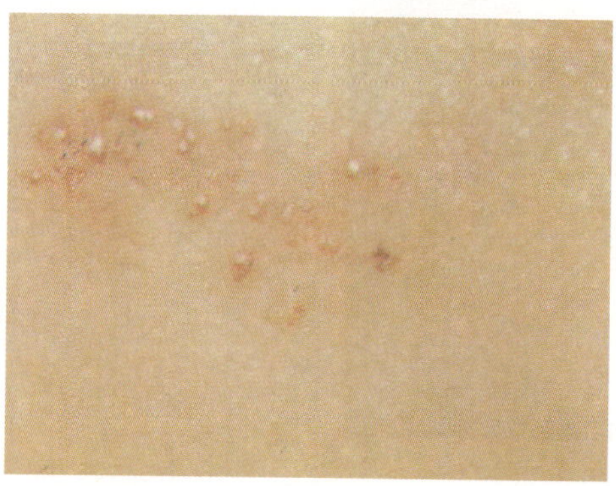

Fig. 27.4: Cystic hygroma with lymphangioma circumscriptum

The simplex type: It consists of a diffuse, elastic swelling which may involve the lips (macrocheilia), tongue (macroglossia) or the genitalia. If superficial vesicles are present; they may rupture and discharge lymph fluid which is straw-coloured and watery. Lymphangioma simplex is prone to secondary infection. Surgery may help some cases, but on the whole, the treatment is unsatisfactory.

The cystic type (hygroma): It consists of multilocular cysts seen most frequently in the neck. The treatment is surgical.

The cavernous circumscribed type (lymphangioma circumscriptum): The sites commonly affected are the axillae, scapular region, arms, neck and buttocks. Lymphangioma is present at birth or appears soon after. It may grow with age or become stationary. It never disappears spontaneously. Clinically, lymphangioma circumscriptum is characterized by irregular shaped, grouped, deep-seated, thick-walled vesicles, which are pinkish or flesh-coloured and firm in consistency. When punctured, these vesicles ooze lymph intermittently or continuously. The condition is painless unless secondarily infected. Lymphangioma may be associated with haemangioma or fibrous naevi. The treatment consists of wide, surgical excision and radiotherapy. Electrocoagulation and CO_2 snow may be helpful at times. Podophyllin paint has also been used with success.

NEUROFIBROMATOSIS

These consist of congenital naevoid, soft tumours developing early in life from connective tissue in relation to nerves or undifferentiated nerve elements. These tumours occur along nerves or as small swellings, on the surface of the skin or as large pendulous masses.

They are painless except when causing pressure on the nerve. The sites commonly affected are the front and back of the trunk, limbs and less so, the face (Fig. 27.5). The small tumours can be made to disappear through small, ring-shaped holes in the skin. Incompletely developed tumours are seen as skin tags (forme fruste).

von-Recklinghausen's disease: This is heredo-familial disease consisting of neurofibromatosis and pigmented freckles, cafe-au-lait macules and patches. Besides, extra-cutaneous lesions may be present along the auditory nerve, optic nerve, near the suprarenals, in the vertebrae, alimentary tract and in the brain. These extracutaneous

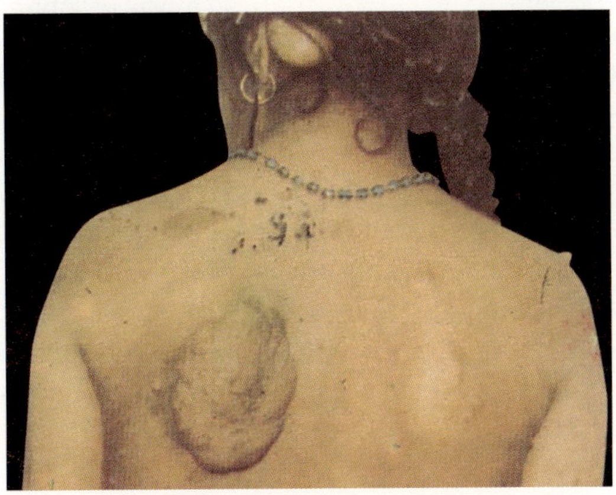

Fig. 27.5: Neurofibromatosis

lesions may cause pressure symptoms; this must be borne in mind. Lesions of von-Reck linghausen's disease start developing in childhood about the age of 8–10 years and keep on increasing till about the age of 30–40. Occasionally neurofibromatosis becomes malignant.

The treatment is surgical and is indicated for three reasons:

1. Pressure symptoms.
2. Suspicion of malignancy.
3. Cosmetic disability.

ADENOMA SEBACEUM

It is a benign naevoid condition, of sebaceous glands, hair follicles, capillaries and collagen. Lesions are mainly present on the central part of the face. They are bilaterally symmetrical. Sides of the nose and adjoining parts of the cheeks are the sites of predilection.

Lesions are pin-head to split-pea sized, firm, yellowish-red papules or nodules. Their surface may show minute capillaries. Besides, periungual warty fibromata and flesh coloured, raised, rough plaques (Shagreen patches—collagen naevi) may be seen. Fitzpatrick has focused attention on leafy hypopigmented macules as the earliest sign of the disorder.

Lesions appear in early childhood from 3 to 7 years of age; they keep on increasing till puberty. Several members of one family and several generations may be affected.

Adenoma sebaceum (angiofibroma) is rare compared to other naevi. Sometimes it forms a part of a clinical syndrome named 'EPILOIA' (Tuberous sclerosis complex). Its other features are mental deficiency, epileptic fits and paralysis (due to tuberous sclerosis of the brain), vascular naevi, pigmented patches, fibromata of the skin, kidneys and eyes, etc.

Treatment: It is unsatisfactory. For cosmetic reasons small lesions may be electro-coagulated or dermabraded. CO_2 Laser is also helpful.

SEBACEOUS CYST

Synonym: Wens, Steatoma.

Clinically the disorder consists of firm, but elastic, well-defined, round or irregular shaped, flesh-coloured or yellowish swellings on the skin attached to it, but movable on the underlying tissues. They vary in size being anywhere between as small as peas to as big as almonds. Sebaceous cysts are usually multiple, but may occur singly. They increase slowly and may become infected causing pain and tenderness. Pus may be discharged. Lesions are mainly present on the face, neck, chest, scalp and the scrotum.

Some sebaceous cysts are naevoid in origin; others are due to retention of keratin and sebaceous material as in acne vulgaris.

The disorder starts at about the age of fifteen, and new lesions continue to appear till about middle age. Usually the lesions are painless. Scrotal lesions may be complicated by mild to severe pruritus.

Treatment: It consists of excision of the cyst including the sac. If the latter is not completely removed, there is risk of recurrence.

Cysts can also be obliterated by destruction; the exact procedure consists of puncture, expression of contents and cauterization of the cyst wall with phenol and curettage. In extreme case of scrotal involvement, the whole of the scrotum skin may have to be excised.

STEATOCYSTOMA MULTIPLEX

It is an uncommon, may be heredo-familial condition originating as a epidermal cyst often incorporating appendages. The condition is seen mainly in young men on the chest and proximal parts of limbs. Clinically the lesions consist of smooth, globoid, pin-head to pea-sized, flesh-coloured or yellowish, slightly elevated, soft or firm, papulo-nodules. They can be freely moved on the underlying structures. No opening is discernible; on puncturing, white oil-like material can be expressed (Fig. 27.6). There is no association with seborrhoea or acne. The condition is asymptomatic unless secondarily infected. Treatment consists of incision or aspiration of an individual lesion, if desired.

CYLINDROMA (TURBAN TUMOUR)

It is a rare, benign, naevoid, epithelial tumour originating from the matrices of the hair follicle. Lesions are mainly confined to the scalp and forehead (turban area). Typical lesions consist of solitary or multiple flesh-coloured or reddish, pea- to walnut-sized tumours. They slowly enlarge.

Histopathology is characterized by masses of pale basal cells surrounded by hyaline connective tissue

Treatment is surgical excision.

BLUE NAEVUS

It is a rare naevoid tumour consisting of spindle-shaped, mesodermal melanoblasts in the deeper part of the dermis. It usually occurs singly, and the face is the site of choice, though it has been seen on the scalp and limbs. Clinically, it is characterized by well-defined, round or oval, firm papule or nodule of blue or bluish-black colour (Fig. 27.7).

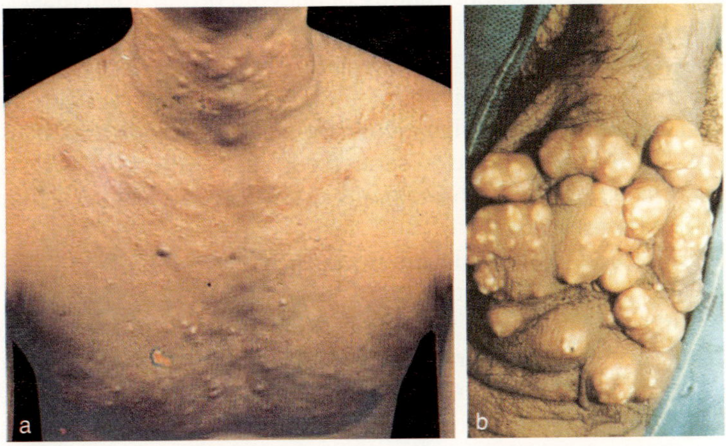

Fig. 27.6: Steatocystoma multiplex. (a) Multiple smooth dermal cysts over trunk; (b) Sebaceous cysts–scrotum

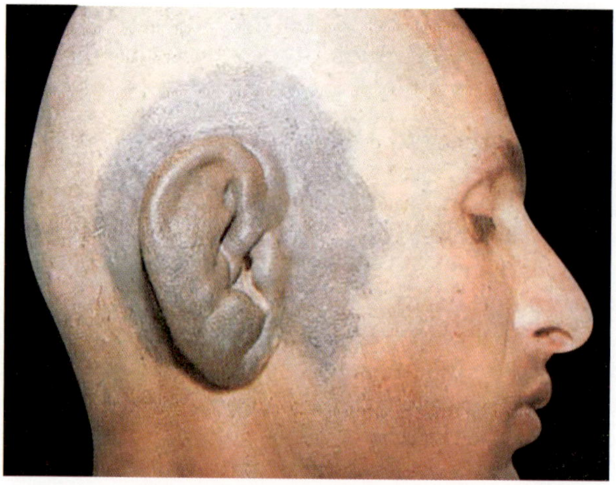

Fig. 27.7: Congenital blue nevus

It develops in infancy or early childhood; once developed, the size is stationary. It does not disappear spontaneously. It rarely becomes malignant.

Treatment consists of surgical excision, being indicated for cosmetic reasons or when there is suspicion of malignancy.

MONGOLIAN SPOT

It is a congenital, bluish, pigmented macule or plaque on the sacral region; there is no induration or infiltration. It is present at birth, and tends to disappear before the age of about 5. It is more common amongst Asiatics than Europeans. Like a blue naevus, a Mongolian spot consists of scattered, spindle-shaped melanocytes in the lower corium.

Since it disappears spontaneously, no treatment, except reassurance, is indicated.

URTICARIA PIGMENTOSA

It is a rare familial cutaneous disorder, mainly of naevoid origin, from mast cells. There are two varieties: (a) childhood and (b) adult variety; the former is far more common than the latter.

The disorder starts in infancy, and is characterized by brownish (in different shades) macules and dermal nodules (mast cell naevus); the size varies from that of a split pea to a one rupee piece. The lesions urticate on scratching, i.e. they become red, swollen and enlarged when scratched lightly with the point of a forceps. It is a very characteristic. sign, but it may not be present in the adult variety. The sites of choice are the front and back of the trunk, less commonly the neck, face and limbs **(Fig. 27.8)**. At times, bullae may develop in infants. Generalized dermographism may be present in many cases; so is generalized flushing due to release of large quantities of histamine. Fresh lesions continue to appear in crops from time to time; ultimately they may disappear spontaneously leaving behind pigmentation which may also fade. Mast cell naevus may be seen as a solitary nodule.

The only subjective complaint is itching which is variable. The histology is diagnostic. Polychrome methylene blue positive mast cells are characteristic.

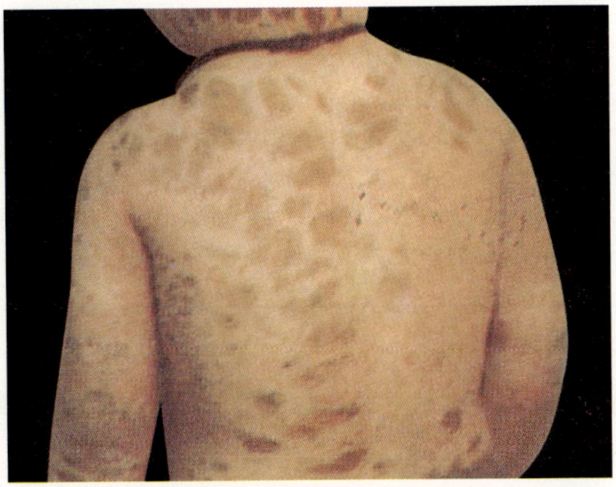

Fig. 27.8: Urticaria pigmentosa

Differential diagnosis: It is from other causes of urticaria, pigmentation and nodules depending upon the clinical variety. Nodular variety causes confusion with xanthomatosis. Other varieties of mastocytosis must be borne in mind.

Treatment: It is unsatisfactory; antihistaminics may help to control the itching and urticaria. Steroids are generally not recommended. *Rauwolfia serpentina* is helpful in controlling generalized flushing.

NAEVUS ACHROMICUS

Synonym: Naevus depigmentosus.

It is rather an uncommon naevoid condition characterized by the absence or hypoplasia of melanocytes, resulting in circumscribed patch of depigmentation. The condition is present at birth, or may appear shortly after; it may increase slowly with age, and then become stationary **(Fig. 27.9)**. It is usually unilateral. The depigmented patch

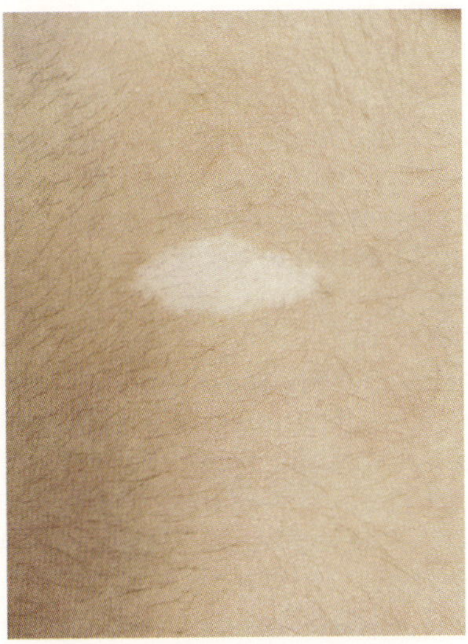

Fig. 27.9: Nevus achromicus

does not have the hyperpigmentary border of vitiligo. Hair in the depigmented patch may be white. There is another type of hypoplastic naevus called naevus anaemicus in which pale or whitish macules occur; these macules do not turn red when warmth is applied, and the flare reaction of Lewis is smaller and disappears more slowly in them than the rest of the skin.

The treatment for both these conditions is unsatisfactory. "Cover-up" (P) helps temporarily, and plastic surgery, permanently.

ALBINISM

It is characterized by the congenital absence of pigment from the integument. Albinism may be complete or incomplete. It consists of well-defined areas of depigmentation seen anywhere on the body; there is no hyperpigmentary border. The hair in depigmented areas are white. The patches remain stationary. At times, it is very difficult to distinguish incomplete albinism from naevus achromicus and vitiligo in infancy. The course of these conditions helps to differentiate them. While the former two are stationary, vitiligo has a progressive but enigmatic course. Further, the latter develops a hyperpigmentary border and even pigmentation inside the patches on treatment.

Complete albinism (albino): It consists of complete and universal depigmentation of the skin, the hair and even the eyes. Albinos are very sensitive to the sun and UVR; their skins burn easily because the protective pigment is absent. The eyes show lack of pigment in the iris and choroid; hence photophobia and nystagmus are common amongst them. Albinos may be physically and mentally backward.

Albinism is often a heredo-familial disorder. There is no satisfactory treatment yet found. Anti-actinic creams, and suitable clothing which gives adequate protection from the sun's rays, sunshades, etc. do help.

ICHTHYOSIS

It is a congenital, often heredo-familial, cutaneous affection consisting of dryness, roughness and scaliness of the integument resulting from deficient secretions and abnormal keratinization. The condition appears at birth, and is aggravated in the cold of winter, clearing up when the weather becomes warmer. The extensor surfaces of the trunk and extremities are selectively involved but the whole integument exhibits some degree of dryness. Its clinical manifestations vary from simple dryness to bullous erythroderma, resulting in a great confusion of terminology. This is exaggerated by heredo-familial variations and linkage to sex. Due to poor skin defences and dryness, patients are prone to develop pyodermas, fungal affections and eczemas (discoid, crackle and infective varieties).

i. ***Xeroderma***. The mild form of ichthyosis is termed xeroderma (xero means dry, and derma means skin, dry skin). The integument is light-grey in colour, dry to the touch and has furfuraceous scaling. There may be slight itching. Climatic, senile and artificial xerosis (due to frequent scrubbing with soap and hot water; avoidance of greasy applications) must be excluded. Treatment consists of use of superfatted soaps and oil massage.

ii. ***Ichthyosis vulgaris***. The severe form of this condition is called sauroderma (crocodile skin) being characterized by skin that is greyish in colour, with plate-like,

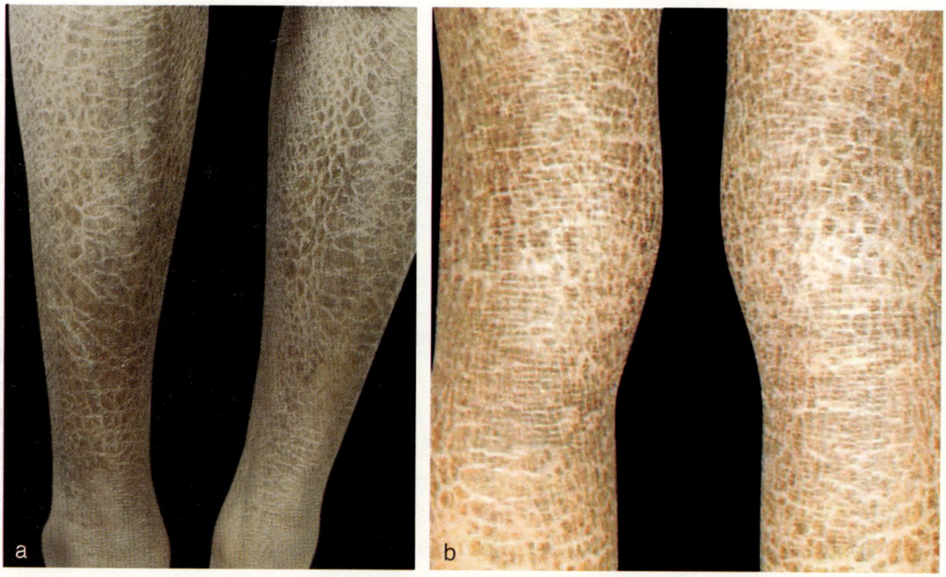

Fig. 27.10: (a) Ichthyosis; (b) X-linked ichthyosis

quadrilateral, thin scales attached at the centre and free at the periphery. There is dryness and harshness **(Fig. 27.10)**. Flexors like the cubital fossae, popliteal fossae, groins and axillae are selectively spared except in the very severe forms of this condition. Follicular, horny plugs may be present on the back of arms and the lateral sides of thighs. The palms and the soles may also show hyperkeratosis.

Ichthyosis is symptomless except for a dry, uncomfortable feeling which becomes worse in winter when natural sweating is reduced and the skin needs extra lubrication. There may be mild itching. Appalling look of the skin causes mental stress, particularly in young females. There is no association with atopy. Complications like chronic folliculitis and eczemas are fairly common. Severe erythrodermic variety of ichthyosis is called congenital ichthyosiform erythroderma (*see* Chapter 20).

Histology consists of thick corneal and granular layers with moderate acanthosis and mild dermal infiltrate of round cells. Pigment is increased. Sebaceous and sweat glands are reduced.

Diagnosis: Typical case hardly presents any difficulty in diagnosis. Onset of the disease in adult warrants a thorough search for an acquired cause, e.g. reticuloses, leprosy and drugs.

Prognosis: The malady progresses to a certain degree till puberty when it becomes stationary. There is no spontaneous recovery. Though the condition cannot be cured, it can be considerably alleviated with systemic and local measures.

Treatment

1. The patient should live in a warm climate which is to a certain degree, humid.
2. His general health should be kept at an optimum level. Vitamin A in large doses helps some cases. Thyroid and injection pilocarpine may also benefit temporarily.

3. Local treatment ameliorates the condition considerably. It consists of:
   a. A daily warm bath.
   b. A warm oil or ghee massage as often as possible.
   c. Superfatted soap only is to be used.
   d. 10% urea and 5% lactic acid ointment in eucerine or vaseline base or coconut oil.
   e. Sunbaths and UVR exposures may help some cases temporarily.
4. Because of proneness to pyodermas and eczemas, patients must be properly advised regarding selection of suitable occupation.

HARLEQUIN FOETUS

Synonym: Ichthyosis congenita.

It is a very rare affection in which either (1) the infant is born with a collodion-like covering over the entire cutaneous surface which is, in reality, the epitrichial layer of the embryo that should have been shed, but persists, or (2) the skin is thick and horny like an armour; it is accompanied by other monstrosities. In the latter type, the infant dies while in the former, the collodion covering exfoliates terminating in simple ichthyosis and the child recovers. The outlook is usually bad.

Ichthyosis hystrix is a hard epidermal naevus (see under naevi).

ICHTHYOSIS FOLLICULARIS

It is a very rare congenital ichthyotic disorder in which hair is replaced by follicular, flesh-colored papules with horny spines on extensor surfaces like the arms, the neck and the trunk. There is moderate itching. This condition should be distinguished from keratosis pilaris (*see* Chapter 25).

DARIER'S DISEASE

Synonym: Keratosis follicularis

It is a rare hereditary (autosomal dominant) disorder. It is worldwide in distribution. Clinically, the typical lesions consist of follicular and interfollicular keratotic, flesh coloured papules covered with greyish crust and also papillomatous tumours and vegetations. Seborrhoeic sites are most affected. The integument may become pigmented. Eruption may have localized or zosteriform distribution. Mucous membrane involvement is seen only occasionally and in severe form may mimic leukoplakia . Nails are brittle, hyperkeratotic and striated longitudinally. Associated pulmonary lesions have been described. General health of the patient remains unaffected except in severe cases. Many patients complain of itching. Disease is chronic and intractable. The course is progressive. Pathogenesis of the disease remains unknown but pathology is characteristic and diagnostic. Typical histopathology consists of dyskeratosis, acanthosis, intra-epidermal lacunae, 'corps ronds' and 'grains of Darier'.

Treatment is only symptomatic consisting of local keratolytic agents like salicylic acid, etc. Huge doses of vitamin A do not help and have side-effects. Fractional Grenz-ray therapy may help to control itching. Dermabrasion may be of some help in case of disfiguring lesions on face. Vitamin A ointment and milk cream massage may be useful. Retinoids are a useful standby.

KERATODERMA

Synonym: Tylosis.

It is a congenital condition which is often heredo-familial. Some patients develop the disorder several years after birth, some at puberty. Commonly seen condition, it is usually of autosomal dominant inheritance.

The palms of the hands and the soles of the feet are bilaterally and symmetrically involved; the disease rarely involves the dorsal surface. Usually, the keratoderma process stops sharply at the lateral edges of the hands and feet **(Fig. 27.11)**. The condition is usually asymptomatic, but there may be an uncomfortable feeling present in advanced cases with itching, burning and even pain. Patterns seen are the diffuse, punctate and circumscript types.

In the diffuse variety, the skin is uniformly dry, rough, thick and covered by flesh-coloured (or darker) plate-like or branny scales. The integument may crack and become fissured, the surface being either smooth or pitted. The margin of the affected area is well-defined, and there is no erythematous halo nor any evidence of inflammation. It becomes disabling in winters due to painful fissures or cracks. In some cases, in the summer months, there is some amelioration but itching may be complained of.

Punctate type is characterized by pin-point (or larger) keratotic papules on the palms of the hands and soles of the feet. It is less often seen than the diffuse type. Various nail deformities have been reported. The condition starts in or after the first decade. Circumscript variety shows circumscribed patches of thickened scaly areas particularly on the pressure sites of the soles of the feet.

Differential diagnosis: Keratoderma congenitale palmaris et plantaris may be associated with ichthyosis or some other ectodermal defect, or may occur by itself. It must be distinguished from other causes of keratoderma.

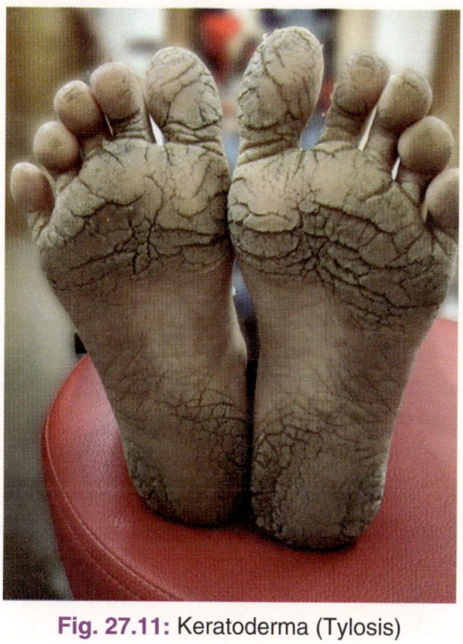

Fig. 27.11: Keratoderma (Tylosis)

The acquired type is associated with hyperhidrosis, sodden skin and an erythematous halo. Besides hyperhidrosis, malnutrition may account for some acquired cases; but in the majority of acquired cases no definite cause can be established (idiopathic cases). Occupational keratoderma of the hands is common in manual workers. The integument of the soles of the feet of people who walk bare-footed becomes coarse, rough and hyperkeratotic producing cracks and even sulci.

Keratoderma is a common feature in arsenical intoxication, chronic eczema, fungus infection (the chronic hyperkeratotic variety of the hands and the feet), pityriasis rubra pilaris, psoriasis, exfoliative dermatitis, syphilis, yaws, gonorrhoea and Reiter's syndrome (keratoderma blennorrhagica). Keratoderma climactericum is a frequent complaint in menopausal women. Deficiency of oestrogens and thyroid is supposed to account for it. Majority of the cases of keratoderma palmaris et plantaris between the ages of 10–40 are due to dyshidrosis sicca, eczematoid keratoderma associated with discoid dermatitis, neurodermatitis and tinea infections. After the age of 40, particularly in females, climacteric is a common cause.

Dyshidrosis sicca is characterized by insidious onset, history of dyshidrosis, demonstration of an occasional vesicle despite keratodermic lesions.

In eczematoid keratoderma, well- or ill-defined crusted patches on erythematous bases on the sides of feet and instep are seen along with typical discoid patches on the legs and forearms. There may be slight oozing. Itching is moderate. Lesions of neurodermatitis resembling keratoderma are typical and the history is obvious. There is more lichenification accompanied by severe itching than in true keratoderma.

Psoriasis especially psoriasis inversus only rarely causes confusion with congenital keratoderma. Typical well-defined lesions with silvery scaling and also lesions on other parts of the body are characteristic.

Course: It is a persistent condition noticed at birth or later in childhood increasing till puberty to become stationary. It never regresses spontaneously.

Treatment: It is unsatisfactory. If associated with hyperhidrosis, the latter should be treated as such. Warm climates suit tylotic but not hyperhidrotic individuals. The measures which may help are:

1. Local use of emollients containing salicylic acid (occlusive bandage).
2. Peeling of the skin with salicylic acid plaster, formalin, 5% lactic acid and 10% urea ointment; in extreme cases by dermabrasion.
3. Grenz-ray therapy may help some cases esp. dyshidrosis sicca and eczematoid keratodermas. In extreme cases, grafts are useful.
4. Vitamin A and E may be beneficial. Thyroid and oestrogens are useful in cases of keratoderma climactericum; penicillin in syphilis and yaws; griseofulvin in hyperkeratotic tinea; injection sodium thiosulphate or Lomodex (P) in cases of heavy metal or drug intoxication .

   Soda bicarbonate soaks followed by emollients application helps to soften the skin.

EPIDERMOLYSIS BULLOSA

It is a rare genodermatosis characterized by bullous eruptions. Depending on the mode of hereditary transmission and the severity of clinical symptoms it has been classified into: (i) Simplex type (autosomal dominant) and (ii) Dystrophic and lethalis types (recessive).

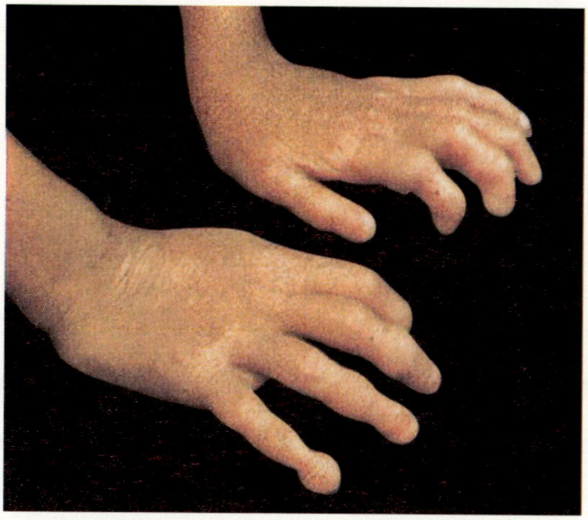

Fig. 27.12: Epidermolysis bullosa

Because of faulty development of cohesiveness in the integument, there is easy vulnerability to trauma and irritation resulting in bullous formation on the exposed body parts, i.e. on the hands, feet and knees. In the simplex variety, bullae follow trauma and leave pigmentation after healing. In dystrophic variety, bullae may appear independent of frictional trauma and involve mucous membranes and the whole integument. On healing are left behind scars of keloids, milia, mutilations and strictures **(Fig. 27.12)**. Diagnosis is not difficult in a typical case; it is made on clinical grounds.

Pathology: Primary site of bulla formation varies with the severity. In simplex type, it is suprabasal while in lethalis type it is intradermal. Underlying pathology is not known but elastic tissue is said to be defective.

Prognosis: Infants with severe variety of epidermolysis bullosa and buccal involvement have a bad prognosis. Mild, simplex variety tends to subside at puberty. In the absence of a specific remedy, prognosis on the whole is not good.

Treatment: It is unsatisfactory. Trauma and irritation should be avoided. Steroids are the mainstay in severe dystrophic and lethalis types. Reconstructive surgery may help to a limited extent in a few cases. Vitamin E is helpful in dystrophic epidermolysis bullosa. Dosage is 200–400 mg daily for at least 3 months or longer.

Chapter

28

Tumours of the Skin

Tumours of skin are classified on the basis of the tissues. Tables 28.1 and 28.2 depict classifications of skin tumours of epidermal and dermal tissues, respectively.

BENIGN TUMOURS

They are very common, much more so than the other types. They are usually symptomless; only a few produce itching (keloids), pain (neuromas, neurofibromas) and pressure symptoms. Treatment may be necessary for cosmetic reasons. Benign tumours, however, rarely become malignant.

Fibromas

They are well-defined, connective tissue tumours composed of connective tissue cells and fibres. They may be single or multiple, soft or hard, sessile or pedunculated, and of varying sizes. They are usually flesh-coloured, but may have a reddish-blue hue. They may occur anywhere on the body. Congenital fibromas usually form a feature of classical neurofibromatosis; acquired ones occur without pigmentation and are less profuse in number. Nodular subepidermal fibrosis is a fibroma-like nodule usually seen on the legs following trauma.

Treatment consists of surgical excision indicated either for cosmetic reasons or if the fibroma assumes large proportions.

Knuckle Pads

They are produced by hyperplasia and accumulation of fibrous tissue resulting in thickening of the skin over the knuckles of the hands and feet. The condition is asymptomatic.

Cutaneous Tags

Synonym: Fibroma fruste.

It is a very common, asymptomatic, harmless, benign problem seen mostly on the neck and axillae in women, less so in obese men, as small, flesh-coloured, pin-head to lentil-sized, sessile and pedunculated growths (Fig. 28.1). Treatment, if at all necessary, is by surgical excision-snipping with sharp scissors and electro-desiccating the base. Procedure is almost painless and leaves little scarring.

Keloid

It is an irregular, fibrous growth of the dermis, resembling an exaggerated hypertrophic scar which grows beyond its limits. In clinical practice, two varieties of keloids are seen:

Tabfe 28.1: Classification of common skin tumours (epidermal tissues)

	Epithelium	*Sebaceous glands*	*Hair follicle*	*Melanogenic system*	*Sweat gland*
Congenital	Epidermal naevi-verrucous naevus	Naevus sebaceous	Hair follicle naevus	• Cellular naevi • Pigmented naevi • Blue naevus • Halo naevus • Mongolian spot	• Eccrine naevus • Syringoma
Benign or tumour-like	• Seborrhoeic warts • Acanthoma • Kerato-acanthoma • Keratosis • Epithelial cyst	• Sebaceous adenoma • Sebaceous cyst • Rhinophyma	• Trichofolliculoma • Trichoepithelioma	• Lentigines • Freckles	• Hidrocystoma • Syringocystadenoma papilliferum • Spiradenoma
Malignant	• Basal cell epithelioma • Squamous cell epithelioma • Intraepidermal epithelioma • Paget's disease • Bowen's disease	• Carcinoma of sebaceous gland		• Malignant melanoma	• Adeno-carcinoma of sweat gland Hidradeno-carcinoma

Majority of these tumours are difficult to distinguish clinically; diagnosis is essentially based on histology. Confusion has been multiplied by stress on degree of differentiation of cells and their interpretation. Since clinical distinction is difficult and treatment is essentially the same for majority of the benign tumours, a practitioner of dermatology should try to avoid getting confused with nomenclature. These tables have been re-arranged because of prevalent confusion in the literature created by microscopist investigators.

Table 28.2: Classification of common skin tumours (dermal tissues)

	Vascular	*Lymphatic*	*Fibrous tissue*	*Miscellaneous—Fat, nerves, muscle, etc.*
Congenital	• Haemangiomas • Angiokeratoma	Lymphangiomas	Fibroma	Neurofibroma Urticaria pigmentosa
Benign	• Glomus tumour • Telangiectasis • Granuloma pyogenicum	Lymphangiomas	• Fibroma • Keloid • Skin tags (Fig. 28.1) • Knuckle pads • Dermatofibroma	• Lipoma • Neuroma • Leiomyoma • Xanthomas • Myxoma • Osteoma • Mastocytosis • Lymphocytosis
Malignant	• Malignant angiosarcoma • Kaposi's idiopathic haemorrhagic sarcoma	Lymphangiomas	Fibrosarcoma	• Mycosis fungiodes • Liposarcoma • Leiomyosarcoma • Reticulosis (malignant lymphomas)

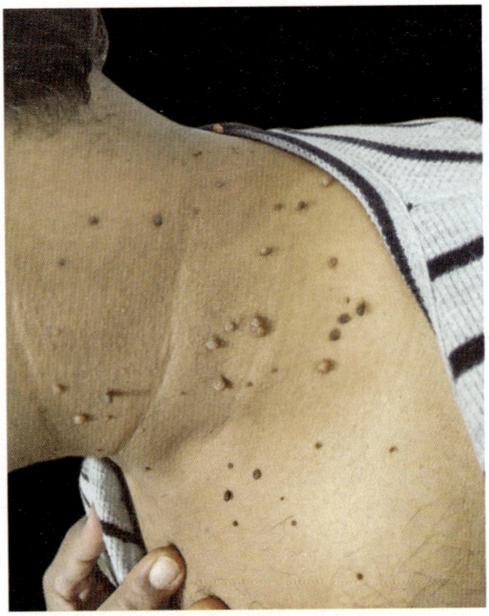

Fig. 28.1: Skin tags (Acrochordon)

1. The cicatricial variety arising from previous injury, burns, bites, pyodermas, acne or scars. An acne keloid is a specific entity in itself (*see* Chapter 11).
2. ***Spontaneous***. Some authorities doubt their spontaneous origin, and feel that primary wounds being very minute, escape notice. Trauma is caused, in such cases, by mosquito bites, scratching, friction, pressure, bruising, etc.

Certain races have an inherent predisposition to keloids, e.g. Blacks and Indians, and so also certain families and individuals. The sites of choice are the sternal region and the shoulders, though keloids can develop anywhere on the body.

Clinical features: The lesion is elevated; there are claw-like projections from the edge of the lesion; its colour varies from flesh-colour to pinky red; the lesion has a firm consistency, a smooth, shiny surface and tendency to grow beyond the limits of the primary scar or injury (in this respect, it differs from a hypertrophic scar) **(Fig. 28.2)**. After a certain degree of growth, a keloid becomes stationary; it seldom undergoes spontaneous resorption. Keloids may be asymptomatic, but usually tend to produce itching and severe pain.

Prognosis: Keloids are troublesome. The symptoms can be very annoying, even agonizing. The prognosis is good in small keloids, but bad in extensive or multiple ones because treatment in such cases is unsatisfactory.

Treatment

Prophylactic: In susceptible individuals, every suspicious wound, burn, etc. should be properly treated. Wounds tending to heal by secondary intention should be grafted. Fresh localized scars should be massaged with betamethasone ointment.

Extensive scars need systemic corticosteroids. In the authors' opinion, it helps to prevent many keloids, and even abort early ones.

Curative

1. Injections of hyaluronidase 600–1500 IU with 25 mg per ml of the intra-articular variety of soluble hydrocortisone or 10–40 mg triamcinolone. The mixture is injected into the keloid with a dental syringe or dermojet; 1–5 ml may be required depending upon the size. Injections are given once in 2–3 weeks for 3–5 times. Soft and early keloids may flatten while hard ones become soft and asymptomatic. Occlusive corticosteroid dressings are also beneficial.
2. Excision followed by X-ray therapy. Surgical excision alone, produces recurrence; hence radiotherapy should be commenced immediately. The dosage varies from

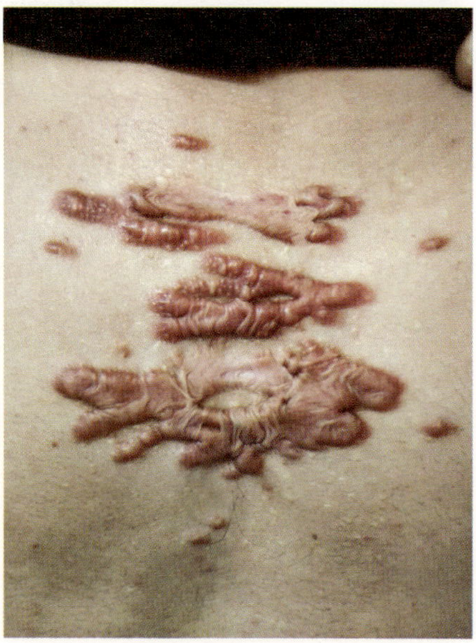

Fig. 28.2: Keloid

800 to 1200 r. While the wound is healing, it should be dressed with betamethasone lotion or ointment. CO_2 Laser is very useful.

3. Tetra-hydroxy-quinone orally has been successfully tried in some cases of extensive keloids (Kelley and Pinkus). Thio-tepa 0.5% has been used topically after excision of the keloid with success. *Centella asiatica* has also been beneficially employed, orally, topically and intralesionally. Silicone gel or oil with compression bandage is very beneficial in contracting and flattening keloids. It is much cheaper and effective than silicone sheets.

Lipomas

They are well-defined, rounded, soft, lobulated and often fluctuating tumours arising from the adipose tissue in the subcutaneous layer of the skin. They vary in size being anywhere between as small as a split pea to as big as walnuts (even bigger). They may be single or multiple. They move freely on the underlying structures, but may not be adherent to the overlying epidermis. They could occur anywhere on the body, but are usually seen on the limbs, back and shoulders. The differential diagnosis is made from other tumours of the skin; sometimes the diagnosis is clinched on histopathology. Treatment consists of surgical removal. Dercum' s disease is a condition of diffuse or nodular lipomatosis of the trunk and limbs in middle-aged women.

Leiomyoma

It develops from the arrector pili muscle, and is very rare. Multiple, cutaneous tumours occur as brownish, papular lesions on the face, neck and extensor surfaces of the limbs, while the subcutaneous tumour originating from the dartos muscle of the scrotum occurs as a large, single lesion. Leiomyomata are usually painful. Histopathology consists of interlacing bundles of smooth muscle fibres with elongated nuclei. Treatment is unsatisfactory. Punch grafts may sometimes be helpful. Solitary lesion can be excised.

Neuroma

It develops from the nerve or ganglion cells, nerve fibres or the perineural sheath. It is usually a single nodule occurring along a nerve, flesh- or reddish-coloured, and tender to the touch. A neuroma is often accompanied by radiating pain. The differential diagnosis is made from neurofibromatosis. Histopathology exhibits numerous bundles of myelinated nerves in the dermis surrounded by fibrous tissue. The treatment consists in removing the neuroma surgically; only an expert surgeon should do this lest the nerve be cut accidentally.

Glomus Tumour

It is a rare tumour. It is usually seen as a single, small, well-defined, bluish-red, painful tumour arising from the glomus body (neuro-myoarterial organ surrounding thearterio-venous junction which is supposed to regulate blood pressure and temperature). Pain is periodic, sharp and spontaneous which may radiate. The site of choice is the subungual region at the tip of the finger. Histopathology essentially consists of numerous small vascular lumina and masses of glomus cells. The latter have faintly eosinophilic cytoplasm and large pale nuclei. Treatment consists of surgical excision, or electro-coagulation with diathermy.

Seborrhoeic Warts

Synonym: Senile warts.

They are very common, and one usually comes across them in adults past middle age. They are more common in males than females. The sites frequently affected are the trunk (chest, sides and back), the face, the neck, and less so, the extremities; the palms of hands and soles of feet are always spared.

Clinical features: A seborrhoeic wart is characterized by a raised, verrucous or flat surface, well-defined margins, a brownish or greyish colour, soft consistency and "stuck-on-the-skin" appearance. They are usually multiple. A seborrhoeic wart is usually about the size of a split pea, sometimes smaller. There is no induration or infiltration of the base; if there is, malignancy should be suspected. Seborrhoeic warts increase slowly in size and number **(Fig. 28.3)**.

Histology: It is characterized by hyperkeratosis and irregular acanthosis. There are no mitotic cells, and dermal infiltration is absent.

Prognosis: It is good. The lesions are asymptomatic, and only cause a cosmetic problem.

Etiology: It is unknown. No virus or any relationship to the sebaceous glands has been demonstrated. They represent a kind of senile, benign epidermal hyperplasia.

Differential diagnosis: It is from moles, solar keratoses and verruca. Age of the patient, multiple number, "stuck-on-the-skin" appearance and duration of the lesions are diagnostic. Histopathology is conclusive.

Treatment: None is usually indicated except when there is fear of malignancy, or treatment is considered necessary for cosmetic reasons. The authors have achieved good results with dermabrasive surgery. In its absence, electro-desiccation or 5% acid salicylic or fluorouracil ointment may be tried.

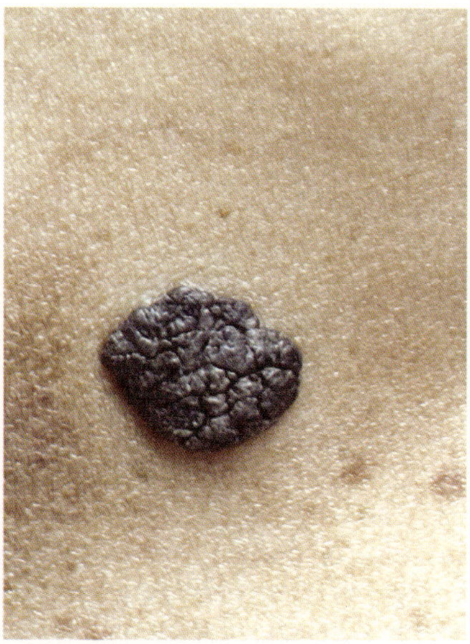

Fig. 28.3: Senile warts

Keratoses

They are of three types: (1) senile (2) arsenical and (3) actinic. Keratoses may also be seen in association with xeroderma pigmentosum and also in tar workers. Keratoses are comparatively more common among the white races than the coloured. Amongst Indians, however, they are rather uncommon.

Senile keratoses occur in elderly people with senile atrophy of the skin. They are seen on the exposed parts of the body, particularly the face and the dorsum of hands. They are usually multiple. Clinically they are characterized by irregular shape; firm or hard consistency; grey or brown colour; crusts or scales that are dry, hard, firmly adherent and cannot be rubbed off easily. Senile keratoses have an embedded nature. The size varies from that of one split pea to that of a 5–10 cm diameter, even bigger. Keratosis may take a conical or horny shape; when this happens, it is called cutaneous horn. Keratosis has a tendency to become raised; there is induration at the base or signs of inflammation appear. In such cases an excision biopsy should be done to establish the diagnosis and exclude malignancy.

Keratosis develops prematurely in the sun-burnt skin (actinic keratoses), radiodermatitis, xeroderma pigmentosum and in tar workers. Clinical features of such keratoses are the same as those of senile keratosis.

Arsenical keratoses are seen on the palms of the hands, soles of the feet and on the trunk in association with arsenical pigmentation, keratoderma and other features of arsenical intoxication. They are very prone to malignancy.

Differential diagnosis: It is made from seborrhoeic warts, epitheliomas, skin tags, warts and other benign tumours. An attempt should be made to establish the causative condition and exclude malignancy in every case before the lesions are labelled as keratoses.

Treatment

A. Prophylactic as for senile skin, solar dermatitis, etc. Cream massage and vitamin A are also helpful.

B. Curative
   1. For superficial ones, electrodesiccation followed by curettage under local anaesthesia.
   2. Electro-excision or surgical excision for large lesions.
   3. Destruction with CO_2 snow, trichloracetic acid, etc.

The authors prefer excision biopsy, because the histopathology can be studied. Dermabrasion has also given very good results.

Keratoacanthoma

It is a pseudo-carcinomatous hyperplasia, sort of transition between benign keratosis and definite epithelioma. Its incidence is low in India. It consists usually of a solitary lesion; multiplex and generalized varieties have been described.

Typical keratoacanthoma is seen on the face or dorsum of hands, as a rapidly growing (1–2 cm in 1–2 months), firm, hemispherical nodule with a central crater covered by a keratinous crust. There is spontaneous resolution within a couple of months leaving a puckered scar **(Fig. 28.4)**.

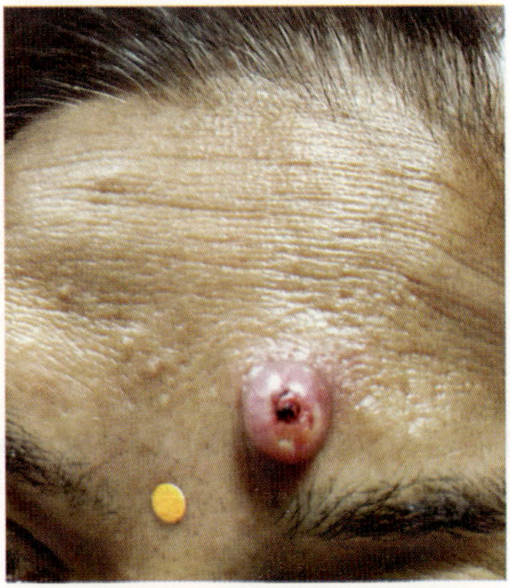

Fig. 28.4: Keratoacanthoma

Histopathology is characteristic. It consists of a crater filled with keratinous material, epithelial hyperplasia with marked keratinization (keratinous pearls) and dense inflammatory infiltrate.

Treatment is surgical excision or electro-cauterization. Though the disorder is self-healing, treatment is recommended in order to be safe and to get good cosmetic results.

Cystic Tumours

Congenital

1. Dermoid cyst.
2. Pilonidal cyst (*see* Chapter 2).
3. Benign cystic epithelioma (epithelioma adenoides cysticum).
4. Syringoma (Hidradenomes eruptifis).

Acquired

1. Traumatic or implantation cyst.
2. Sebaceous cyst (*see* Chapter 27)
3. Milium.
4. Mucous cyst (*see* Chapter 35)
5. Hydrocystoma (*see* Chapter 34)

Dermoid Cyst

It is seen at the sites of fusion of branchial clefts and develops due to inclusion of embryonic epidermal structures in the subcutaneous tissue. It consists of a cystic tumour containing hair, hair follicles and sebaceous glands, etc. Treatment is surgical excision.

Implantation Cyst

Synonym: Traumatic cyst.

It is formed by accidental implantation of epidermis in the underlying tissue after injury. Common sites are the fingers and hands. A cystic growth develops. The course is progressive. It is painless, at least in the early stages. Treatment is surgical excision.

Multiple Benign Cystic Epithelioma

Synonym: Epithelioma adenoides cysticum (Brook).

It is a rare hereditary disorder. Onset is at puberty. Lesions are mostly confined to the central part of the face and temples, distributed usually bilaterally symmetrically.

Typically, lesions consist of asymptomatic, discrete pin-head to pea-sized, pearly, pale-pinkish, solid, round or oval papulo-nodules embedded in the skin; they are only slightly raised above the surface. They develop for a few years and then become stationary. Only rarely do they ulcerate or become malignant.

Histology consists of proliferation of mature basal cells from outer walls of hair follicles forming strands and cysts. No mitotic figures are seen.

Treatment is surgical. Dermabrasion, liquid N_2 or CO_2 laser may benefit in some cases.

Syringoma

Synonym: Hidradenomes eruptifis

It is a rare naevoid disorder presumed to develop from embryonic sweat glands or ducts. According to many authorities, adenoma sebaceum, syringoma, multiple benign cystic epithelioma and cylindroma are variants of the same condition.

Typical syringoma lesions are seen mainly on the face, especially the eyelids, neck and upper trunk in young women as pin-head to split-pea-sized, soft, flesh or yellowish coloured, globoid, discrete or grouped, papulo-nodules, almost embedded in the skin. Histopathology is diagnostic. It shows cystic sweat ducts lined by several layers of epithelial cells, comma-like tails to the cysts and also bands of epithelial cells.

Treatment is surgical or electro-desiccation.

Milium

It is a very common disorder. It usually occurs in large numbers on the face and less so on the genitalia. In the former case, milia occur on the eyelids, below the eyes, cheeks, temples and forehead.

Clinical features: They are multiple in number, and about the size of pin-head or millet seed, being pearly-white in colour. They are globoid in shape, have a firm consistency and are slightly elevated. When punctured, a whitish substance is expelled resembling the kernel of rice. The lesions are asymptomatic; even so, they can become a problem with sensitive people who consider them cosmetic blemishes.

Etiology: The cause is unknown. They are considered to be simple epithelial cysts or represent the encysted retention of sebum and hair cells. Milia are commonly seen on the scars of epidermolysis bullosa and pemphigus, etc. They occur in infancy or middle-age.

Differential diagnosis: It is made from vesicles, acne comedones, molluscum contagiosum and other cystic tumours.

Prognosis: It is fair.

Treatment: It is necessary only in sensitive people who are self-conscious. It consists in:
1. Puncturing the cystic tumour with a fine needle and pressing out the contents.
2. Destruction by electrolysis needle.

Granuloma Pyogenicum

It is a rapidly growing, vascular, fleshy, granulomatous nodule (sessile or pedunculated) which may occur anywhere on the body. The lesion may be smooth or ulcerated and is bathed in sero-purulent secretion. Its size varies from that of a pea to an almond **(Fig. 28.5)**. Trauma and pyogenic infection are the probable causes. According to Crocker, it is an exaggeration of proud flesh. Treatment consists of surgical removal and/or electrocauterization.

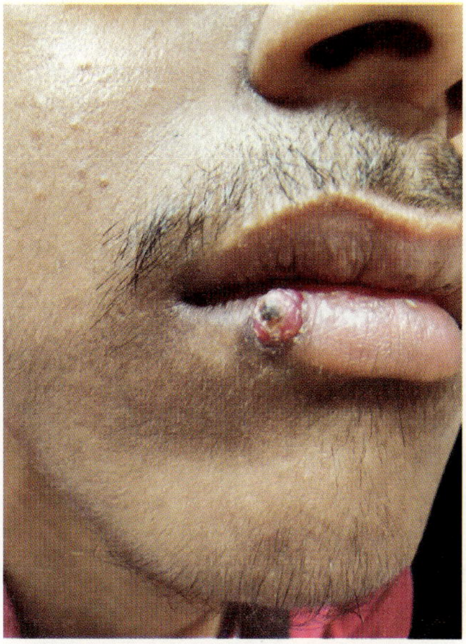

Fig. 28.5: Pyogenic granuloma

MALIGNANT TUMOURS

Carcinomas

Basal cell epithelioma	Squamous cell epithelioma
Intra-epidermal epithelioma	Paget's disease
Melano-carcinoma	Secondary metastases

Sarcomas

Sarcoma	Kaposi's idiopathic multiple haemorrhagic sarcoma

Reticuloses

CANCER OF THE SKIN

The skin, being a superficial structure, has the advantage of showing up the beginning of a cancer, making it apparent at an early stage, only if, due attention is given to the examination of a skin lesion. Patients must be educated to seek dermatological advice for all lumps, bumps and ulcers of the skin that tend to grow fast or to destroy the skin. The incidence of skin cancer is very low in India.

Etiology: The exact causation is still obscure but many factors are known to predispose, excite or contribute to the development of a skin cancer.

Age: Uncommon before the age of 40.

Heredity: May predispose to cancer development.

Race: White people who reside for long periods in tropical climates tend to develop cancer much more easily than dark people in similar circumstances. That is why skin cancers are so common in Australia and parts of America.

Individual: More common in persons with fair, sensitive skins and also in blondes.

Irritation factors: Sunlight, X-rays, smoking, constant trauma or irritation as by ragged teeth and tobacco chewing.

Occupation: Chimney sweepers, mule spinners, Kangri burns common among Kashmiri labourers, tar workers.

Precancerous dermatoses: Xeroderma pigmentosum, keratoses, leukoplakia, erythroplasia of Queyrat, chronic ulcers.

Skin cancers originate from the epidermis; malignant tumours of the dermal appendages are very rare. A single injury or insult to the skin may determine the development of carcinoma; though long, continued exposure to irritants is the more potent cause. A combination of several irritant effects is more carcinogenic than a single agent; hence trauma to a scar or mole, X-rays to lupus vulgaris and other similar combinations must be avoided. For the same reason, those people who have skins that are recognizably prone to cancer should avoid the known habitual, occupational and climatic hazards. Furthermore, skin cancers are relatively benign and easily curable, if treated early and efficiently. This is not true of cancers involving the muco-cutaneous junctions and malignant melanomas. Malignant tumours are characterized by local destruction, infiltrative growths, recurrence after removal and tendency to local or distant metastases.

Basal Cell Epithelioma

Synonym: Rodent ulcer.

Clinical features: It develops from the basal cell layer of the epidermis and also from the pilo-sebaceous apparatus. It is relatively benign, and is usually only locally malignant, without any tendency to metastasize. The tumour is characterized by slow growth, and the presence of a pearly nodule or ulcer with a rolled edge. Ulceration occurs late in the basal cell epithelioma **(Fig. 28.6)**.

The site most commonly affected is the upper part of the face; the lower part of the face, the hands and the trunk are less commonly affected. The lesion is usually single. A typical lesion starts as a firm papule which grows slowly into a nodule or a flat, raised plaque. In the course of time, the plaque shows a depression in the centre and more pearly papules at its periphery. Later, the centre breaks down to form an ulcer with a rolled edge which may also show firm pearly papules (rodent ulcer). The ulcer enlarges slowly; in the process, it destroys the local structures. The course usually extends over years; this fact should be brought out during history-taking.

Besides the typical lesion described above, one may come across several atypical varieties: the nodular type; the invasive destructive type; the scarring type (atrophic,

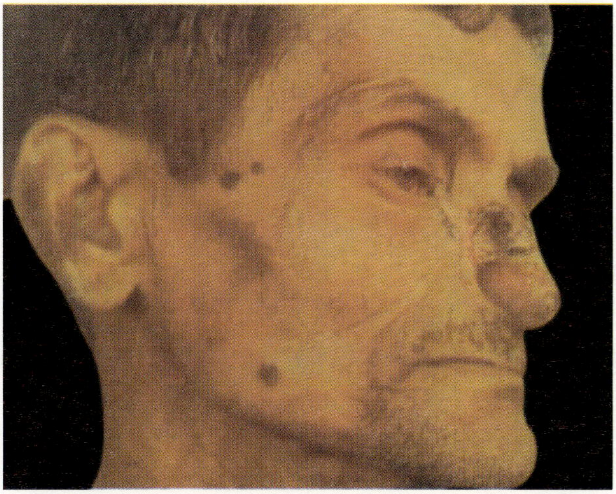

Fig. 28.6: Extensive basal cell carcinoma

smooth shiny patch); the cystic type (pea- to nut-sized translucent pearly tumour); the multiple superficial type (well-defined reddish-brown patches with thin pearly margin seen usually on the trunk) and the pigmented variety. Some of the features of the typical basal cell epithelioma can be discerned in these atypical varieties. Some basal cell epitheliomas may grow into squamous cell carcinomas.

Pathology: The typical features are downward projections of the basal cell layer; strands and islands of epidermal cells surrounded by a palisade of typical columnar basal cells containing a large nucleus; deep bluish staining and inflammatory reaction in the corium which is more marked at the periphery of the lesion.

Diagnosis: It is based upon: (1) the typical site, (2) a slowly growing lesion. The history usually extends over years. (3) a typical pearly nodule or ulcer with rolled edge, and (4) histopathological characteristics.

Differential diagnosis: It is made from keratoacanthoma, squamous cell epithelioma and chronic granulomas, particularly lupus vulgaris and lupus erythematosus, and tertiary syphilis. The latter produces confusion in scarring and superficial varieties of basal cell epitheliomas.

Keratoacanthoma	It grows rapidly; is self-healing; has a keratinous crater. Histopathology is characteristic.
Squamous cell carcinoma	It grows faster; history is in months. Convex surface in early stages; later. ulcer with indurated border, everted margins and granular base. More opaque and solid than basal cell epithelioma.
Lupus vulgaris	Onset is in childhood. History is in years. Typical reddish-brown patch with apple jelly nodules. No pearly border. Tissue paper wrinkled scar on healing.
Lupus erythematosus	Exposed parts; butterfly distribution; multiple patches; adherent scaly, follicular plugging.
Tertiary syphilide	History of syphilis and earlier rashes; rapid and bigger ulceration; punched out ulcer; positive serology.

Prognosis: It is good with a high percentage of cures. Recurrences and relapses are seen especially in cases where removal is incomplete. In sensitive persons, new lesions keep on developing on exposed parts from time to time.

Treatment: The patient should not be frightened with the name cancer since the growth is mainly benign. It is perferable to use the word rodent ulcer when explaining the disease process to the patient.

There is no mass approach to treatment. Every case should be individualized. The usual lines of therapy are:

1. X-ray therapy gives good cosmetic results as the basal cell epitheliomas are radio-sensitive. The dose is from 2,500 to 4,000 r in fractional or massive doses. It is contraindicated in recurrent lesions, in lesions near the eyes, on bones, tendons and cartilages. The authors prefer to employ preliminary cauterization and curettage followed by fractionated X-ray therapy. There is an initial inflammatory reaction followed by separation of the crust, and healing takes place in about 6–8 weeks. Radium plates have also been successfully employed.
2. Excision surgically or by diathermy and curettage. At least 5 mm all around should be excised. Scar can be repaired by plastic surgery. Mohs' chemosurgery or electro-surgery is used by many workers. Small lesions have been successfully treated with liquid nitrogen and topical cytotoxic agents. Every case should be watched for about 3 years because of the likelihood of recurrence.

Squamous Cell Epithelioma

Clinical features: It develops from the prickle tells of 'the epidermis. The tumour is characterized by rapid growth, early ulceration, absence of the pearly nodule of the basal cell epithelioma, a prickle cell histopathology and a tendency to metastasize **(Fig. 28.7)**.

The sites of choice are the dorsal aspects of the hands, the face, the muco-cutaneous junctions and the mucous membranes of the mouth and the genitalia, though lesions can occur anywhere.

Epithelioma may arise as such, or may complicate dermatoses like keratosis, cutaneous horn, leukoplakia, chronic ulcer, lupus vulgaris, etc. The second mode of origin is more common than the first.

When it starts *de novo*, it is seen first as a nodule or a firm, thickened plaque which undergoes ulceration within a few weeks. The ulcer is well-defined with an indurated, everted border. The base is granular, papillomatous or even fungating and is covered by a crust. Sometimes one may come across a cauliflower-like tumour. The lesion bleeds easily when the epithelioma complicates a primary condition; in such cases the precancerous lesion shows rapid growth, signs of inflammation, induration and ulceration as evidence of malignant change.

The regional lymph glands may show enlargement due to metastases. Hence, they should always be palpated. Metastases usually occur within 6–12 months.

Pathology: It is characterized by marked hyperplasia of the polygonal, eosinophilic staining prickle cells in irregular masses in the corium, cell nests and inflammatory reaction. The epidermal cells show abundant mitoses. The histopathological features are helpful in deciding about the degree of malignancy (grading).

Occasionally, it can be difficult to distinguish pseudo-epitheliomatous hyperplasia from early squamous cell epithelioma.

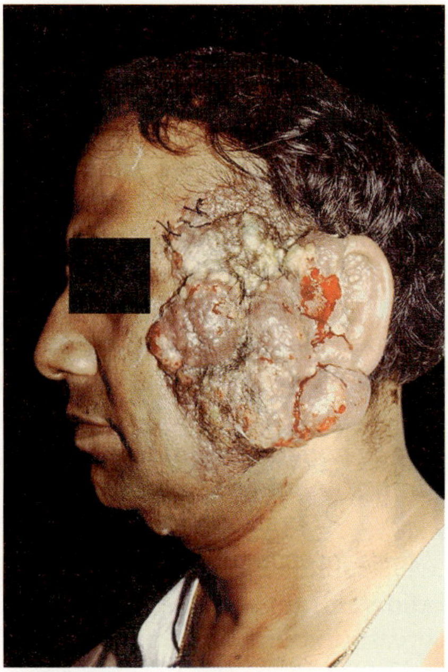

Fig. 28.7: Squamous cell carcinoma

Course: It is rapid and extends over weeks and months. It is locally destructive to the cartilages, bones and other structures like, for instance, the eyes. First, the metastases occur in the regional lymph glands, and later there is dissemination to the other glands and by bloodstream to the other viscera.

Diagnosis: It is based upon:

1. A fast-growing lesion in a person past middle-age.
2. The presence of precancerous dermatosis.
3. An ulcer with an indurated border, everted margins and a granular base.
4. Biopsy and histopathological features.

Differential diagnosis: It is made mainly from basal cell epithelioma, keratoacanthoma and tertiary syphilides. For details, see under basal cell epithelioma. Mixed types of baso-squamous cell epitheliomas do occur; this intermediate variety can be recognized through the microscope. When in doubt, it is a good principle to excise and examine histopathologically. Penile warts can sometimes cause confusion.

Prognosis: It is fair if the case is diagnosed early. The outlook becomes poor once the metastases have occurred. Deep lesions, adherent and destructive lesions, and lesions on the mucous membranes or the muco-cutaneous junctions have grave prognosis.

Treatment: It varies with the individual. X-ray therapy (3,600–6,000 r) in divided doses and wide surgical excision are the two known methods of treatment used. In advanced cases, regional lymph glands should be excised. Exact treatment, however, should only be undertaken after there has been a consultation between a dermatologist, surgeon and pathologist. Mohs' chemosurgery or electro-surgery gives good results in expert hands.

Intra-epidermal Epithelioma

Synonym: Bowen's disease.

It is rare, slowly growing tumour in thc cpidcrmis. Tumour cells grow sidewards and upwards remaining within the epidermis for years; the tumour may later develop into a basal or squamous cell epithelioma. Hence, it is usually considered as a precancerous dermatosis. Clinically, it starts as a firm, pale-red papule which develops into a crusted plaque. Under the crust, there may be oozing and a red surface that is granular or papillomatous **(Fig. 28.8)**.

Histology: It may either be by diathermy or by surgical excision. X-ray therapy is contraindicated.

Paget's Disease

It is an intra-epidermal and intra-ductal epithelioma affecting the areola and nipple of the female breast; it may also be seen in males, and on other sites of the body like the genitalia and umbilicus.

It is seen typically as a well-defined patch of erythema and scaling or oozing with gradual induration, infiltration and retraction of the nipple. In the course of time, a palpable carcinoma of the breast becomes discernible.

Histology: It is characterized by (1) acanthosis, (2) a disorganized epidermis inclusive of the basal cell layer, (3) the presence of typical, large pale-staining Paget's cells in the epidermis, the walls of the hair follicles and the lactiferous ducts.

Diagnosis: It is based upon the demonstration of a sharply-defined, indurated lesion around the nipple which may be retracted. Paget's disease usually affects one nipple. The differential diagnosis is made mainly from contact or infective eczematoid dermatitis of the nipples. Eczema occurs at any age, is bilateral, there is oozing and crusting accompanied by itching, edges are ill-defined. Further, it has no induration and nipples are not retracted. History is chronic with periods of complete remission.

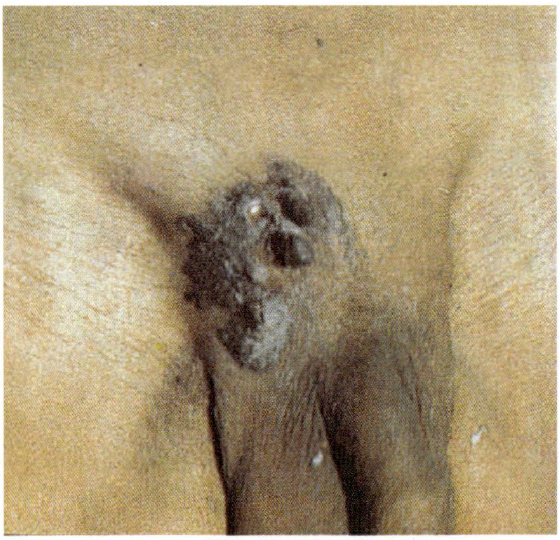

Fig. 28.8: Hyperkeratotic lesions of Bowen's disease

Prognosis: It depends upon the stage at which the diagnosis is made. It is similar to cancer of the breast.

Treatment: It consists of radical surgery of the breast and the lymph glands with or without radiotherapy.

Malignant Melanoma

It is the most malignant and dangerous of all skin tumours. It appears at any age but usually in elderly people. Its incidence is on the increase in white coloured people who have to sit in the sun or have frequent UVR exposure.

Clinical features: It is precipitated by irritation, pressure or interference. The indications of malignancy in a mole are enlargement of size, deepening of colour, induration, itching, easy bleeding and radiating lines of pigment in the lymphatics **(Fig. 28.9)**. Though such melanomas are often pigmented they need not be so. They may originate from:

Xeroderma pigmentosum: Lentigines become malignant neoplasms. This origin is not common in practice because firstly, xeroderma pigmentosum is rare, and secondly, the keratoses which occur in this condition usually develop into squamous cell epitheliomas. But sometimes, though rarely, malignant melanomas may also develop from senile pigmented macules. The common site is the face.

Normal skin: The common sites are the feet, nail-beds and the face. It starts as a blue black or non-pigmented nodule and whitlow which proceeds to grow rapidly.

Malignant melanomas metastasize rapidly first to the regional lymph glands, and later, to other parts of the integument, the liver, lungs and brain.

Histopathology: It is characteristic and consists of anaplastic naevus cells, deep, irregular infiltration and inflammatory reaction. Pigment can usually be demonstrated.

Prognosis: It is usually grave, more so, if metastases have occurred.

Treatment

Prophylactic in pigmented naevi: They should not be interfered with half-heartedly. If likely to be irritated by trauma or pressure, they should be excised completely by surgery.

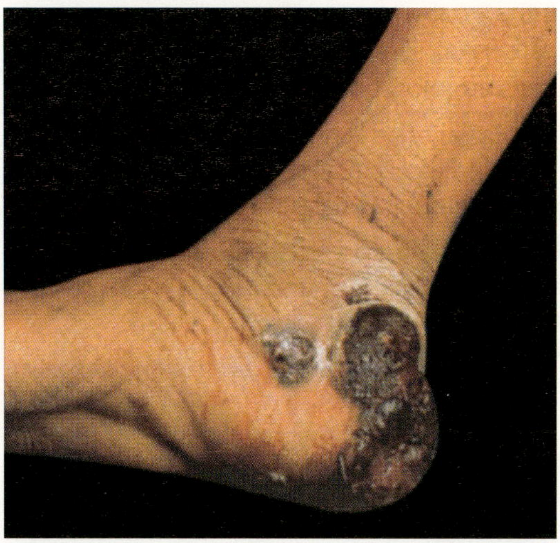

Fig. 28.9: Malignant melanoma—Invasion of the reticular dermis

Curative: Wide and deep excision is most important. Regional lymph glands and lymphatics must be dissected. Radiotherapy is only palliative in non-operable cases. Metastatic melanomas are treated with chemotherapy (decarbazine, nitrosoureas and methotrexate) and immunotherapy with BCG vaccine.

Secondary metastases in the skin: They result from primary carcinomas situated in the systemic organs reaching the skin by direct spread through the lymphatics or the blood stream. The common primary carcinomas which metastasize to the skin are those that occur in the breast, liver, prostate, gastrointestinal tract, and melanomas. Secondary metastases develop suddenly as solitary or multiple, firm, and discrete nodules, less so, as infiltrated plaques. They are usually freely movable in the early stages, and become adherent to the overlying skin by reactionary inflammation and ulceration. They are usually painless and asymptomatic.

SARCOMA OF THE SKIN

Sarcomas

It is rather a rare, malignant cutaneous neoplasm. Primary sarcoma can be of various types: lymphosarcoma, reticulum cell sarcoma, melanosarcoma from blue naevus, angiosarcoma, etc. Secondary sarcomas develop by extension from primary, systemic ones. A primary sarcoma usually starts as a purplish, smooth and firm nodule which grows slowly, terminating in ulceration or a fungoid growth. The histopathology helps in establishing the diagnosis. Surgical removal is the treatment of choice.

Kaposi's Idiopathic Haemorrhagic Sarcoma

It is rare condition. Seen on the hands and feet of adults as reddish-brown nodules, it may result in infiltrated plaques associated with telangiectasia, soft tumours and purpuric, cystic and bullous lesions. It may involute into atrophic, pigmented scars. The lesions are painful and itchy. Metastases occur everywhere. The histology is characteristic. The treatment is unsatisfactory. Radiotherapy and excision are useful in small localized areas. Where there is extensive involvement, chemotherapy with nitrogen mustard and vinblastine can be used.

RETICULOSES

This is the group name given to malignant conditions arising from the reticulo-endothelial tissues. They include many systemic diseases of the leukemia group; others may affect the skin only. The etiology remains unknown. According to Semenov, chronic dermatoses may get transformed into reticuloses. Parapsoriasis can be a premycotic condition. Histologically, they are either monomorphous or polymorphous. In the practice of dermatology, the latter group is more important, comprising mycosis fungoides and Hodgkin's disease. Only these two conditions will be described here in detail.

Mycosis Fungoides

Its incidence is low in India. Starting as a non-specific symptom or lesions, it takes a very chronic course, extending over years, to terminate fatally (Fig. 28.10). Its clinical evolution passes through three phases, viz., premycotic or non-specific stage, infiltrative stage and the tumour stage. Clinical and histological features of these stages are

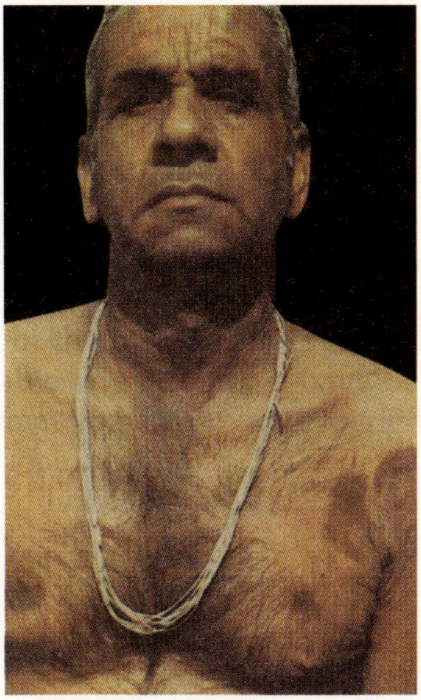

Fig. 28.10: Mycosis fungoides

Table 28.3: Mycosis fungoides

Stage	*Clinical features*	*Histology*
Premycotic	Pruritus; erythematous urticarial, eczematous, psoriasiform, erythema multiforme-like lesions, pityriasis rubra pilaris-like, etc. Distribution generalized. Characteristic multiforme and vivid colours.	Non-specific inflammation specially in deeper dermis.
Infiltrative	Pre-existing lesions getting infiltrated. Mucous membranes also affected. Erythroderma more often seen in this stage. Lesions may ulcerate.	1. Pleomorphism 2. Mycosis cells 3. Mitotic figures 4. Pautrier's abscesses 5. Abundant infiltrate
Tumour	Infiltrated lesions gaining in size to form tumours. Sometimes *de novo* origin. The ulcer formed is deep, base covered with greyish crust; margins may be rolled.	All the features of the infiltrative stage are much more pronounced.

summarized in Table 28.3. Organs connected with the reticular system, i.e. liver, spleen and lymph glands may also be affected.

Diagnosis: It may not be easy especially in the early stages since clinical and histological features are non-specific but in elderly persons, mycosis fungoides should always be considered in differential diagnosis.

Treatment of choice in mycosis fungoides is radiotherapy and steroids. These modalities bring subjective and symptomatic remissions without affecting the ultimate course. Methotrexate has been tried successfully by many. Infusions of monoclonal antibodies may help (Miller).

Hodgkin's Disease

Usually it starts in the lymph nodes and then involves the skin. Lesions may be specific or non-specific. The specific lesions consist of crops of papules or nodules on the trunk and limbs. Some of them may show urtication and others ulceration; few develop central necrosis. Itching may be marked. Glands are enlarged. Acquired erythroderma, pigmentation of Addison's type, pruritus and alopecia are frequently seen. Extensive and fulminating herpes zoster is sometimes a skin marker.

Histology: Histology reveals, in addition to pleomorphism common to all reticuloses, a special type of giant cell—Dorothy–Reed cell.

Prognosis: It is not favourable. A detailed systemic examination should be undertaken to assess visceral involvement.

Treatment: It is palliative. It consists of radiotherapy, steroids, hormones and chemotherapy.

THERAPY OF SKIN MALIGNANCIES

Available modes of therapy are: (i) Surgery-scalpel, cryosurgery, electro-surgery, chemo-surgery; (ii) Radiation; and (iii) Cytotoxic agents (Table 28.4).

Cytotoxic agents: The systemic use of these agents is indicated only in malignant lymphomas, i.e. mycosis fungoides, leukaemia cutis and Hodgkin's disease. Many such drugs have been synthesized and the available ones are classified as follows:

In the common varieties of skin surface malignancies, the systemic antineoplastic drugs have no place. Attempts to find a substance with a selective lethal effect on cancerous tissue have met with failure till now. Lately therapy with local cytotoxic agents has been found beneficial (Table 28.5).

Table 28.4: Cytotoxic agents

1. Alkylating agents	Nitrogen mustard, ethyleneimine, fluorouracil, cyclophosphamide
2. Anti-metabolites	8-azaguinine, 6-mercaptopurine, aminopterin, methotrexate
3. Antibiotics	Sarcomycin, actinomycin, carcinophyrin, mitomycin-C, chromomycin, bleomycin, vinblastine
4. Hormones	Sex hormones, ACTH; corticosteroids
5. Radio-isotopes	P 32, I 131, Co 60, Au 190
6. Plant derivatives	Podophyllin, colchicine, milkweed, *Abrus precatorius*

Table 28.5: Chemotherapy of skin cancers

Agents	*Concentration (%)*	*Indication*	*Side-effects*
1. Fluorouracil	1	Actinic keratoses, Bowen's disease, erythroplasia of Queyrat	Mild transitory dermatitis
2. Demecolcine	0.5	Rodent carcinoma, Bowen's disease, leukoplakia and keratoacanthoma. No effect on squamous cell carcinoma.	Irritation of surrounding skin.
3. Methotrexate	0.5	Similar to 2, but less effective	

Besides these, chloroquine (5%) and steroids have also been used. Battley demostrated remarkable success with 20% podophyllin in rodent ulcer.

Chemo-surgery: Introduced by Frederic E Mohs, it consists of freezing the tissue with zinc chloride and scraping off the malignant cells. It requires repeated and careful histological examination before cure is claimed and treatment terminated.

Present modified Mohs' surgery uses a knife or diathermy needle to achieve the same result. Neoplasm is removed completely; frozen sections are studied to see if any malignant cells exist at the edge or base. If they do, further resection is undertaken till the neoplasm is completely eradicated and edges and base are free of neoplastic cells.

Chapter

29

Pruritus

INTRODUCTION

The Hindustani equivalent for pruritus is *'kharish'* or *'khujli'*. It is a symptom, and scratch marks are its sign. The amount of advertisements this symptom has inspired, and the number of panaceas it has brought forth, indicates what a common and annoying condition it must be. Pruritus interferes with activity and sleep; so it becomes a social problem . The intensity of itching excited by a stimulus varies with the sensitivity of the skin and the mind, from person to person. Tramps, for instance, hardly feel mosquito bites; people with morbid minds, on the other hand, may start scratching at a mere suggestion. The skin and the nervous system are closely related because of their common origin in the embryo; for this reason, mental stress can not only start itching, but also complicate several skin disorders, particularly pruritus.

The exact mode in which pruritus is produced still remains obscure, but it is believed that pruritus is produced by the activation of the nerve endings of pain, which are present in the papillary layer of the corium, due to summation of sub-threshold stimuli. In comparison, intermittent stimulation results in tickling and threshold stimuli produce pain. There are no known special nerve endings concerned specifically with itching. The itch sensation terminates centrally in the thalamus; that is why comatose patients itch and people scratch in dreams.

Pathophysiology of pruritus still eludes satisfactory explanation and understanding. Histamine and certain proteoses (and enzymes) whether introduced from outside or liberated as a consequence of antigen-antibody reaction evoke pruritus. Threshold of pruritus is lowered in thin-skinned individuals under emotional stress and loneliness. People prone to sense of heat (*see* Chapter 3) are more prone to pruritus.

Results of Itching

Local	Scratch marks. Broken hair.
	Excoriations. Polished nails.
	May be secondary pyoderma, eczematization and even ulceration. Lichenification.
	Pigmentation and even depigmentation.
General	Interference with physical and social activities. Irritability.
	Insomnia.
	Exhaustion and wasting.

Causes of Pruritus

A. Physical and physiological.

1. Rough clothing, wool next to skin, tight clothes.
2. Heat, cold, dryness, humidity. Hot and cold baths also produce itching.
3. An unclean body, dirt and dust accumulated in the absence of frequent bathing.
4. Hot, spicy food and alcohol causing cutaneous flushing.

B. Itching dermatoses (Itching caused by a skin disease or infection)

1. Animal parasites—scabies, pediculoses, insect bites, fleas, bugs, mites, mosquitoes, etc. (Refer to Chapter 13)
2. Ringworm (Refer to Chapter 12)
3. Dermatitis and eczema (Refer to Chapter 10)
4. Urticaria, angioneurotic oedema (Refer to Chapter 9)
5. Lichen planus (Refer to Chapter 20)
6. Neurodermatitis-localized and disseminated (Refer to Chapter 10)
7. Prurigo simplex, nodularis, atopic
8. Psoriasis patients itch in tropical climate (Refer to Chapter 20)
9. Mycosis fungoides and reticuloses (Refer to Chapter 28)
10. Erythrodermas (Refer to Chapter 20)
11. Prickly heat (Refer to Chapter 34)
12. Dermatitis herpetiformis (Refer to Chapter 22)
13. Local stasis, Schamberg's disease (Refer to Chapter 25)

C. Local irritation by discharges, etc.

D. Systemic disorders producing itching, but perhaps no skin lesions

1. Hepatic diseases.
2. Renal diseases.
3. Diabetes, myxoedema.
4. Drugs—morphine, cocaine, barbiturates.
5. Animal parasites—intestinal worms, trichiniasis, onchocerciasis.
6. Anaemia and leukaemias.
7. Senility.
8. Pregnancy and oral contraceptives.
9. Internal malignancy.

E. Psychogenic

1. Neurasthenia.
2. Neurodermatitis.
3. Acarophobia.
4. Prurigo.

General Discussion

Syphilides hardly ever itch except when present in moist areas or when they are scrofulosorum in type. Besides the above list of causes of pruritus, regarding which information can be obtained in the respective chapters dealing with them, there are some special varieties of pruritus: pruritus ani, pruritus vulvae and pruritus scrotum.

Before proceeding to describe the different varieties (Fig. 29.1), we shall discuss the method of tackling a case of pruritus laying emphasis on the following:

1. One should look for evidence of dermatoses, insect bites, etc. The majority of cases of itching fit in the group of itching dermatoses. The patient must be completely unclothed, examined fully in natural or fluorescent light; the clothes should also be scrutinized for lice and other parasites. The distribution of pruritus and the nature of the lesions decide the exact etiological diagnosis.
2. Physical factors like heat, cold, clothing, diet, etc. should not be forgotten. Even if a physical factor is not the primary cause, common experience has shown that in almost all patients, pruritus is aggravated by exposure to the sun, change of temperature, movement of air, by a cold or hot bath and peripheral vascular dilatation resulting from the intake of alcohol and hot spicy food.
3. When pruritus is present without skin lesions, a complete systemic examination including rectal and vaginal examinations should be undertaken along with an examination of the urine for sugar, albumin, etc.; stool test; haemogram; blood

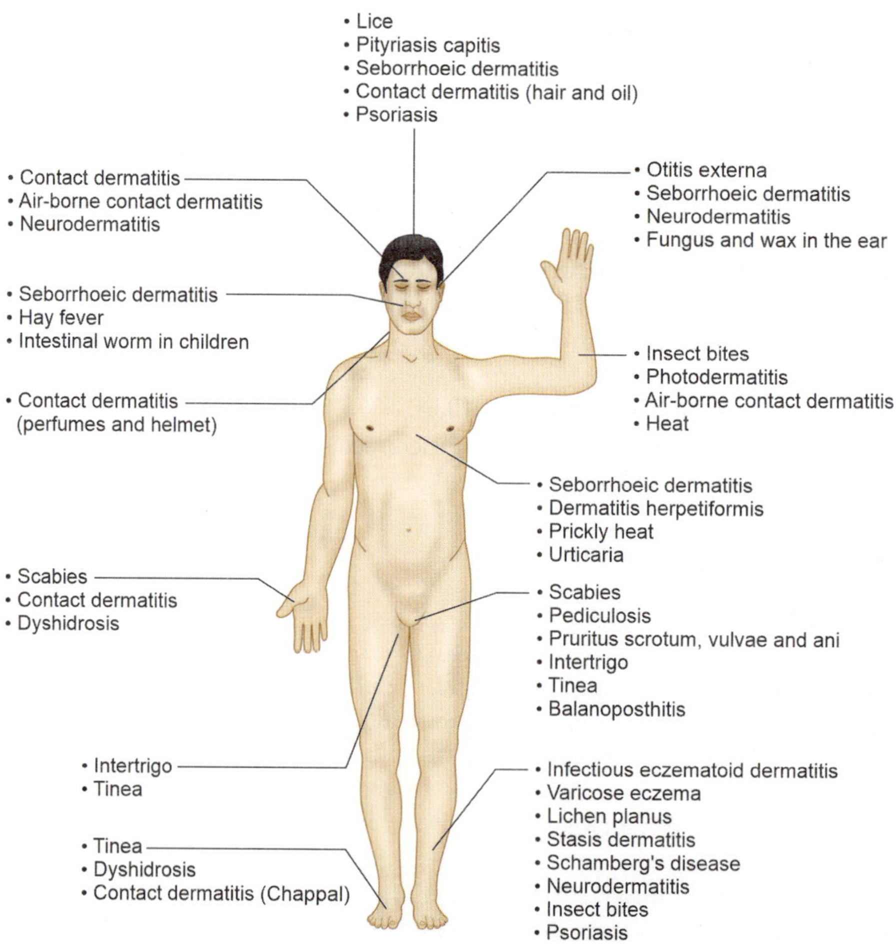

Fig. 29.1: Common itching dermatoses

sugar, cholesterol, urea, uric acid; liver function tests, X-ray of the chest and bones; psychiatric and emotional assessment.
4. Any drug habit or association must be brought out in the history.
5. Only in the absence of the above factors and in the presence of definite evidence of psychogenic involvement, must a diagnosis of psychogenic pruritus be accepted. It must be borne in mind that any pruritus can become worse or exaggerated due to secondary mental involvement establishing a vicious circle.

General Treatment

It consists in:
1. Eliminating the cause.
2. Removing the exciting factors. The patient must be properly clothed; avoid sudden changes of temperature; indulge in luke-warm baths; take simple bland food and avoid excess of tea, coffee and alcohol. The bowels must be kept clean.
3. Reassurance.
4. Palliative therapeutic measures:
   a. Antihistaminics are also good antipruritics.
   b. Sedatives; hypnotics and tranquillizers depending upon individual needs *Andropogon muricatus* (Khas) infusion/syrup.
   c. Bran baths.
   d. Local soothing treatment. The local antipruritics generally employed are: camphor, menthol, chloral hydras, pix liquida, liq. picis carb. and ichthammol in lotion, cream or ointment form. Cocaine and antihistaminic derivatives are useful but tend to produce local sensitization. Hence they should, as far as possible, be avoided.
   e. X-ray therapy is helpful in lichenified eczema, neurodermatitis and prurigo.
   f. Corticosteroids are useful in allergic dermatoses, erythroderma, acute lichen planus, etc.
   g. Calcium gluconate and Sandosten (P) are also helpful.
   h. Sex hormones, oestrogens in females and androgens in males, are sometimes helpful, particularly in middle and old age.

SENILE PRURITUS

Strictly speaking, the term implies generalized itching in elderly people, usually past the age of 50 or 60, with senile, atrophic, dry skin; itching is precipitated by rough or woollen clothing, sudden changes in temperature, baths etc. The other known causes of pruritus and itching dermatoses are absent. Though itching becomes generalized sooner or later, to begin with, it may be confined to the trunk or the lower extremities. The course is usually progressive, and the outlook is rather poor. The treatment consists in:
1. Massage with oil, Nivea cream (P) or pure animal fat like butter or ghee; 2–5% camphor may be added.
2. Protection from the physical exciting causes.
3. Course of oestrogens in females and androgens in males.
4. Palliative treatment on the lines mentioned above.

SUMMER PRURITUS

It is a fairly common complaint during the summer months in the hotter parts of tropical countries. In northern India, it is seen in between the months of April and August, but it occurs in its worst form during the monsoon. Dry heat frequently causes pruritus, but the other more common causes of summer pruritus are: profuse perspiration which results in clothes sticking to the body; dusty environment; uncleanliness; heat spots and prickly heat. It is more common in people who are overweight and overclothed for the climate.

The treatment should lay emphasis on correcting the responsible causes, improving the general health of the patient, encouraging them to use thin clothing, to live and work in cool hygienic environment. Air-conditioning, if possible, is very helpful. A talcum dusting powder massage is also beneficial. For an extreme case, a holiday at a cool hill station is the answer.

WINTER PRURITUS

It implies itching in the cold winter months in certain individuals; the itching disappears with the onset of the warm weather; other known causes of pruritus are absent. Itching occurs mostly on the trunk, thighs and arms on undressing. Exposure to cold weather is the precipitating cause, though dry skin, a run-down condition, the use of strong alkaline soaps, a very cold or very hot bath and woollen clothes tend to cause pruritus. The treatment consists in correcting the exciting and predisposing causes, in bathing properly, clothing the body suitably and improving the general health. The palliative treatment is the same as discussed above.

PRURITUS ANI

It may occur as such, or be associated with pruritus vulvae and scrotum. It is a fairly common complaint seen as simple pruritus with a sodden anal skin, but sooner or later, sequelae of pruritus like excoriations, pyoderma, lichenification and eczematization develop to complicate matters. Pruritus ani is more common in males than females. It is common in Asiatic countries because of heat and perspiration causing maceration, frequent gastrointestinal disorders, hot spicy food and the high incidence of intestinal worms, etc.

Etiology: The common causes of pruritus ani are:

a. Local causes (Inside the anus)	Threadworms
	Fissure in ano
	Haemorrhoids, polypi and fistula
	Moist anus due to improper drying
	Chronic constipation or diarrhoea
	Hot spicy or sensitising foods.
b. Skin diseases	Tinea, monilial infection, intertrigo
	Condylomata lata and acuminatum
	Seborrhoeic dermatitis
	Psoriasis, eczema
	Pediculoses

	Lichen sclerosus et atrophicus
	Contact dermatitis to toilet paper, enemas
c. Systemic	Use of antibiotics and other drugs
	Diabetes
	Achlorhydria
	Reticuloses
	Senility
d. Spread of pruritus from vulval area	Also from the scroto-penile region in conditions like diabetes, leucorrhea, pelvic tumours
e. Psychogenic pruritus neurodermatitis	

Diagnosis: In pruritus ani, the diagnosis is mainly etiological; hence before any treatment is instituted, the patient must be subjected to a thorough examination and investigation to establish the cause. Firstly, cutaneous diseases and the possibility of pruritus having spread from neighbouring areas must be ruled out. If both these groups of causes are absent, the gastrointestinal tract must be completely investigated by history-taking, repeated stool examinations, a rectal swab, a proctoscopic examination, etc. Only when no etiological factor is identified, may primary psychogenic causes be considered as producing the neurodermatitis.

Treatment consists in:

1. Reassurance.
2. Eradication of causes. In early and mild cases, this alone is enough. The diet should be simple, light and wholesome. All indigestible food-stuffs, chillies, condiments, curries and alcohol must be withheld. Anal region should be lubricated with oil at bath time.
3. The affected part must be kept clean, cool and dry. Underwears should be of cotton and loose.
4. An anti-pruritic cream or lotion on the lines mentioned above.
5. Antihistaminics and sedatives as the need arises. *Andropogon muricatus* (Khas) in infusion, syrup form internally and paste topically.
6. In resistant cases:
   a. Peri-anal infiltration with proctocaine or decadron which may also be injected around the anal canal.
   b. Grenz-ray therapy small, fractional exposures.
7. Psychogenic therapy in idiopathic and neurodermatitis cases.

PRURITUS VULVAE

It is a common and often very distressing form of localized pruritus occurring by itself or in association with pruritus ani or itching of the groins and adjacent parts of the thighs. Itching may either be confined to the vulval skin or include the vaginal walls and urethral orifice. Simple pruritus soon gets complicated by excoriations, lichenification, eczematization and pyoderma (Fig. 29.2). It is common in married women, 30–50 years of age. Occasionally, it is come across in children and adolescents.

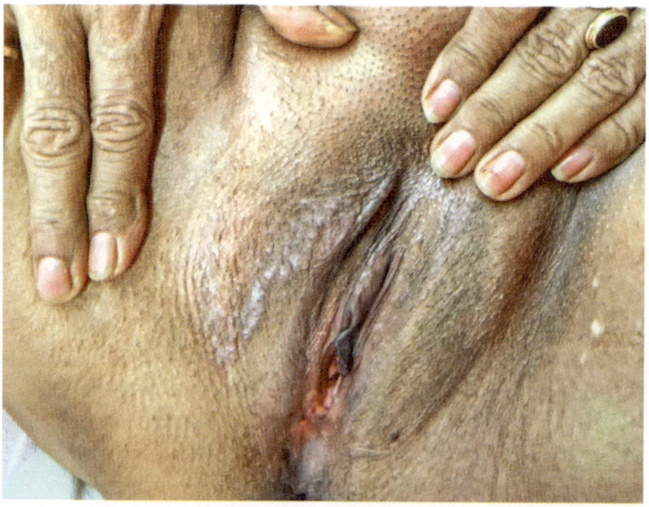

Fig. 29.2: Pruritus vulvae

Etiology

a. ***Cutaneous diseases of the vulval region***

Scabies, pediculoses.

Tinea

Contact dermatitis due to contraceptives, douches, pessaries, medicated sanitary pads, toilet paper and local medicaments.

Lichen planus

Psoriasis

Herpes progenitalis

Intertrigo, infective eczema, seborrhoeic dermatitis

Condylomata lata and acuminatum

Lichen sclerosus et atrophicus, leukoplakia

Senile vulvitis and kraurosis vulvae.

Filariasis-elephantiasis, and schistosomiasis

Lymphogranuloma venereum causing esthiomene

Fox Fordyce's disease.

b. ***Local causes in the vaginal and urinary tract***

Vaginal discharge-monilial or trichomonas infection

Cystitis, vaginitis and cervicitis

Acid urine and also urinary incontinence

Urethral stones

Pregnancy and pelvic congestion

c. ***Spread from neighbouring areas***

Anus—threadworms and pruritus ani (other causes).

Thighs—tinea, intertrigo, etc.

d. ***Systemic***

Diabetes

Drug eruptions especially antibiotics
Achlorhydria
Senility
Liver disease
Malignancy
Reticuloses

e. ***Psychogenic***
Neurodermatitis is due to sexual frustration, perversion, sex guilt or fear of venereal disease.

Diagnosis: Since the diagnosis is mainly etiological, emphasis should be laid on eliciting the cause before prescribing any treatment. A complete examination should be made of the skin of the vulval region for cutaneous disease, and also of the uro-genital tract, the anus, and the neighbouring regions. Routine investigations include examination of urine for sugar and acidity; of stools for ova and vaginal discharge for infective flora. Though mental and emotional factors are responsible for a great deal of chronic pruritus vulvae (both primarily and secondarily), physical organic causes must first be excluded. The help of a psychoanalyst and a social worker may prove useful in tracking down the psychogenic causes.

Prognosis: Pruritus vulvae can be most distressing; in a small percentage of cases, it becomes an obstinate complaint.

Treatment: The basic principles of treatment are almost the same as those applied in general pruritus and pruritus ani. They consist of:

1. Reassurance, particularly about the absence of cancer, or any contagious diseases.
2. Eliminating the causes and giving a treatment appropriate to the disease. Flagyl (P), Viozol (P), or Clotrimazole (P) pessaries for discharge per vaginum are useful.
3. Keeping the affected part clean, dry and lubricated.
4. Using an antipruritic cream, lotion or powder.
5. *Systemic:* Antihistaminics, sedatives, hypnotics, etc. Oestrogens in cases of kraurosis vulvae, senile vulvitis and menopausal women. Progesterone sometimes helps in prutitus caused by pregnancy.
6. In resistant cases:
   a. Grenz ray therapy in small fractional doses.
   b. Infiltration with Proctocaine (P) 5–30 cc or hydrocortisone.
   c. Vulvectomy in chronic obstinate cases with leukoplakia complication. It is to be done as a last resort.
   d. Psychotherapy. It should be given only by an expert psychotherapist.

PRURITUS SCROTUM AND PENIS

It is a fairly common complaint in young or middle-aged persons in tropical countries. According to the authors' experience, pruritus of the male genital organs is more common than pruritus vulvae in India. The reasons for this may be that:

1. Shy women do not come forward for consultation as men do.
2. Nutritional deficiencies affect the scrotum causing itching.

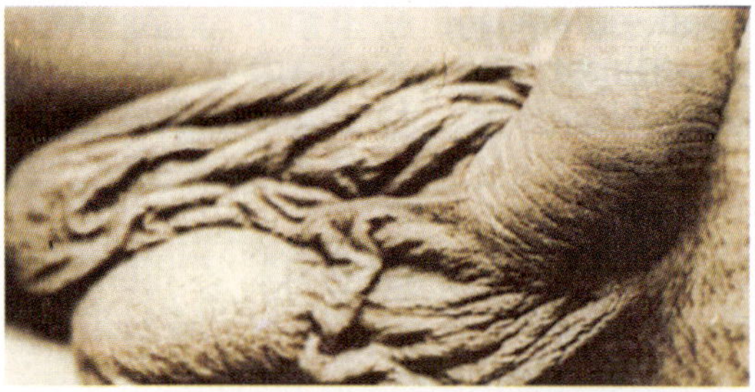

Fig. 29.3: Scrotal dermatitis

Itching may be mild, moderate, or very severe and distressing. The skin becomes thickened, rugose, excoriated and lichenified (Fig. 29.3).

There may be a secondary complication of pyoderma; and itching from the scrotum or anus may also spread to the perineum.

The common causes are:

1. Pruritus on the penis
   a. Glycosuria.
   b. Herpes progenitalis.
   c. Pediculoses, scabies, tinea.
   d. Contact dermatitis due to contraceptives, suppositories, etc.
   e. Irritation by vaginal discharges after unprotected sex.
   f. Prostatic affections.
   g. Neurodermatitis.
   h. Spread of itching from neighbouring areas, other cutaneous diseases, etc.
2. Pruritus on the scrotum
   a. Scabies, pediculoses.
   b. Contact dermatitis due to contraceptive, irritation by vaginal discharges, etc.
   c. Excessive sweating.
   d. Intertrigo starts at the junction of the penis with the scrotum.
   e. Chaffing by underwear, loin cloth or suspensory bandage.
   f. Tinea cruris.
   g. Nutritional deficiency.
   h. Use of broad-spectrum antibiotics.
   i. Neurodermatitis.
   j. Spread of itching from neighbouring areas and other cutaneous diseases including sebaceous cysts.

Treatment is similar to that employed in pruritus vulvae and ani.

PRURITUS IN PREGNANCY

Besides the usual causes of pruritus, there is a small group of dermatoses characterized by pruritic papules and urticarial plaques that occur predominantly, if not exclusively, during pregnancies, clearing up on delivery and recurrence with subsequent pregnancies. There are nine conditions, and of these, four stand out as distinct entities either because their pathogenic mechanism is now elucidated (herpes gestationis, pruritus gravidarum, auto-immune progesterone dermatitis of pregnancy) or because of unique clinical and laboratory findings (impetigo herpetiformis).

Prurigo gravidarum is the commonest in this group. There is generalized itching resulting from cholestasis. Jaundice may occur in severe cases. Cholestyramine, a non-absorbable synthetic ion-exchange resin adequately relieves pruritus in most of the cases. Liv 52 (P), phenobarbitone and vitamin K supplements may also help.

PRURIGO

It is a rare heterogenous group of itching dermatoses accompanied by the formation of papules or nodules. The term prurigo is an example of a symptom labelled as a disease. The etiology is different in each prurigo. It varies from insect bites to atopy and psychogenic stresses. More emphasis should be on etiological diagnosis rather than on the morphological and clinical labelling. Many of these prurigo are heredo-familial.

The common types of prurigo are:

1. Besnier's prurigo-asthma—eczema syndrome or atopic dermatitis (*see* Chapter 10).
2. Summer prurigo—aggravated form of summer pruritus.
3. Common prurigo—lichenification or neurodermatitis (*see* Chapters 10 and 30).
4. Idiopathic prurigo (Hebra).
5. Prurigo nodularis.

Idiopathic prurigo (Hebra): It is a very rare, chronic, itching dermatosis. The cause is unknown, but it may be brought about by psychogenic factors or sensitization to food-stuffs and focal sepsis (Sequira). The condition starts in childhood and continues to adulthood, though a spontaneous resolution may occur at any time, particularly at puberty. Clinically, the features are: Urticarial papules, thickening of the integument which becomes rough and coarse, excoriations and scratch marks; secondary eczematization and pyodermas may also be seen. The sites typically involved are the extensor surfaces of the limbs, and, less frequently, the trunk; the face is usually spared. The patient looks nervous, irritable and miserable. Though his general health is normal to begin with, in the later stages, there is wasting and emaciation.

The prognosis is usually bad, and the treatment unsatisfactory. Tar applications, antihistaminics, corticosteroids and X-ray therapy may bring good results in some cases.

Prurigo nodularis: It is characterized by discrete, indurated papules and nodules erupting mainly on the limbs, accompanied by severe itching. Adult females are selectively affected; in its early stages, it resembles lichen simplex and later (due to its dark verrucous surface) to lichen planus hypertrophicus **(Fig. 29.4)**. Histopathology helps to clinch the diagnosis (thick corneal layer, tremendous hyperplasia of malpighian cells, massive dermal lymphocytic infiltrate particularly around nerves). The exact cause is unknown though it is supposed to be caused by psychogenic disorders. The course is chronic, and the treatment is unsatisfactory. Crude tar, radio-therapy, derm-abrasion and infiltration with hydrocortisone preparations are helpful, along with other symptomatic therapies.

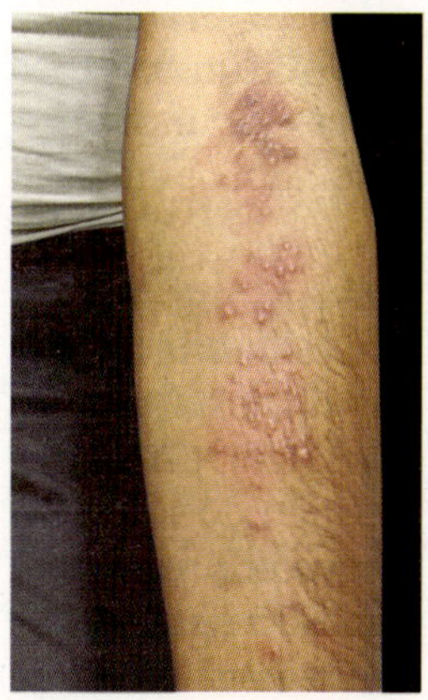

Fig. 29.4: Prurigo nodularis

Chapter

30

Psychodermatology—The Mind and the Skin

Basic Facts

1. Embryologically, both the skin and brain are derived from the ectoderm.
2. Close psychological relationship between the mind and the skin.
3. Skin is an important part of individual's development, behaviour and ego.
4. Skin health, beauty and cosmetics are an important part of sex appeal.
5. Skin is the canvas for reflection of emotions like fear, anger, happiness, despair.
6. Skin is the expression of social and biological transactions in the daily life.

Usually pigment loss or increase, scales, crusts and ulcers have an ugly look and provoke fear of contagion. Many people harbour the belief that itching, irrespective of the cause, is due to dirt. So, they keep away from a patient with a skin disease. From childhood onwards he or she is the target of rejection, withdrawal of affection, ridicule and sexual isolation. He cannot mix with people truly, cannot participate in group sports and recreational activities; his colleagues at work complain about him; his (more so in the case of a girl) chances of marriage are adversely affected, and chances of marital discord increase. This social background of patients with diseased skins must be borne in mind by every physician who handles them.

Sir Jonathan Hutchinson remarked in 1884 that while the old physicians laid stress on temperament and diathesis, the modern ones have become victims of pathology. These remarks are as true today as they were over 140 years ago.

Wittkower opines, "It is a reasonable estimate that emotional factors are of significant etiological importance in something between one quarter and one-half of all skin diseases." In our experience in India, psychological factors are responsible for skin diseases in about 10–15% of cases affecting mainly the educated, economically well-off classes. Poor, uneducated people are relatively free from them. Hence the importance of emotional factors in the etiology of skin diseases varies considerably in hospital and private practice.

In recent years, there has been an increasing awareness on the part of physicians about this close relationship between "Psyche" (mind) and "Soma" (body), and in every branch of medicine (including dermatology) a large group of chronic illnesses are being designated as "psychosomatic."

Wittkower has summarized the direct and indirect influence of the mind on the skin:

1. The symptoms or signs may be completely psychogenic, e.g. some cases of pruritus and hyperhidrosis, etc.

2. The emotional factor is often the most important feature in reactions of hypersensitivity, e.g. some cases of pruritus, eczema, urticaria, prurigo, etc.
3. A normal emotional manifestation in the skin may occur too easily and be maintained, e.g. rosacea, hyperhidrosis.
4. Emotion may be one of the excitants setting off or aggravating virus and other infections, e.g. recurrent herpes, sycosis barbae.
5. Emotional disturbances may predispose to skin infections, e.g. hyperhidrosis leading to tinea pedis, and various infections.
6. Emotional conflicts may increase the risk of exposure to venereal diseases, or increase the chance of drug intoxication or increase the risk of dermatitis, e.g. compulsive neurosis leading to excessive use of soap or antiseptics.
7. The gratification of itching if inhibited in one skin area, may be satisfied elsewhere, because one area is less forbidden than another, e.g. some cases of neuro dermatitis, flexural prurigo and excoriated eruptions.

The above list of skin–mind relationship at once makes us aware that skin diseases cannot always be treated as superficial, somatic lesions; they are, in fact, multifactorial in origin, and are conditioned by varied constitutional and environmental factors.

Explanations for site and type of cutaneous affection:

1. Genetic vulnerability of the area.
2. Intermittent insults (traumas) received over the years have made the areas vulnerable.
3. Personality traits.

The skin lesion (or the organ system) itself symbolically represents the type of psychological conflict.

While dealing with a patient, answer the following:

1. "What kind of person am I idealing with"—inherited and acquired characters, physical and mental constitution.
2. "What has he met'—germs, allergens, emotionally disturbing experiences, etc.
3. "What happened"—the physiologic mechanism and the psycho-pathogenesis.

So, history and observation of behaviour assume vital importance. The physician must necessarily be "inquisitive", alert to all visible evidence, watchful of every statement made by the patient. Above all, he must know what to look for. "The eyes do not see what the mind does not know." This point needs emphasis.

CLINICAL EXAMINATION

For good clinical examination from psychiatric angle, one should study the following features:

History-taking	Family history of psychiatric problems
	Childhood neurosis
	Emotional background
Examination	Bearing
	Mannerisms
	Vasomotor reactions
Observation	Presenting symptoms and their relationship with lesions

There are certain signs and symptoms which should act as clues to the experienced physician when he labels a case as psychosomatic in origin. Kelly mentions some valuable clues: inexplicable fluctuations in the intensity of an illness, transient improvement to every new form of treatment, flare-up of lesions in the morning suggesting that they had been produced consciously or unconsciously by rubbing at night, change of environment (hospitalization or going out of station) causing improvement of symptoms and a recurrence immediately on return.

DIAGNOSIS

The six postulates (Weiss and English) which need to be satisfied before an illness can be designated as psychosomatic **(Table 30.1)** are as follows:

1. A family history of psychological difficulties (heredity and pseudoheredity).
2. Evidence of a childhood neurosis.
3. Sensitivity to specific emotional factors at crucial life periods (puberty, marriage, child-birth, climacteric, etc.)
4. A specific personality structure (other evidence of neurosis or character disturbances).
5. Demonstration of a specific behaviour while the history is taken (the examination becomes an artificial exposure to a conflict situation).
6. Hyposensitization by psychotherapy or the avoidance of the provocative situation.

Table 30.1: Summary of skin conditions caused by emotional factors (Sneddon, modified by Behl)
A. Always psychic in origin • Dermatitis artefacta • Acarophobia • Trichotillomania • Neurotic excoriations.
B. Dermatoses with large psychogenic factor • Rosacea • Atopic eczema • Alopecia areata • Acne neurotica • Neurodermatitis • Pruritus ani and vulvae • Prurigo
C. Dermatoses which may be precipitated by psychogenic factors • Pompholyx • Canities • Psoriasis • Urticaria • Hyperhidrosis • Lichen planus
D. Psychogenic overlay in an otherwise non-psychogenic problem occupational dermatitis. • Eczema • Acne vulgaris • Vitiligo • Hypertrichosis

The above discussion amply reveals to us that the concept of psychosomatic relationship is a precise one, and it should not be used by a physician to ascribe any inflammatory dermatosis of unknown origin to psychological conflicts and tensions.

Sulzberger and Baer have rightly pointed out the danger of yielding to the temptation of finding an escape from diagnostic dilemmas into vague psychological conjectures. This tendency is also provoked by many patients who would rather welcome a vague, long-winded diagnosis rather than a clear-cut one and frequently give a history of "nerves" as the cause of their illness. Such explanations "serve as face-saving devices" of the precipitating factors like loss of love or loss of self-esteem, etc. So the physician must not accept voluntary information at its face value.

TREATMENT

It must be realized that diagnosis and treatment cannot be reviewed separately in psychogenic problems. Subtle forces of therapy are already at work, when the patient hears about the reputation of a physician, and finally steps into his clinic. The rapport is easily established and each of the conscious or unconscious gestures of the physician, even his personality and bearing, his touch, his word, influence the course of the therapy. The intelligent physician must know his technique and understand the importance of suggestibility in the uncovering of deep-seated causes, and its value in the amelioration of symptoms. So, diagnosis and treatment proceed concurrently from the first interview onwards. The following specific measures are adopted.

Supportive psychotherapy: The objective in this process is to suppress the patient's symptoms; this is done by reassurance, advice, re-education, by helping the patient to make minor adjustments in domestic relationships or if necessary, in his occupation, by rest, distraction, hypnotism, etc. No attempt is made to unearth the deep-seated underlying causes; rather, the assets of the patient's personality are strengthened. This is possible when the personality is more or less intact, and the causes of maladjustment are superficial and easily accessible. This method is within the reach of every family physician, because it is he, who comes in contact with the patient first and has the best chances of establishing rapport with him and influencing the course of his recovery. However, this method is ineffective in severely disturbed patients, or in such patients "who are too fragile psychologically to be tampered with, too inflexible to be capable of real personality alterations, or too defective to have an active insight".

Analytical psychotherapy: It may be brief and intense, or prolonged depending on the individual case. The patient is encouraged to re-live past experiences. During this process , the doctor helps the patient to gain and learn to re-adjust his style and goal of living in accordance with his assets and liabilities. Obviously, this is a long drawn-out, costly and highly technical art which calls for special training on the part of the doctor, and on the part of the patient, a little above-average intelligence, and a capacity for introspection. Again, it cannot be undertaken when the patients are acutely ill or too old to change. It is like a major operation and should be undertaken only by a trained psychiatrist.

Abreaction: Methods of abreaction by intravenous pentothal sodium injection or methylamphetamine injection or inhalation of carbon dioxide 30% and oxygen 70% are used to lessen inhibition and facilitate emotional release.

Table 30.2: Psychotropic drugs in dermatology

Antidepressants
• Alprazolam 0.25–2 mg/day
• Hydroxyzine 25 mg three times a day
• Imipramine 100–300 mg daily
• Amitriptyline HCl 25–75 mg HS
• Buspirone 5–10 mg three times a day
• Doxepin 25–50 mg three times a day
• For obsessive or compulsive symptoms
• Clomipramine 10 mg increasing to 30–150 mg/day. Elderly 75 mg/day
• Fluoxetine 20–40 mg/day.
Antipsychotics
• Benzodiazepines
• Diazepam 2.5–10 mg/day
• Lorazepam 1–3 mg/day
• Nitrazepam 10 mg/day
• Flurazepam 15 mg/day

Group psychotherapy: Because of its easy administrative and financial advantages, this method is being used in various institutions.

Relaxation: Krafchill, Moller and others have reported good results with a system of relaxing exercises. Particularly beneficial are some of the Indian techniques of Yogic exercises.

Drug and physical treatment: It consists of administration of sedatives, hypnotics, tranquillizers **(Table 30.2)** and electroconvulsive therapy depending on the nature and intensity of the mental symptoms accompanying the skin disorders. Many exaggerated claims have been made by various doctors who are biased about one form of treatment or the other. But it is more or less accepted by all that physical and drug treatment, unless accompanied by psychotherapy, produces only temporary benefit.

Chapter

31

Diseases Associated with Sebaceous Glands

Basic Facts

1. Seborrhoeic state is constitutional, may be heredo-familial (Table 31.1).
2. It is influenced by:
   a. Sex hormones
   b. Psychogenic stresses
   c. Dietary errors like beverages, starches, oils, alcohol, synthetic/junk foods.
   d. Digestive upsets especially constipation
   e. Climate
3. Seborrhoeic state favours the growth of organisms like *pityrosporon* or *malassezia, staphylococcus albus* and acne bacillus.
4. It is aggravated by air pollution, sudden changes of temperature, general health and drugs.
5. It mainly affects seborrhoeic sites like the scalp, face (esp. the nose, eyebrows and retro-auricular area), neck, chest (sternal region, shoulders, back-interscapular region) and flexures. Palms and soles are never affected.

General Management Measures

1. Frequent washing with soap and water.
2. Avoiding cream and powder or other greasy application.
3. Cleansing with astringent lotion or spirit 25% in rose water.
4. Personal hygiene, active life and balanced diet.

SEBORRHOEA OLEOSA

It signifies over-secretion from the sebaceous glands and also change in the composition of sebum. As a temporary event, it is seen at puberty in many persons but as a permanent feature, it is pathological. Clinically, seborrhoea is characterized by greasy sticky hair and an oily shiny skin. These features are noticeable mostly in the evening under artificial light. Thread-like, cheesy plugs, looking like greyish worms can be readily expressed from the patulous pilo-sebaceous openings on the skin. These features are visible mainly on the forehead, nose, ears, and cheeks.

CRADLE CAP

Synonym: Milk crusts.

Table 31.1: Conditions associated with sebaceous disorders

Infancy	Cradle cap. Infantile seborrhoeic dermatitis Infantile acne Infectious eczema Leiner's disease
Puberty	Pityriasis capitis Seborrhoeic dermatitis Seborrhoeids Acne vulgaris Fordyce's spots Nevus sebaceous Sebaceous cysts
Middle age	Exfoliative dermatitis in immuno-compromized, AIDS
Pregnancy	Sebaceous gland hypertrophy
Miscellaneous	Drugs—Anti-epileptic Spinal cord injury Parkinsonism Unhygienic persons Cerebrovascular accident

It is seen in newborn infants within a week or two after birth. It is a special form of pityriasis capitis. Dirty, yellowish, thin or thick crusts on the vertex of the scalp are typical of this condition. There is little itching and no inflammation or oozing unless complicated by seborrhoeic dermatitis. Dried vernix caseosa can resemble this condition, but it can be excluded by the persistence of the condition after thorough cleaning of the scalp after birth. Complicating seborrhoeic dermatitis must be differentiated from infantile eczema. The latter affects the cheeks initially, there is frank oozing and spasms of pruritus, while seborrhoeic dermatitis starts on the scalp, oozing is little and crusting is more pronounced (*see* Chapter 10).

Prognosis: It is usually good and the condition tends to subside in a couple of months unless complicated by infection and dermatitis.

Treatment: It consists of frequent washing with Cetavlon (P) or Savlon (P) lotion and application of Vioform (P) or 1% sulfur ointment in non-greasy emulsifying base. 1% hydrocortisone with bacitacin or soframycin cream (P) are recommended in cases complicated by infective eczema or seborrhoeic dermatitis. Strong antiseptics or medicaments must be avoided in infants.

PITYRIASIS CAPITIS

Synonym: Dandruff, *Scurf* in Hindustani: sikri or *bafa*.

Clinical features: The condition is seen as diffuse scaliness of the scalp. In reality, there are two distinct varieties of pityriasis capitis: dry (sicca) and greasy (steatoides) **(Table 31.2)**.

Transitory scaliness or scurf of the scalp comes across in an intercurrent illness. In conditions like erythroderma or disseminated eczema, persistent pityriasis capitis

Table 31.2: Pityriasis capitis	
Dry variety	*Greasy variety*
1. Scales are white, fine and furfuraceous dry and greyish; scales fall freely on shoulders.	1. Waxy, greasy, yellowish thick scales and crusts; scalp may be pale red.
2. Hair dry and lustreless	2. Hair greasy and may be matted; tendency to thinning.
3. Mild or no itching	3. Itching moderate. If severe, secondary eczematization or seborrhoeic dermatitis should be suspected.
4. Common in dry cold weather	4. Common in hot and humid weather. But may be seen in cold weather.
5. Affects people reluctant to use oil on the scalp resulting in exaggeration of normal exfoliation of hairy areas.	5. Affects seborrhoeic individuals.
6. Outlook better. Improves with oil application.	6. Outlook not so good.

seen as a part of the general affection. It is also seen in pityriasis rubra pilaris, Darier's disease and pemphigus erythematoides. In nutritional disorders, scaliness of the scalp is exaggerated.

Treatment: In all cases, an attempt should be made to correct the etiological factors. The palliative treatment is mainly local; it consists of:

1. Frequent washing and shampooing. Simple forms will respond to this measure alone. The shampoos preferably employed are: Ketoconazole, Cetavlon (P), Savlon (P), Tetmosol (P) and Selsun suspension (P). In the presence of even slight irritation or dermatitis, shampoos must be avoided.

   Some indigenous preparations have been successfully employed by the authors; amongst these, particular mention should be made of ritha, amla, trifala, and *aloe vera*.
2. Greasy dressings should be avoided except in the pityriasis sicca variety. If secondary eczematization or infection has set in, use Hydrocortisone or Betamethasone lotion or cream with neomycin or framycetin or vioform. Ketoconazole cream has its advantages. However, avoid application of medicated ointments and shampoos if unwarranted.
3. Topical application of sulphur, acid salicylic, resorcinol and ammoniated mercury, etc. Sulphur should not be employed in lotion form since it does not dissolve. It should be mixed with unguentum emulsificans aquosus. Resorcinol should not be used for blondes, as it turns fair hair to metallic green; in such people, mercuric chloride can be employed. Furthermore, women do not, as a rule, like ointments on the scalp. Hence the principle should be to employ lotions in women and ointments in men. In the initial stages of treatment, loose, impoverished hair may fall; the patient should be warned about this. Topical ointment/lotion is recommended in the initial stages of chronic cases only; once the condition is brought under control, treatment with medicated shampoo can be carried on indefinitely without much discomfort.

Examples of common prescriptions for dandruff are:

Resorcinol	2 g
or Hydrag perchlor	0.1 g
Acid salicylic	2 g
Ol. ricini	2–5 cc
Ol. lavendulae	QS
Spt. methylated/eau de cologne to	100 cc

Sig: To be applied on scalp surface in the night twice a week after parting the hair at different places. Next morning, the scalp is washed.

Cetavlon (P)	0.5 g
Acid salicylic	2 g
Sulphur	N_2 g
Ung emulsificans aquosus to	100 g

Sig: To be rubbed into the scalp every night.

4. Improve general health; balanced diet; cut down tea, coffee, alcohol, heavy food. Exercises in fresh air need to be encouraged.

SEBORRHOEIC DERMATITIS

Since it is a constitutional disease with disturbed sebaceous secretion, the name dys-seborrhoeic is more appropriate. Its incidence is fairly high but varies between hospital and private practice.

The transition from seborrhoea of both forms, the oily and the dry type, into seborrhoeic dermatitis is a rather common occurrence since an inflammatory reaction very often complicates the seborrhoeic state. It affects the areas of the body where the sebaceous glands are abundant or hairy regions and flexures **(Fig. 31.1)**. The usual uncomplicated seborrhoeic dermatitis is characterized by two types of lesions: (i) Scaly erythematous plaques. (ii) Follicular papules. There is little oedema; in place of redness, there is a peculiar yellowish colour; if papules develop, they are very small. Vesicles are entirely lacking, and consequently there may be little or no weeping; abundant scaling and crusting do not originate from bursting vesicles. Pruritus is minimal or troublesome.

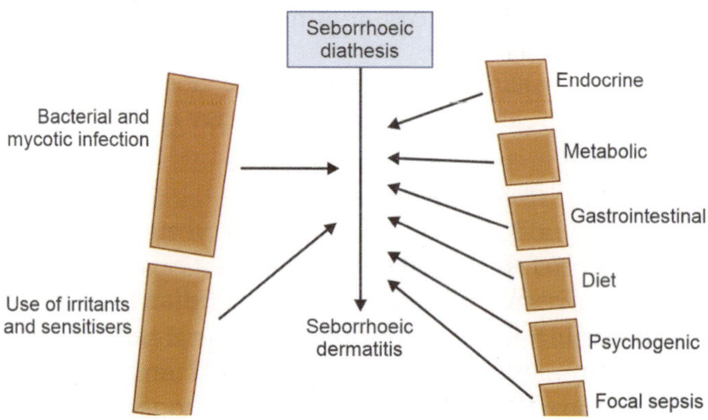

Fig. 31.1: Factors responsible for causation of seborrhoeic dermatitis

Altogether, the eczema is chronic in appearance from the beginning. Patient usually has sedentary habits, a sallow look and constipation. Features of seborrhoeic diathesis are usually present (Table 31.3).

Clinical Features

A. ***Scalp***: The disease usually starts on the scalp and consists of patchy or diffuse reddish areas covered with fine, loosely adherent, greasy, yellowish scales or crusts. Oozing is slight unless there is complication by infective or chemical eczema (Fig. 31.2).

B. ***Face***: Besides the involvement of naso-labial folds, itchy otitis externa and marginal blepharitis, there is redness and crusting of eyebrows. On the cheeks and forehead, itchy reddish scaly patches may be encountered. Beard region shows diffuse erythema, mild oedema and follicular pustules and crusting. On the sides of neck, similar erythemato-squamous patches may be seen.

C. ***Trunk:*** The sternal region is very frequently involved, especially in the males. The eruption here has a characteristic pattern: Annular, circinate or gyrate, discrete or confluent, scaly macules, reddish at the borders and fawn-coloured at the centre. Similar lesions are seen on upper back and interscapular region. The condition is ordinarily asymptomatic and often remains unnoticed in individuals with hairy

Table 31.3: Differential diagnosis of seborrhoeic dermatitis

Seborrhoea oleosa	Absence of itching and inflammation
Atopic dermatitis in children	Mainly on cheeks and less on scalp Severe paroxysms of itching Marked oozing Family history of asthma, eczema or allergy
Adults	Involvement of flexures chiefly Marked itching Tendency to lichenification
Psoriasis	Patches of erythema with silvery scales Typical distribution Little oozing and itching Pinpoint bleeding on removing scales If not sure, term sebopsoriasis is used
Pityriasis rosea	Herald patch Medallion-like lesions on back with scales pointing towards the centre Distribution along the ribs Limited course of 6–12 weeks
Discoid lupus erythematosus	Butterfly distribution Well-defined erythematous macules with adherent scales, follicular plugging and scarring. Aggravation by sunlight
Tinea corporis	Well-defined macules Inflammatory border and central clearing Marked itching Microscopic examination shows fungal hyphae

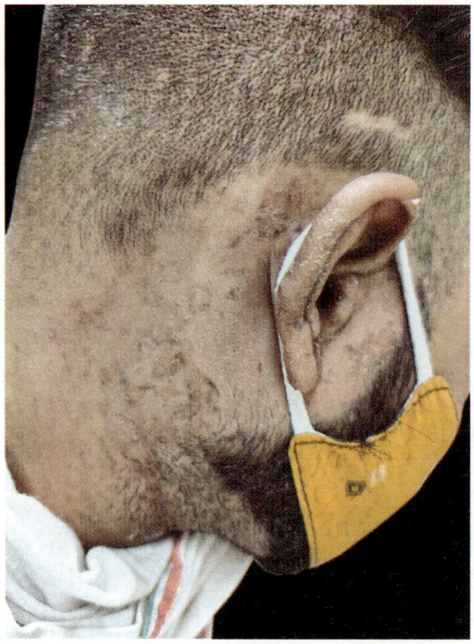

Fig. 31.2: Seborrhoeic dermatitis

chests. In some cases, the disease spreads and affects large areas of the trunk and extremities-seborrhoea corporis. The term 'Seborrhoeide' is sometimes used. Occasionally, seborrhoeic dermatitis develops a psoriasiform pattern.

D. *Flexures:* In the intertriginous folds such as the retro-auricular, sub-mammary, umbilical, axillary and anogenitocrural areas, the clinical picture of seborrhoeic dermatitis shows a deviation. Scaling is not prominent and sometimes even lacking; the yellowish tinge gets more reddish; moisture, fissuring and crusting may develop causing pain.

E. ***Folliculitis.*** Seborrhoeic folliculitis is frequently seen on the legs. Itching is troublesome some. Similar lesions may be seen on the thighs, pubic area, arms and beard region.

Eczema seborrhoeicum is very common in early childhood; it differs, however, considerably from the adult type showing acuteness and a tendency to disseminate over large areas. It also starts on the scalp, but usually spreads to the face, neck, the intertriginous folds and their adjacent areas. Rarely does an almost universal involvement occur, exhibiting the picture of an exfoliative dermatitis (Leiner's disease).

Seborrhoeic dermatitis is characterized by its diminished resistance to bacterial and yeast infection.

Histopathology: It is not typical. The changes are somewhat between eczema and psoriasis; epidermis shows hyperkeratosis, parakeratosis and intra- and extracellular oedema. In the cutis, there is a perivascular infiltration consisting mainly of lymphocytes and polymorphs.

Diagnosis: It is based upon:

1. Demonstration of a seborrhoeic state.
2. Distribution of eruption.
3. Mildness of the dermatitis.
4. Chronicity from the beginning.

5. Typical erythematous plaques with scales or greasy crusts and slight oozing, accompanied by mild to severe itching.

Tinea amiantacea can be described as a special type of seborrhoea capitis. It is characterized by presentation of asbestos-like, rather thick scales which mat the proximal portion of the hair like a sheath. There is no alopecia, but bundles of hair bound by scales can readily and painlessly be extracted.

Prognosis: It is good in mild cases. Severe extensive cases are troublesome, resistant and recurrent, though with newer corticosteroid creams, eruption may be kept in check. Chances of permanent cure are poor.

Treatment: There is no specific treatment. Open air life, exposure of the integument to fresh air, mild exercise, bland well-balanced diet (cutting down of carbohydrates, fats and beverages) and mental relaxation are very beneficial. General health of the patient must be improved. A nice relaxing holiday sometimes does the trick. Mainly, the treatment is the same as in pityriasis capitis.

In the acute stage, silver nitrate lotion 1%, or hydrocortisone with neomycin lotion or soframycin are useful; ointments should not be used at this stage. Silver nitrate lotion is painted every 4 hours during the day for the first 24–48 hours. Burrow's solution or alum lotion are also useful. In chronic cases, a cream is rubbed in twice a day.

Infected seborrhoeic lesions generally respond quickly to the systemic use of antibiotics like erythromycin or doxycycline, locally neomycin, soframycin, bacitracin and fusidin are very effective. In intertriginous areas, 1% aqueous solution of gentian violet will help to control the frequently accompanying monilial infection. For stubborn, circumscribed seborrhoeic eruptions, betamethasone cream in the strength of 0.1–0.5% is helpful.

On the scalp and trunk, ultra-violet therapy is sometimes of benefit especially when combined with liquor picis carb paint. In obstinate cases of eczema seborrhoeicum of the face and glabrous skin, fractional roentgen ray treatment is of great value. Extract of *Aloe vera* has also been successfully used.

Internal: Antihistaminics are useful in controlling troublesome itching. Use of antibiotics should be restricted to grossly infected cases. Non-specific stimulant therapy in the form of autohaemotherapy, zinc, B-complex, *Swertia chirata* are a useful stand-by in resistant cases. Corticosteroids are also effective against widespread, acute seborrhoeic dermatitis but should be used with discretion.

ACNE VULGARIS

Synonyms: Pimples; in Hindustani: *Kil, Muhase.*

Introduction: Acne vulgaris is one of the most common dermatoses. It develops at puberty (teenage) when the sebaceous glands are the most active. In the pre-adolescent period, seborrhoea oleosa and some comedones frequently appear as fore-runners of the disease. In pregnancy, it gradually decreases, and is again seen especially in women at a later age (post-adolescent acne), due to family planning and periods may become scanty by that age. It occurs in both girls and boys; in the latter, in a somewhat severer form.

For the development of acne, besides seborrhoea, the hyperkeratosis of the pilo-sebaceous ostia is an important pathogenic factor. A keratinous-cum-sebaceous plug is formed in the follicular neck resulting in the narrowing and sometimes blocking of the canal. In general, a well-developed growing hair interferes with the collection of keratinous and sebaceous material. The growing hair plays the role, as it were, of a needle. That is why acne never occurs on the scalp, and only rarely, on the beard region despite seborrhoea being present in these areas.

Clinical features: The main localization of acne is the face; then follows the neck, the upper part of the chest, the shoulders and the back. Occasionally, acne is seen on the thighs and buttocks. The distribution is usually bilaterally symmetrical. Seborrhoea oleosa is prominent on the face, and the openings of the sebaceous glands-the pores-are distinctly visible and patulous.

The primary lesion of acne is the comedo; it signifies a plug composed of dried sebum, epithelial cells and keratinous scales; it fills the pilosebaceous canal (Fig. 31.3). On the surface of the skin, it appears as a slightly elevated white dot, called whitehead; with the passage of time the sulphur constituent of sebum soon gets converted into sulphide turning the whitehead into a black dot, called a blackhead. With a comedone extractor, the entire comedone can be readily squeezed out as a yellowish, cheesy-looking, worm-like mass. Some comedones may persist and remain unchanged, but often an inflammatory reaction occurs. The first stage is erythema which surrounds or engulfs the comedone, and a papule develops-*acne papulosa*. The comedone is transformed into a moderately firm hemispheric, lentil to bean-sized papule of rose-red colour. Most of these papules gradually involute leaving no trace; others suppurate to form pustules resulting from the action of secondary invading microorganisms, chiefly staphylococci-*acne pustulosa*. The suppuration may be superficial or deep-seated. The deep-seated pustules take time to involute. *Acne indurata* is characterized by rather firm, perifollicular nodules of bluish-red colour. They persist for a long time. Many of them eventually become completely or partially absorbed, others transform into cysts-*acne cystica* (Fig. 31.4). They, however, also tend to persist, discharging from time to time a thin, purulent fluid.

Scarring, usually pitted, is a common sequel of acne, being most marked when the lesions are nodular and suppurative. Sometimes the pits are closely aggregated giving rise to a worm-eaten appearance.

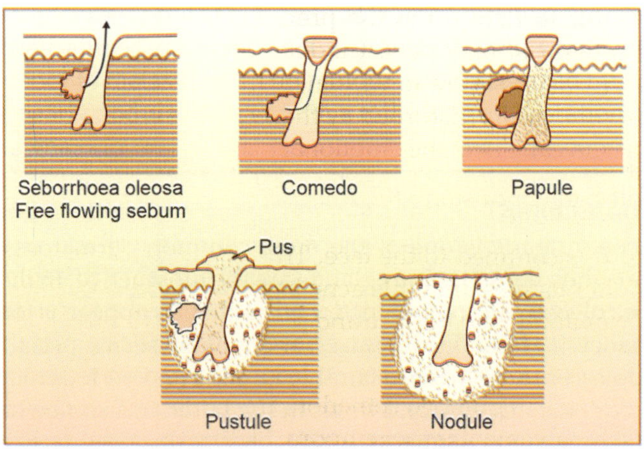

Fig. 31.3: Different acne lesions

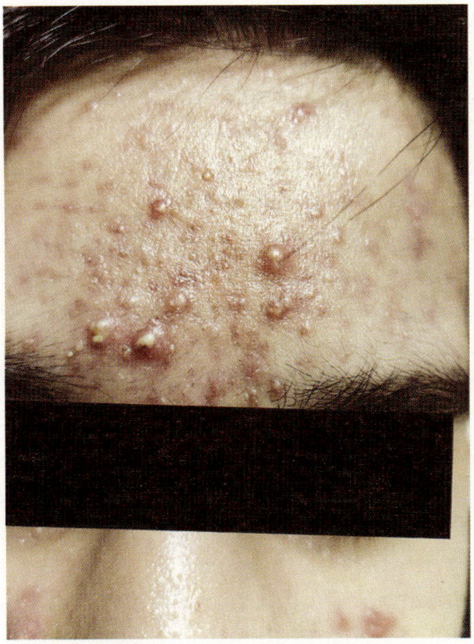

Fig. 31.4: Acne vulgaris

Hypertrophic scars are rarely encountered on the face; they are more frequent on the chest and nape of the neck. Occasionally, these scars become keloidal.

In an ordinary case of acne of moderate severity, various types of lesions may occur ranging from non-inflammatory (Grade I) comedones to indurated or suppurating abscesses, inflammatory papules and pustules (Grade III) and residual scars, although it is entirely possible that a particular kind of lesion may predominate in an individual case. As a rule acne lesions are asymptomatic; only the deeply suppurating ones are somewhat tender or painful. The excoriations seen on the faces of some acne patients, particularly girls, are the results of the bad habit of picking or neurotic scratching of the lesions.

Course: The course of the disease is chronic with frequent remissions and exacerbations. There is a tendency to flare up in the premenstrual period. Acne tends to subside in the early twenties, but may persist indefinitely. The mild form is not particularly troublesome. In its more severe form, acne becomes a source of great anxiety to the young. They are profoundly disturbed by the disfiguring scars and the new "pimples", hence this condition can affect the emotional state of a patient.

Special Varieties of Acne

Acne in infants: It is confined to the face. The main lesions are comedones with only a few papules and pustules. Infantile acne is probably caused by maternal hormones, but oily substances applied to the face and scalp can also produce grouped comedones in children.

Acne in the aged: Single or grouped comedones are frequently seen in the elderly people. The main seat of involvement is the temporal and the periocular regions. They usually persist unaltered, only occasionally showing a tendency to become inflamed.

Acne conglobata: This is a very severe type of acne; lesions originate in comedones but eventually assume considerable size. It affects adolescents and adults, chiefly men, and is widespread over the face, trunk and extremities. The individual lesions are big, fluctuating, dark red, cyst-like abscesses which persist for a long time. Some of them rupture-forming sinuses; others become ulcerated resembling scrofuloderma. They cause destruction of tissues, but finally heal, leaving hypertrophic, often bridged scars.

Occupational acne: Certain chemical substances plug, irritate and block the pilo-sebaceous apparatus causing acne-like lesions. Workers handling chlorine, oils and greases are particularly prone to this condition (chlor-acne and oil acne). The lesions occur on the exposed, and less so, on the covered areas of the body through impregnation of the clothes. The authors have seen the use of indigenous medicated oils for hair dressing and facial lubrication producing comedones and even papulo-pustules.

Acneiform drug eruptions: Certain drugs, particularly iodides and bromides produce eruptions resembling ordinary acne (Iatrogenic acne). No comedones develop; the eruption is frequently associated with mild pruritus. Bromides and iodides may sometimes aggravate the withdrawal of drugs.

ACTH, androgens and anabolic hormones may produce acneiform eruption unconnected with comedones, but frequently accompanied by hypertrichosis. Such cases are often seen in women who receive high doses of testosterone propionate for cancer of the breast and ACTH for rheumatoid arthritis.

Tropical acne: It is characterized by (a) its sudden development among white people visiting the tropics; (b) a severe eruption of large pustules and abscesses, which leave disfiguring scars; (c) affection of the chest, back, buttocks and thighs (the face is comparatively clear); (d) the eruption subsides dramatically when the patient leaves the tropics.

Etiology: Acne is a common occurrence at puberty. With the increased production of sex hormones, the sebaceous glands become hyperactive. Androgen and progesterone are responsible for the hyperplasia of the oil glands. Eunuchs do not have oily skins, nor do they suffer from acne, but testosterone given to castrates may produce acne lesions. The usual premenstrual flare-up is explained by some observers as occurring during the period when the normal androgen-oestrogen balance in the blood is altered in favour of androgen. Hence hormonal imbalance is held responsible for causing acne.

Besides seborrhoeic diathesis and hormonal imbalance, other factors which aggravate acne are a diet rich in fats and starches; intestinal stasis, especially constipation; a sedentary life; excessive use of greasy cosmetics, pomade, detergents and mechanical rubbing. Acne vulgaris usually runs in families. Psychogenic stresses, particularly the habit of picking pimples, makes them worse.

Treatment: It is not very satisfactory, because there is no specific remedy. Undoubtedly, many cases of minimal acne can be controlled by simple hygienic measures.

The patient often takes this disorder very seriously. He feels unhappy, and hence needs medical advice and reassurance.

Internal Treatment

Oestrogens: Oestrogen therapy is only warranted in severe acne. If there is history of dysmenorrhoea or premenstrual aggravation of acne, stilbestrol 1 mg should be given daily for 10 days before the expected onset of the menses. Boys and girls with very severe acne sometimes benefit from cyproterone acetate, anti-androgen hormone. A few courses of contraceptive pills would help girls with menstrual disorders and bad acne.

Antibiotics and other drugs: Long-acting sulphonamides and minocyline, doxycycline, erythromycin are effective in acute as well as chronic cases. They should be used judiciously. Starting with a dose of 100 mg daily of doxycycline. It can be reduced to 100 mg twice a week and maintained for months. Retinoids are useful in cystic, nodular, resistant cases of acne vulgaris. It has to be continued for months. The cost is prohibitive. Zinc sulphate by mouth 200 mg daily is also useful in some cases. Indian herbs, *Swertia Chiraita*, 1–2 g a day, is very useful in mild and moderate acne.

External Therapy

Lotions containing 2–3% salicylic acid in combination with 1–5% resorcinol are applied overnight and removed in the morning. The lotion may be used for three nights in succession, and then followed by rest of one day.

A very good and pleasant shake-lotion for acne is:

Potassa sulphurata	3–8 g
Zinc sulphate	3–8 g
Calamine prep.	5–10 g
Spirit rectified	30 cc
Aqua calcis	to 100 cc

Benzoyl peroxide (2.5 or 5%) and Azelaic acid are the potent external agents.

This lotion may be applied by women also during the day as "make up" powder if liquor ferrichlorate is added in quantities adjusted to the different complexion. Some cases of acne with multiple comedones, with severe lesions and residual scars which fail to respond to ordinary therapy, require peeling with Lassar's peeling paste:

Beta naphthol	2 g
Sulphur sublimis	4 g
Soft soap	12.0 g
Vaseline	12.0 g

The paste is rubbed into the skin at night for 2–3 days till hyperemia and desquamation occur. This procedure may be repeated after a few days rest. Two to three such courses are usually enough.

Vitamin A acid (Retinoic acid), topically is a good keratolytic agent and gives fair to excellent results. There are dozens of medicines, both external and internal, marketed for treatment of acne; none of them is a panacea. All are, more or less, designated on the lines discussed above. In acne therapy, there should be simultaneous treatment of accompanying seborrhoeic condition of the scalp.

Physical Treatment

Comedone removal with a comedone extractor. The hole is placed over the blackhead, and with some pressure the entire comedone is expressed into the cup. Hot compresses should precede the procedure. The extraction should be made at intervals and on different areas to avoid irritation.

Artificial ultraviolet radiation may be used in countries or regions where sunlight is not available. Instead of peeling pastes, some dermatologists use the cold quartz lamp for peeling; others give only small doses to achieve slight erythema and minimal peeling.

Roentgen-ray therapy is an effective measure employed in resistant cases of severe acne. It should not, however, be used indiscriminately, and should be given only by an experienced dermatologist (*see* Chapter 6).

Surgical incision and curetting of cysts and abscesses should be done properly. They should be drained completely to prevent them from refilling. Intralesional steroids may help cysts and keloids.

Dermabrasive surgery is required to deal with acne scarring (*see* Chapter 6).

Management of Acne

1. General measures:
   a. Proper cleansing
   b. Avoid use of cosmetics
   c. Avoid picking of pimples
   d. Relaxation
   e. Avoid constipation
   f. Diet rich in salads and fruits
   g. In tropical towns, the air is often polluted, so the face must be cleaned on returning from work and also when changing from hot to cold places.
2. *Internal:*
   a. *Swertia chiretta* or *Azadirichta indica* capsules or powder in grade I and grade II.
   b. Antibiotics like doxycycline or minocycline in grade III and may be grade II acne.
   c. Stock or Auto Vaccine in infected cases
   d. Use of vitamin A, zinc.
   e. Oestrogen, spironolactone or cyproterone acetate (Diane—35–50).
   f. Retinoids as a last resort because of severe side-effects. Avoid pregnancy during and after treatment for at least 1 years.

ROSACEA

Rosacea is a chronic disease which develops gradually in middle and advanced age. It is limited to the face affecting the flush areas of the central part of the face, especially the lower part of the forehead, the nose, the cheeks and the chin. As the name indicates, it is characterized by a special redness. In the beginning, flushing appears under certain circumstances such as emotional stress, exposure to intensive cold, heat, the sun's rays or after alcoholic drinks; this flushing lasts longer than usual. In due course, the hyperemic state tends to persist and eventually becomes permanent **(Fig. 31.5)**. It varies in intensity, with individuals and different times, from pinkish to dull-red. Simultaneously or later, the blood vessels become dilated. The telangiectasia presents an important feature of the disease, and often dominates the clinical picture. Acne lesions develop frequently on seborrhoeic soil. The follicular openings are prominent, but acne lesions of the papular, indurated or pustular type may appear without originating from comedones.

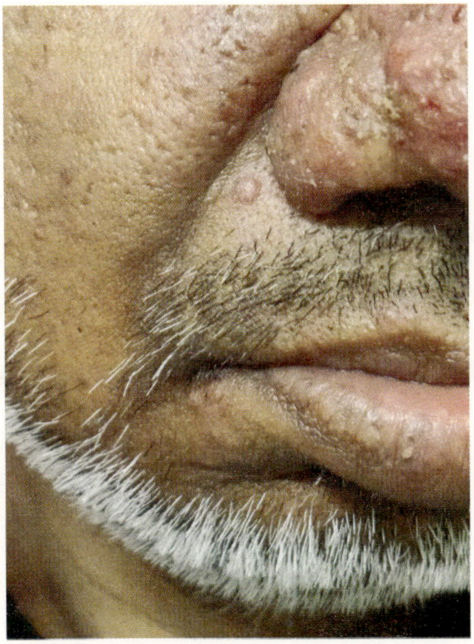

Fig. 31.5: Rosacea

In acne rosacea, infiltration and hypertrophy may increase considerably, particularly on the nose. In men, a clinical picture develops which is called rhinophyma. The nose is enormously enlarged and often lobulated. The pores are widened and oily masses can be readily expressed.

Ocular involvement is not rare; it is seen as blepharitis, conjunctivitis or keratitis.

Etiology: Rosacea is an example of multi-causal dermatosis. Many factors precipitate the disease, such as atmospheric influences, exposure to cold, heat, strong sunlight; dietetic errors, excessive consumption of hot and strong tea, coffee, alcoholic drinks; gastrointestinal troubles; pelvic and menstrual disturbances in women and emotional stresses. The psychogenic factor plays a significant role not only in aggravating but also in causing the disease. Its incidence is low in India. Women are more frequently affected than men. Patients complain of sense of heat (SOH), quick temper and easy excitability.

Diagnosis: It is generally not difficult, and is based upon the following features: (1) Age-middle-age, usually after 30 years of age. (2) Distribution-central part of the face. (3) Seborrhoeic skin. (4) Redness, telangiectasia and acneiform lesions without blackheads.

It is distinguished from acne vulgaris by the age of the patient, the lack of comedones, the presence of telangiectasia and the limitation of the disease to the central part of the face. Some patchy lesions may resemble lupus erythematosus. But the absence of infiltration, hyperkeratosis and atrophy help to eliminate lupus in the differential diagnosis.

Prognosis: It is a chronic disease with a tendency to progressive aggravation.

Response to treatment is not very satisfactory.

Treatment: Rosacea should be treated both internally and locally. The systemic treatment aims at correcting the causes. The diet should be light and simple. Foods like hot tea, coffee, alcohol and spicy foods which cause flushing of the face should be strictly avoided. Vegetarian food is encouraged. Exposure to sudden alterations in temperature should be minimized. Every effort should be made to relieve nervous tension.

Local treatment is similar in principle to that used for acne vulgaris, stress being laid on shake lotions. Dilated vessels can be successfully obliterated by superficial electrodessication, or injection of 25% saline into the vessels with a very thin needle. Patches with closely aggregated telangiectases can be favourably treated by freezing with CO_2 snow for 10 seconds under moderate pressure. Massage of the skin with an astringent lotion is often beneficial. In resistant cases, X-ray therapy is indicated. Rhinophyma is treated by dermabrasive surgery, by the surgical removal of the excessive skin or X-ray therapy. The advice of an ophthalmologist should be sought for ocular lesions.

Tetracyclines are useful in resistant cases, more so in cases with rosaceous keratitis. The latter warrants early and prolonged treatment with tetracyclines. Some patients have shown good results with metronidazole. The authors have reported very good results with khas (*Andropogon muricatus*) decoction three times a day for six weeks or so. Zinc sulphate orally (200 mg capsule) may be helpful. Retinoids do give good results.

Chapter **32**

Diseases of the Hair and Scalp

Clinical examination consists of the study of the distribution of hair on the body and the examination of hair for length, density, colour, lustre, greasiness or dryness, consistency, breaking, splitting and any other abnormalities. The hair should be examined in good, natural light. For complete examination of the scalp, all hair clips, pins, ribbons, etc. should be removed, and the hair parted at intervals. The underlying skin should also be studied in detail, so also, the regional glands in cases of infection and tumour.

HYPERTRICHOSIS

Hypertrichosis implies excessive hair and/or on abnormal regions. A typical example would be hypertrichosis of young women with excessive hair on the beard region.

Causes

Congenital

1. Generalized—Dog or ape-man.
2. Localized—Hairy naevus, spina bifida.

Acquired

1. Localized—Use of irritants
2. Generalized, or regional or only on faces of women.
   a. Endocrine—Virilism due to hyperplasia of the adrenal cortex; pituitary adenomas or hyperplasia; tumour of the ovaries (arrhenoblastoma).
      Menopausal—artificial or natural; use of androgens and ACTH; hypogonadism.
   b. Nutritional—Anorexia nervosa.
   c. Idiopathic—Usually heredo-familial.

Diagnosis: Congenital and localized acquired cases resulting from local irritation are straight forward cases, and usually do not pose diagnostic problems. To avoid confusion, it is better to confine the term "Hirsutism" to androgen-controlled excessive hair growth **(Fig. 32.1)**. In virilism of females, a search must be made for endocrine tumours. In such cases, menstruation is upset, the genitalia are atrophic, the clitoris is enlarged, the integument becomes coarse and, besides, there is a masculine type of hypertrichosis. X-ray of the skull, ultrasound examination of suprarenals and ovaries, pyelography, a pelvic examination for ovarian tumours, and 17-ketosteroid/cortisol, oestrogen, progesterone, prolactin studies are helpful. Menopausal cases are typical; the hypertrichosis is usually of a mild nature. In the majority of females having excessive hair on the beard region, to begin with, the hair is thin and downy, but gradually become thicker and pigmented;

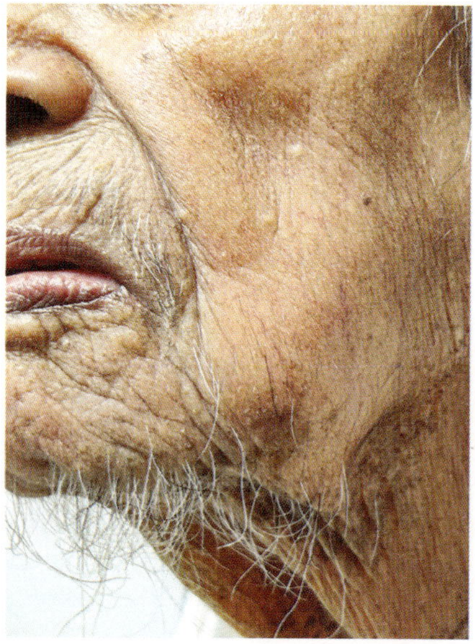

Fig. 32.1: Hirsutism in an 80-year-old woman

no definite causation can be established. Hypertrichosis starts between the ages of 15 and 20, and slowly progresses till the age of 30 or so. Some of these patients show some degree of hypogonadism, thick coarse skin, big pores, acne and scanty menstruation; others only show heredo-familial tendencies but no definite etiology. These idiopathic cases are difficult to handle in practice. It must be emphasized that in every case of hypertrichosis, a complete physical examination should be undertaken with the help of a general physician or endocrinologist; furthermore, laboratory investigations will help to rule out the important group of endocrine disorders.

Prognosis: It is usually unsatisfactory unless the cause is removable. A young woman often develops an inferiority complex and even psychosis; besides there will be matrimonial problems.

Treatment: It consists in:

1. Elimination and treatment of the cause.
   a. Surgery or irradiation for endocrine tumours.
   b. In idiopathic cases of young women, a course of serum gonadotrophin or oestrogens may be beneficial, particularly if there is evidence of hypogonadism or scanty menstruation. Cyproterone acetate and spironolactone is worth a trial in severe cases. *Shatawari* (a local herb) is sometimes very useful.
   c. The general nutritional state should be improved with tonics.
2. Symptomatic removal of superfluous hair.
   a. Electrolysis/thermolysis.
   b. Waxing of the hair, bleaching with pure hydrogen peroxide.

   Electrolysis is an ideal method and gives the best results in the long run. Waxing gives temporary results, and has to be repeated every 7–15 days. The hair must be long enough to be caught in the wax. Pumice stone, threading, chemical depilatories;

clipping, plucking and shaving, radium, X-ray and thallium acetate are other methods of removing hair; since these give bad results in the long run, their use is to be strongly discouraged.

3. Bleaching of the hair with pure hydrogen peroxide. The hair becomes less conspicuous. Hydrogen peroxide is useful in cases of excessive, thin hair which bleach easily; thick, coarse hair usually do not.

ALOPECIA

Synonym: Baldness.

Causes

Non-cicatricial	*Cicatricial*
Localized Alopecia areata Syphilis (Chapter 18) Tinea (Chapter 12) Traction alopecia	*Primary* Pseudo pelade Folliculitis decalvans
Diffuse A. Congenital B. Premature 1. Alopecia steatoides 2. Symptomatic a. Post-febrile b. Debility and emaciation c. Syphilis d. During lactation e. Endocrine: Simmond's disease, myxoderma f. Stresses and strains g. Drugs like thallium acetate, hydantoin, cytotoxic drugs, hormones, etc. 3. Idiopathic: Probable causes in such cases are: masculinity or heredity or stress of civilization. C. Senile	*Secondary* Injury Favus and kerion (Tinea) Lupus vulgaris Lupus erythematosus Gumma Leprosy Dissecting cellulitis X-ray burn Scleroderma

General diagnosis: The above classification is based upon clinical experience. It helps in easy and correct etiological diagnosis. Examination for whether there is atrophy or scarring, and then if the alopecia is non-cicatricial, whether it is localized or diffuse helps to narrow down the differential diagnosis. Scarring of the scalp is seen as a shining surface, diminution or absence of hair pores, loss of skin elasticity and wrinkling; it feels like thickened, scarred tissue when palpated. Atrophy is seen as wrinkling, thinning and loss of elasticity and normal shine of the integument. In non-cicatricial alopecias, the skin looks and feels normal but the hair is lost. The differential diagnosis is discussed further under the respective group headings.

The above classification is further helpful in forecasting the prognosis and treatment; in cicatricial cases, hair never grow back, while in non-cicatricial cases, they do, if the cause can be controlled and treated.

FALLING OF HAIR

Synonym: Diffuse hair loss, Defluvium capillorum.

Diffuse loss of hair is a very common complaint in practice and patients are often seriously concerned about it. Patient notices hair entangled in comb or brush; he notices thinning of the scalp hair but not complete baldness. Defluvium capillorum is the first stage of alopecia. It is of two types: Anagen effluvium and telogen effluvium **(Fig. 32.2)**.

Etiology: Important causes are as follows: Run-down state; change of climate and shifting of residence; poor diet or crash dieting; over-work; pregnancy; delivery; loss of blood due to other causes; typhoid or other febrile illnesses; acute mental strain; debilitating diseases; drugs like methotrexate, other cytotoxic drugs like thallium, colchicine, diuretics, anticoagulants, hypervitaminosis A, bismuth, borax, mepacrine; seborrhoea oleosa, seborrhoeic dermatitis and extensive skin diseases especially erythroderma, pemphigus, etc.

A thorough search should be made for the cause or causes. Here it should be noted that at a time, 80–90% of hair are in the anagen phase and rest 10–20% in the telogen/catagen phase of hair cycle and hence the falling of few hair daily is within physiological limits.

Treatment consists in finding the cause and its elimination, reassurance and improvement of general health with good nourishing diet, liver extract, vitamins and minerals. In debilitated individuals, anabolic hormones can be given. A quiet relaxing holiday is very beneficial. Local treatment consists in:

1. Avoid repeated and too frequent combing and shampooing.
2. Avoid excessive use of oil and oily preparations especially in seborrhoeic individuals.
3. Light massage of the scalp with any of the following preparations: Flucort (P) or Betnovate-lotion (P) or the following formulations:

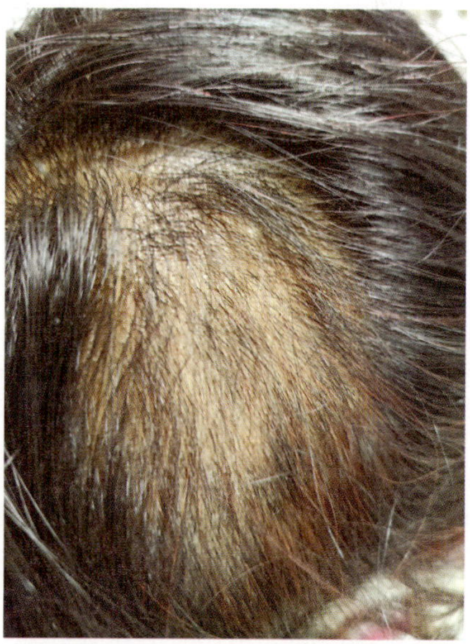

Fig. 32.2: Telogen effluvium

a. Active phase when hair are falling:

Stilboestrol	50 mg
Prednisolone	50 mg
Ung emulsificans aquosus Ft ung	100 g

Sig/Rub into the scalp lightly every night.

b. Quiescent phase when hair fall has become stationary and regrowth is desired: Tinct K5 (P), Alopex (P) or the following formulations:

1. Tinct. capsicum	12.0 cc
Sol of cantharidine	12.0 cc
Spt of Rosemary	QS
Ol.ricini	5.0 cc
Aqua to	100 cc
mft mist	

Sig/Lightly rub into scalp 2–3 times a week.

2. Oil of bergamot	3.0 cc
Oil of babchi	3.0 cc
Tinct. cantharidine	12.0 cc
Ung. emulsificans aquosus to	100 g
Ft ung	

Sig./To be rubbed into the scalp 2–3 times a week

ALOPECIA AREATA

It is a very common condition in the practice of dermatology. Incidence is on the increase.

Clinical features: It affects selectively the scalp and the beard region, though it may also affect the other hairy regions of the body. It can occur at any age, but is usually seen in young adults and children. The disorder is characterized by round or oval, circumscribed patches of alopecia without any signs of inflammation, scarring or atrophy. The integument is shiny, slightly thin and depressed. The hair pores are visible. The onset is usually sudden; one or more patches may develop at the same time; by peripheral extension and confluence, irregular areas may be formed. Hair is loose at the periphery in a spreading, active patch; but is, on the other hand, firmly attached in a stationary one. In a patch where the hair is tending to grow back, it is seen typically in the shape of an exclamation mark. An exclamation mark hair has a thin lower portion and a thick stump; this is so, because the newly growing hair is thin, and the portion of old hair which has broken off is thick **(Fig. 32.3)**. There are no subjective symptoms.

Alopecia areata may become widespread and lead to total loss of hair on the scalp (Alopecia totalis); in an universal case, even the hair from the eyebrows, eyelashes, beard region and all the hairy portions of the body may fall (Alopecia universalis).

The course is slow and variable. The hair usually grows back in two months to two years. The new hair is usually first downy, and then grey; it takes time to come back to normal. In a bad case, the hair may not grow back, and eventually atrophy of the skin may ensure. In a case of moderate intensity, the new hair may stay grey. Alopecia areata may be accompanied by pitting, shedding or atrophy of the nails.

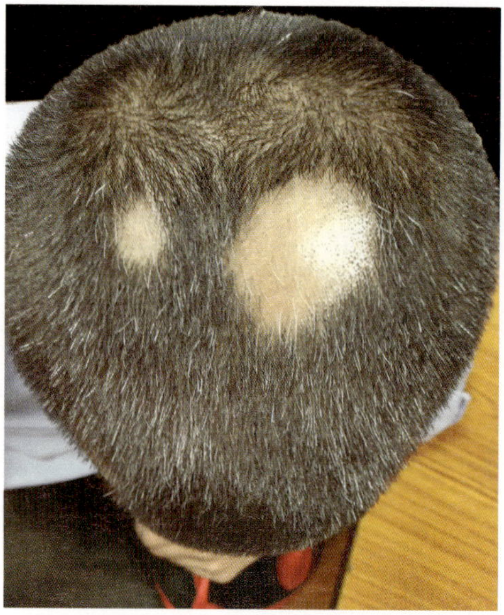

Fig. 32.3: Alopecia areata

Etiology: The exact cause is unknown. The consensus of opinion is that alopecia areata is the result of acute physical or emotional stress in a sensitive individual (trophoneurosis). This is true in the majority of cases. The condition is certainly not caused by any infective microorganism or virus; toxins from sore throat or any septic focus may be the cause in some cases. Some workers blame auto-immune mechanism, as by chemicals, drugs and infections.

Differential diagnosis: It is usually made from other causes of localized, non-cicatricial alopecias.

Tinea capitis	Well-defined patches of alopecia with dull broken hair, greyish scales; Wood's lamp shows fluorescence, and potassium hydroxide preparation shows fungus. Black-dot type cases may cause difficulty, but a microscopic examination is conclusive.
Syphilis	The occipital and temporal regions are usually involved. Patches are irregular and ill-defined; hair appear moth-eaten. Other stigmata of syphilis are present.
Trichotillomania	Neurotic temperament; itching sensations precede alopecia; furthermore, the patches are irregular in shape. Irregularly broken hair and so also tangled masses of twisted hair may be visible.

If the patches become widespread, the condition must be distinguished from conditions causing diffuse alopecia. Grey hair in recovering alopecia patches must be differentiated from other causes of canities and vitiligo. Inflammatory diseases like contact and seborrhoeic dermatitis may produce localized or diffuse alopecia; the cause is usually obvious in such cases.

Prognosis: It depends upon:

1. *The age of the patient:* The outlook is better in younger patients.

2. *Duration:* The shorter the duration, the better the prognosis. In old-standing cases, the hair may not grow back. Repeated attacks and recurrence of alopecia implies bad prognosis.
3. The size of the patch: The outlook is better in smaller patches.
4. "Exclamation-mark hair" signifies recovery; firmly implanted hair present at the periphery means that the alopecia has become stationary, while loose hair at the periphery implies that the disease is still active.
5. General health of the patient and other trophic/auto-immune disease.

Treatment: It consists in:

1. Reassurance.
2. Improving the general health with diet, tonics, etc.
3. Removing the active causes like nervous or physical strain, septic focus, etc. Avoiding the use of chemicals and junk food. A quiet holiday in a congenial environment is very beneficial.
4. Symptomatic.
   a. *Internal*
      a Sedatives in nervous patients with active disease.
      b. Stimulants like Orabolin (P), Dianabol (P).
      c. ACTH or steroids in resistant, widespread cases.
      d. Levamisole 150 mg once a week for 6–8 weeks.
      e. *Andropogon muricatus* and *Withania somnifera* herbs are very beneficial.
   b. *External*
      a. Steroid cream like Flucort (P) in active phase.
      b. Only when it has become stationary, must local stimulants be used , like 10% cantharidine solution, Tincture K5 (P), Alopex (P), *Ammi majus oil*, tincture iodi mitis, UVR, etc. Irritants should be strictly avoided.
      c. Local infiltration with hydrocortisone, triamcinolone is helpful in resistant cases.
      d. DNCB 0.5–1% in obstinate cases.

TRACTION ALOPECIA

A characteristic pattern of hair loss is seen in Rajasthani females and Sikh males who tie their hair in traditional knots and apply excessive traction in the process. The frontal hair line which is normally sharp becomes unsightly, irregular and receding. Stumps of broken hair with mild erythema and inflammation around the follicular opening can be seen. Hair population is thin in these areas. Skin of the area is not atrophic but if the traction continues for a long time, cicatrization may follow.

Treatment consists of avoiding traction.

CONGENITAL ALOPECIA

It is very rare. Hair may not be present at birth, and will not grow at all later. In some cases, the hair may be poorly formed or downy, growing sparsely. In others, a good growth may be present at birth, but later, the hair may fall and not grow back. Congenital alopecia may occur alone or be accompanied by other congenital ectodermal defects of the skin, nails, teeth, etc.

ALOPECIA STEATOIDES

It affects young adults. It is characterized by seborrhoeic diathesis, constant dandruff-like scaling from the scalp, accompanied by moderate itching, the presence of short, poorly formed hair and by the slowly progressive loss of hair from the vertex and temples.

There may or may not be frank seborrhoeic dermatitis.

The condition is progressive and rather resistant to treatment. The latter consists of therapy for pityriasis capitis and mild, stimulant topical preparations such as mentioned for alopecia areata. Scalp should be washed with Selsun suspension (P), or Cetavlon lotion (P) followed by the rubbing in Flucort (P) lotion or any of the following ointments:

Ointment for males

1. Oil of cade	10 g
Acid salicylic	2 g
Ung. emulsificans aquosus	to 100 g
Ft ung	

Sig. to be rubbed in at night

2. Acid salicylic	3 g
Sulphur	2 g
Prednisolone	50 mg
Ung. emulsificans aquosus	to 100 g
Ft. ung	

Sig/Rub into the scalp before retiring daily or alternate days or biweekly.

For females, the authors recommend tincture K5 (P) applied twice a week or acid salicylic, sulphur, prednisolone cream.

IDIOPATHIC PREMATURE ALOPECIA

Synonym: Masculine alopecia, androgenetic alopeia.

It is a fairly common problem in practice. It usually affects young male adults. The onset is gradual. It commences between 20 and 40 years of age. It starts with a receding hair margin and with widening of the forehead, thinning of the hair which become atrophic and lustreless; later, the hair from the vertex, frontal regions, temples and even the whole of the scalp may fall completely. The distribution of alopecia is symmetrical. A few lanugo hair may keep on growing but these lack quality for full growth and vigour.

The exact cause is unknown. In most cases, there is heredo-familial predisposition to alopecia. The patients are usually males, intelligent and the sedentary type. The fact that the eunuchs do not get bald proves that the androgens are greatly responsible for this condition. Some authorities consider it as a disease of civilization. Artificial menopause may produce a somewhat similar alopecia. Recently, similar alopecia has been reported amongst females from some advanced countries.

The treatment is unsatisfactory. Oestrogen and prednisolone ointment rubbed in locally into the scalp may be helpful. Minoxidil lotion 2% may give satisfactory results.

Hair transplantation with or without scalp reduction is helpful in covering the defect in baldies. A wig may be tried as a last resort.

SENILE ALOPECIA

It is characterized by symmetrical thinning or loss of hair in old age giving the patient a dignified look. The vertex, frontal region, temples or even the occipital region may be involved. Atrophic changes that take place with age are also present in the integument. Some of the causes responsible for idiopathic, premature alopecia may be contributory factors.

Senile alopecia is seen at any age after 45–50 years, but some old people can retain a good growth of hair. Being a degenerative process, no treatment is satisfactory.

PRIMARY CICATRICIAL ALOPECIA

Synonym: Pseudo-pelade.

It is a rare disease of the scalp, and is characterized by ill-defined, round or oval areas of alopecia; the skin appears white, shining, atrophic or scarred without any signs of inflammation or subjective symptoms. Cicatricial alopecia patches appear like footprints in the snow across the scalp. The onset is insidious, and the course variably fluctuating. The disease affects mainly young adults; it is more common in males than females. The exact etiology is unknown, but factors, like syphilis, focal sepsis and local infection should be excluded **(Fig. 32.4)**.

Differential diagnosis: It is made from all other causes of secondary cicatricial alopecia; but is mainly from the following conditions:

Folliculitis decalvans: Follicular pustules and small abscesses; irregular areas of scarring and alopecia which may become confluent; signs of inflammation, especially on the periphery of the bald patches; some degree of pain. The treatment is with antibiotics and local antiseptics.

Dissecting cellulitis of the scalp: Synonym-Perifolliculitis capitis androgenetic et suffodiens. It is an exaggerated form of folliculitis decalvans. The characteristic features

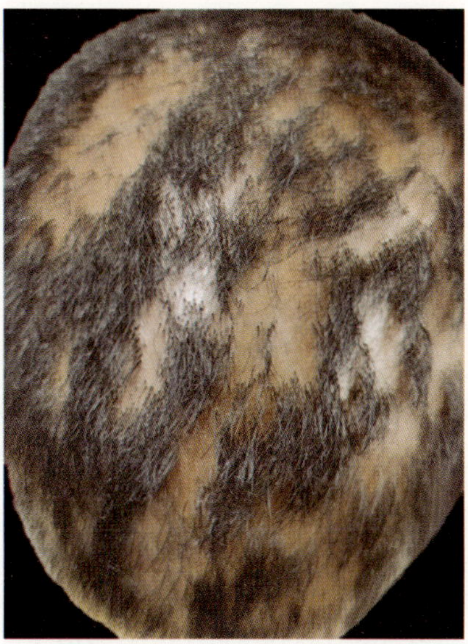

Fig. 32.4: Cicatricial alopecia

are: Nodules and abscesses which communicate with each other under the skin; patches of cicatricial alopecia; sinuses and crust formation. The condition is caused by pyogenic cocci. The treatment consists in administering antibiotics, in surgical incisions of the abscesses, in applying local antiseptic dressings and in the use of autovaccine.

Prognosis: It is gloomy; the alopecia is permanent. The whole of the scalp is seldom involved. The course is unpredictable and variable.

Treatment: It is unsatisfactory. A course of broad-spectrum antibiotics and local infiltration of the alopecia patches with hydrocortisone or, prednisone and hyaluronidase is worth trying. These measures may not stimulate the regrowth of hair, but they may help to check the extension of the disease process.

GREYING OF HAIR

Synonyms: Canities, white hair.

Causes

A. Localized patches of grey hair
   1. Congenital
   2. Vitiligo
   3. Alopecia areata
   4. Naevus depigmentosus

B. Generalized and diffuse greying
   1. Senility
   2. Chronic diseases, particularly gastro-intestinal, sinusitis and nutritional disorders. Repeated antibiotic therapy
   3. Nervous strain and stress
   4. Heredo-familial
   5. Endocrine-hypopituitarism, Simmond's cachexia and hypothyroidism
   6. Use of chemicals on the hair in the form of medicated oils
   7. Organic nervous affections, migraine, etc.
   8. Congenital albinism

Greying of the hair appears in different shades from dirty grey to silvery white. There are three mechanisms usually operating in the production of grey hair (Montgomery and Ormsby), namely: the loss of pigment situated in the matrix of the hair; unevenness of the surface of the hair, this leads to the refraction of light; appearance of air bubbles in rapidly developing canities.

Depending upon the cause, greying may be localized and stationary, or widespread and progressive. Usually the greying of hair is a permanent feature, but the authors have seen grey hair revert to black colour with treatment, particularly in people suffering from vitiligo with leucotrichia. Cases of premature, generalized and diffuse canities are important in dermatological practice. Most of these cases are chronic and insidious. Sometimes, though rarely, one comes across cases of sudden greying. These are caused by acute nervous strain or shock, accident or wasting disease. In senile cases, canities begin in localized patches, and soon become symmetrical; the beard and temple regions are usually the first to be affected.

Diagnosis: The main emphasis should be laid on a complete physical examination, a nutritional and endocrinal survey, a study of the organic nervous causes and also a study of the local bleaching factors.

Prognosis: It is usually unfavourable, though elimination of the causes and nutritional "building up" may help to check further progress.

Treatment: It consists in:

1. Reassurance.
2. Elimination of causes. Avoid excessive use of antibiotics.
3. Improvement of general health; the administration of iron, liver extract, vitamins synthetic or predigested proteins, aminoacids, copper, zinc, Orabolin (P) or Placental extract injection, calcium pantothenate 200 mg daily.
4. Ammi majus lotion or ointment, and UVR exposures (similar to the treatment for vitiligo) may be beneficial.
5. Dyeing is often the only effective method of changing the colour of grey hair. A patch test must be done to detect sensitization. Dyeing has to be repeated every 15 days to one month, depending upon the growth of the hair. Dyes, must be properly applied to prevent injury to the hair. The commonly used dyes are: vegetable dyes—henna (especially Black Egyptian henna), camomile, indigo; metallic dyes-silver nitrate and lead acetate; chemical dyes—paraphenyldiamine and its different derivatives. Loma, Trutone and Lady Grecian are some of the patent dyes available.

ATROPHY OF THE HAIR

The hair becomes thin, short, dry, lustreless and friable; it may split or break easily, or curl in abnormal directions. Atrophy of the hair is common condition in dermatological practice. Mild splitting of the terminal ends is a normal feature with long hair. The common causes of atrophy are:

A. Symptomatic
   a. *Localized:* Tinea, favus, lice, impetigo.
   b. *Generalized:* Pityriasis capitis and seborrhoeic dermatitis. Chronic wasting diseases. Poor nutritional state.

B. Idiopathic

The supposed active factors are too frequent and rough combing and brushing, the use of hairpins and other ornaments, drying with hot blasts of air, the neglect of proper oiling after washing, the use of strong alkaline soaps and shampoos and the use of dyes. In these cases, the nutritional state of the hair is below par; furthermore, very often the hair is subjected to repeated mechanical and chemical injuries.

The treatment consists in improving the general health, correcting the causative factors and proper hygienic care (for details *see* Chapter 7). A light massage with a bland oil like olive or coconut oil and mild stimulant lotion is beneficial.

TRICHORRHEXIS NODOSA

It is a rare dystrophy of the hair. It occurs chiefly on the scalp and male beard, and is characterized by nodes on the shaft of the hair; transverse fractures occur at these sites. The cause is unknown but it may be associated with follicular keratosis and pruritic dermatoses. Occasionally trauma, UVR, and brushing may bring about this anomaly. Rarely it is congenital. Treatment is unsatisfactory. Nutrition of the hair should be improved, as in atrophy of the hair, and associated causes tackled.

MONILETHERIX

It occurs on the scalp of children. It is characterized by nodes and rings on the hair accompanied by broken and lustreless hair. It is a rare, dystrophic condition of a trophoneurotic nature. Children usually grow out of it by puberty.

INGROWING HAIR

It is a rare disorder. It occurs commonly on the beard region or on the back of the neck. Because of anatomical defects and foreign body reaction, painful papules, pustules and keloids may be produced. Close shaving is the most common cause. The condition is persistent. The treatment consists of shaving correctly, using an electric razor or electrolysis of these ingrowing hair.

TRICHORRHEXIS SPINULOSA

It is also called "bundle bush hair". Instead of one hair protruding from a hair follicle, bundle or bush of hair come out of a single follicle. It has no pathological significance.

Chapter 33

Diseases of the Nails

The anatomy of the nail has been described in Chapter 2. Though nails are vestigial organs comparable to claws and hoofs of lower animals, they have a cosmetic importance in man. Good, healthy nails are objects of admiration. They also protect the terminals of the limbs and the delicate tissues contained at these sites. The whole of the nail grows in about five months; in one month the growth is about 1/8th of an inch.

The study of the nail includes: examination of the shape, contour, colour, glossiness, translucency, consistency, deformity and structure. The latter should include a study of the nail folds (both the posterior and the lateral), the nail bed, the plate consisting of the root, the lunula and the body proper.

Though nail changes can be tell-tale signs of a patient's occupation, a systemic disease, of vascular and neurogenic disorders, of the patient's nutritional state and dermatological affections, these changes are not always true indications in every case, since each sign can be the product of several causes; hence dogmatic deductions can often be misleading. This point will be illustrated presently. Furthermore, numerous tongue-twisting terms have been employed in the past in describing diseases of the nails; this has tended to create confusion as well as frustration. Since their importance is very limited, an attempt is being made to curtail terms drastically.

SPECIAL TERMS AND DISEASES

Anonychia	Complete absence of nails. It is usually congenital or traumatic.
Atrophy of nails	It is seen as thinning, shedding, fragility, fragmentation or splitting. The nail may become lustreless, discoloured or worm-eaten. The common causes are trauma, vascular or neural disorders, systemic diseases, infections of the posterior nail fold or dermatological affections.
Beau's lines	Transverse lines or furrows on the nail plate due to disturbed nail growth caused by a systemic or local disease. By measuring its distance from root of the nail and calculating in terms of monthly nail growth, the date of the causative illness can be ascertained.
Clubbing	The nail is curved from the top downwards; the angle at the junction of the nail with the rest of the finger becomes acute and the tip of the finger looks like a drumstick. It is presumed that the condition is caused by anoxaemia

resulting from cardiovascular and pulmonary disease. It can also be familial (Pachydermo-periostosis).

Claw nails Overgrown, hypertrophied nails which are distorted like claws. Usually seen on the big toes, but may affect other toes and fingers as well. *Causes:* Trauma by ill-fitting shoes, neglect, acromegaly.

Dystrophy Signifies disordered development or growth. It may be seen as splitting, fragility, fragmentation or discoloration **(Fig. 33.1)**. The causes are similar to those operating in the atrophy of nails, particularly psoriasis, eczema, syphilis, tinea, paronychia, too frequent manicuring. A rare type of nail dystrophy characterized by a longitudinal nail groove or a ridge in the nail plate is called Dystrophia unguium canaliformis mediana.

Egg-shell nails The free edges of these nails are curved upwards. The causes are similar to those operating in the dystrophy of nails.

Hypertrophy Overgrown nails without distortion. It is seen in acromegaly, gigantism, repeated local trauma and irritation.

Haemorrhages Seen in traumatic haematoma, trichinosis and subacute bacterial endocarditis.

Ingrowing nails As the name signifies, the nail appears to grow into the soft tissues at its free edge with the walls of the lateral fold growing over it. Foreign body reaction produces inflammation, granulomatous sore, and possibly, secondary infection ; hence the pain. Causes: the faulty cutting of nails which produces sharp angles rather than rounded border; clipping the nails too short; badly fitting shoes. Treatment is surgical avulsion of the affected part of

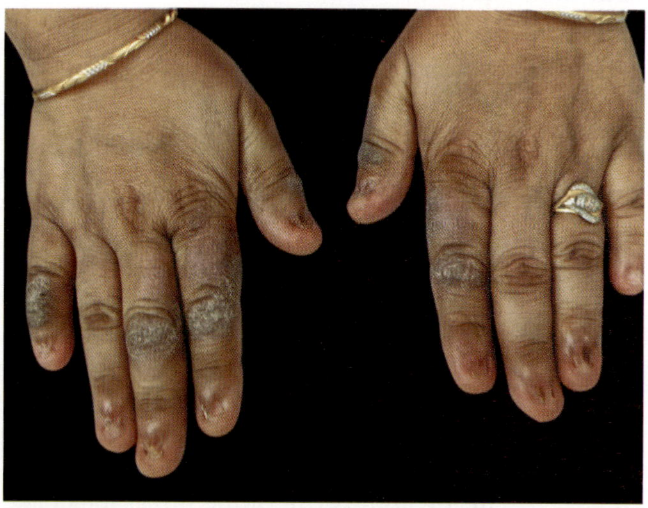

Fig. 33.1: Twenty-nail dystrophy in hands

	the nail folds, under local anaesthesia in case of infection and severe pain; otherwise, a conservative lifting of the ingrowing edge everyday to help it to grow over the overgrown walls is resorted to, along with correcting the causative factors.
Koilonychia	The concave upper surface of the nail plate making it look like a spoon. Causes: anaemia (Plummer–Vinson's syndrome), cachexia, hyperthyroidism and occupational immersion of the hands in alkalis. It starts on the index finger of one hand, and then extends to the other nails. The authors have seen a few cases of congenital koilonychia.
Leuconychia	White spots (also called gift spots), streaks or bands on the nail plate due to imperfect keratinization. Causes: local trauma, systemic disease, psychogenic stresses and also disturbed nutrition.
Nail biting	The free edge is absent or disfigured; it may also be secondarily infected. The picking of nails may produce similar picture. Cause: neurosis or neurasthenia. Treatment consists of psychotherapy and the application of bitters to stop the habit.
Pachyonychia	A thickened plate-like nail. *Causes:* Congenital, hyperparathyroidism and vitamin D therapy.
Paronychia	Inflammation of the posterior nail fold, and the formation of an abscess in between the posterior nail fold and the root of the nail. Seen as a tender, boggy swelling with discharge; it results in dystrophy of the nail. Causes: monilia, pyogenic organisms, and possibly, syphilis. It is rarely caused by sensitization dermatitis from handling local anaesthetics used by dentists. Predisposing causes: trauma by faulty manicuring, frequent washing, wet work etc. Treatment. Acute: Surgical opening and antibiotics. Chronic: *See* Chapter 12.
Pitted nails	Shallow depressions in the form of pits on the surface of the nail plate **(Fig. 33.2)**. The most common causes: psoriasis, also seen in alopecia areata. At times it may be familial without any other pathology.
Pterygium of the nails	Hypertrophy of the eponychium leading to covering of the lunula and part of the body of the nail plate. Lichen planus and impaired circulation are the important causes.
Pruritic nails	Polished and worn-down nails in people with chronic pruritus. Seen particularly in erythrodermas.
Pigmentation	Haematoma due to trauma producing colour changes as in bruise; slate-blue nails in argyria; white bands in mepacrine intoxication; bluish pigmentation due to atabrine; also pigmentation due to phenolphthalein ingestion, antibiotics (tetracycline), X-ray therapy,

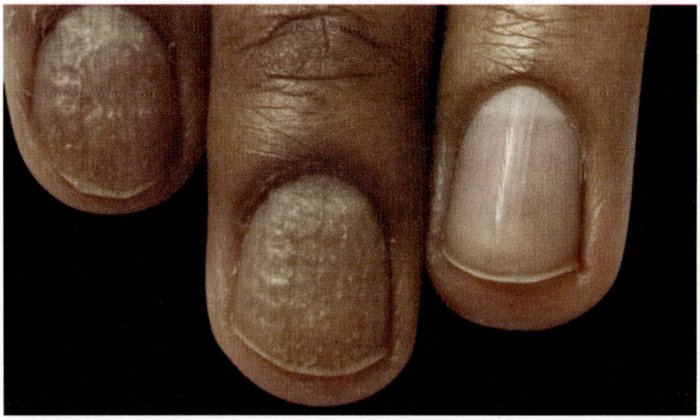

Fig. 33.2: Nail pitting

	the use of hair dyes, mercury lotions and the result of various dermatoses; pallor in anaemia and bluish tinge in cyanosis, yellowish tinge in jaundice and carotinemia.
Onycholysis	Separation of nails: A nail separates from the nail bed at its distal end with the formation of a free space but may still be attached at its root. It may be complete or partial. Causes: psoriasis, eczemas, syphilis, tinea, subungual tumours, chronic trauma and cosmetics.
Shedding of nails	The nail separates at the lunula or matrix, and is shed completely or partially. Causes: Systemic, neurogenic or vascular disorders; paronychia and other dermatoses around the nails.
Splitting of nails	Onychorrhexis. Longitudinal cracks or fractures of the nail plate. It may accompany other features of dystrophy, or may occur alone. Causes: psoriasis, eczema, paronychia, nutritional upsets, systemic illnesses and old age.
Subungual hyperkeratosis	Heaped-up, hyperkeratotic debris under the free edge of the nail. Common causes: tinea, psoriasis, trauma, manicuring, eczema.
Tumours	They are rare. Subungual warts and corns. Subungual fibromas in association with adenoma sebaceum. Melanotic whitlow. Glomus tumour.

ETIOLOGICAL DISCUSSION

The common causes of nail disorders are:

1. *Congenital:* Anonychia, pachyonychia, koilonychia. They occur as such, or in association with other congenital ectodermal defects.
2. *Systemic diseases:* Beau's lines, shedding of the nails, brittle nails, leuconychia, koilonychia, pigmentation, atrophy, debilitating disease or acute psychogenic stress may produce these lesions. Subacute bacterial endocarditis and trichinosis produce subungual haemorrhages. In acromegaly and gigantism, the nails are hypertrophied, while in anaemia, myxodema and hypoparathyroidism, the nails are dry, brittle, thin

and lustreless. Dystrophy of the nails may be seen in chronic arthritis; pulmonary tuberculosis produces Beau's lines, leuconychia and clubbing.

3. *Skin diseases:* The common ones are psoriasis, eczemas, leprosy, syphilis, tinea, erythroderma, alopecia areata and paronychia. They usually produce dystrophy of the nails.
4. *Occupation:* Soft or spoon-shaped nails in chemical workers particularly, when there is constant immersion in alkalies. Pigmentation may also be seen.
5. *Trauma:* Both physical and chemical. Subungual haematoma, ingrowing nails, claw nails, pterygium, and so forth, are produced by physical trauma. Immersion of nails in alkalis may cause softening, even koilonychia. Ill-fitting shoes and manicuring are responsible for many a disorder.
6. *Vascular and neurogenic disorders:* These interfere with the nutrition and growth of the nails; hence, dystrophic changes, e.g., leprosy, syringomyelia, tabes, Raynaud's disease, etc.
7. *Infections:* Tinea, monilial, pyogenic and syphilis.
8. *Nutritional:* In malnutrition and avitaminosis, the nails become thin and brittle, and may also be shed.
9. *Psychogenic:* Nail biting, pitting, koilonychia and shedding of nails may be seen in acute psychogenic stresses. In the latter, it may accompany alopecia areata totalis.
10. *Drugs:* Usually produce pigmentary changes, viz., silver, arsenic, mepacrine, phenolphthalein, tetracycline, etc.
11. *New growths:* Subungual and periungual warts, fibromas, melanoma and glomus tumour.

Most of these Causes Act on Either of the Three Sites

1. Posterior nail fold—Its affection influences the structure of the matrix. Most dermatoses, particularly paronychia, act in this manner. Dystrophic changes are first seen at the proximal end, and then, they slowly extend forwards.
2. Matrix—Systemic, neurological, vascular and nutritional causes usually act at this site. The newly-formed nail is deformed; with time, changes extend peripherally.
3. Nail bed—Physical and chemical trauma, occupational dermatoses, drugs and pompholyx may directly affect the nail bed. The deformity is first seen on the nail plate proper rather than at the root.

MANIFESTATIONS OF COMMON DERMATOSES

1. Tinea unguium—*see* Chapter 12.
2. Psoriasis—*see* Chapter 20.
3. Eczema—Contact dermatitis of the nail folds and pompholyx produce dystrophic changes in the nails in the form of brittleness, splitting, separation, shedding, discoloration, loss of lustre, etc. These manifestations are produced by secondary affection of the matrix or the posterior nail fold. It is believed by several authorities that pompholyx and secondary dystrophy of the nails are responsible for secondary contamination by fungus and other microorganisms. Nail polish, polish remover and artificial cuticle cause allergic contact dermatitis; primary trauma may lead to softening and deformities of the nails.

4. Exfoliative dermatitis and erythrodermas—these produce first dystrophy which results in deformed, brittle nails with subungual debris, and later, shedding and even atrophy of the nail. Chronic pruritus in these dermatoses results in the nails becoming polished and worn-out; with recovery from these conditions, the healthy nail grows slowly from the proximal end.
5. Syphilis—Primary: Rare. Chancre on the nail fold. Induration is present. The supra-trochlear glands are enlarged. Secondary: There may be splitting, separation and shedding of the nails. Tertiary: Rarely gumma. Congenital: Rarely paronchia.
6. Leprosy—Nail changes are frequent in neural leprosy. Nails are deformed or even shed due to trophic changes.
7. Paronychia—*see* Chapter 12.
8. Alopecia areata—By itself, it does not affect the nails directly, but auto-immune and emotional stresses which are responsible for alopecia areata may manifest themselves in nail dystrophies consisting of leuconychia (gift spots), Beau's lines, brittle and thin nails. There may also be total or partial shedding of the nails.

GENERAL REMARKS ABOUT DIAGNOSIS AND TREATMENT

1. First of all, identify the clinical manifestation in the nail, and then try to gauge whether it is starting proximally or from the free edge. It is important to establish these facts besides making sure whether all the nails on hands and feet are involved, or there is unilateral affection, or only a single nail is affected. Single nail involvement is usually due to some local cause; unilateral involvement is usually due to neurological or circulatory involvement, while bilateral, symmetrical involvement is due to a systemic cause or generalized dermatosis. The above statement is somewhat of a generalization, and exceptions do occur.
2. Since most nail disorders are not disease entities, and very many causes can produce the same manifestation, one must be careful in jumping to rash conclusions. Moreover, a cause can produce different manifestations, hence, the difficulty in establishing the cause.
3. Try to sort out the exact cause by history and a complete physical examination dermatological , systemic, psychogenic, nutritional, etc.
4. Local causes in the form of trauma, manicuring and dermatoses are very important; hence, they must be considered before a systemic etiology is presumed.
5. In treatment, emphasis should be laid on the correction of etiological factors; local treatment is rather unsatisfactory. Calcium administration, contrary to general belief, does not help. Use of gelatin by mouth is sometimes helpful. The authors have used thyroid and anabolic steroid like Dianabol (P) with success in stimulating the growth of nails in nail dystrophies. General health of the patient must be improved by nourishing diet, supplementary vitamins, balanced work, exercise and mental relaxation. Local antiseptics and fungicides are used according to the type of suspected infection. Planning with dental burrs help some cases of dystrophia unguium (See nail surgery, Chapter 6.)

The outlook is rather gloomy in most nail affections, unless the primary cause can be corrected. Even then, enough time should be allowed for the new nail to grow. A simple olive oil massage helps to bring back the shine and lustre of nails.

Chapter **34**

Diseases of the Sweat Glands

The anatomy and physiology of the sweat glands has been described in detail in Chapter 2. The special terms used in the different affections of the sweat glands are as follows:

Anhidrosis	Absence or reduced sweating.
Bromhidrosis	Foul sweating.
Chromhidrosis	Coloured sweating, viz., blue, black or red.
Dyshidrosis	Disturbed sweating. In practice, it implies vesicular dermatitis of the hands and feet. Synonym: pompholyx. *See* Chapter 10.
Fox–Fordyce's disease	Papular itching eruption of the apocrine glands in the axillae or around nipple.
Hidradenitis suppurativa	Pyogenic infection of the apocrine sweat glands particularly in the axiliae. *See* Chapter 11.
Hidrocystoma	Dermal cyst due to retention of sweat. Related to miliaria profunda.
Hyperhidrosis	Excessive sweating which may be localized or generalized.
Granulosis rubra nasi	Red, papular eruption on the nose in children with acrocyanosis and sweating of the nose.
Miliaria	Group name for sweat retention dermatoses. Synonym: sudamina. *Types:* Crystallina, rubra, profunda and pustulosa.
Periporitis	Pyogenic inflammation of sweat pore. *Synonym:* Miliaria pustulosa. May result in abscesses of sweat glands.
Syringoma	Naevoid tumour of sweat duct.
Tropical anhidrotic asthenia	*Synonyms:* Sweat retention syndrome, thermogenic anhidrosis. Failure of the sweating mechanism, common in tropical countries, resulting in sweat retention, surface anhidrosis, asthenia, fever, alkalosis, etc.
Urhidrosis	Excessive excretion by sweat of urea and other waste products as in renal failure.

Common Disorders of the Sweat Apparatus

Functional	Hyperhidrosis, anhidrosis, bromhidrosis, chromhidrosis, dyshidrosis.
Infection	Periporitis, abscesses, hidradenitis suppurativa.
Inflammatory and sweat retention	Miliaria, Fox–Fordyce's disease, dyshidrosis exfoliativa. Cystic-hydrocystoma.
Tumours	Naevoid-syringoma. Rare Malignant tumours.

HYPERHIDROSIS

It may be generalized or localized, physiological or pathological, transient or permanent. Besides being uncomfortable, hyperhidrosis may interfere with social and occupational activities. Furthermore, exaggerated sweating predisposes to maceration of the skin, growth of fungus (dermatophytes, monilia and *Microsporum furfur*), miliaria, intertrigo, secondary dermatitis, contact eczema and keratoderma. The causes of hyperhidrosis are:

Generalized

1. Physiological	Exertion, emotional embarrassment. High atmospheric temperature combined with humidity. Alcohol, tea, spicy food (Gustatory). Drugs like pilocarpine.
2. Pathological	Fevers like malaria. Shock—cold, clammy sweats. Endocrine—thyrotoxicosis, acromegaly. Debility and wasting diseases (diabetes, tuberculosis).

Localized

The common sites are: the palms and the soles, the axillae, the groins and the forehead. The causes are: Heredity, autonomic imbalance, emotional stresses, neurasthenia, local deformity, e.g. flat feet; sense of heat (SOH), excessive use of alcohol and tea. Palmar and plantar hyperhidrosis can be distressing. It may be complicated by bromhidrosis (on the feet, due to bacterial decomposition), keratoderma (the palms and the soles), ringworm (feet), contact dermatitis (particularly on the feet due to the sweat dissolving the chemicals from footwear), and dyshidrosis (the palms and the soles). In the flexures, particularly the axillae, the groins and the ano-genital region, hyperhidrosis tends to cause intertrigo, contact dermatitis (in the axillae from clothing), dermatitis (scrotum) and monilial infection (groins and infra-mammary regions).

Prognosis: It is uncertain. There is a remote possibility of spontaneous resolution; otherwise the outlook is poor. Condition persists until the cause is removed.

Treatment: It consists in:

1. Improving the general, physical and mental health of the patient; also of cutting down hot spicy food, tea, alcohol and tobacco. Living in the cool, fresh air, in loose thin clothing which allows evaporation of sweat, should be encouraged. Constant emotional stresses, strains and excitement must be avoided and physical exertion reduced.

2. The cause or causes must be removed. For instance, in localized hyperhidrosis of the feet, deformities like flat-footedness should be corrected; if there is obesity, the weight should be reduced.
3. Symptomatic treatment. It is important in the localized type of hyperhidrosis.

Internal

a. Pro-banthine for severe cases of hyperhidrosis of the hands and feet. The dose is 50 mg. QID till the symptoms are controlled, and then maintained with 50 mg or so daily. Side-effects of pro-banthine are dryness of the mouth, interference with ocular accommodation, loss of libido and dizziness.
b. Belladona and sedatives for neurotic patients.

External

a. Wiping the skin dry as often as permissible.
b. Clothing—loose garments.
   Sleeveless shirts for axillary hyperhidrosis. Sandals or chappals or open-type shoes. Socks should be changed twice a day in case of hyperhidrosis of the feet. Avoid nylon or woollen socks.
c. Deodorants or ammonium chloride solution 25% for topical use in the axillae.
d. The feet and the palms.
   25% ammonium chloride solution dabbed on the parts. Tea water soaks for feet. Alum is also useful.
   Potassium permanganate, 1 in 4,000 solution soaks for 5–10 minutes daily. Aluminium salts and glutaraldehyde.
   2–5%. Formalin soaks. Topical propantheline bromide.
   Iontophoresis with 0.5% soluble glycopyrrolate (Robinul-P) solution repeatedly (do not use during pregnancy) for 10–20 minutes, 10–20 mA bi-weekly.

Powder for Feet

R/Sodium hexametaphosphate	4 g
Calomel	4 g
Acid salicylic	1 g
Talcum	50 g
Pulv cret gallae add to	100 g

e. In resistant and distressing cases:
   1. X-ray therapy in localized hyperhidrosis. Its usefulness is limited as the dose which would affect the deep lying sweat glands would do damage to the overlying epidermis and dermis.
   2. Preganglionic sympathectomy for palmar hyperhidrosis; it is not so beneficial in plantar hyperhidrosis.
   3. Excision of sweat glands in axillary hyperhidrosis.

BROMHIDROSIS

Foul-smelling sweat is usually confined to the feet, and less often, to the axillae and the genitalia. It usually results from hyperhidrosis and bacterial decomposition of sweat.

It may also be produced by the intake of valerian, asfoetida, onions and garlic in food and, occasionally, in diseases like gout and diabetes. The treatment is similar to that employed for localized hyperhidrosis, namely: sterilization of clothing and socks by boiling, of shoes by formalin, frequent changes of clothes and footwear, and the wearing of open chappals. Locally, sodium hexametaphosphate powder or Dequadin (P) or Mycoderm (P) powder is useful; so also 2–5% chromic acid paint once a week has been successfully used . Cetrilak (P) soap may be used.

ANHIDROSIS

Diminished sweating is more common than complete absence of sweating. It is uncomfortable for two reasons: (1) The patient feels a sense of dryness of the integument. (2) The patient cannot tolerate heat easily, and there is danger of hyperpyrexia and heat stroke. The common causes are: congenital xeroderma, ichthyosis and atrophy of the skin and congenital ectodermal defects.

Localized anhidrosis is seen in patients after they have been affected by sympathectomy, Horner's syndrome, leprosy and other neurogenic disorders. Destruction of sweat glands in radiodermatitis and scleroderma also produces localized anhidrosis. In atopic dermatitis, blocking of sweat ducts may also produce partial or complete anhidrosis. The treatment consists in correcting the causative factors.

Generalized anhidrosis can be treated with warm baths, mild exposures to the sun and pilocarpine injections.

CHROMHIDROSIS

It is very rare. Most of the patients seen are cases of fraud. The main causes of coloured sweating are: (1) Injection of iodides, copper, phosphorus, iron, or elimination of products of metabolism like indicans in the sweat; (2) mixture with colouring organisms, e.g., special forms of Leptothrix: (3) dyes and chemicals from clothing, cosmetics, shoes, etc. (Fig. 34.1).

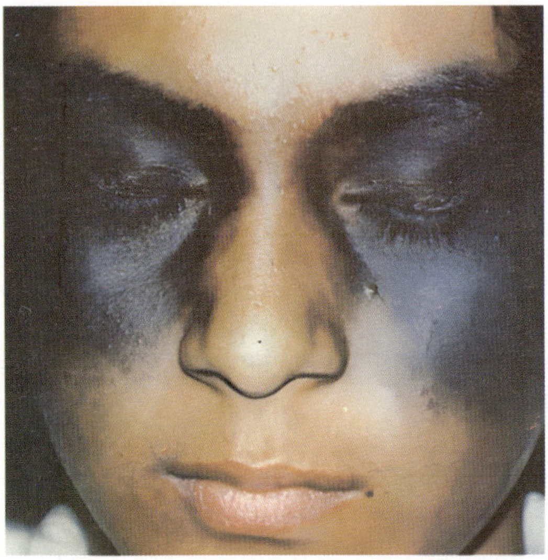

Fig. 34.1: Facial pseudochromhidrosis

MILIARIA

It is a group of dermatoses characterized by sweating, but obstruction of discharge results in the sweat getting trapped inside the skin. According to Shelley and Simons, sweat is secreted into, instead of onto the skin. Depending upon the sites at which the sweat is retained. There are four types of miliaria: crystallina, rubra, profunda and pustulosa.

Miliaria Crystallina

Synonym: Sudamina.

Sweat retention occurs in the stratum corneum with the production of discrete but agglomerated, superficial (almost on the surface of the skin), pin-point, crystal-clear, translucent vesicles which can be easily rubbed off. There are no signs of inflammation. Lesions are transitory, appearing suddenly and disappearing rapidly by fine desquamation. The common causes are:

a. Generalized—Seen on the trunk in acute fevers, and after steam baths.
b. Localized—in sunburn, sticking plaster application, wet hot fomentation, in the use of irritants like croton oil.

The diagnosis is straightforward. Treatment is with talcum powder massage, or application of calamine lotion.

Miliaria Rubra

Synonym: Prickly heat.

All practitioners in tropical countries are familiar with this common malady in which sweat retention occurs in the epidermis with the production of pin-head-sized papulo-vesicles and vesicles with erythematous halo. The lesions are discrete. When they involute, desquamation is produced. The common sites of affection are the trunk, neck, cubital and popliteal fossae, and less so the face and limbs. The palms and the soles are always spared. The condition lasts for a few days, weeks or months; lesions develop in recurrent crops. The condition becomes aggravated when sweating is exaggerated, and *vice versa*—basis of the atropine test.

The common accompanying complaints are burning, tingling and itching. To begin with, there is hyperhidrosis; later, the skin surface shows anhidrosis resulting from the retention of sweat. Scratching may result in excoriations, pyoderma and eczematization.

Etiology: Prickly heat is very common in the hot and humid parts of tropical countries. High atmospheric temperature, and more so, high humidity are responsible for prickly heat. Hence, it is seen more in the monsoon than in the dry, hot weather. Though it can occur in any individual, some people are more prone to it than others. Besides this individual proneness, prickly heat occurs in people who sweat profusely, are obese, have sensitive skins and are run-down. Local friction or maceration also predisposes to prickly heat. Overclothing and nylon garments tend to invite prickly heat.

It is common in people working in hot, stuffy rooms without proper ventilation. To sum up, increased sweating and maceration which causes the blocking of sweat pores are responsible for the production of prickly heat.

Diagnosis: In a typical case, the diagnosis is easy. It is based upon: seasonal appearance; typical papulo-vesicles; characteristic distribution; symptoms of tingling, burning and itching; aggravation by exaggerated sweating.

Eczema can be ruled out by the absence of uniform vesiculation, oozing, crusting, the distribution of the lesions and the history. Varicella is characterized by the lack of subjective symptoms, by centripetal distribution of polymorphous lesions and typical papules involuting into pustules.

Treatment: It consists in:

A. Prevention of excessive sweating by:

1. Reduced physical exertion.
2. Working and living in air-conditioned rooms; failing which, proper ventilation and fans should be employed.
3. Light diet, avoidance of alcohol, tea, coffee and hot, spicy foods. Consumption of meat, eggs, etc. should be restricted.
4. Proper, light and loose cotton clothing. Nylon garments should be strictly avoided in the hot weather.
5. Frequent cold baths, followed by thorough drying and talcum powder massage. In the author's experience, light oil application to the skin is very beneficial.

B. Vitamin A 50,000 IU twice a day for a month may be helpful.

C. Keratolytic local lotion

Acid salicylic	3.0 g
Camphor	2.0 g
Menthol	1.0 g
Spt. rectified	50.0 cc
Glycerine	5.0 cc
Aqua to	100.0 cc

To be dabbed on the affected regions, twice a day for about a week. Alternatively, calamine lotion or hydrocortisone lotion may be employed in cases of localized, prickly heat. The authors have tried with success catechu lotion, and Fuller's earth (Gachani).

Medicated powders and strong lotions should be avoided for they may produce secondary eczemas.

Miliaria Profunda

Sweat retention occurs in the dermis with the production of flesh-coloured, dermal papules localized around a sweat pore (not follicular). The lesions are discrete and multiple; they are seen best when viewed from an oblique angle. The papules increase in size as the sweating increases, but the surface stays dry. When punctured, sweat can be demonstrated. The lesions occur mainly on the trunk and extremities. It takes several weeks or months for the lesions to involute. There are no subjective symptoms.

Miliaria profunda lesions occur in *anhidrotic tropical asthenia*, a disease characterized by a severe degree of miliaria profunda, fever, surface anhidrosis of the trunk but hyperhidrosis of the face, asthenia and exhaustion. Even death may occur. The condition is seen after exposure to sunlight and physical exertion. Air-conditioning and proper nursing help to cure the condition.

Miliaria Pustulosa

It is pustular sweat retention in the epidermis and is characterized by non-follicular, superficial, discrete pustules with whitish purulent material **(Fig. 34.2)**. The condition

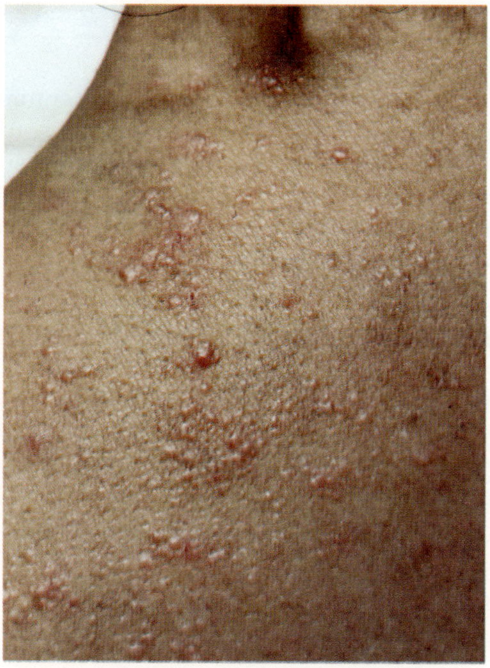

Fig. 34.2: Miliaria pustulosa

is pruritic: Miliaria pustulosa is usually produced by increased sweating on any skin disease like dermatitis, intertrigo, etc. that interferes with sweat secretion. It is found in the areas of the. body where primary skin diseases occur. The condition must be distinguistied from folliculitis; here the lesions are follicular, yellowish, deeper pustules. Usually, the condition is benign; secondary infection with *Staphylococcus aureus* results in abscesses of the sweat glands (Periporitis). Treatment consists in adopting measures to reduce sweating, and in therapy for primary dermatosis responsible for miliaria pustulosa.

FOX–FORDYCE'S DISEASE

It is also called chronic itching papular eruption of the axillae and pubis. It is a rare affection seen mainly in young females, and is characterized by multiple discrete, pin-head to lentil-sized, firm, flesh-coloured, translucent papules; occasionaliy, a punctum or crust may be seen on the papule. Lesions are accompanied by marked pruritus. The most common site of affection is the axillae; less frequently, the pubes and the breasts may be involved.

The etiology is unknown. The feeling amongst authorities is that it is either an obstruction of the apocrine glands, an endocrine disorder or a toxic manifestation. A bout of itching is precipiated by emotional upset and not so much by heat.

Treatment is unsatisfactory. Good results have been reported with X-ray therapy and/or oestrogens and progesterone. In resistant cases, the surgical excision of the skin may have to be resorted to. Good results with oral contraceptive-Enovid (P), have been reported.

DYSHIDROSIS EXFOLIATIVA

Synonym: Keratolysis exfoliativa.

It is a common, self-limited condition occurring in the summer weather in tropical countries. It is characterized by superficial, tiny, delicate, dry scales on the palms and the palmar surfaces of the fingers. There are no symptoms nor any signs of inflammation or vesicles. A similar condition occurs at the time when the weather changes. The treatment consists of lanoline massage, if the skin is dry, and 1–2% acid salicylic in alcohol or eau de cologne if there is hyperhidrosis.

HYDROCYSTOMA

It implies non-inflammatory, cystic retention of sweat in the dermis, and hence it is related to miliaria profunda. The condition is seen in housewives, washerwomen and cooks who come in contact with steam. The condition is characterized by a chronic, symmetrical eruption on the face, consisting of multiple, discrete, deep-seated, pin-head to lentil-sized, translucent, flesh-coloured vesicles. When punctured, clear sweat can be demonstrated. Hyperhidrosis is usually present. The lesions may involute spontaneously.

Treatment: It consists in:

1. Removal of precipitating causes like hyperhidrosis, working with steam, etc.
2. Puncturing the lesions with a fine, sterilized pin followed by dabbing with methylated spirit.
3. Dermabrasion as a last resort in cases with widespread, persistent affection.

GRANULOSIS RUBRA NASI

It is a rare affection seen on the cartilaginous portion of noses of children. The typical features are: a run-down condition, acrocyanosis, over-sweating of the nose and pin-head sized, red papules. The treatment consists in improving the health and in the local use of an astringent lotion. The malady usually disappears at puberty.

Chapter 35

Diseases of the Mucous Membranes (Mouth and Genitalia)

Diseases of the mucous membranes in proximity with the skin are described, in their varied aspects, in books of internal medicine, surgery, otorhinolaryngology, gynaecology and venereology. Because patients with such diseases often seek the help of dermatologists, and also because cutaneous diseases occasionally involve the mucous membranes as well, some basic knowledge of them is essential in the practice of dermatology. Particular emphasis is laid here on their relationship with skin diseases and their diagnostic significance.

DISEASES OF THE LIPS

Primary or independent
- Chapped lips
- Cheilitis—contact, glandular, exfoliative
- Fordyce's disease
- Macrocheilia
- Mucous cysts

Systemic diseases
- Avitaminosis — *See* Chapter 25
- Perleche — *See* Chapter 11

Cutaneous diseases
- Herpes simplex — *See* Chapter 14
- Lichen planus — *See* Chapter 20
- Lupus erythematosus — *See* Chapter 24
- Syphilis — *See* Chapter 18
- Tubercular ulcers — *See* Chapter 15
- Pemphigus — *See* Chapter 22
- Muco-cutaneo-ocular syndrome. *See* under "Diseases of the Mouth"
- Pigmentary anomalies—vitiligo, melanoderma — *See* Chapter 23
- Drug eruptions — *See* Chapter 21
- Tumours—keratosis, warts, epithelioma — *See* Chapter 28

CHAPPED LIPS

It implies dryness, roughness and peeling of the mucous membrane of the lips. It may occur in association with dryness of the integument or independently. The common causes of chapped lips are dry and cold weather (North Indian winter), cold wind, exposure to the strong sun as in desert conditions, a run-down state, malnutrition, fever etc. This condition is common in people living in dry climates. The sufferer complains of an uncomfortable feeling.

The treatment consists in: protecting the affected part against cold winds, boro-glycerinated amyli, butter or ghee, lanoline, chapstick, etc.

CHEILITIS

It implies inflammation of the lips, and is characterized by erythema, swelling and scaling or crusting **(Fig. 35.1)**. The common subjective complaints are: burning, pain and tenderness often precipitated by eating, drinking and exposure to the sun or wind. Cheilitis may be acute, subacute or chronic. The common causes are:

1. ***Contact cheilitis.*** It is due to sensitizing, offending agents, namely: lipstick, toothpaste and powder; fruits and vegetables, particularly mangoes, tomatoes, strawberry; cigarettes and cigarette holders; mouthwashes; nail varnish; rubber balloons, etc.
2. ***Cheilitis glandularis.*** It affects chiefly the lower lips which swell and show pin-point pores discharging mucoid or muco-purulent fluid which tends to glue the lips, especially in the morning.

   Palpation of the lips may show enlarged, nodular, mucous glands under the surface. The condition resembles dyshidrosis or cheiropompholyx. It is quite a common malady in India. It is caused by nervous stress, poor dental hygiene, focal sepsis, the chewing of tobacco and the use of strong condiments in food.
3. ***Cheilitis exfoliativa.*** It is characterized by chronic inflammation of the mucous membrane of one or both lips, usually the lower, exhibiting itself as continuous or

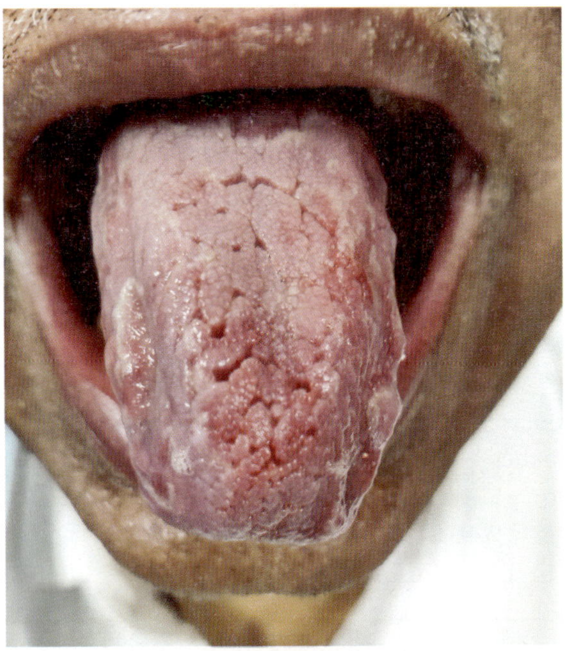

Fig. 35.1: Cheilitis and glossitis

recurrent exfoliative scaling and crusting. When the scale is removed, a red, moist, smooth fissured surface is seen. It is accompanied by burning, tenderness and pain. The exact cause is unknown. According to some authorities, it bears resemblance to seborrhoeic dermatitis. Nervous stress, exposure to the sun, the eating of chillies and condiments tend to aggravate the condition.

The treatment consists in removing the cause or causes, using soothing, local preparation like glycerinated amyli, hydrocortisone lotion or ointment. In chronic and resistant cases, Grenz-ray therapy is very helpful.

FORDYCE'S DISEASE

It is a chronic but benign malady affecting the mucous membrance of the lips (vermilion portion), and sometimes, the buccal mucosa. It is characterized by discrete, pin-head-sized, superficial, light or yellow milium-like, maculo-papular lesions without any subjective sensations. It is more common in males than females. The condition usually appears at puberty. It is a type of sebaceous, naevoid condition resembling milium. No treatment is usually necessary.

MACROCHEILIA

It signifies a chronic, non-pitting swelling of the lips due to recurrent lymphangitis resulting in lymphatic obstruction, hyperplasia and hypertrophy. It may be accompanied by fever and pain **(Fig. 35.2)**. Lymphangioma must be excluded in the differential diagnosis. The treatment is unsatisfactory in advanced cases. It can be treated in the same way as elephantiasis with antibiotics, medical diathermy, etc.

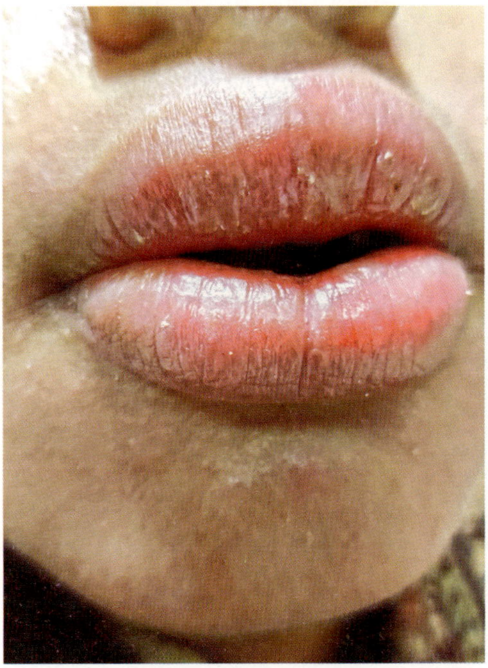

Fig. 35.2: Macrocheilia

MUCOUS CYSTS

They are retention cysts of mucous glands seen on the lips, tongue or buccal mucosa. Mucous cysts are seen as small, lentil to pea-sized protuberances; when punctured mucoid or straw-coloured fluid is discharged. The treatment consists of surgical excision or cauterization of the whole cyst including the lining membrane with phenol or electric cautery.

DISEASES OF THE MOUTH

Primary or Independent

- Stomatitis
- Oral moniliasis
- Fordyce's disease
- Ulcers in the mouth
- Leukoplakia

Systemic Diseases

- Avitaminosis
  - Angular stomatitis
  - Bleeding gums as in scurvy
- Stomatitis in leukaemia, aplastic anaemia, drug eruption.

Cutaneous Diseases

- Lichen planus *See* Chapter 20
- Syphilis *See* Chapter 18
- Pemphigus *See* Chapter 22
- Pigmentary anomalies *See* Chapter 23
- Tumours *See* Chapter 28
- Muco-cutaneo-ocular syndrome.

STOMATITIS

It implies inflammation of the buccal mucosa, and is characterized by erythema, swelling and superficial erosions accompanied by subjective complaints of burning, pain and tenderness which interfere with talking, drinking and eating. The symptoms are always more severe than the visible signs of stomatitis. The common causes of stomatitis are:

Aphthous stomatitis
Contact stomatitis
Dyspepsia
Monilial stomatitis *See* Chapter 12
Tuberculosis *See* Chapter 15
Diphtheritic stomatitis
Syphilis *See* Chapter 18
Oral sepsis—pyorrhoea alveolaris
Vincent's angina

Infectious fevers — *See* Chapter 26
Deficiency diseases—scurvy, pellagra — *See* Chapter 25
Mercurial stomatitis. Also due to lead, arsenic and bismuth
Muco-cutaneo-ocular syndrome
Stomatitis due to drugs-stomatitis medicamentosa
Gangrenous stomatitis (Noma)
Sclerosing stomatitis
Blood disorders like leukaemia, aplastic anaemia

Aphthous stomatitis: It is presumed to be caused by virus. The lesion is a superficial, yellowish vesicle on an erythematous base. The roof of the vesicle soon gets rubbed off, and a shallow erosion is generally seen. The lesions are multiple and are distributed all over the mouth, tongue and lips **(Fig. 35.3)**. The eruption takes about a week to 10 days to clear up. Like herpes simplex, aphthous stomatitis is an acute condition; it may take a chronic, recurrent form which continues for periods varying from months to years. In the latter type, precipitating causes like oral sepsis, psychogenic stresses and gastro-intestinal disturbances must be excluded.

Contact stomatitis: The common offending agents are: mouthwashes; dental cream and powder; dentures and tooth fillings; antibiotic; lozenges; cigarettes and tobacco; hot condiments; foods like strawberries, mangoes, yam (*jimikand*), candy and chewing gum.

Dyspepsia: It may be the sole cause of stomatitis, but generally, it predisposes to aphthous stomatitis. Sprue may also produce stomatitis.

Vincent's angina: It is an acute condition caused by *B. fusiformis* and Vincent's spirochaetes. According to many authorities, these organisms are saprophytes, and

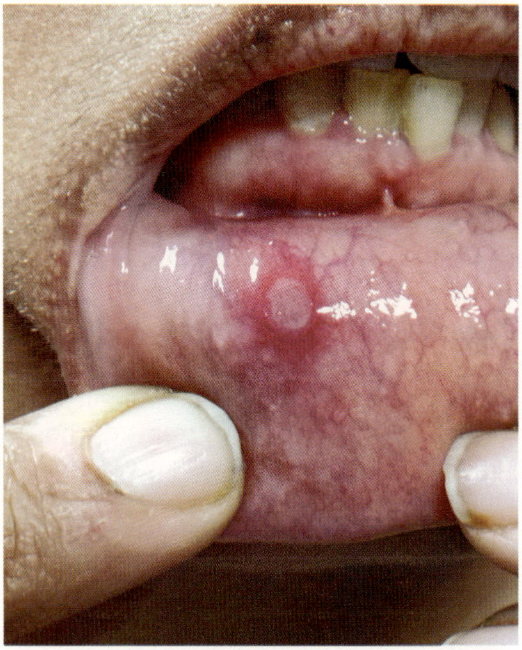

Fig. 35.3: Aphthous ulcers

become pathogenic when the local resistance is lowered by some disease process. It is seen most frequently in young adults. The clinical features are characteristic and consist of superficial, non-indurated ulcers covered by dirty, greyish membrane, and surrounded by dull redness. The ulcers bleed easily. Lesions usually occur on the buccal mucosa, throat and gums. The regional glands may be enlarged. Severe cases are accompanied by constitutional symptoms like fever, headache, malaise, etc.

The diagnosis is confirmed by the demonstration of organisms under the microscope, but since Vincent's angina can occur secondarily to glandular fever (infectious mononucleosis), leukaemia, aplastic anaemia, etc. great care should be exercised in the diagnosis.

The specific treatment consists of penicillin systemically, and an antiseptic paint locally. In resistant cases, broad-spectrum antibiotics are good standbys. The general health of the patient must be improved and the primary causes tackled in every case.

Mercurial stomatitis: It is not common these days since penicillin has replaced mercurials in the treatment of syphilis. The common complaints are: a mercurial taste in the mouth, gingivitis, salivation and generalized stomatitis. Similarly, stomatitis may develop with arsenic, bismuth and lead. Blue bismuth line and bluish-black lead line on the gums are typical of bismuth and lead poisoning; generalized stomatitis in these two conditions is uncommon.

Behcet's syndrome: Muco-cutaneo-ocular syndrome is a loose term implying several allied disorders. To avoid confusion, this term is being dropped. Stevens–Johnson Syndrome is an acute fulminating variety of erythema multiforme. Behcet's syndrome is characterized by a chronic, recurrent eruption on the mucous membranes of the mouth and genitalia, lesions on the skin and involvement of the eyes. The eruption in the mouth is in the nature of aphthous stomatitis; the genitalia show erosions, ulcerations and chancroid-like lesions; on the skin pustules, papules and sometimes small nodules are seen; the eyes show blepharitis, conjunctivitis and ulcers.

Presumably, the cause of Behcet's syndrome is a virus resembling that of aphthous stomatitis. The specific treatment is unsatisfactory; broad-spectrum antibiotics and corticosteroids are helpful in acute cases.

Diphtheritic stomatitis: It usually affects the pharynx and the tonsillar area. The typical feature is an adherent, yellowish-white membrane surrounded by an erythematous halo. Typical organisms can be demonstrated in the smear. The treatment consists of administration of penicillin and anti-diphtheritic serum.

Stomatitis medicamentosa: The common offending drugs are penicillin, aureomycin and other broad-spectrum antibiotics; heavy metals like mercury, lead, bismuth and arsenic; diphenylhydantoin (Dilantin) and the aminopterin group of drugs used in the treatment of reticuloses. The clinical features vary from vesicles, ulcerations to erythema and angioneurotic oedema. Penicillin usually produces a furred tongue, erythemato-ulcerative lesions and angioneurotic oedema. Broad-spectrum antibiotics cause monilial infection, features of avitaminosis and ulceration. Dilantin is responsible for typical gingival hypertrophy.

Sclerosing stomatitis (submucosal fibrosis): It is a fairly common problem in practice. Some cases start primarily as such; others develop as a complication of recurrent aphthous stomatitis, lymphogranuloma venereum, tobacco and betel nut chewing, and systemic sclerosis. The clinical features consist of diffuse, greyish-white, firm thickening of the mucous membrane which may break from time to time to produce ulcers. It causes difficulty in opening the mouth and in mastication. The condition resembles scleroderma. The treatment is unsatisfactory; repeated triamcinolone and hyaluronidase infiltration of the affected mucosa may help some patients. Orabolin (P) 2 mg daily may help to control the progress of disease. Treatment of stomatitis consists in:

1. Elimination or correction of causes.
2. Mouth rinses with potassium permanganate or hydrogen peroxide or Binaca (P) or Amosan (P).
3. Painting the ulcers with 5–10% silver nitrate or alum stick or cocaine 5–10%.
4. Painting boroglycerine, or 1% gentian violet (aqueous). Tyrothricin lozenges are also helpful.
5. Broad-spectrum antibiotics in cases of severe aphthous stomatitis, Vincent's, angina, gangrenous stomatitis or in cases with secondary infection. Tetracycline and corticosteroid sprays are being beneficially used.

ULCERS IN THE MOUTH AND ON THE TONGUE

The common causes are:

- Ulcerative stomatitis—aphthous, contact, Vincent's angina, dyspepsia, pemphigus, erythema multiforme, etc.
- Dental ulcers
- Tuberculosis orificialis
- Syphilitic ulcers and rarely granuloma venereum.
- Neoplastic carcinomas.

The features of stomatitis have been described in the preceding pages. Superficial erosions must be differentated from ulcers. The latter are deep and have definite length and breadth. Pemphigus, erythema multiforme, aphthous stomatitis and viral affections usually produce erosions rather than ulcers. Dyspeptic ulcers are usually multiple, round and small. They are present mainly on the dorsum and edges of the tongue. The history shows definite relationship between digestive upsets and the development of ulcers.

A dental ulcer is usually single; it is situated on the side of the tongue opposite a jagged tooth. The ulcer is small and superficial. It heals rapidly when the cause is corrected **(Fig. 35.3)**.

Tubercular ulcers usually accompany pulmonary and laryngeal tuberculosis. They may be single or multiple; they are present on the tip of the tongue or the buccal mucosa. A tubercular ulcer is irregular in shape; it has thin, undermined edges and pale granulations on the base which may be caseous. It is usually painful.

Syphilitic ulcers are of several types; primary chancre, secondary serpiginous ulcers and tertiary gummatous ulcers. It is the gummatous ulcer which often creates confusion, especially when it is accompanied by syphilitic leukoplakia and glossitis.

Carcinomatous ulcers are more common amongst men about 40–50 years of age. They are usually deep, well-defined and indurated with raised nodular everted edges. In a suspected case, a biopsy must be done to confirm the diagnosis.

LEUKOPLAKIA

It signifies chronic, hypertrophic and hyperkeratotic affection of the mucous membrane, especially of the buccal mucosa and the tongue. It affects persons past middle age. In the mouth, it is more commonly seen in males, and in females, the vulvar region. The causes of buccal leukoplakia are: chronic smoking especially pipe smoking, tobacco chewing, poor hygiene and strong alcohol. Dental caries and jagged teeth are the most common causes of leukoplakia of the margin of the tongue.

Clinically, it is characterized by the formation of small reddish areas which gradually develop into dry, milky-white, irregular-shaped, but well-defined patches which may be smooth, raised or verrucous. It has a typical, leathery feel. Leukoplakia has a tendency to malignant change. The biopsy characteristically shows hyperkeratosis, acanthosis, spongiosis and slight cellular infiltration.

On the glans penis and vulva, well-defined brilliant red areas with velvety surface are seen—Erythroplasia of Queyrat. This is supposed to represent the moist stage of leukoplakia.

If the condition is diagnosed at an early stage, and the causative factors eliminated, leukoplakia may disappear spontaneously. If it is advanced, a carcinomatous change should be suspected. In every case of leukoplakia, a blood serology for syphilis and a biopsy to rule out malignancy are indicated.

The condition must be distinguished from lichen planus and syphilitic mucous patches (for the differential diagnosis, *see* Chapter 18).

The treatment consists in correcting the causes like tobacco smoking, stop alcohol and control oral sepsis. Caustics and irritants should be avoided. Presently, leukoplakia is excised either surgically or by diathermy or laser. Surgical advice should be sought if there is suspicion of cancer.

DISEASES OF THE TONGUE

Primary and Independent

- Glossitis and ulcers—discussed under stomatitis
- Functional burning tongue
- Geographical tongue
- Black hairy tongue
- Scrotal tongue
- Möhler's glossitis
- Glossitis rhombica mediana
- Smooth atrophy of the tongue

Systemic Diseases

- Sprue
- Anaemia, Plummer–Vinson syndrome. Avitaminosis
- Leukaemia, aplastic anaemia, etc.

Cutaneous Diseases

Lichen planus *See* Chapter 20

Tuberculosis	*See* Chapter 15
Syphilis	*See* Chapter 18
Pemphigus	*See* Chapter 22
Muco-cutaneo-ocular syndrome	*See* under "Diseases of the Mouth"
Warts	*See* Chapter 14
Leucoderma and pigmentary disease	*See* Chapter 23
Tumours	*See* Chapter 28

BURNING TONGUE

It implies a burning sensation of part or whole of the tongue without any visible changes in the structure or features. The common causes are: pellagra, neurosis, over-indulgence in smoking and drinking, gastritis, and sometimes, though rarely lingual tonsillitis. Neuritis of the lingual nerve should be excluded. The treatment consists of correction of the causes, soothing mouthwashes and vitamin-B complex by mouth. Sedatives and tranquillizers are used for resistant cases of neurotic origin.

GEOGRAPHICAL TONGUE

It is a peculiar, symptomless shedding of the surface epithelium of the mucous membrane of the tongue resulting in a slowly extending patch which is smooth, red, bald with a well-defined, but irregular, figurate edge. It is found on the tip or dorsum of the tongue **(Fig. 35.4)**. The condition is benign: the exact cause is still obscure. The course is enigmatic, and is marked by ups and downs. It is always difficult to predict the prognosis. The differential diagnosis is made from mucous patches of syphilis, lichen planus, avitaminosis and leukoplakia. The treatment consists of: giving reassurance to

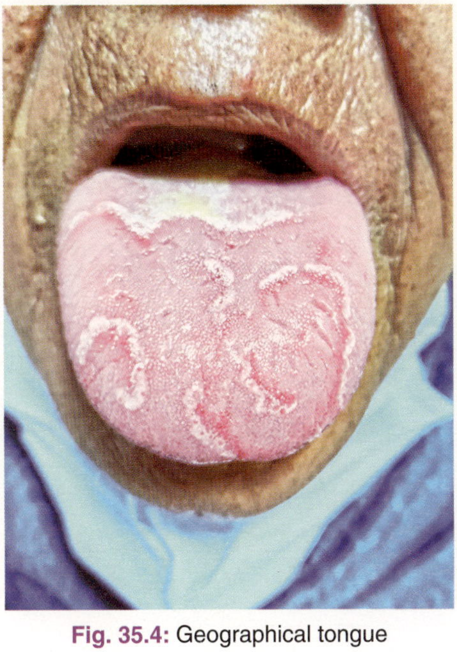

Fig. 35.4: Geographical tongue

the patient, improving his general health, improving oral hygiene and giving vitamin B complex in large doses. Locally, boroglycerine or tannic acid glycerine, etc. is usually prescribed. Smoking and drinking should be cut down, or completely avoided.

BLACK HAIRY TONGUE

It is a rare affection seen on the mid-line of the dorsum of the tongue as a brownish-black plush due to hypertrophy of the epithelium of the filiform papillae and secondary infection with yeast-like organisms. The exact etiology is obscure. The course is unpredictable, but the condition has tendency to clear up spontaneously. The treatment consists of scraping or shaving off of the affected portion and applying mild caustics.

SCROTAL TONGUE

It usually signifies congenital hypertrophy of the tongue, resulting in a rather large tongue with superficial and deep furrows and a glazed surface; the picture resembles scrotal skin **(Fig. 35.5)**. Secondary glossitis is common complication resulting from collection of food and debris in the sulci. The treatment is unsatisfactory.

MÖHLER'S GLOSSITIS

This uncommon condition is a chronic, superficial inflammation of the tongue resulting in painful, well-defined, very red, raw patches. The etiology is obscure. The course is slow and chronic, marked by cyclic variations. The treatment is unsatisfactory. Broad-spectrum antibiotics and corticosteroids are worth trying. Topical Flucort (P) lotion and ghee massage are helpful.

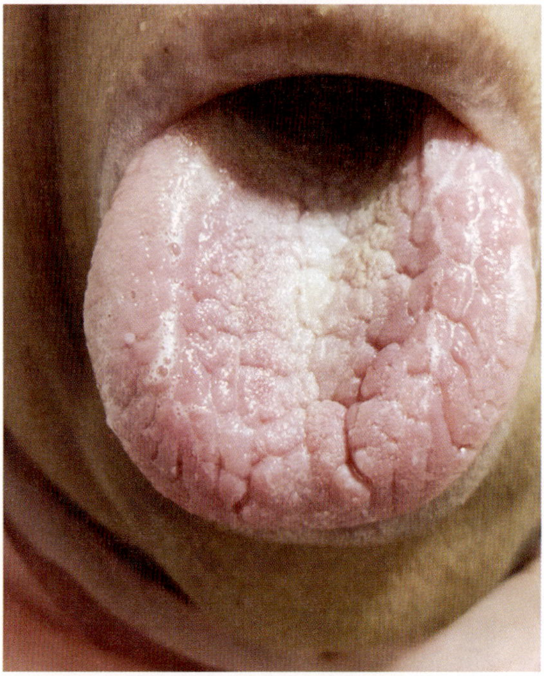

Fig. 35.5: Scrotal tongue

GLOSSITIS RHOMBICA MEDIANA

It is a chronic, symptomless, fibrosing inflammation of the tongue characterized by oval, red, smooth, shiny plaques with moderate induration on the dorsum of the middle of the tongue. Adults are selectively affected. The etiology is obscure. There is no specific treatment.

SMOOTH ATROPHY OF THE TONGUE

There are two main types of smooth atrophy of the tongue:

1. With fibrosis as seen in syphilis.
2. Without fibrosis, viz., in hypochromic anaemia, avitaminosis, etc.

In pernicious anaemia and pellagra, the tongue is bright red. In Plummer–Vinson syndrome, the mucous membranes of the tongue and the pharynx are atrophic causing dysphagia. This symptom is accompanied by spoon-shaped nails (koilonychia).

DISEASES OF THE VULVA

Independent and Primary

Gonorrheal and pyogenic vulvitis	*See* Chapter 19
Chancroid	*See* Chapter 19
Syphilis	*See* Chapter 18
Lymphogranuloma venereum	*See* Chapter 19
Granuloma venereum	*See* Chapter 19
Leukoplakia	*See* under "Diseases of the Mouth"
Kraurosis vulvae	*See* Chapter 25

Elephantiasis due to lymphogranuloma venereum, tuberculosis, lymphangioma, chronic lymphangitis, cellulitis and filariasis.

Prolapse of the uterus

Systemic Diseases

Diabetes mellitus

Deficiency diseases–malnutrition syndrome

Cutaneous Diseases

Contact dermatitis due to contraceptives, pessaries, douches, sanitary pads and toilet paper	*See* Chapter 10
Tinea and moniliasis	*See* Chapter 12
Pruritus vulvae	*See* Chapter 29
Herpes progenitalis	*See* Chapter 14
Scabies and pediculoses	*See* Chapter 13
Lichen planus.	*See* Chapter 20
Verruca acuminata and warts	*See* Chapter 14
Psoriasis	*See* Chapter 20
Drug eruptions, especially fixed drug eruption	*See* Chapter 21
Neurodermatitis	*See* Chapter 10

Lichen sclerosus et atrophicus	*See* Chapter 20
Tumours—benign and malignant	*See* Chapter 28
Leucoderma and pigmentary anomalies	*See* Chapter 23
Cutaneous tuberculosis.	*See* Chapter 15
Muco-cutaneo-ocular syndrome	*See* "Diseases of the Mouth"
Pemphigus	*See* Chapter 22
Oxyuriasis and amoebic infection	*See* Chapters 11 and 13

The above-mentioned conditions have been described in detail in the preceding chapters. Here, they have been grouped together for emphasis, and for facilitating differential diagnosis.

DISEASES OF THE MALE GENITALIA

On the glans penis and scrotum almost identical conditions occur. The common ones are listed below:

Syphilis	*See* Chapter 18
Chancroid	*See* Chapter 19
Granuloma venereum	*See* Chapter 19
Lymphogranuloma venereum	*See* Chapter 19
Gonorrhea	*See* Chapter 19
Phagedena	
Contact dermatitis	*See* Chapter 10
Moniliasis	*See* Chapter 12
Diabetes	*See* Chapter 25
Scrotal pruritus	*See* Chapter 29
Lichen planus	*See* Chapter 20
Drug eruptions	*See* Chapter 21
Scabies	*See* Chapter 13
Verrucae	*See* Chapter 14
Leucoderma and vitiligo	*See* Chapter 23
Pediculoses	*See* Chapter 13
Leukoplakia	*See* under "Diseases of the Mouth"
Carcinoma	*See* Chapter 28
Pemphigus	*See* Chapter 22
Tuberculosis	*See* Chapter 15
Herpes	*See* Chapter 14
Lichen nitidus	*See* Chapter 20
Balanitis xerotica obliterans	*See* Chapter 25

Diseases of the Anus

Pruritus ani	*See* Chapter 29
Condyloma acuminatum	*See* Chapter 14
Condyloma lata	*See* Chapter 18
Moniliasis	*See* Chapter 12

Anal fistula and sinuses	
Amoebiasis cutis	*See* Chapter 11
Tinea	*See* Chapter 12
Esthiomene	*See* Chapter 19
Carcinoma	*See* Chapter 28
Oxyuriasis	*See* Chapter 13
Contact dermatitis	*See* Chapter 10
Tuberculosis	*See* Chapter 15

PEARLY PENILE PAPULES

These are discrete, acuminate, flesh coloured tiny papules, distributed circumferentially around the coronal sulcus in 1–3 rows usually. They vary in size from 1 to 4 mm. They portray the moustache around the mouth. They should be differentiated from penile warts. The latter are asymmetrical, multiple, filiform growths on the prepuce and glans developing after exposure.

Histology of pearly penile papule is characteristic of young fibroblastic proliferation entrapping vascular channels.

No treatment is warranted.

Chapter

36

Pediatric, Geriatric and Occupational Dermatology

PEDIATRIC DERMATOLOGY

Since about 20–30% problems in infants and children pertain to dermatology, lot of interest has developed in the field of pediatric dermatology. At this stage of life, the integument differs from that of adults in important essentials; hence the proneness and development of disease varies in several respects viz. genodermatoses exhibit; infections are common; atrophies, hypertrophies and tumours are uncommon; ecological exposure is different because of sheltered and protected lives; immunological development is incomplete and psychosomatic system immature and unstable.

Integument is thinner; stratum corneum (Barrier layer) js poorly developed. There is weak cohesion of cells both epidermal and epidermodermal; hence blister formation is common. Eccrine and sebaceous secretions are less. Hair are also less. There is increased susceptibility to trauma, irritants and infections. There is depressed contact allergen reactivity. Percutaneous absorption is increased only in the premature, damaged and scrotal skin.

Dermatological Problems

These have been discussed in earlier chapters. Here they are being grouped for the convenience of the reader interested in the subspeciality.

a. **Newborn (neonatal)**

Toxic erythema	Due to coccal toxins and/or drugs.
Birth trauma	Caput succedaneum, pressure trauma, suction blisters.
Nevi and genodermatoses	(See under hereditary dermatoses)
Toxic dermatoses	Toxic epidermal necrolysis. Ritter's and Leiner's syndrome. Dermatitis medicamentosa (Drugs given to mother during delivery or late pregnancy).
Infections	Impetigo neonatorum, syphilis, herpes simplex and varicella zoster
Exanthemata	Toxoplasmosis
	Sclerema neonatorum and fat necrosis
Vascular	Cutis marmorata, harlequin colour changes
Diaper rash	Friction, irritation due to soap, etc. and *Candida* infection.
Seborrhoeic	Cradle cap, congenital acne, seborrhoeic dermatitis. Pityriasis capitis.
Miscellaneous	Letterer Siwe disease, granuloma gluteale infantum.

Climate	Acrodermatitis enteropathica Miliaria

b. **Hereditary/genodermatoses/heredo-familial disorders**
Ichthyosis
Epidermolysis bullosa
Keratoderma
Ectodermal defect
Albinism
Incontinentia pigmenti
Lentigines
Elastosis cutis and Ehler–Danlos syndrome
Angiokeratoma
Pachyonychia congenita
Hereditary haemorrhagic telangiectasis (Osler's syndrome)

c. **Developmental (congenital)**
Naevi (Birthmarks)—Epidermal, cellular, haemangioma, lymphangioma
Mongolian spot
Lipoma
Adenoma sebaceum
Cylindroma
Syringoma
Urticaria pigmentosa

d. **Eczematous**
Atopic, Infantile and Seborrhoeic dermatitis. Contact dermatitis is over-diagnosed. Recently researchers have shown that important pathogenic factors in atopic dermatitis are beta-blocker derangement and imbalance of autonomic nervous system—components of excessive irritability.

e. **Infections**
Pyoderma, viral warts, scabies, candida infection and pediculosis. In the tropics, lupus vulgaris, dermal leishmaniasis, and leprosy are fairly common.

f. **Erythematosquamous**
About 10% patients develop psoriasis before the age of 10 and 25% before the age of 20. Lichen planus is very uncommon and so is pityriasis rubra pilaris.

g. **Hair disorders**
Alopecia, hirsutism and dystrophies.

h. **Seborrhoeic**
Acne may be seen as early as 8–9 years of age. Seborrhoeic dermatitis is common both in infants and children.

i. **Nail disorders**
Congenital, tinea.

j. **Bullous eruptions**
Common because of poor cohesion of cells. Juvenile dermatitis herpetiformis and pemphigoid are the two common conditions besides impetigo which tends to be bullous.

k. *Papular urticaria* and may be angioncurotic oedema are common.

l. **Pigmentary**

Vitiligo is uncommon before the age of one year. What is often seen is naevus achromicus, pityriasis alba and seborrhoeides in infancy.

m. **Tropical problems**

Kwashiorkor	Tropical ulcer
Noma	Anthrax
Lupus vulgaris	Leprosy
Onchocerciasis	Tinea
Maggots	Dermal leishmaniasis

Management

Treatment of dermatoses in infants and children is more or less on the same lines as discussed in earlier pages. Proper handling of these tiny tots may be difficult. They may refuse examination and they are often unable to relate their symptoms. Parents are anxious; they need discrete and diplomatic handling.

Prognosis should be properly explained to get their cooperation. Besides usual reassurance, they must be frankly told about infectivity, time needed to control, curability, recurrence, scarring, heredity, etc.

All infective cases especially impetigo neonatorum must be isolated and barrier nursing implemented.

Diet diary is very useful in patients with allergy and atopic dermatitis.

One must be careful in the use of drugs; dosage for age must be properly calculated. At all costs, over-drugging and over-treatment should be avoided especially with antihistaminics, steroids and antibiotics. Even the steroids should not be used topically for long periods for obvious reasons.

Itching must be controlled. Phenergan (P) syrup is helpful because of its sedative side-effect. Mittens, stockings, tight long pyjamas and sleeves help in protecting the part. Infants and children do not relish injections; hence they should be used only in very essential cases.

GENETIC COUNSELLING

Genetic counselling consists of provision of information about the risk of disease in the parents, their children and members of their family. Exact advice is about reproductive practice which is based on the following basis:

1. Accurate diagnosis.
2. Constructing a pedigree of the patient's family.
3. Knowledge of principles of genetics and determination of risk to the patients and family.
   a. *Autosomal dominant inheritance*. Recurrence rate 40–50% (because of incomplete penetration of gene).
   b. *X-Iinked inheritance*. Female—Sons and daughters. Male—only to daughters.
   c. *X-linked recessive inheritance*. Males in maternal line affected; daughters carriers in 50%. Mutation possible.

d. *X-linked dominant inheritance.* Similar to that of autosomal dominant except that male to male transmission is rare.
e. *Multifactorial inheritance.* Interaction between alleles at different loci, each contributing a small effect and variation, combination of multiple effects and environmental factors resulting in a disease pattern.

4. Special studies
   a. Chromosomal studies
   b. Trans-abdominal amniocentesis (study of foetal cells in amniotic fluid and determination of sex). It can also help in detection of disease.
   c. Heterozygote detection for X-linked or autosomal recessive genes especially when a single isolated case comes across.

GERIATRIC DERMATOLOGY

With the increasing span of life, number of aged persons is steadily rising and so is the problem of dermatoses in the aged. Integument exhibits forcibly and vividly the advance of old age. Skin becomes transparent, pale, dry, inelastic and wrinkled. Lower eyelids becomes baggy. There may be increase of hair on the pinna of ears and eyebrows may become bushy. The vascular and mesenchymal system of the skin bear the brunt of advancing age; other changes are the consequence. Epidermis shows reduction in water content, thinning and diminished life span, flattening of junction and leucomelanosis. Changes in the dermis consist of atrophy, disintegration of collagen and elastic tissue and decreased sebaceous secretion. Hair show decrease in number, atrophy and greying Nails grow slowly or deformed or show overgrowth. There is decrease in cell-mediated and humoral immunity. Blood vessels becomes thickened and circulation shows signs of slowing. Wound healing is slow, linear decrease in hormones, increase in gamma globulins, reduction in RNA content and decrease in enzymes.

Besides the cutaneous affection, the aged person may have unsuspected and undiagnosed systemic diseases. Skin may also exhibit markers of systemic disorders and malignancy. Hence, a thorough cutaneous and systemic examination and detailed investigations are essential.

Dermatological Problems

a. ***Universal problems of all ages*** viz. infections, erythematosquamous eruption, dermatitis and eczema, urticaria, drug eruption, etc.
b. ***Senile atrophy*** of the integument is a common feature in practice. On this senile atrophic skin, develop seborrhoeic warts, horns, keratoses, senile ectasis (de Morgan's spots), white anetoderma, lentigenes (liver spots), epitheliomas **(Fig. 36.1)**.
c. ***Senile pruritus*** is occasionally seen. Other causes of pruritus, both cutaneous and systemic have to be thoroughly excluded before labelling a case as true senile pruritus. The course is usually progressive and the outlook is rather poor. Testosterone in the males and oestrogens in the females may be useful.
d. Other common problems in the aged are: (i) Proneness to infections especially Pyoderma, fungi, herpes (Post-herpetic neuralgia is severe in the aged). (ii) Stasis ulcers. (iii) Bullous pemphigoid. (iv) Rosacea, rhinophyma. (v) Gangrene—Atherosclerotic, diabetic. (vi) Tumours—Both benign and malignant. (vii) Reticulosis. (viii) Erythrodermas.

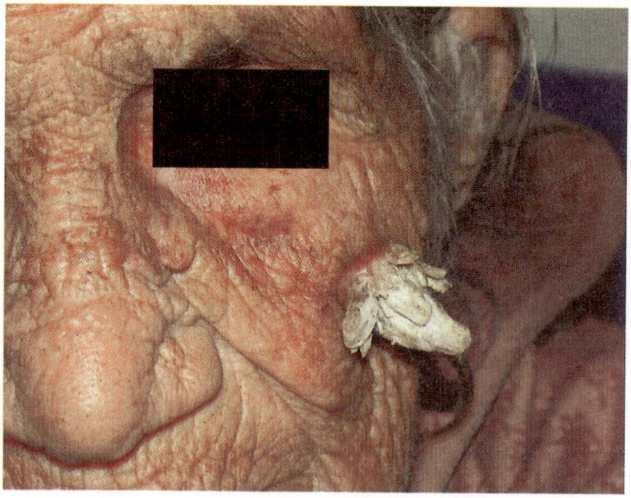

Fig. 36.1: Cornu cutaneum in an 89-year-old woman originating from a basal cell carcinoma

Skin tumours like leukoplakia, basal cell epithelioma, squamous cell epithelioma, malignant melanoma and sarcoma are commoner in the aged persons. White people living in the sunny tropics frequently present themselves with skin tumours. Incidence of skin tumours is the highest in Australia, New Zealand, California, etc. All lumps, bumps, ulcers and infiltrative lesions in the aged should be critically examined to exclude malignancy. Histopathological examination is extremely helpful in such cases.

On the vascular scene, stasis ulcers and gangrene are common. Their causes should be meticulously investigated and controlled. Change in living habits like cooking while standing, sitting on chairs for long hours, use of synthetic material stockings, elastic garters etc. are often responsible for stasis and Schamberg's disease. Underlying diabetes and atherosclerosis should be taken into consideration while investigating gangrene.

Management

Main emphasis should be on slowing down the wear and tear of the ageing process as it cannot be completely prevented. Maintaining good health, avoiding excessive exposure to climatic extremes and the strong sun, regulated exercises and massage, optimum mental and emotional health help considerably. Retinoic acid topically, vitamin E by mouth or topically and pregnenolone help very little, despite commercial claims. Hydration with urea and lubrication with emollients of skin are useful. Massage with milk cream and 'Upvatnas' (Gram flour and milk cream, etc.) help towards proper toning.

Chemical peel, dermabrasive surgery, cryosurgery, electrosurgery and face lift have limited usefulness. Skin cancers and tumours are treated on usual lines. Stasis ulcers warrant strict avoidance of stasis and improving the circulation by proper exercises, etc.

OCCUPATIONAL HEALTH AND DERMATOLOGY

In the present days world, medical men are mostly involved in doctoring patients with ill-health; they are spending less and less time on creating positive health. Besides, there is rapidly increasing number of ecological onslaughts to which we are often immune till a tragedy strike. Incidence of industrial and occupational diseases is steadily rising with the increasing pace of development. It is vital to take note of this sea-change. Incidence of occupational dermatoses is very high; according to many workers, it overshadows other organ involvement.

In India and many Asian countries, no reliable statistics are available because the labour is not fully organised . Agricultural sector is backward and ignored and because of communication gaps, all the cases of occupational dermatoses are not reported. According to Schwartz, et al. (1947), 72% of all occupational diseases pertain to skin; 1–2% of all workers have occupational dermatitis and 2–10% of all skin diseases are occupational in origin.

Since Bernardino Ramazzini' s book (year 1714) 'De Morbis Artificium Diatriba', the nature of occupational dermatoses has changed radically. At his time and age, common occupational skin diseases affected bakers (swollen, painful, fissured hands). Millers (Itch mite), washerman (Lye dermatitis), salt mixers (leg ulcers), etc. Since then Percival Scott (England), Alibert (France), Hebra (Germany), Schwartz, Tulipan (USA), etc. and many other workers have worked in this field of dermatology and published their findings. In India, this sub-speciality of work is not sufficiently studied and documented.

The topic of occupational health and dermatology has three components:

1. **Occupational**
   a. Industry (coal, petro-chemicals, chemical, rubber, textile, etc).
   b. Agricultural (plants, insecticides, fertilizers, etc).
   c. Others (painters, polishers, pharmacists, medicos, builders, photographers, etc.).
2. **Health**—Skin and systemic.
3. **Dermatology occupational accidents, burns, dermatitis.**
   a. Physical agents—Dust, heat, cold, friction.
   b. Biological (Infections).
   c. Irritants—Turpentine, kerosene, acids, alkalies, coal-tar products, cutting oil.
   d. Sensitizers—Epoxy resins, acrylic compound, polymers, salicylanilides.
   e. Toxic chemicals.
   f. Miscellaneous—Pigmentary, neoplastic, Raynaud's syndrome, miliaria, maceration, emotional, hair disorders, nail disorders.

Besides the subject would involve study of epidermiology, ecology and consumer effects to complete the picture.

Diagnosis

In establishment of correct etiological diagnosis, the emphasis should be laid on the following aspects:

1. Chalk out the worksheet. Seven days in a week consists of 168 hours. Out of this, 35–50 hours should be spent on occupational work, 75–80 hours on non-occupational work like hobbies. domestic chores, second jobs, diversions, weekend and off time including vacation activities and rest of the time on sleep.
2. Job title and details. In some countries, job directory is available. Patient must be thoroughly questioned as to exact work, materials and plants handled. Further the influence of weekend and vacation should be elucidated. Allergic history—both personal and family—should be taken.

3. Physical examination should stress examination of location, on onset, spread, description of dermatitis, involvement of other workers, occupational site survey, use of cleansing facilities and detergents, etc. Dermatologist has a useful role to play in investigating occupational skin diseases **(Flowchart 36.1)**. He is a useful member of the team, looking after the industrial and occupational health of one community. His importance can be assessed from **Flowchart 36.2**.
4. Patch tests with materials and contact allergens (standard and special battery) may be used to confirm diagnosis. They should not be done so long as the disease is active.

Flowchart 36.1: Usefulness of dermatologist in industrial projects

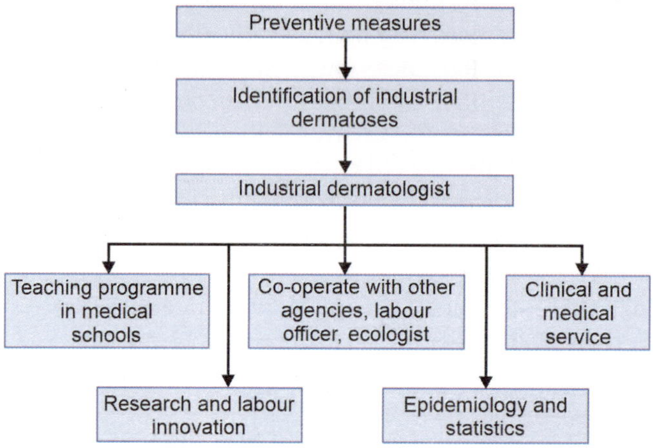

Flowchart 36.2: Investigations of occupational skin diseases

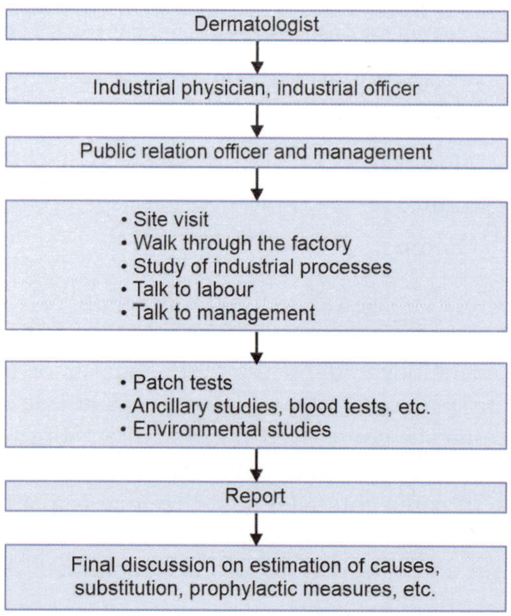

Examples of Occupational Dermatitis

Infections:

Anthrax	Butchers
Brucellosis	Cattle and sheep handlers and breeders
Erysipeloid	Butchers
Glanders	Horse handlers and breeders
Tularemia	Foresters, butchers
Tuberculosis	Butchers, anatomists
Dermatomycosis	Farmers, cattle breeders
Erysipelothrix	Fishermen (also urticaria and anaphylactic shock)
Mite and tick infestation	Farmers; grocers, etc.
Insects	Poultry farmers, honey-bee keepers
Helminthes	Farmers, dog and pig breeders

Causes of Environmental Acne

- Crude oil and fraction, cutting oil
- Coal tar products—Coal tar, pitch, creosote. Halogenated compounds (Chloracne).
- Miscellaneous—Heat, friction, harsh detergents, pomade, drugs.

Chemicals Causing Depigmentation

Hydroquinone, MBEH, butylalcohol, amylphenol, glutaraldehyde, octylphenol.

Causes of Hyperpigmentation

Chemical and thermal burns. Post-inflammatory reaction to irritants and sensitisers. Photo-sensitivity to asphalt, pitch, tar, psoralens, figs.

Photo-Allergic Contact Dermatitis

Halogenated Salicylanilides—tetrachlorsalicylanilide, tribromosalicylanilide, hexachlorophene, buclosamide, sulphonamide, phenothiazine, diphenylhydramine, optical brightners. Plants like ragweed. Sunscreen, methyl-coumarin, glyceryl p-aminobenzoic acid.

Industrial Hair Disorders

Alopecia: Thallium, chloroprene dimers, ionizing radiation, thermal burns, mechanical trauma, chemical burns.

Accidental discoloration: Green (copper), blue (cobalt and indigo), yellow (picric acid), red brown (TNT), red (soda ash).

Nail Disorders

Paronychia: Bar tenders, housewives, laundry workers.
Discoloration: Photographic chemicals, radiation.

Management of Occupational Disease of the Skin

A—Prevention

1. Avoiding contact with injurious chemicals by designing of factories.

2. Cleanliness at site and afterwards.
3. Air-conditioning and humidifiers.
4. Pre-employment examination: (a) General health, (b) Proneness to diseases–dryness, seborrhoea, allergy.
5. Maintaining systemic, skin, social and mental health.
6. Safety measures at site against possible hazards.
7. Orientation of workers and proper training.
8. Exploring risk factors. Maintaining directory of occupational job titles and their hazards with constant revision.
9. Protection—clothing, gloves, shoes.
10. Barrier cream—silicone, lanoline, shellac, beeswax.
11. Industrial skin cleansers—soap, solvent, wetting agents.
12. Avoiding sensitising medicaments and drugs.
13. Training and orientation of medical personnel.

B—Curative

1. Removal of cause.
2. Reassurance.
3. Symptomatic/palliative
4. a. Cleaning.
   b. Topical medicaments with lotions, creams, ointments, etc.
   c. Systemic treatment with antihistaminics, antibiotics, steroids, etc. on the usual lines (*see* Chapter 5 for details).

Chapter 37

Plant Dermatology

Plants are integral part of human environment. They constitute an important and major part of human beings—both for survival as well as sustainance. However, this close interaction may sometime cause some adverse reactions. In India, dermatoses causes by plants (phytodermatoses) are fairly commonly encountered in the practice of dermatology. Because of the jungle of terminology—both botanical and dermatological and confusion in the identification of plants and weeds by an average practitioner or a dermatologist, the task of correct diagnosis and correlation of the offending plant to dermatoses can indeed be difficult. This difficulty is further increased due to the fact that many plants have different local, provincial, linguistic and national names. To overcome this difficulty, different vernacular names have been added wherever the information is available.

INCIDENCE

There are no statistics available to establish the correct incidence of phyto-dermatoses. The impression amongst experts is that the problem is much more common than is realized, for the simple reason that poor farmers, foresters, etc. do not get the opportunity to reach the specialist, and because there is a great shortage of qualified and trained dermatologists.

There was little knowledge of the frequency of "Dhobi mark dermatitis" till several dozens of cases in foreign visitors to Delhi reported with this allergy to marking nut. The incidence of "cashew-nut dermatitis" was unknown in south India, but on visiting a cashew-nut farm, the workers showed contact allergy on their hands. Further, a poor peasant-woman explained how common the dermatitis due to the plant was amongst her family members and colleagues. Because of the distance of about 20 miles to town, they did not have the time or the money to go there for treatment. According to Raghavan (1975), 80,000 cashew workers are exposed to the hazard of contact dermatitis in Kerala. In the last 20 years or so, congress grass is reported to have caused severe dermatitis in Pune, Delhi and is fast spreading to other areas. These instances help to demonstrate the importance of phyto-dermatoses in practice, which often are grossly under-reported.

POPULAR NAMES

Contrary to the established practice, popular names have been given preference over botanical names as headings, to facilitate the task of a practising dermatologist, and a general practitioner. In taking the history of a case, the medical practice is to note down the patient's ideas of the cause in the patient's own language. Similarly, the etiological diagnosis is built on the information given by the patient about the plants he handles. Since an average patient has little idea of botanical names of plants, he can only tell the doctor the popular names. Hence, the emphasis given on popular names. The authors are well aware of the pitfalls in the use of popular names, viz., the same popular name may be used in different areas for different plants and scientific inexactitudes in description may creep in. But, to facilitate the practice of dermatology rather than increase theoretical knowledge, we have stuck to popular names wherever available.

BOTANICAL INFORMATION

Literature on the botanical aspects of plants is voluminous and confusing, while information on indigenous plant-dermatoses is very meagre from the dermatological point of view. According to Rook (1961) some knowledge of elementary botanical principles will often enable the dermatologist to pick out the probable offender among the plants to which his patient is exposed; to predict the probability of cross-sensitization; and to plan his patch testing logically and scientifically, making allowance for the variable biological factors which may influence his results.

Since plants are usually propagated by seeds, they are not necessarily identical. From the clinical point of view, it is important to remember that there is a diurnal variation in the metabolic activity of the plant as well as the more obvious seasonal changes. When considering the possible irritant or sensitizing capacity of an unknown plant, the dermatologist should study the records of its near relations with the diligence of a geneticist seeking a bride. Further, cross-sensitization between several plants (e.g. mango, poison ivy and marking-nut) must be borne in mind.

Of course, it would be ideal if the suspected offending plants were accurately identified and the correct, scientific, botanical names given to it. This however, is usually beyond the scope of the practising dermatologist; nor is it always imperative. In majority of the cases, a rough recognition of the plant is all that is necessary. Our brief botanical note can only help, together with its illustrations and geographical distribution, to facilitate the task of the dermatologist, to roughly recognize the offending plant. Our two publications—'*Sensitizing and Irritant Plants of India*' and '*Herbs Useful in Dermatologic Therapy*' are recommended for a better understanding of various plants important for a practicing dermatologist. The broad botanical features of irritant plants found in India have been provided in the simplest, as far as possible, non-technical language, along with suitable indexes and a glossary explaining the inevitable botanical terminology employed. Some plants are very distinctive indeed, and can be identified at a glance. The accompanying illustrations should help in their identification. No claim to originality is made either in the botanical description or the illustrations which have been taken from standard Indian floras (Wight, Roxburgh, Brandis), Kirtikar and Basu's Indian Medicinal Plants or from sources indicated below the illustration. If however, for proper diagnosis it is necessary to have the offending plant accurately identified, help of a professional botanist or botanical institute should be sought.

Despite the many advances in botany, it must be admitted that all the cultivated and wild plants have not been identified. Horticultural varieties and species do occur and so does the sensitivity to such single sub-varieties. Further, the literature on the subject is bulky, and many facts unknown. Besides, most of the substances responsible for sensitization dermatitis have not been identified.

For a plant to cause sensitization dermatitis, it must contain potential sensitizers which must gain directly or indirectly through mediaries, the practising physician must not only be acquainted with the geographical distribution of the plant, the season of flowering, known folk-lore, chemical constituents, but also be well-acquainted with the distribution of the sensitizing substances throughout the different parts of the plants and their manner of re lease to gain access to the patient's skin.

CHEMICAL ASPECTS OF PLANTS

To understand the pathogenesis of phytodermatoses, some elementary knowledge of the biochemistry and chemical aspects of plants is essential. A few fundamental facts are introduced here:

Chemicals in plants can be grouped under two main headings:

1. Growth hormones, e.g. chlorogenic acid
2. Secretions and excretions–essential oils, balsams, plant chemicals, like phenolic compounds, benzene compounds, furocoumarins, glucosides, alkaloids, etc.

Chlorogenic acid is allergenic under certain conditions. Coffee beans, apples, oranges, grapefruits and chrysanthemums are rich in it. Urticaria, dermatitis and allergic rhinitis have been attributed to coffee-bean chaff in persons engaged in sorting, milling or roasting coffee-beans. Patch test can show a positive result in in over 60% of the affected workers.

Secretions from the glandular hairs of plants as well as secretions following injury (balsams) contain cutaneous irritants and sensitizers; the content and quality vary with part of the plant, the season, the area where the plant grows, etc.

Essential oils: They are volatile substances responsible for smell, taste, fragrance, etc. They are composed of carbon chains. Essential oils are complex mixtures of terpenes, phenolics (phenol, catechol, resorcinol and hydro-quinone) and coumarins. They contain most of the sensitizing substances so far identified. They occur predominantly in the flowers (lavender), the fruits (citrus fruits), leaves (eucalyptus), bark (cinnamon), wood (sandalwood). An oil may possess different compositions in different parts of the plant.

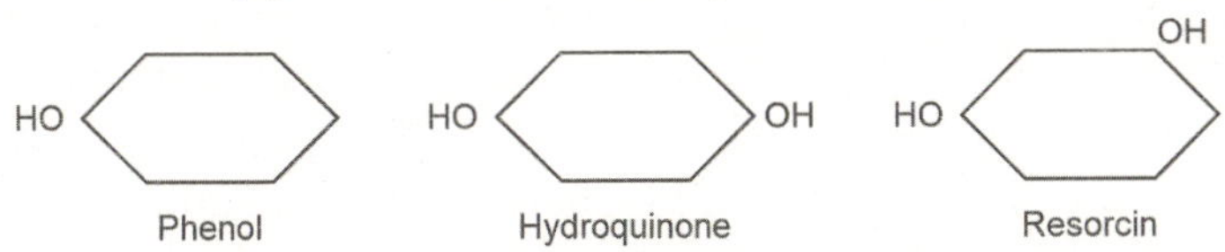

Balsams: They represent abnormal, pathological, secretions following injury to the plant. They contain essential oils and polymers, e.g. Balsam of Peru from *Myroxylon*.

Oleo-resins: They are sticky substances composed of polymers and phenolics.

Resins: They are acidic substances occurring either as amorphous vitreous solids or solution in essential oils. Some are phenolic derivatives, but others are polymerization and oxidization products of terpenes, e.g. the residue of crude turpentine oil distillate is resin. An example of a plant exudate which is a mixture of true gum, oil and resin is *Asafoetida*.

Glucosides: A phenolic (phenol compound) consisting of a benzene ring with OH group attached, coupled with glucose forms a glucoside, e.g. primulin in *Primula*.

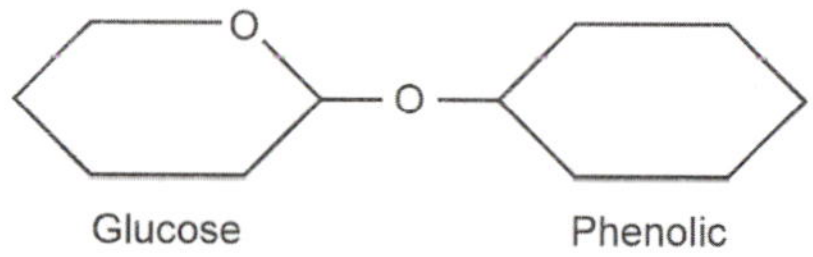

Furocoumarins: These are phenolics with the long side chains hooked up forming curious cyclic compounds. They are fluorescent compounds with a capacity to absorb light rays (ultraviolet) and producing photo-sensitization.

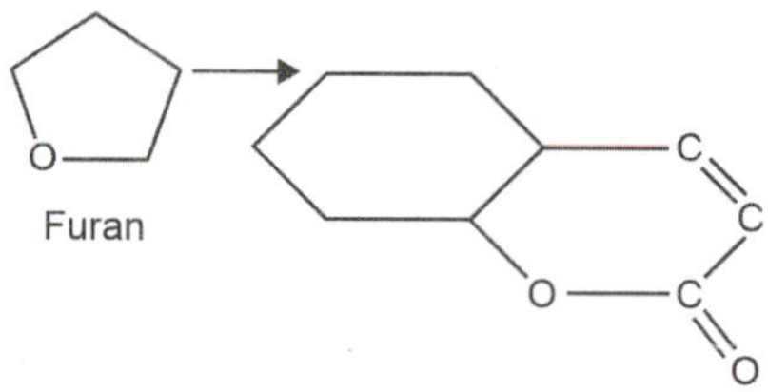

Furocoumarins

Terpenes: These are made up of multiple isoprene (C_5H_8) units. They are often associated with phenolics in balsams and essential oils.

$$CH_2{=}\underset{}{\overset{CH_3}{\overset{|}{C}}}{-}CH{=}CH_2$$

These are responsible for sensitization dermatitis caused by citrus fruits, celery and turpentine. Terpenes are present in many essential oils of plant origin used in the cosmetic industry.

The presence of cross-sensitization between two or more plant species provides clear evidence of the presence in all of common antigenic substances or of substances closely related chemically. Experience with patch testing suggests that the great majority of patients sensitive to a particular plant are sensitized by the same or a closely related compounds but there is evidence that this is not invariably true.

DERMATOLOGICAL ASPECTS OF PLANT

Irritant and sensitizing properties of plants have long been known to Indian, Chinese and Arab physicians. The old Indian barber has made use of the irritant properties of certain plants for cauterization of skin diseases; the photo-sensitizing properties of *Psoralea* seeds have been described in Charaka Samhita, and the Sushrut several centuries before Christ. Beggars and malingering servants have long used plant juices to produce sores.

On coming in contact with the skin, plants produce different reactions depending upon the nature of the plant (sensitizer or irritant), the type of skin, and other varying factors. Further, it must be realised that a certain plant causes irritation at one time and sensitization or photo-sensitization at another, depending upon the amount and concentration of the irritant and other environmental factors. Hence, the classification of plant dermatitis is often arbitrary. For practical purposes, the following classification is useful.

1. Mechanical Irritation

a. Wounds from thorns and large spines—roses, citrus, bouganvilleas.

b. Erythema or urticaria from T-shaped hairs of dogwood.
c. Scabies-like sabra dermatitis from palms, pears and other cacti (spicules).
d. Urticarial papules due to different grasses (*Gramineae*)—barley, millet, rice (spicules on awn).
e. Cotton grass, Spanish needles, spear grass also cause mechanical irritation (Maheshwari-personal communication).

2. Mechanical and Chemical Irritation

Glandular hairs present on some plants are specialised structures for intradermal injection of irritants. Hence the mode of the irritant action of such plants is both mechanical and chemical (histamine, acetyl-choline, formic acid, etc.).

Local reaction is usually urticarial accompanied by severe itching and burning. Rash develops in small or large patches and lasts from a few minutes to several hours leaving behind no traces.

Common incriminating plants are nettles and other stinging plants (*Urticaria, Laportea, Girardinia, Tragia, Fleurya*, etc.).

What happens in the case of such plants is that on contact with the plant, the very fragile ends of the hairs penetrate the skin and are broken off. The irritating principle from inside the hair is brought in contact with the tissues and an uncomfortable, itchy urticarial reaction is set up. Dilute ammonia, one's own saliva or some *Rumex* spp. growing near the nettles are helpful in controlling the reaction.

3. Chemical Irritation

Primary irritants set up, on contact, dermatitis in the form of redness, blisters or even ulcers; the causative agent being chemical rather than mechanical. These chemicals are primary chemical irritants. Common examples of such plants are marking-nut (Bhilawa), cashew-nut, the Euphorbias, buttercups, anemones, delphinium, ak, mustards (*Brassica* spp.), radish, lobelia and podophyllum. Turpentine is also a primary chemical irritant. Being primary chemical irritants, diagnosis is usually not difficult. Local medicine are very familiar with these plants.

4. Allergic Sensitization

Contact dermatitis occurs only in susceptible or sensitive individuals. Skin reaction consists of typical eczematous lesions varying from erythema to violent vesiculation, oedema, pustulation, oozing and crusting accompanied by marked itching. The sticky sap of plants containing phenolic oily resins or like substances is usually responsible. Toxicodendrol present in some of the foreign *Rhus* spp. is not volatile, but it may be conveyed to some distance in the soot, in the smoke of burning plants, and perhaps on dust. It may be conveyed by the hands or clothing from one person to another, as if it were contagious.

Travellers in the Himalayan forests often meet villagers having similar beliefs regarding the Indian species of *Rhus*. Villagers will not touch the *Rhus* trees or have anything to do with them; some of them actually avoid passing under them. Even the smoke, smell or sight, they say, will cause swelling and vesiculation of the skin. And yet it has been observed that many individuals are immune to these plants.

Plants responsible for sensitizing dermatitis are many and the etiological diagnosis can be difficult indeed, unless this fact is borne in mind. Contact dermatitis usually occurs on exposed parts, particularly the face and hands.

Well known examples of such plants are: *Anacardiaceae* (marking-nut, cashew-nut, mango, *Rhus, Holigarna*); *Euphorbiaceae* (binding tree, castor-oil plant, purging-nut, Euphorbias); *Asclepiadaceae* (Ak); *Compositae* (ragweed, chrysanthemums); *Primulaceae* (Primula); *Liliaceae* (Tulip); *Amaryllidaceae* (Daffodil, Narcissus).

Sometimes, allergic dermatitis is produced by inhalant allergies from pollens and moulds. Acute recurrences of dermatitis are observed on the head, neck, limbs and hands which do not correspond to direct external contact; even parts covered by clothes may be affected by inhalant allergens. Occasionally, generalised erythroderma may be produced. Interesting features are swelling of the eyes, history of rhinitis or asthma and cutaneous lesions resembling disseminated neurodermatitis. Pollen dermatitis is seasonal and the patient can be helped by moving to other places. Common causes are oleoresins and water soluble antigens from pollen of ragweed, box elder, poplar, maple, ash, elm, cocklebur, mare's tail, marsh elder and cherry blossoms.

5. Phyto-photodermatitis

It means photo-sensitisation of the skin after contact with plants which have either phototoxic and/or photo-allergic action. The actual incriminating principles are ammoidin and heraculin. The same condition has been described under different headings as Dermatitis bullosa striata pratensis, and Berloque dermatitis. Clinically, the lesions consist of erythematous bullous rash which heals in a week or two. On healing, pigmentation is left behind which takes several months to disappear. Rash develops after contact with the plant during, or followed by exposure to sunlight **(Fig. 37.1)**.

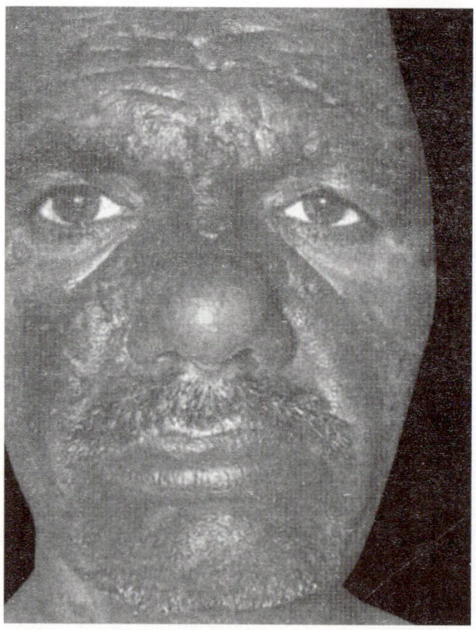

Fig. 37.1: Phytophotodermatitis due to *Parthenium hysterophobus* in a male 40 years old, confirmed by patch test

Phyto-photodermatitis has been known to Indian physicians for centuries; the use of *Psoralea corylifolia* (Babchi) has been described in *Charaka Samhita* and by *Sushrut* several centuries before Christ.

Plants known to cause photo-sensitization are as follows:

Umbelliferae: *Pastinaca sativa* (Parsnip); *Heracleum* spp. (Cow parsnip); *Angelica* spp.-(Angelica); *Ammi majus; Apium graveolens* (Celery).

Rutaceae: *Ruta graveolens* (Rue); *Dictamnus albus* (Gas plant); *Citrus* spp. (Oranges).

Moraceae: *Ficus* **(Fig. 37.2)**.

Leguminosae: *Psoralea corylifolia* (Babchi); *Medicago denticulata* (Bur clover).

The furocoumarins, psoralene, bergaptene (5-methoxy-psoralene) and xanthotoxin (8-methoxy-psoralene) show a powerful photo-sensitizing action while the remaining 29 furocoumarins that have so far been found in nature, have a slight, or, in most cases, no such effect.

The occurrence or non-occurrence of phytophotodermatitis in an individual case is decided by the following factors: (i) The amount of furocoumarins with photo-sensitizing action on the skin that are present; (ii) The dose and composition of the light with which the skin area is irradiated; (iii) The condition of moisture of the skin; (iv) The thickness of the horny layer and in some cases; (v) The pigmentation of the skin. Factors (iv) and (v) are somewhat responsible for the reduced incidence of phytophotodermatitis among Indians.

There exists another cause of photo-sensitization–ingestion of some plants such as *Fagopyrum esculentum* and *Hypericum perforatum*. This condition affects cattle and laboratory animals only. Among human beings, certain individuals are known to be sensitive to buckwheat, cow parsley, cow parsnip, taramira (*Euroa sativa*), figs, babchi (*Psoralea corylifolia*) and *Ammi majus* (used in the treatment of vitiligo). Hence, ingestion

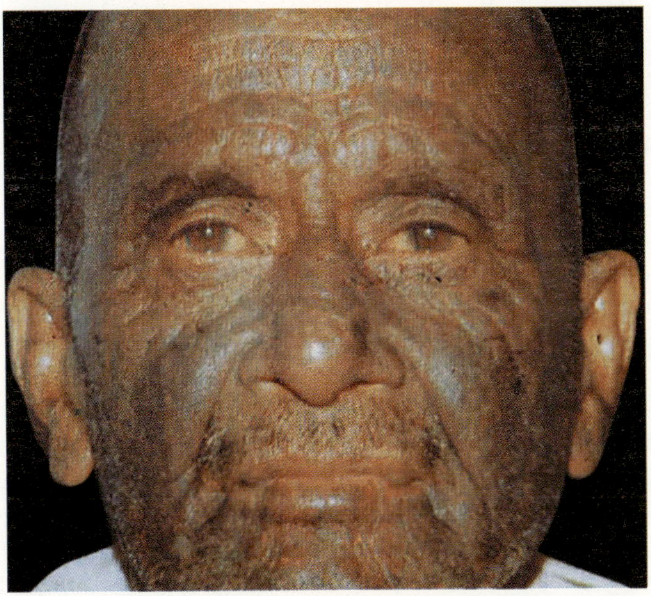

Fig. 37.2: ABCD—Parthenium black face

of these plants as such, or, as adulterants of foodstuffs, may be responsible for causing photo-dermatitis of exposed parts followed by melanosis. In the present state of the country's economy and with prevailing business standards in the country, adulteration is rampant. The authors feel that this must be borne in mind in investigating so-called idiopathic photo-dermatoses and melanoses.

Pseudo-phytodermatitis: Dermatitis due apparently to plants, but really to adventitious factors associated with plants are conveniently labelled pseudo-phytodermatitis (wood, 1962). These adventitious factors are as follows:

i. Parasites, like cantharides, chiggers, *Trombicula irritans, pediculoides ventricusos,* batala louse, copra mite, jute mite, cotton mite and acarus are often responsible for skin irritation when the plant is blamed. Lesions are usually in the form of papular urticaria. These mites are found in stored grain, linseed, dried fruits, bulbs, copra, tea, cottonseed, common ivy and gosseberries. Caterpillars have been suggested as a cause of timber dermatitis.
ii. Smuts and rusts on cereals and related plants are potent sensitizers.
iii. Insecticides , fungicides, chemical fertilizers and farm-yard manure are often blamed for dermatitis. They must be kept in view while trying to trace the cause of dermatitis in persons known to the handling plant-material.
iv. *Dyes:* Azo dyes or cardols used to disguise the colour of fruits are often responsible for dermatoses. Fortunately, this problem is so far unknown to Indian farmers and horticulturists. The so-called jute dermatitis is due to aniline dyes or mineral oils.
v. Allergic dermatitis on ingestion of plants and fruits, e.g. urticaria after eating strawberries or zaminkand, etc. is in reality not phyto-dermatitis. Hence, this condition is not further dealt with here.

DIAGNOSIS AND MANAGEMENT

The following criteria underline the diagnosis of phyto-dermatitis:

i. *Seasonal incidence:* Phyto-dermatitis is usually a seasonal dermatitis.
ii. *Distribution:* Exposed parts like the face, dorsum of the hands and the legs are affected; the genitals and even other parts of the body may be affected by secondary transfer from the hand or by scratching. Less often, the feet, ankles and knees may be affected. In case of pollens, grasses and weeds, eruption usually occurs on the face, but stops sharply at the collar line.
iii. *Eruption:* It is usually acute, and consists of erythema, oedema and vesicles.
iv. Burning and itching are usually marked.
v. *Course:* Dermatitis may last for weeks, depending upon the sensitivity or irritation.
vi. History of previous attacks or sensitization.
vii. Diagnosis is confirmed by patch testing in the case of sensitizers. Otherwise, the irritant nature of the plant suggests the diagnosis.

Patch testing: The following recommendations have been made:

i. Patch test, whenever possible, with the actual plant to which the patient has been exposed. Where this is not practicable; use well-grown, healthy specimens of the same species or horticultural variety.
ii. Test initially with leaf. If this be positive, test with flower and pollen of the same species or variety.

iii. Test with botanically related species of any plant to which a positive reaction is obtained and in case of horticultural varieties, with other varieties of the species or hybrid.
iv. In the case of species whose primary irritant properties are unknown, carry out control patch tests on normal subjects.
v. Ensure that all plants giving positive reactions are accurately identified and the correct botanical nomenclature is employed in all case reports.
vi. Juices, sap, resins, terpenes and oils may also be employed in patch testing under controlled conditions. In case of marking ink (Bhilawa), cloth with the ink mark should be used for patch testing.

Prognosis: Phyto-dermatitis usually is an acute problem, but tends to become chronic unless the exciting, offending plants have been detected and eliminated from contact; otherwise, dermatitis continues with exacerbations and remissions throughout the season. It spreads to other parts by transfer or may become disseminated due to auto-sensitization. Due to secondary infection, impetiginization, pyoderma or infective eczematization may take place.

Lichenified eczemas take a long time to clear up even after the cause has been eliminated, because of anatomical and functional changes in the skin. These cases respond well to corticosteroids, occlusive bandages and superficial roentgen therapy.

Melanosis, in cases of phyto-photodermatitis, takes several months to clear up. In some individuals, the affected integument becomes so sensitive to the sun's rays, that it becomes itchy on exposure to the sun even after the cause has been withdrawn.

ROUTINE TREATMENT AND PROPHYLAXIS

a. Prevention

i. People with a past history of plant dermatitis should be careful in handling plants to which they are sensitive and also to botanically and chemically allied plants. The best prophylactic is to avoid contact. Known primary irritants, both mechanical and chemical, should not be touched. If they have to be handled, leather gloves should be worn.
ii. Field workers with a sensitive skin should wear long trousers, long sleeves and gloves. Similarly, housewives with sensitive fingers should not clean irritating vegetables and should avoid gardening except with gloves on.
iii. Protective ointments for people who cannot wear gloves. There is no fool-proof ointment available for all the plants. Barrier creams usually vary with the nature of the plant. A good protective ointment is as follows:

Shellac	10
Alcohol	55
Sod. perborate	10
Carbital	5
Talc	20

It dries on the skin leaving a film which gives physical protection and sodium perborate gives chemical protection.

iv. People with a history of poison ivy dermatitis, should be careful while residing in the tropics. Washerman (Dhobies) should be told not to use Indian marking ink (*Semecarpus anacardium*) on their clothes. Further, they should be careful in handling mangoes, cashew-nuts, etc.
v. After returning from the field, garden, hunting, cleaning vegetables, etc. the exposed parts should be cleaned with soap and water. If clothes are contaminated, they may be decontaminated with calcium hypochlorite 1% for 15 minutes, and then laundered. Fresh clothes should be put on. Tools should be decontaminated.
vi. Hyposensitization, subcutaneous or oral may be tried. Results have not been very impressive according to the experience of many. It has been particularly tried in cases of poison ivy dermatitis in the USA. Acute glomerulonephritis has been reported following administration of *Rhus* toxin, so one must be careful in its use.

b. Curative

i. Wash the part immediately with soap and water.
ii. Clean with alcohol and rupture all the vesicles.
iii. Wet compresses soaked with 10% solution of tannic acid for 30 minutes.
iv. Use of calamine lotion or Burrow's solution or hydrocortisone lotion or cream. Do not use phenolated medications, particularly in poison ivy and related plant dermatoses.
v. Oral antihistaminics in moderately severe cases.
vi. Corticosteroids by mouth in extensive and severe cases.
vii. Protection from sunlight in phyto-photodermatoses using sunscreens.

Skin Formulary

SOLUTIONS AND SOAKS

Indications: For acute, swollen, weeping or crusted lesions.

Technique:
- Paint 2–3 times daily.
- Wet soaks-use towel and keep it wet.
- Do not use lotions for more than 48 hours without removing the crust or switching on to cream or paste.

Name	*Action*	*Concentration*
1. Aluminium subacetate solution (Burrow's solution)	Astringent	1–5%
2. Silver nitrate lotion	Astringent. antiseptic and caustic	0.5–5%
3. Gentian violet lotion	Astringent , antiseptic and fungicide (*Monilia*)	0.5–1%
4. Potassium permanganate solution (Condy's solution)	Antiseptic, astringent and oxidizing	0.01–0.1%
5. Saline soaks	Soothing and cleansing	1%
6. Sodium bicarbonate soaks	Soothing and cleansing	3%
7. Sodium thiosulphate solution	Useful in tinea versicolor	10–20%
8. Hydrogen peroxide solution	Bleaching agent for superfluous hair	Pure or half strength

LOTIONS

Indications: Acute, subacute and chronic conditions.

Technique: Once or twice a day. Clean before re-application if a crust has formed. Stop use, if any complaint of undesirable dryness.

Name	*Prescription*		*Instructions and remarks*
1. Calamine lotion Soothing and drying	Calamine prep	10.0	Phenol, sulphur, boric acid, paramino-benzoic acid, etc. can be added to modify action.
	Zinc oxide	5.0	
	Glycerine	5.0	
	Aqua calcis ad	100.0	

Name	*Prescription*		*Instructions and remarks*
2. Alba lotion. Drying and keratolytic	Pot. sulphurata	4–8	Useful for acne. Apply at night time after washing with soap and hot water.
	Zinc sulphate	4–8	
	Calamine prep	5.0	
	Spt. methylated	65.0	
	Aqua calcis ad	100.0	
3. Tannic acid lotion. Astringent, antiseptic and tanning.	Tannic acid	5:0	Useful in chronic folliculitis and resistant dermatitis
	Hydrarg perchlor	0.5	
	Spt. methylated	65.0	
	Aqua ad	100.0	
4. Alopecia lotion Stimulating	Tinct. capsicum	12.0	Used in cases of quiescent alopecia. Avoid if hair fall is active. Avoid irritation
	Sol. of cantharidine	12.0	
	Ol. ricini	5.0	
	Aqua ad	100.0	
5. Sun-screen lotion. Sun-protective.	Para-aminobenzoic acid	5–10	Useful for photosensitive dermatoses. Apply during the day before exposure to sun.
	Calamine lotion ad	100	
6. Coal tar lotion. Soothing, kerato-plastic and mildy stimulating.	Solution of coal tar	5–10	Apply at night and clean in the morning. Do not use on acute or infected lesions or hairy regions.
	Calamine lotion ad	100	
7. Oily lotion. Soothing and drying but also lubricating.	Olive or coconut oil	5–20	Apply 2–3 times a day. Less drying than calamine lotion. Useful in subacute dermatitis.
	Zinc oxide	10.0	
	Aqua calcis ad	100.0	
8. Benzyl bensoas emulsion	Benzyl benzoas	12–25	Scabicide. To be rubbed in throughly after a hot bath. 2–3 applications Wash at the completion of treatment.
	Emulsion base ad	100.0	
9. DDT emulsion	DDT (chlorophenothane)	2–5	Effective against pediculosis To be rubbed into the scalp or skin; wash after 12 hours.
	Emulsion base ad	100.0	
10. Anti-perspirant lotion	Aluminium chloride	10–20	Useful anti-perspirant for armpits and soles of feet.
	Glycerine	5.0	
	Distilled water ad	100.0	
11. Acid salicylic. resorcinol lotion	Acid salicylic	2.0	Useful for dandruff. Do not use for blondes. Also useful in acne vulgaris-dilute with water to 3/4 strength.
	Resorcinol	2.0	
	Ol. ricini	Q.S.	
	Spt. methylated	100.0	

PAINTS AND TINCTURES

Spiritous lotions for better application of medicinal agents.
Do not use on acute or inflamed lesions.

Name	*Prescription*		*Instructions and remarks*
1. Liq. picis carb.	Full strength		Coal tar liquid extract. Useful in psoriasis and seborrhoeic dermatitis.
2. Tinct. iodi special paint	Tinct. iodi fortis	6.0	Useful in chronic paronychia. Dispense about 30 cc.
	Phenol	3.0	
	Spt. rectified ad	100.0	
3. Chrysorabin paint	Chrysorabin	4.0	Useful in monilial paronychia.
	Tinct. chlorof. ad	100.0	
4. Sun screen paint	Paramino-benzoic acid	5.0	Very effective sunblocking agent.
	Ethanol 50% ad	100.0	
5. Spiritous gentian violet.	Gentian violet	1	Antiseptic and hardening agent. Paint twice a day. Use in chronic folliculitis.
	Spirit 75% ad	100.0	
6. Tinct. benzoin cc.	Full strength		Useful in erosions, abrasions, fissures and ulcers.
7. Modified Whitfield's paint	Acid salicylic	3.0	Effective fungicide. Useful also in pityriasis versicolor
	Acid benzoic	5.0	
	Copper sulphate	0.5	
	Spt. methylated	65.0	
	Glycerine	5.0	
	Aqua ad	100.0	
8. Crude tar varnish	Pix liquida or crude coal tar		Useful in chronic eczema, lichenification and chronic folliculitis. Apply cream or paste over it after 12 hours or so.
9. Castellani's paint	Boric acid	1.0	Useful in fungal infection Because of its staining properties, it is not liked.
	Resorcinol	10.0	
	Acetone	5.0	
	Ziehl–Neelsen's Carbol fucshin ad	100.0	

CREAMS AND PASTES

Creams are soothing agents for subacute dermatitis.
Pastes provide physical protection and less medicament penetration.
Peeling paste causes peeling of skin.

Name	*Prescription*		*Instructions and remarks*
1. Calamine cream	Calamine prep. Wool fat Paraffin molle Arachis oil Aqua calcis	20.0 20.0 20.0 20.0 20.0	Soothing and midly astrigent. Phenol/or brilliant green can be added to get antipruritic or antiseptic action.
2. Lassar's paste (Zinc oxide paste)	Zinc oxide Starch Vaseline ad	20.0 20.0 100.0	Useful protective application in subacute dermatitis Active medicament penetration is poor. Brilliant green can be added to make it antiseptic.
3. Tar paste	Pix liquida Zinc oxide Vaseline ad	5.0 20.0 100.0	Useful in chronic dermatitis Soothing and keratolytic.
4. Peeling paste	Beta-naphthol Sulphur sublimis Soft soap Vaseline ad	7.0 13.0 40.0 100.0	Useful peeling agent in acne scarring and comedonicus. Do not use for more than 2–3 nights at a time and then wait till the
peeling			completely subsides.
5. Bis. subgallas paste	Bis. subgallas Amylum Vaseline ad	20.0 20.0 100 0	Useful astringent and soothing agent for sub acute eczemas.
6. Unna's paste	Zinc oxide Gelatin Glycerine Aqua ad	25.0 35.0 20.0 100.0	Useful in neurodermatitis. Liquify before use by putting the jar in boiling water. Paint with brush on affected lesion when reasonably cool.
7. Glycerinated amyli (BP)	Amylum Glycerine	10.0 100.00	Useful in cheilitis and mouth erosions, etc.

OINTMENTS

Indications:

1. To apply active medicaments.
2. To provide physical protection to diseased areas.
3. To keep skin greasy.

Contraindications: Vesicular, oozing or acutely inflamed lesions.

Name	*Prescription*		*Instructions and remarks*
1. Whitfield's ointment (modified Formula)	Acid salicylic	3.0	Useful fungicide. Also useful in pityriasis versicolor. Avoid on acutely inflamed areas.
	Acid benzoic	5.0	
	Copper sulphate	0.5	
	Ung. emulsificans aquosus	100	Can be diluted to 1/2 strength.
2. Acid salicylic and ammoniated mercury ointment	Acid salicylic	2.0	Useful in scaly lesions esp. psoriasis. Also mild fungicide.
	Hydrarg ammon	5.0	
	Lanolin or vaseline ad	100.0	
3. Acid salicylic and sulphur ointment	Acid salicylic	2.0	Useful in scaly lesions esp. psoriasis. Also mild fungicide. In emulsifying or Brylcream (P) base, it is useful in seb. dermatitis of the scalp.
	Sulphur	2.0	
	Lanolin or vaseline ad	100.0	
4. Alopecia ointment	Oil of Bergamot	3.0	Useful in alopecia areata and other alopecias. Dilute, if irritating.
	Oil of Babchi	3.0	
	Tinct. cantharidine	12.0	
	Ung. emulsificans ad	100.0	
5. Burrows' ointment (Aluminium acetate ointment)	Aluminium acetate	10.0	Useful for subacute dermatitis. Astringent and soothing. Prednisolone, antiseptic and other agents can be added as need be.
	Zinc oxide	20.0	
	Wool fat ad	100.0	
6. Sulphur ointment	Precipitated sulphur	5 to 10	Useful in scabies.
	Lanolin or Vaseline ad	100.0	
7. Dithranol ointment	Dithranol or	0.5 to 2	Use in chronic discoid psoriasis. Also useful fungicide.
	Chrysorabin	0.5 to 8	
	Acid salicylic	2.0	
	Sulphur	2.0	
	Lanolin or vaseline ad	100.0	

Useful bases for ointments

Inert oil bases	Theobroma oil (Cocoa butter)
	Mineral oil
	White yellow paraffin (Petrolatum or Vaseline).
Water in oil bases (W/O)	Eucerin
	Petrolatum hydrophylic
	Hydrous lanolin
	Wool fat (anhydrous)
	Nivea cream (P)
	Cold cream

Oil in water bases (O/W)	Ung. emulsificans aquosus Brylcream (P)
Water miscible bases and emulsifying agents	Carbowax Propylene glycol Lanette wax Parabens Polyoxyl stearate

POWDERS

Soothing agents for dry lesions. Adsorb moisture.
Easy to apply. Integument must be dried before applying it.

Indications:

1. Intertrigo.
2. Macerated areas.
3. Prickly heat, etc.

Name	Prescription		Instructions and remarks
1. Talcum powder	Talcum		Simple dusting powder.
2. Nystatin powder	Nystatin	100,000 iu	Useful in monilial infection.
	Dusting powder ad	10 g	
3. Boric acid powder	Boric acid	1.0	Mildly antiseptic.
	Dusting powder ad	100.0	
4. DDT powder	DDT	1.0	Useful in pediculosis corporis and pubis. Dust on inside of underclothing and on the skin.
	Talcum ad	100.0	
5. Anti-perspriant powder	Sod.hexameta phosphate	4.0	Useful in troublesome hyperhidrosis.
	Calomel	4.0	
	Acid salicylic	1.0	
	Talcum	50.0	
	Pulv. cret. gallae ad	100.0	

List of Reference Books

A. General Textbooks

1. *Diseases of the Skin*, Andrews, GC: Philadelphia WB Saunders Co, 2018.
2. *Dermatology Vol I & II*, Moschella, Pilsbury and Hurley, Philadelphia WB. Saunders Co., 2016.
3. *Skin, Other Diseases.* Fox and Farquhar: London, Churchill & Co., 1976.
4. *Dermatology, Diagnosis* and *Treatment*, Sulzburger MB, et al.: Chicago, The Year Book publishers, 1961.
5. *Manual of Skin Diseases*, Sauer GC: Philadelphia, JB Lippincott Co.
6. *Text Book of Dermatology*, Rook, Wilkinson & Ebling: Oxford & Edinburgh, Blackwell Scientific publications, 2002.
7. *Skin Diseases in Arabian Countries* M El. Zawahry: Cairo, 1967.
8. *An Introduction to Dermatology*, Percival GH: Edinburgh & London E & S Living stone Ltd., 1967.
9. *Fitzpatrick's Dermatology in General Medicine*, 8th Edition, Eds. Goldsmith et al: New York. MacGraw Hill Book Corporation, 2012.
10. *Practical Pediatric Dermatology*, WL Weston: Boston-Little Brown & Co., 1979.
11. *Practical Dermatology*, 3rd Ed. IB Sneddon: London, Edward Arnold & Co., 1977.

B. Skin Tumours

1. *Tumours of the Skin*, Eller & Eller: London, Henry Kimpton, 1951.
2. *Atlas of Tumours of Skin*, Koff, Bart, Andrade, London, WB Saunders & Co., 1979.

C. Dermatology and Internal Medicine

1. *Skin Manifestations of Internal Disorders*, Wiener K: St. Louis, The CV Mosby Co.,1947.
2. *Systemic Associations and Treatment of Diseases*, Weiner K: St. Louis, The CV Mobsy Co., 1955.
3. *Dermatology Clues to Internal Diseases*, Behrman, HT: New York, Grune, 1967.
4. *The Cutaneous Manifestations of Systemic Diseases*, Downing JG: Springfield, III, Charles C. Thomas, 1974.

D. Atlases

1. *Atlas of the Common Skin Diseases*, Semon & Moritz: Bristol , John Wright & Sons, 1975.
2. *Atlas of Histopathology of the Skin*, Percival GH, et al.: Edinburgh, E & S Livingstone, 1967.
3. *A Colour Atlas of Dermatology*, GM. Levene: London, Wolfe Medical Publicationas, 1979.

E. Skin Pathology

1. *Histopathology of the Skin*, Lever WF: Philadelphia JB. Lippincott Co., 2018.
2. *Dermatopathology, Vol I & II*, Montgomery H: New York, Harper & Row, 1967.
3. *An Introduction to the Diagnostic Histopathology of Skin*, JA Milne: London, Edward Arnold, 1972.
4. *Dermal Pathology*, James H. Graham: et al. New York Harper & Row, 1972.
5. *Gross and Microscopic Pathology of Skin*, 2 Vols, Milton R, Okun and Leon M. Edelstein: Boston-Dermatopathology Foundation Press, 1976.
6. *A Guide to Dermatohistopathology*, 3rd Ed. Pinkus H & Mehregan AH, New York, Appleton Century, 1980.

F. Mycology

1. *Manual of Clinical Mycology*, Conant NF, et al: Philadelphia, Military Medical Manu als, WB. Saunders Co., 1974.
2. *Medical Mycology*, Dey NC: Calcutta, 1968.
3. *Medical Mycology*, 3rd Ed. CW. Emmons: Philadelphia, Lea & Febiger, 1979.

G. Psychosomatic Dermatology

1. *Emotional Factors in Skin Diseases*, Witikower E & Russel B: New York, Paul B. Hoeber, 1953.
2. *Psychocutaneous Dermatology*, Obermayer ME: Springfield, III Charles C. Thomas, 1955.

H. Chemistry and Microbiology

1. *Practical Survey of Chemistry and Metabolism of the Skin*, Markowitz M: Philadelphia, Blakiston's Son & Co., Inc., 1962.
2. *Physiology and Biochemistry of the Skin*, Rothman S: The University of Chicago Press, 1974.
3. *Textbook of Microbiology*, Burrows W: Philadelphia WB. Saunders Co., 1976.

I. Historial Aspects of Dermatology

1. *The History of Dermatology*, Pussey, WA: Springfield, IIICharles C. Thomas, 1953.
2. *Classics in Clinical Dermatology*, Shelley WB & Grissey JT: Springfield, III., Charles C. Thomas, 1953.

J. Venereal Disease and AIDS

1. *Management of Venereal Diseases*, US Dept of Health, Education and Welfare, Wash ington DC.
2. *Modern Diagnosis and Treatment of the Minor Venereal Diseases*, Canizares O. Springfield III, Charles C. Thomas, 1973.
3. *Venereal Diseases*, King A and Nicol C: London, Bailliere Tindall & Cassell, 1980.
4. *AIDS-Diagnosis, Treatment and Prevention*. Kotia and Srivastava, CBS Publishers and Distributors, New Delhi, 1995.

K. Allergy

1. *Allergy*, Urbach E and Guttlieb PM: London, William Heinemann, 1963.

2. *A Manual of Clinical Allergy*, Sheldon, Lovell and Mathews: London WB. Saunders Co., 1964.
3. *Practice of Allergy*, Vaughan WT: St. Louis, The CV Mosby Co., 1966.

L. Special Dermatoses

1. *Handbook of Tropical Dermatology*, Simons RDG. Ph: Houston, Elsevier Pub!. Co. Inc., 1952.
2. *Occupational Diseases of the Skin*, Schwartz, Tulipan and Peck: London, Henry Kimpton, 1947.
3. *Viral and Rickettsial Diseases of the Skin*, Eye and Mucous Membranes of Man, Blank, H and Rake G: Boston, Little Brown & Co., 1955.
4. *Non-venereal Diseases of the Genitals*, Callomon & Wilson: Springfield III, Charles C. Thomas, 1956.
5. *Donovanosis*, Rajam and Rangiah Geneva, WHO, 1954.
6. *Skin Surgery*, Epstein E, Philadelphia, Lee and Febiger, 1979.
7. *Eczemas*, Loewenthal, LJA, Edinburgh E & S Livingstone, 1954.
8. *Oral Diagnosis and Treatment*, Miller SC: New York, McGraw-Hill Book Co., 1957.
9. *The Management of Oral Disease*, Bernier JL: St. Louis, The CV Mosby Co., 1955.
10. *Dermatology and Venereology for Nurses*, Behl, P.N.: Delhi, Skin Institute, 1957.
11. *Contact Dermatitis*, Fisher AA, Philadelphia, Lee and Febiger publishers, 1999.
12. *Leprosy in Theory and Practice*, Cochrane RG and Davey TF: Bristol, John Wright & Sons, 1964.
13. *Appendage Tumours of the Skin*, Hashimoto K and Lever WF: Springfield, Charles C. Thomas Publishers.
14. *Essays on Tropical Dermatology*, Simons RDG Ph and Marshall J: Hauge, Mouton & Co., 1969.
15. *Peripheral Vascular Diseases*, Winsor & Hyman: Philadelphia; Lee & FebigerPublishers, 1965.
16. *Comparative Physiology and Pathology of the Skin*, Rook AJ & Walton GS: Oxford, Blackwell, 1965.
17. *Leprosy for Practitioners*, Yawalkar SJ: Bombay, Popular Prakashan, 1980.
18. *Skin Irritant and Sensitizing Plants found in India*, 3rdnd Edn. Behl, Srivastava: New Delhi, Chand & Co., 2002.
19. *Clinical Genodermatology*, Butterworth & Strean: Baltimore, Williams & Williams & Wilkins, 1962.
20. *Skin Diseases–Teaching aids for Nurses and Medical Auxilaries*, Behl PN: New Delhi, Skin Institute, 1976.

M. Diseases of the Scalp

1. *The Scalp in Health and Disease*, Behrman HT: St. Louis, The CV Mosby Co., 1952.
2. *The Hair and the Scalp*, Savill A: London, Edward Arnold & Co., 1952.

N. Review of Dermatological Interest

1. *Recent Advances in Dermatology*, Goldsmith WN and Hellier FF: London, Churchill & Co., 1954.
2. *The Year Book af Dermatology and Syphilogy*: Chicago, Year Book Publishers, 1954 to 1980.

O. Cosmetology

1. *Handbook of Cosmetic Materials*, Greenberg & Lester. New York, Interscience Publishers, 1954.
2. *Modern Cosmeticology*, Harry RG: London, Leonard Hill, 1955.

P. Therapy of Skin Disorders

1. *Skin Therapeutics*, Poland MK: Houston, Elsevier Publ. Co., Inc., 1952.
2. *Modern Dermatological Therapy*, Strenberg & Newcomer: New York, McGraw-Hill Book Co., 1959.
3. *The Indian Pharmaceutical Codex Vol. I & II. Indigenous* Drugs, Mukerjee B: New Delhi, Council of Scientific and Industrial Research, 1953.
4. *Electro-surgical Apparatus and their Application in Dermatology*, Burdick KH: Spring field, Charles C. Thomas publishers, 1969.
5. *Plastic Surgery, A concise Guide to Clinical Practice*, Graff WG & Smith JW: Boston, Little Brown & Co., 1967.

Q. Journals and Abstracts

1. *Excerpta Medica. Ill*, Kelverstraat, Amsterdam.
2. *The British Journal of Dermatology*, 136 Gower St., London, WC 1, England.
3. *The Journal of Investigative Dermatology*, Mt. Royal and Guilford Aves., Baltimore 2. Md, USA.
4. *AMA Archives of Dermatology*, 535 N. Dearborn Street, Chicago 10, Illinois, USA.
5. *Indian Journal of Dermatology*, Venerology and Leprology, Vellore (India).
6. *International Journal of Dermatology*, JB Lippincot Company, Philadelphia, Toronto.
7. *Journal of Cutaneous Pathology*, Muknsgaard, Copenhagen.
8. *The Journal of Dermatologic Surgery and Oncology*, Park Avenue South, New York.
9. *International Journal of Leprosy and Other Mycobacterial Diseases*, 1262 Broad St. Bloom field, New Jersey, USA.
10. *Leprosy in India*, Hind Kusht Nivaran Sangh, 1 Red Cross Road, New Delhi.
11. *International Dermatology News*, 275 Madison Avenue, New York.
12. *Dermatology Times*, Skin Institute, Greater Kailash I, New Delhi.

R. X-ray and Radium Therapy

1. *X-rays and Radium in the Treatment of Diseases of the Skin*, Mackee, GM and Cipollaro AC: London, Henry Kimpton, 1946.

S. Technique

1. *Investigative Techniques in Dermatology*, Edit R Mark: London, Blackwell Scientific Publications, 1979.
2. *Office Techniques in Diagrwsis of Skin Diseases*, William Eggleson and David Pairse: Year Book Medical Publishers, Chicago, 1979.

Index